How well do you know your anatomy?
Use our online study aid to find out.

- **Test yourself with:**
  - 400 USMLE-style questions with explanatory answers (200 from the book, plus 200 additional questions)
  - Over 500 anatomical illustrations with "labels on, labels off" functionality

- **Get immediate feedback**, quickly identifying areas needing further study

Get started today!

Scratch off the panel below to reveal your access code and then log on to www.WinkingSkull.com to get started.

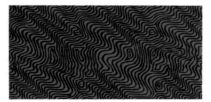

This book cannot be returned if the access code panel is scratched off.

Anatomy
An Essential Textbook

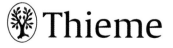

Anatomy
An Essential Textbook

Anne M. Gilroy, MA
Associate Professor
Departments of Cell Biology and of Surgery
University of Massachusetts Medical School
Worcester, Massachusetts

Illustrations by
Marcus Voll
Karl Wesker

Thieme
New York • Stuttgart

Thieme Medical Publishers, Inc.
333 Seventh Ave.
New York, NY 10001

Vice President and Editorial Director,
Educational Products: Anne T. Vinnicombe
Development editor: Marjorie Singer Anderson
Production Editor: Megan C. Conway
Editorial Assistant: Renee Kestenbaum
Senior Vice President, Editorial and
E-Product Development: Cornelia Schulze
Chief Financial Officer: Sarah Vanderbilt
President: Brian D. Scanlan
Compositor: Manila Typesetting Company
Printer: Everbest Printing Co. Ltd.
Illustrations: Markus Voll and Karl Wesker

Library of Congress Cataloging-in-Publication Data

Gilroy, Anne M.
  Anatomy : an essential textbook / Anne M Gilroy.
    p. ; cm.
  Includes index.
    ISBN 978-1-60406-207-6 (pbk.) — ISBN 978-1-60406-208-3 (e-ISBN)
  I. Title.
  [DNLM: 1. Anatomy—Atlases. 2. Anatomy—Examination Questions. QS 18.2]

  612.0076--dc23
                      2012049133

Copyright ©2013 by Thieme Medical Publishers, Inc. This book, including
all parts thereof, is legally protected by copyright. Any use, exploitation, or
commercialization outside the narrow limits set by copyright legislation
without the publisher's consent is illegal and liable to prosecution. This
applies in particular to photostat reproduction, copying, mimeographing
or duplication of any kind, translating, preparation of microfilms, and
electronic data processing and storage.

Important note: Medical knowledge is ever-changing. As new research
and clinical experience broaden our knowledge, changes in treatment and
drug therapy may be required. The authors and editors of the material
herein have consulted sources believed to be reliable in their efforts to
provide information that is complete and in accord with the standards
accepted at the time of publication. However, in view of the possibility
of human error by the authors, editors, or publisher of the work herein
or changes in medical knowledge, neither the authors, editors, nor
publisher, nor any other party who has been involved in the preparation
of this work, warrants that the information contained herein is in every
respect accurate or complete, and they are not responsible for any errors
or omissions or for the results obtained from use of such information.
Readers are encouraged to confirm the information contained herein
with other sources. For example, readers are advised to check the product
information sheet included in the package of each drug they plan to
administer to be certain that the information contained in this publication
is accurate and that changes have not been made in the recommended
dose or in the contraindications for administration. This recommendation
is of particular importance in connection with new or infrequently used
drugs.

Some of the product names, patents, and registered designs referred to
in this book are in fact registered trademarks or proprietary names even
though specific reference to this fact is not always made in the text.
Therefore, the appearance of a name without designation as proprietary
is not to be construed as a representation by the publisher that it is in the
public domain.

Printed in China
5 4 3 2 1
ISBN 978-1-60406-207-6

To my mother, Mary Gilroy, a woman of courage and love;
To Colin and Bryan, my strength and sanity;
And once more, to my Dad.

Contents

Acknowledgements

Special thanks to authors Michael Schuenke, Erik Schulte, and Udo Schumacher of the award-winning three-volume *Thieme Atlas of Anatomy* and illustrators Marcus Voll and Karl Wesker for their work over the course of many years

For their careful and thoughtful review of the manuscript, thanks to

Brian R. MacPherson, PhD
Department of Anatomy and
Neurobiology
University of Kentucky School of
Medicine
Lexington, KY

Carmen E. Rexach, PhD
Department of Biological Sciences
Mount San Antonio College
Walnut, CA

Lawrence M. Ross, MD, PhD
Department of Neurobiology and
Anatomy
University of Texas Medical School
Houston, TX

For their contributions to the problems sets, thanks to

Frank J. Daly, PhD
Department of Biomedical Sciences
University of New England
School of Osteopathic Medicine
Biddeford, ME

Geoffrey Guttman, PhD
Department of Cell Biology and Anatomy
University of North Texas Health Science Center
Texas College of Osteopathic Medicine
Fort Worth, TX

Krista S. Johansen, MD
Department of Cell Biology
University of Massachusetts Medical
School
Worcester, MA

Michelle Lazarus, PhD
Department of Neural and
Behavioral Sciences
Pennsylvania State College of
Medicine
Hershey, PA

Preface

Medical education continues to undergo innovative reform that challenges students, educators, and publishers. As curricula in the first two years of medical school have become increasingly multidisciplinary, the market for review-style textbooks has blossomed. Students are often presented with concepts in anatomy, physiology, histology, embryology, radiology, and even basic pathology and immunology in a single course. Despite the excitement that integrated courses generate, an unfortunate consequence is that students have even less time to devote to mastery of each subject by pouring over the large single-subject textbooks, which were the standard learning tools of the past. While these books are often the most relied upon references for practitioners and educators, students now gravitate towards concise texts that provide clinical context and allow for rapid review and self-testing. Such concise texts, together with dissection guides and atlases, are the go-to resources for today's anatomy students. Our challenge has been to provide adequate content in a format that fits this new learning style. Living up to that challenge has been our goal as we developed *Anatomy – An Essential Textbook*.

The introductory chapter provides clear explanations of anatomic terminology, concepts, and systems that will be especially useful for first-year students. The remainder of the book is organized into units by region (Back, Thorax, Abdomen, Pelvis/Perineum, Upper Limb, Lower Limb and Head and Neck). Each unit begins with an overview chapter that summarizes important regional concepts as well as the details of skeletal, vascular, and nervous system components of that region. Subsequent chapters focus on organ and functional anatomy, often by key subregions.

The book is generously populated with over 450 outstanding images and 95 tables (including many of the well-received muscle facts tables and schematics) from Thieme's award winning *Atlas of Anatomy*. In addition, over 165 clinical correlations are incorporated into the text. Each unit is followed by an extensive USMLE-style question set that tests basic knowledge of that region's anatomy and its clinical application, a total of over 400 for the book. We hope that this unique combination of regional and systemic approaches presented via prioritized bulleted explanations, supported by summary tables, carefully coordinated visuals, clinical correlations, and self-testing will appeal to students as they journey through the world of anatomy.

I am grateful to so many colleagues for their contributions and expertise in completing this project. Most importantly, my editor, Anne Vinnicombe has guided, encouraged, and supported me throughout the process, always knowing when to push hard and when to tread gently. Marjorie S. Anderson, my developmental editor, suffered patiently through many versions of the text, as did editorial assistants Debra Zharnest and Renee Kestenbaum. Megan Conway helped in the layout and production of this volume. Their tireless efforts organized my thoughts into a publishable product. Thank you to developmental editor Julie O'Meara, who did the research on the clinical boxes and my humble and heartfelt thanks go to my valued colleagues Brian MacPherson (University of Kentucky College of Medicine), Larry Ross (University of Texas Medical School at Houston), and Carmen E. Rexach (Mount San Antonio College), who reviewed the manuscript and found and corrected my mistakes and inconsistencies. I'm grateful to Frank Daly (University of New England, College of Osteopathic Medicine), Krista Johansen (University of Massachusetts Medical School), Geoffrey Guttman (University of North Texas Health Center, Texas College of Osteopathic Medicine), and Michelle Lazarus (Pennslyvania State College of Medicine) for their contributions to the extensive question set and to Cathrin Weinstein, who helped in the editing process. I offer special thanks to authors Michael Schuenke, Erik Schulte, and Udo Schumacher of the three-volume *Thieme Atlas of Anatomy* and illustrators Marcus Voll and Karl Wesker for their collaboration, the results of which enrich the pages of this book.

Anne Gilroy
Worchester, Massachusetts
January 2013

1 Introduction to Anatomic Systems and Terminology

1.1 Terms of Location and Direction, Cardinal Planes and Axes

— All locational and directional terms used in anatomy, and in medical practice, refer to the human body in the **anatomic position**, in which the body is upright, arms at the side, with the eyes, palms of the hands, and feet directed forward (**Fig. 1.1, Table 1.1**).

Fig. 1.1 ► **Anatomic position**
Anterior view.

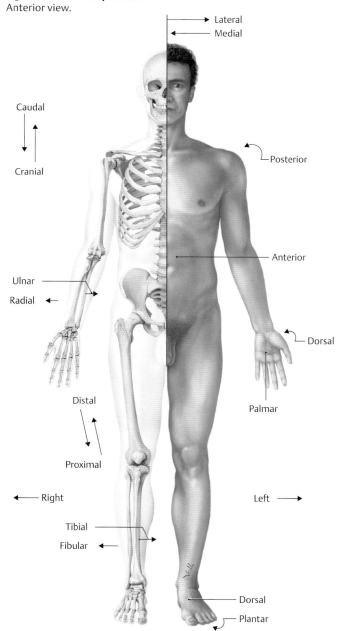

Table 1.1 ► **General Terms of Location and Direction**	
Upper body (head, neck, and trunk)	
Term	**Explanation**
Cranial	Pertaining to, or located toward, the head
Caudal	Pertaining to, or located toward, the tail
Anterior	Pertaining to, or located toward, the front Synonym: Ventral (used for all animals)
Posterior	Pertaining to, or located toward, the back Synonym: Dorsal (used for all animals)
Superior	Upper or above
Inferior	Lower or below
Axial	Pertaining to the axis of a structure
Transverse	Situated at right angles to the long axis of a structure
Longitudinal	Parallel to the long axis of a structure
Horizontal	Parallel to the plane of the horizon
Vertical	Perpendicular to the plane of the horizon
Medial	Toward the median plane
Lateral	Away from the median plane (toward the side)
Median	Situated in the median plane or midline
Peripheral	Situated away from the center
Superficial	Situated near the surface
Deep	Situated deep beneath the surface
External	Outer or lateral
Internal	Inner or medial
Apical	Pertaining to the top or apex
Basal	Pertaining to the bottom or base
Sagittal	Situated parallel to the sagittal suture
Coronal	Situated parallel to the coronal suture (pertaining to the crown of the head)
Limbs	
Term	**Explanation**
Proximal	Close to, or toward, the trunk, or toward the point of origin
Distal	Away from the trunk (toward the end of the limb), or away from the point of origin
Radial	Pertaining to the radius or the lateral side of the forearm
Ulnar	Pertaining to the ulna or the medial side of the forearm
Tibial	Pertaining to the tibia or the medial side of the leg
Fibular	Pertaining to the fibula or the lateral side of the leg
Palmar (volar)	Pertaining to the palm of the hand
Plantar	Pertaining to the sole of the foot
Dorsal	Pertaining to the back of the hand or top of the foot

— Three perpendicular cardinal planes and three axes based on the three spatial coordinates can be drawn through the body (**Fig. 1.2**).

- The **sagittal plane** passes through the body from front to back, dividing it into right and left sides.
- The **coronal plane** passes through the body from side to side, dividing it into front (anterior) and back (posterior) parts.
- The **transverse** (axial, horizontal, cross-sectional) **plane** divides the body into upper and lower parts. A particular transverse section is often given the designation of the corresponding vertebral level, such as *T4*, which passes through the 4th thoracic vertebra.
- The **longitudinal axis** passes along the height of the body in a craniocaudal direction.
- The **sagittal axis** passes from the front to the back (or the back to the front) of the body in an anteroposterior direction.
- The **transverse** (horizontal) **axis** passes through the body from side to side.

1.2 Landmarks and Reference Lines

— In surface anatomy, palpable structures or visible markings on the surface of the body are used to identify the location of underlying structures. **Reference lines** are vertical or transverse planes that connect palpable structures or markings (**Tables 1.2, 1.3,** and **1.4**; see also **Fig. 1.4A** and **B**).

Fig. 1.2 ▶ **Cardinal planes and axes**
Neutral position, left anterolateral view.

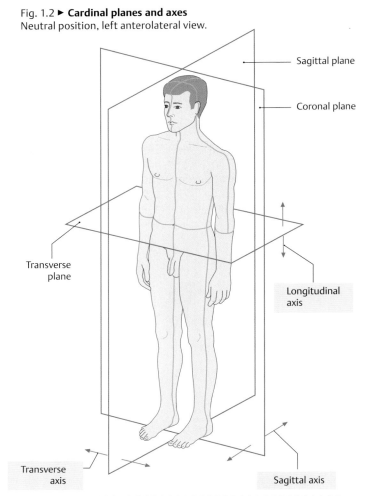

Table 1.2 ▶ Anterior and Lateral Reference Lines on Trunk	
Anterior midline	Passes through the center of the sternum
Sternal line	Passes along the lateral border of the sternum
Midclavicular line	Passes through the midpoint of the clavicle
Parasternal line	Passes through a point midway between the sternal and midclavicular lines
Anterior axillary line	Marks the anterior axillary fold formed by the pectoralis major muscle
Posterior axillary line	Marks the posterior axillary fold formed by the teres major muscle
Midaxillary line	Marks the midpoint between the anterior and posterior axillary lines

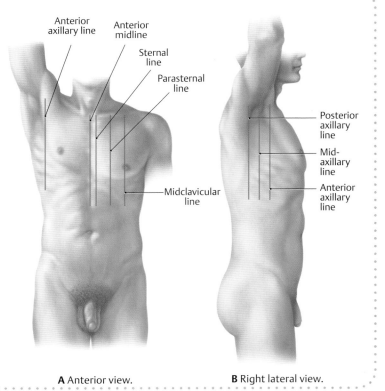

A Anterior view.   **B** Right lateral view.

Table 1.3 ▶ Landmarks and Transverse Planes on the Anterior Trunk	
Jugular notch	Marks the superior border of the manubrium
Sternal angle	Marks the junction of manubrium and body of the sternum
Transpyloric plane	Passes through the midpoint between the jugular notch and pubic symphysis
Subcostal plane	Marks the lowest level of the thoracic cage, the 10th costal cartilage
Supracrestal plane	Connects the top of the iliac crests
Intertubercular plane	Passes through the iliac tubercles
Interspinal plane	Connects the anterior superior iliac crests

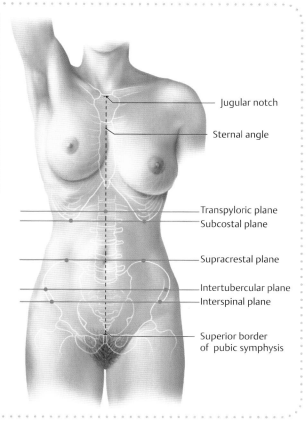

Jugular notch
Sternal angle
Transpyloric plane
Subcostal plane
Supracrestal plane
Intertubercular plane
Interspinal plane
Superior border of pubic symphysis

Table 1.4 ▶ Vertebral Spinous Processes and Posterior Landmarks	
C7	The vertebra prominens
T3	Level of the medial edge of spines of the scapulae
T7	Level of the inferior angles of the scapulae
T12	Level of the lower limit of the thoracic cavity
L4	Level of the iliac crests
S2	Level of the posterior superior iliac spine

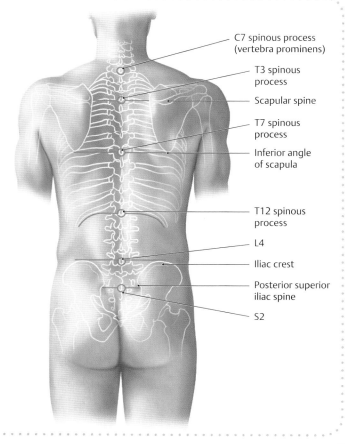

C7 spinous process (vertebra prominens)
T3 spinous process
Scapular spine
T7 spinous process
Inferior angle of scapula
T12 spinous process
L4
Iliac crest
Posterior superior iliac spine
S2

3

1.3 The Integumentary System

The skin (integument), the largest organ of the body, protects underlying tissue from biologic, mechanical, and chemical injury; regulates body temperature; and participates in metabolic processes, such as the synthesis of vitamin D.

— The skin is composed of

- an outer waterproof avascular layer, the **epidermis**, which has a superficial layer of keratinized cells that shed continuously and a deep basal layer of regenerating cells, and
- an inner richly vascularized and innervated layer, the **dermis**, which supports the epidermis and contains hair follicles.

1.4 Fascia

Fascia is a sheet of connective tissue that lies between the skin and underlying muscles and bone (**Fig. 1.3**).

— **Superficial fascia**, a layer of varying thickness that lies deep to the skin, is composed of loose connective tissue and fat. Superficial nerves and vessels traverse this layer.
— **Deep fascia**, a dense connective tissue layer, lies under (deep to) the superficial fascia and is devoid of fat. It forms an investing layer, which envelops neurovascular structures and muscles of the limbs, trunk wall, head, and neck. Invaginations of the deep fascia of the limbs form **intermuscular septa** that separate limb musculature into functional groups (compartments).

Fig. 1.3 ▶ **Fascia**
Cross section through the right arm, proximal view.

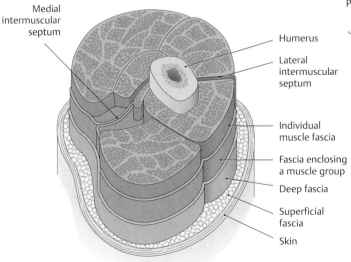

Medial intermuscular septum
Humerus
Lateral intermuscular septum
Individual muscle fascia
Fascia enclosing a muscle group
Deep fascia
Superficial fascia
Skin

1.5 The Skeletal System

The bones and cartilages of the body, which make up the skeletal system, provide leverage for muscles and protect the internal organs. Bone is also the site for calcium storage and blood cell production.

— There are two anatomic divisions of the skeleton (**Fig. 1.4A** and **B**):

Fig. 1.4 ▶ **Human skeleton**
Left forearm is pronated, and both feet are in plantar flexion.

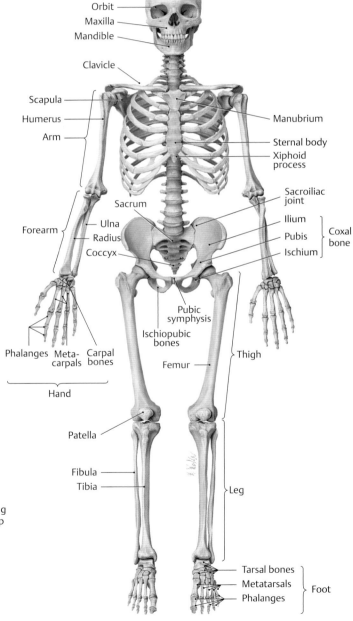

Frontal bone
Orbit
Maxilla
Mandible
Clavicle
Scapula
Humerus
Arm
Manubrium
Sternal body
Xiphoid process
Sacroiliac joint
Sacrum
Ulna
Radius
Coccyx
Forearm
Ilium
Pubis
Ischium
Coxal bone
Pubic symphysis
Ischiopubic bones
Phalanges Meta-carpals Carpal bones
Femur
Thigh
Hand
Patella
Fibula
Tibia
Leg
Tarsal bones
Metatarsals
Phalanges
Foot

A Anterior view.

- The **axial skeleton**, which consists of the skull, vertebrae, sactum, coccyx, ribs, and sternum
- The **appendicular skeleton**, which includes the clavicle and scapula of the pectoral girdle, the coxal bones of the pelvic girdle, and the bones of the upper and lower limbs

— **Periosteum** is a thin layer of fibrous connective tissue that coats the outer surface of each bone (**Fig. 1.5**). **Perichondrium** forms a similar layer around cartilaginous structures. These tissues nourish and assist in the healing of the underlying bone.

— All bones have a superficial layer of dense **compact** (cortical) **bone** that surrounds a less dense **cancellous** (spongy) **bone**. In some areas of the bone, a **medullary cavity** contains yellow (fatty) or red (blood cell or platelet-forming) **bone marrow**.

— Bones develop from **mesenchyme** (embryonic connective tissue) through two processes of ossification (bone formation).

- The clavicle and some bones of the skull develop by **membranous ossification**, in which the bones form through direct ossification of mesenchymal templates that are set down during the embryonic period.
- Most bones, including the long bones of the limbs, develop by **endochondral ossification**, in which a cartilaginous template, formed from mesenchyme, is laid down during the fetal period. Over the first and second decades of life, bone replaces most of the cartilage.
  - Within each bone undergoing endochondral ossification, bone formation occurs first at a **primary ossification center**, which is in the **diaphysis** (shaft) of the long bones. **Secondary ossification centers** appear later at the **epiphyses** (growing ends) of the bones.

— Long bones of the skeleton increase in length through growth of the epiphyses and diaphysis on either side of the **epiphyseal plate**, an intervening cartilaginous area. During childhood and adolescence the epiphyseal plates gradually shorten as they are replaced by bone. In the adult these areas are completely ossified, and only thin **epiphyseal lines** remain.

— **Apophyses**, bony outgrowths that lack their own growth center, serve as attachment sites for ligaments or tendons. Specific apophyses are referred to as condyles, tubercles, spines, crests, trochanters, or processes.

— **Ligaments** are connective tissue bands that connect bones to each other or to cartilage. (Within the body cavities, the term *ligament* refers to folds or condensations of a serous or fibrous membrane that support visceral structures.)

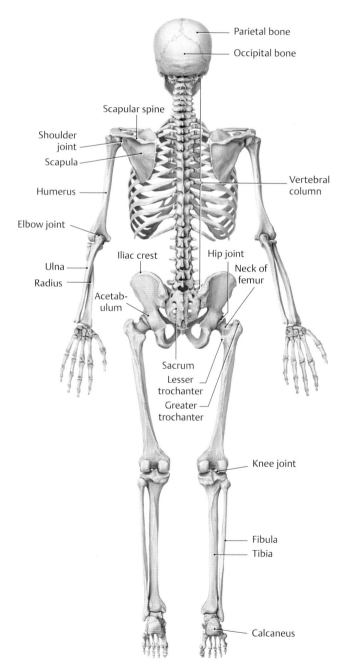

B Posterior view.

Labels on figure:
- Parietal bone
- Occipital bone
- Scapular spine
- Shoulder joint
- Scapula
- Humerus
- Elbow joint
- Ulna
- Radius
- Acetabulum
- Iliac crest
- Hip joint
- Neck of femur
- Vertebral column
- Sacrum
- Lesser trochanter
- Greater trochanter
- Knee joint
- Fibula
- Tibia
- Calcaneus

Fig. 1.5 ► **Structure of a typical long bone**
Illustrated for the femur. Coronal cuts through the proximal and distal parts of an adult femur.

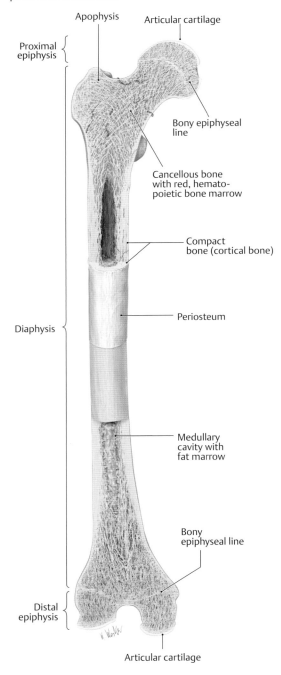

- Joints are classified according to the type of tissue that connects the bones.
  - **Syndesmoses** (fibrous joints), such as those found in the sutures of the skull and interosseous membrane of the forearm, are united by fibrous tissue and allow minimal movement (**Fig. 1.6A and B**).
  - **Synchondroses** (cartilaginous joints) are united either by fibrocartilaginous segments, such as the costal cartilages of the ribs, intervertebral disks, and pubic symphysis (**Fig. 1.7A and B**), or by articular cartilage, often found in temporary joints, such as those that join the ilium, ischium, and pubis of the hip bone (**Fig. 1.7C**). Subsequent fusion of these temporary joints creates **synostoses** (sites of bony fusion) (**Fig. 1.8**).
  - **Synovial joints**, the most common type of joint, allow free movement (**Fig. 1.9**) and typically have
    - a **joint cavity** that is enclosed by a fibrous **joint capsule** and lined by a **synovial membrane**, which secretes a thin film of lubricating **synovial fluid**;
    - articulating ends of the bones that are covered by articular (hyaline) cartilage; and
    - extrinsic ligaments on the outer surface, which reinforce the joints.
    - Some synovial joints also contain intrinsic (intra-articular) ligaments and intervening fibrocartilaginous disks (such as the menisci of the knee joint).
- **Bursae** are closed sacs that contain a thin film of fluid and are lined with a synovial membrane. Commonly found around joints of the limbs, bursae cushion prominent bony processes from external pressure and prevent friction where tendons cross bony surfaces.

Fig. 1.6 ► **Syndesmoses**

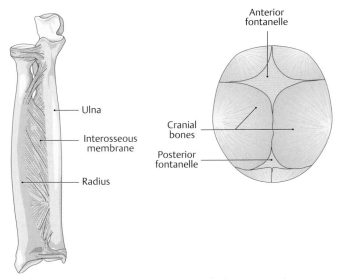

A Interosseous membrane of the forearm, anterior view.

B Skull of a neonate showing open fontanelles, superior view.

Fig. 1.7 ► **Synchondroses**

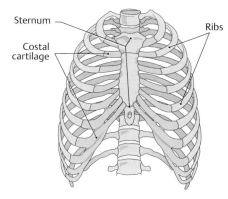

A Costal cartilages.

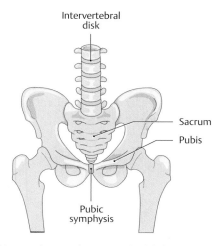

B Pubic symphysis and intervertebral disks.

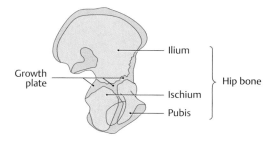

C Hip bone before closure of the growth plates.

Fig. 1.8 ► **Synostoses**
Hip bone (fusion of the ischium, ilium, and pubis).

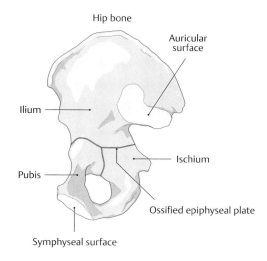

Fig. 1.9 ► **Structure of a synovial joint**

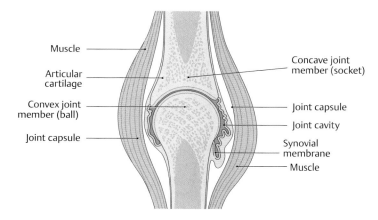

1.6 The Muscular System

The muscular system is composed of muscles and their tendons, which produce movement through contraction of muscle cells.

- **Muscle cells** are the structural units of the muscular system. Connective tissue binds muscle cells (fibers) together to form bundles, which in turn are bound together to form muscles (**Fig. 1.10**).
- **Somatic muscles** move the skeleton and are found in the neck, trunk wall, and limbs; **visceral muscles** alter the shape of internal structures, such as the heart and gastrointestinal tract.
- Muscle tissue is classified by location (somatic or visceral), appearance (striated or nonstriated), and innervation (voluntary or involuntary).
  - **Skeletal muscle**, the most prevalent type of muscle, which is found in the limbs and body wall, is somatic, striated, multinucleated, and voluntary.
  - **Cardiac muscle**, which makes up the thick muscular layer (**myocardium**) of the heart, is visceral, striated, and involuntary.
  - **Smooth muscle**, found in the walls of blood vessels and hollow internal organs, is visceral, nonstriated, and involuntary.
- **Tendons**, dense fibrous bands, connect muscles to their bony attachments. **Aponeuroses** are tendons that form flat sheets and attach muscles to the skeleton or to other muscles.

Fig. 1.10 ► **Structure of a skeletal muscle**
Cross section through a skeletal muscle.

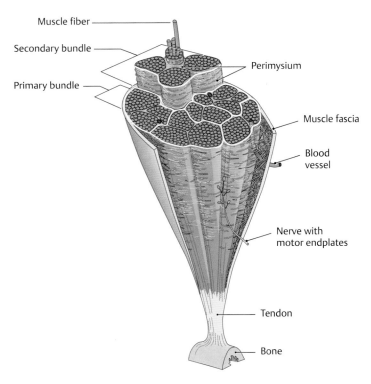

Muscle fiber
Secondary bundle
Primary bundle
Perimysium
Muscle fascia
Blood vessel
Nerve with motor endplates
Tendon
Bone

1.7 The Circulatory System

- The heart and blood vessels, which make up the circulatory system (**Figs. 1.11** and **1.12**), transport blood to tissues of the body for the exchange of gases, waste products, and nutrients.
- The muscular heart provides the pumping action that maintains the flow of blood through the vessels.

Fig. 1.11 ► **Overview of the principal arteries in the systemic circulation** Anterior view.

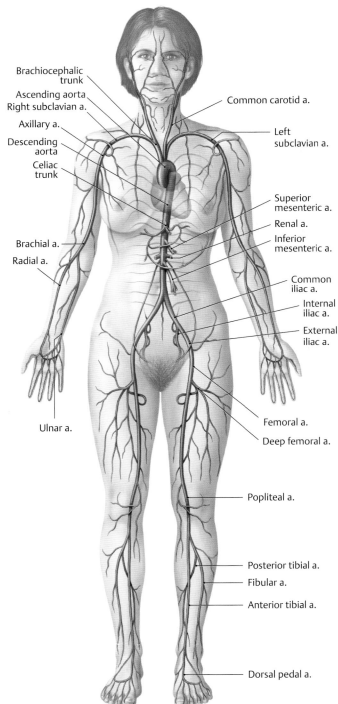

Brachiocephalic trunk
Ascending aorta
Right subclavian a.
Axillary a.
Descending aorta
Celiac trunk
Brachial a.
Radial a.
Ulnar a.
Common carotid a.
Left subclavian a.
Superior mesenteric a.
Renal a.
Inferior mesenteric a.
Common iliac a.
Internal iliac a.
External iliac a.
Femoral a.
Deep femoral a.
Popliteal a.
Posterior tibial a.
Fibular a.
Anterior tibial a.
Dorsal pedal a.

— The blood vessels of the circulatory system (**Fig. 1.13**) are classified as follows:

- **Arteries**, which transport blood away from the heart and branch into many smaller **arterioles**
- **Veins**, which carry blood toward the heart and are formed by the convergence of many small **venules**
  - Many veins, particularly in the limbs, have multiple valves along their length to prevent backward flow due to gravity.
  - The veins are divided into **superficial veins** that travel in the superficial fascia and **deep veins** that accompany the arteries. **Perforator veins** connect the superficial and deep venous circulations.
  - Veins are more numerous and more variable than arteries and often form venous plexuses (networks), which are named for the structure they surround (e.g., uterine venous plexus).
- **Capillaries**, which form networks that intervene between the arteries and veins at the **terminal vascular beds**, where gas, nutrient, and waste exchange occurs
- **Sinusoids**, which are wide, thin-walled vessels that replace capillaries in some organs, such as the liver

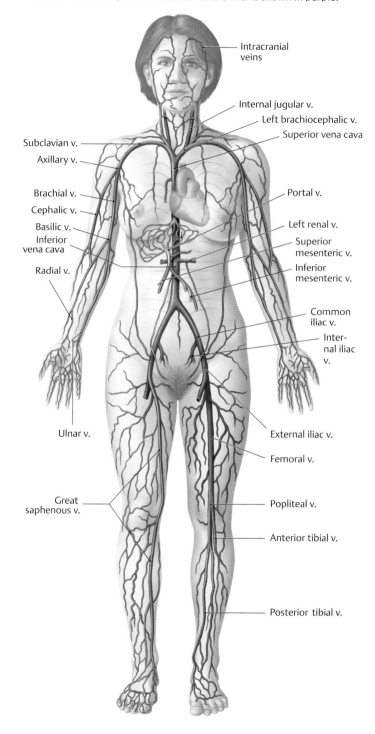

Fig. 1.12 ▶ **Overview of the principal veins in the systemic circulation**
Anterior view. The portal circulation of the liver is shown in purple.

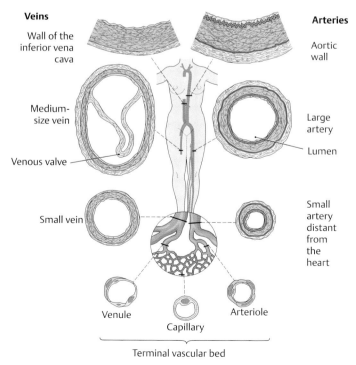

Fig. 1.13 ▶ **Structure of blood vessels**
Blood vessels in different regions of the systemic circulation, shown in cross section.

— The circulatory system has two circuits (**Fig. 1.14**):

    1. The **pulmonary circulation** transports oxygen-poor blood from the right side of the heart to the lungs through **pulmonary arteries**. Oxygen-rich blood from the lungs flows back to the left side of the heart through **pulmonary veins**.

    2. The **systemic circulation** distributes oxygen-rich blood from the left side of the heart to body tissues through the systemic arteries (the **aorta** and its branches). Oxygen-poor blood returns to the heart through the systemic veins (the **superior** and **inferior venae cavae** and their tributaries—sometimes referred to as the **caval system—**and the coronary sinus).

— A **portal circulation** is a route within the systemic circulation that diverts blood to a second capillary network before returning it to the systemic veins. The largest of these, the **portal system** in the liver, diverts blood from the gastrointestinal tract to the capillaries (sinusoids) in the liver before returning it to the systemic veins. A similar portal system is found in the pituitary gland.

— An **anastomosis**, a communication between arteries, allows blood to bypass its normal route and flow through an alternate, or collateral, route. Although blood volume through the anastomosis is usually minimal, it increases when the lumen of vessels along the normal route is obstructed.

— **End arteries** are vessels that lack anastomoses. Gradual narrowing of end arteries stimulates the formation of new vessels, but an abrupt obstruction of an end artery can cause necrosis (death) of the target tissue.

1.8 The Lymphatic System

The lymphatic system, which runs parallel to the circulatory system, consists of lymph, lymphatic vessels, and lymphoid organs.

— The lymphatic system performs the following functions:

    • Drains excess extracellular fluid from body tissues and returns it to veins of the systemic circulation

    • Mounts an immune response in the body

    • Transports fat and large protein molecules that cannot be taken up by venous capillaries

— Lymphoid organs and tissues that are part of the body's immune system include the thymus, bone marrow, spleen, lymph nodes, and tonsils. They also include bronchus-associated lymphatic tissue (BALT) in the airway and gut-associated lymphatic tissue (GALT), such as Peyer's patches and the vermiform appendix, within the gastrointestinal tract (**Fig. 1.15**).

— **Lymph**, extracellular fluid that is extracted by lymph capillaries and transported by lymphatic vessels, is a clear, watery substance similar to blood plasma.

— The conducting vessels of the lymphatic system include

    • blind-ended **lymphatic capillaries** that begin in the tissues and drain to lymphatic vessels;

    • **lymphatic vessels**, which are interposed with lymph nodes along their length and drain to lymphatic trunks; and

    • two major **lymphatic trunks**, the thoracic duct (left lymphatic trunk) and right lymphatic trunk, which drain into large veins of the neck.

— The **thoracic duct** (left lymphatic duct), which arises from the **cisterna chyli** (chyle cistern), a dilated lymphatic vessel in the abdomen, is the larger of the two major lymphatic trunks. It drains lymph from the right and left lower quadrants and left upper quadrant of the body. The smaller **right lymphatic duct** drains only the right upper quadrant of the body (**Fig. 1.16**).

Fig. 1.14 ▶ **Circulation**
Schematic showing the pulmonary and systemic circulations. The portal circulation through the liver is part of the systemic circulation. Arteries are shown in red, veins in blue, and lymphatic vessels in green.

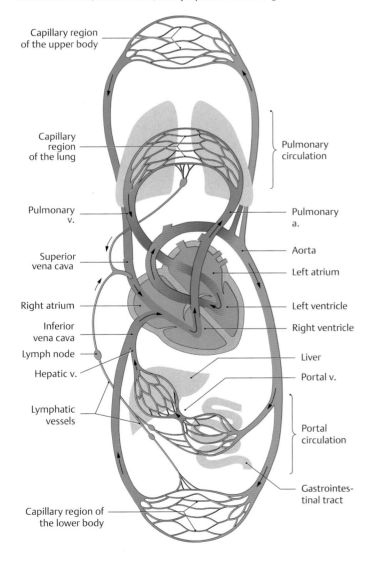

Capillary region of the upper body

Capillary region of the lung

Pulmonary v.

Superior vena cava

Right atrium

Inferior vena cava

Lymph node

Hepatic v.

Lymphatic vessels

Capillary region of the lower body

Pulmonary circulation

Pulmonary a.

Aorta

Left atrium

Left ventricle

Right ventricle

Liver

Portal v.

Portal circulation

Gastrointestinal tract

— Lymph carried by the thoracic duct and right lymphatic duct returns to the systemic venous circulation at the **left** and **right venous angles** (junction of the internal jugular and subclavian veins), also known as the jugulosubclavian junction, in the neck (**Fig. 1.17**).

Fig. 1.15 ▸ **Lymphatic system**
The lymphatic system parallels the veins of the circulatory system and includes lymphatic vessels and lymphatic organs.

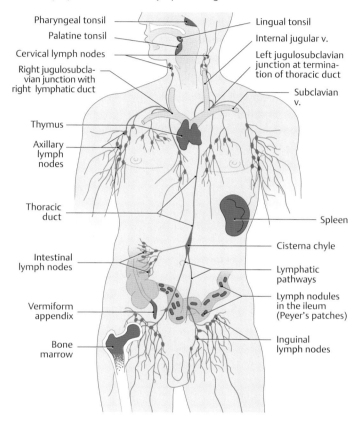

Pharyngeal tonsil
Palatine tonsil
Cervical lymph nodes
Right jugulosubclavian junction with right lymphatic duct
Thymus
Axillary lymph nodes
Thoracic duct
Intestinal lymph nodes
Vermiform appendix
Bone marrow

Lingual tonsil
Internal jugular v.
Left jugulosubclavian junction at termination of thoracic duct
Subclavian v.
Spleen
Cisterna chyle
Lymphatic pathways
Lymph nodules in the ileum (Peyer's patches)
Inguinal lymph nodes

Fig. 1.16 ▸ **Lymphatic drainage by body quadrants**

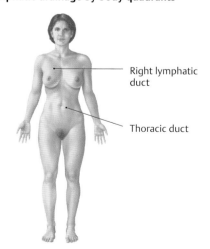

Right lymphatic duct

Thoracic duct

Fig. 1.17 ▸ **Lymphatic pathways**
Anterior view. The right lymphatic duct (~1 cm long) collects lymph from the right upper quadrant of the body and empties into the right venous angle at the junction of the right internal jugular vein with the right subclavian vein. Its major tributaries are

— the right jugular trunk (right half of the head and neck),
— the right subclavian trunk (right upper limb, right side of the chest and back wall), and
— the right bronchomediastinal trunk (organs of the right thoracic cavity).

The thoracic duct is approximately 40 cm long and transports lymph from the entire lower half of the body and left upper quadrant. It empties into the left venous angle between the left internal jugular vein and left subclavian vein. Its main tributaries are

— the left jugular trunk (left half of the head and neck),
— the left subclavian trunk (left upper limb, left side of the chest and back wall),
— the intestinal trunks (abdominal organs), and
— the right and left lumbar trunks (right and left lower limb; pelvic viscera; right and left pelvic, abdominal, and back wall).

The intercostal lymphatic vessels transport lymph from the left and right intercostal spaces to the lymphatic duct.

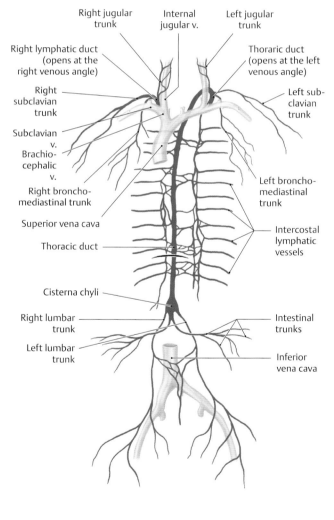

Right jugular trunk
Internal jugular v.
Left jugular trunk
Right lymphatic duct (opens at the right venous angle)
Thoracic duct (opens at the left venous angle)
Right subclavian trunk
Left subclavian trunk
Subclavian v.
Brachiocephalic v.
Right bronchomediastinal trunk
Left bronchomediastinal trunk
Superior vena cava
Intercostal lymphatic vessels
Thoracic duct
Cisterna chyli
Right lumbar trunk
Intestinal trunks
Left lumbar trunk
Inferior vena cava

1.9 The Nervous System

The nervous system receives, transmits, and integrates information throughout the body through the conduction of nerve impulses.

— The nervous system has two major anatomic divisions (**Fig. 1.18**):
  • A **central nervous system** (CNS) that consists of the brain and spinal cord
  • A **peripheral nervous system** (PNS) that consists of 12 pairs of cranial nerves, 31 pairs of spinal nerves, and autonomic (visceral) nerves

Fig. 1.18 ► **Topography of the nervous system**
Posterior view.

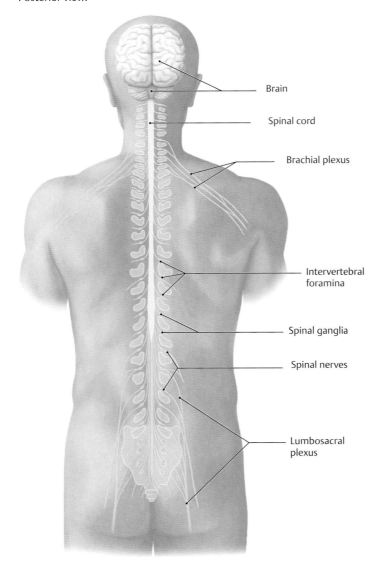

Brain

Spinal cord

Brachial plexus

Intervertebral foramina

Spinal ganglia

Spinal nerves

Lumbosacral plexus

— The nervous system has two functional divisions:
  • The **somatic nervous system**, which controls voluntary functions such as contraction of skeletal muscles
  • The **autonomic nervous system**, which controls involuntary functions such as gland secretion
— There are two classes of cells within the nervous system:
  • **Nerve cells** or **neurons**, the functional unit of the nervous system that are specialized for conducting nerve impulses
  • **Neuroglia,** or **glial** cells, the nonneuronal cellular components of the nervous system that act as supporting cells and perform a variety of metabolic functions
— The **neuron** has a **cell body** (soma) with many short dendrites and a single long axon (**Fig. 1.19**).
  • An aggregate of cell bodies is called a **nucleus** in the CNS and a **ganglion** in the PNS.
  • **Dendrites** receive information and transmit impulses toward the cell body.
  • **Axons**, or nerve fibers, transmit impulses away from the cell body. Bundles of axons in the CNS form **tracts**; bundles of axons in the PNS form **nerves**.
  • A **synapse** is the site at which a neuron communicates with another neuron or with a receptor cell (typically, a cell of a muscle or gland).
  • Many axons are surrounded by a lipid-rich insulating **myelin sheath** that increases the speed of impulse conduction. Myelin is formed by glial cells, which include **Schwann cells** in the PNS and **oligodendrocytes** in the CNS.

Fig. 1.19 ▶ Neurons
The nervous system is composed of neurons (nerve cells) and supporting neuroglial cells, which vastly outnumber neurons (10 to 1). Each neuron contains a cell body (soma) with one axon (projecting segment) and one or more dendrites (receptor segments). The release of neurotransmitters at synapses creates an excitatory or inhibitory postsynaptic potential at the target neuron. If this exceeds the depolarization threshold of the neuron, the axon "fires," initiating the release of a neurotransmitter from its presynaptic terminal (bouton).

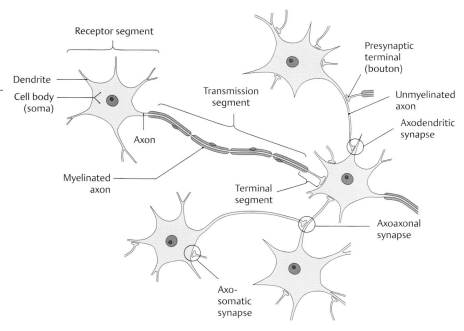

1.9a The Central Nervous System (Fig. 1.20)

— The brain and spinal cord of the central nervous system consist of

- **gray matter** that contains the cell bodies and dendrites of neurons;
- **white matter** that contains the axons of neurons, most of which are surrounded by a myelin sheath; and
- neuroglial cells that are abundant in both white and gray matter.

— The brain resides in the cranial cavity of the skull. Gray matter forms the **cortex**, or outer layer, of the brain and surrounds the inner areas of white matter. Axonal tracts of the white matter link regions of the brain with each other and with the spinal cord.

— The bony vertebral column encloses the spinal cord. Gray matter in the spinal cord is located centrally and is surrounded by the white matter. The gray matter forms an H-shaped area that consists of bilateral **anterior horns**, **posterior horns**, and, in the thoracic and upper lumbar region, **lateral horns**.

Referred pain

Referred pain is a sensation that originates from viscera but is perceived as if coming from an overlying or nearby somatic structure. It occurs because the somatic and visceral sensory fibers converge onto the same spinal cord segment. Diaphragmatic irritation from a splenic abscess, for example, is typically referred to the shoulder because both the diaphragm and the skin over the shoulder convey sensory information to C3–C5 segments of the spinal cord.

Fig. 1.20 ▶ Gray and white matter in the central nervous system
Nerve cell bodies appear gray in gross inspection, whereas nerve cell processes (axons) and their insulating myelin sheaths appear white.

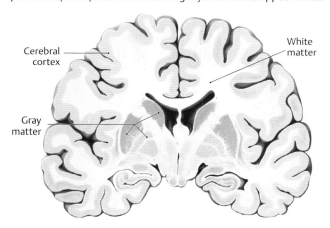

A Coronal section through the brain.

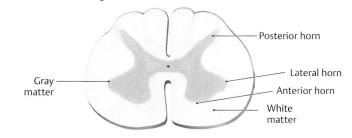

B Transverse section through the spinal cord.

1.9b   The Peripheral Nervous System

— The anatomic components of the peripheral nervous system (**Fig. 1.21**) include the following:

- Twelve pairs of **cranial nerves**, designated by Roman numerals, that arise from the brain and primarily innervate structures of the head and neck. The **vagus nerve** (cranial nerve X) also innervates viscera of the thorax and abdomen.
- Thirty-one pairs of **spinal nerves** that arise from the spinal cord and exit the vertebral column through **intervertebral foramina** (openings between vertebrae). Spinal nerves are named for the section of the spinal cord from which they arise (e.g., T4 is the fourth segment of the thoracic part of the spinal cord).

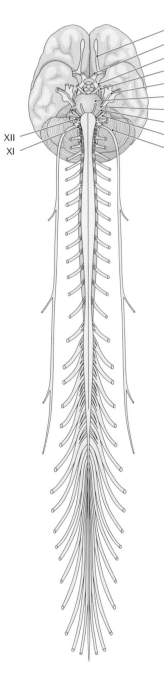

Fig. 1.21 ▶ **Spinal nerves and cranial nerves**
Anterior view. Thirty-one pairs of spinal nerves arise from the spinal cord in the peripheral nervous system, compared with 12 pairs of cranial nerves that arise from the brain. The cranial nerve pairs are traditionally designated by Roman numerals.

— The functional components of the peripheral nervous system (**Fig. 1.22**) include the following:

- **Sensory** (afferent) **nerves**, which carry information regarding pain, temperature, and pressure to the central nervous system (CNS) from peripheral structures. Sensory nerves can contain **somatic sensory fibers**, which transmit the information from skin and skeletal muscles, and **visceral sensory** (visceral afferent) **fibers**, which transmit information from smooth muscle, cardiac muscle, and internal organs.
  - Sensations carried by visceral sensory fibers are vague and poorly localized (such as nausea) in contrast to sensations carried by somatic sensory fibers, which are sharp and localized (such as a paper cut).
- **Motor** (efferent) **nerves**, which transmit impulses from the CNS that elicit responses from peripheral target organs. They can contain **somatic motor fibers**, which innervate skeletal muscles, and **visceral motor fibers**, which innervate smooth muscle, cardiac muscle, and glands.

— Most nerves of the peripheral nervous system are **mixed nerves** that contain motor, sensory, and visceral fibers.
— Spinal nerves originate from the spinal cord and form by the merging of (**Fig. 1.23**)

- an **anterior root** carrying motor fibers whose cell bodies are located in the anterior horn of the spinal cord, and

Fig. 1.22 ▶ **Information flow in the nervous system**
Fibers that carry information to the central nervous system (CNS) are called sensory or afferent fibers; fibers that carry signals away from the CNS are called motor or efferent fibers.

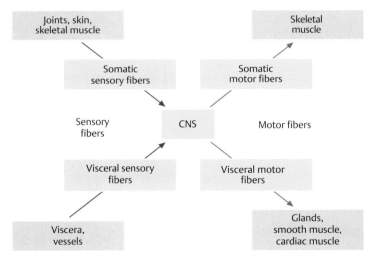

Fig. 1.23 ▶ Topographic and functional organization of a spinal cord segment
Somatic sensory (blue) and visceral sensory (green) fibers pass through the posterior root into the spinal cord and terminate in the posterior horn. Somatic motor fibers (red), originating in the anterior horn, and visceral motor fibers (brown), originating in the lateral horn, pass through the anterior root to the corresponding target organ. Somatic motor fibers synapse directly on their target organs (skeletal muscles), but the visceral motor fibers synapse with other autonomic fibers in discrete sympathetic ganglia or in ganglia embedded within the viscera.

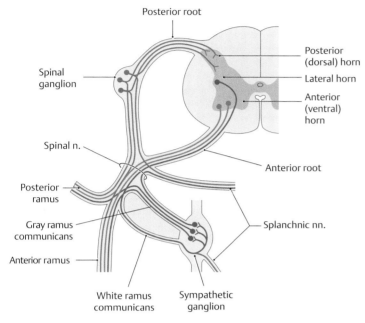

- a **posterior root** carrying sensory fibers whose cell bodies are located in a spinal ganglion located outside the spinal cord.
— Spinal nerves emerge from the intervertebral foramen and split to form
  - **posterior rami** that innervate structures of the back and
  - **anterior rami** that form peripheral nerves and plexuses that innervate the rest of the body.

1.9c   The Autonomic Nervous System

The autonomic nervous system, the visceral part of the peripheral nervous system, innervates blood vessels, glands, smooth muscle, and cardiac muscle.

— The autonomic nervous system consists of two divisions that often have antagonistic effects on the same organ (**Fig. 1.24, Table 1.5**):
  - The **sympathetic division** allows the body to respond to stress ("fight or flight").
  - The **parasympathetic division** allows the body to maintain, or return to, a state of homeostasis ("rest and digest").

Table 1.5 ▶ Effects of the Sympathetic and Parasympathetic Nervous Systems		
Organ	**Sympathetic nervous system**	**Parasympathetic nervous system**
Eye	Pupillary dilation	Pupillary constriction and increased curvature of the lens
Salivary glands	Decreased salivation (scant, viscous)	Increased salivation (copious, watery)
Heart	Elevation of the heart rate	Slowing of the heart rate
Lungs	Decreased bronchial secretions; bronchial dilation	Increased bronchial secretions; bronchial constriction
Gastrointestinal tract	Decreased secretions and motor activity	Increased secretions and motor activity
Pancreas	Decreased secretion from the endocrine part of the gland	Increased secretion
Male sex organs	Ejaculation	Erection
Skin	Vasoconstriction, sweat, secretion, piloerection	No parasympathetic innervation

Fig. 1.24 ▶ **Structure of the autonomic nervous system**

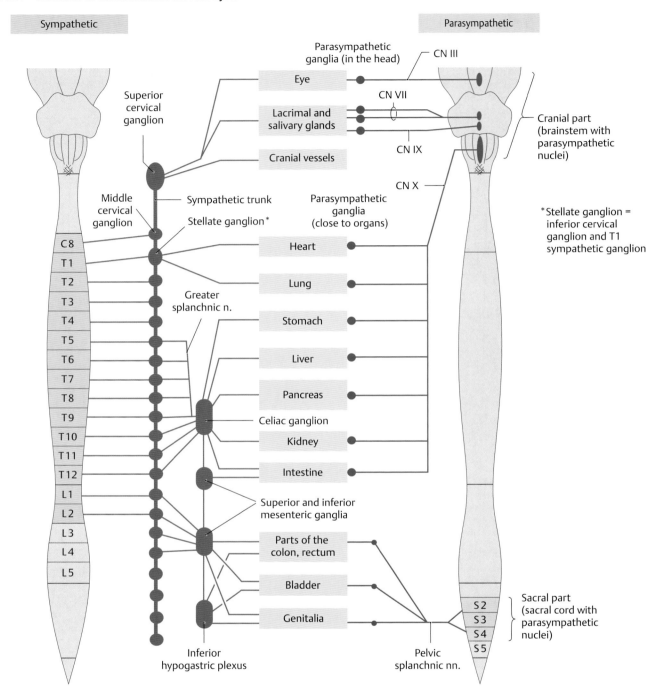

— Nerves of the autonomic nervous system consist of a two-neuron path between the CNS and the target organ: a proximal **preganglionic** (presynaptic) **neuron** and distal **postganglionic** (postsynaptic) **neuron** that synapse in an intervening ganglion (**Fig. 1.25**).

- Sympathetic nerves arise from the thoracic and lumbar spinal cord (T1–L2) and exit the vertebral column with the corresponding spinal nerves.

  ∘ Preganglionic sympathetic fibers leave the spinal nerve via **white rami communicans** to synapse on cell bodies of postganglionic fibers in **paravertebral ganglia**. These ganglia form a chain that runs along each side of the vertebral bodies known as the **sympathetic trunk**. Postganglionic fibers then rejoin the spinal nerve via **gray rami communicans**.

  ∘ Some sympathetic preganglionic fibers form **thoracic**, **lumbar**, and **sacral splanchnic nerves**, autonomic nerves that bypass ganglia of the sympathetic trunk to synapse in **prevertebral ganglia**, such as the celiac ganglion. These nerves contribute to autonomic plexuses in the thorax, abdomen, and pelvis and innervate viscera in those regions.

- Parasympathetic nerves arise from the brain and the S2–S4 segments of the sacral spinal cord.

  ∘ Preganglionic parasympathetic fibers that arise from the brain travel with cranial nerves III, VII, IX, and X and synapse in parasympathetic ganglia of the head (or, in the case of the vagus nerve, ganglia near the target organ).

  ∘ **Pelvic splanchnic nerves** are formed by the preganglionic parasympathetic fibers of the sacral spinal cord. They contribute to autonomic plexuses in the pelvis and abdomen and synapse in small ganglia located close to their target organ.

— The autonomic nervous system is considered to be a visceral motor system, although visceral sensory fibers accompany both sympathetic and parasympathetic nerves.

- Visceral sensory fibers carrying sensations of pain (visceral pain fibers) travel with sympathetic nerves.
- Visceral sensory fibers carrying sensations from physiological processes, such as distension of the bladder, travel with parasympathetic nerves.

1.10 Body Cavities and Internal Organ Systems

— The large organs of the endocrine, respiratory, digestive, urinary, and reproductive systems are housed in the thorax, abdomen, and pelvis.

— A thin serous (fluid-secreting) membrane lines the **thoracic** and **abdominopelvic cavities** of the trunk and their contents. A **parietal layer** forms the outer wall of the cavity and is continuous with a **visceral layer** that reflects from the outer wall to cover, or enclose, the viscera (see **Figs. 12.2** and **12.3A**). Thus the parietal pleura lines the outer wall of the pleural cavity, and the visceral pleura covers the surface of the lung within the cavity.

Fig. 1.25 ▶ **Autonomic nervous system circuitry**
The autonomic nervous system innervates smooth muscle, cardiac muscle, and glands. It is divided into the sympathetic (red) and parasympathetic (blue) nervous systems, which often act in antagonistic ways to regulate blood flow, secretions, and organ function. Sensory (afferent) fibers are shown in green, motor (efferent) fibers are shown in purple.

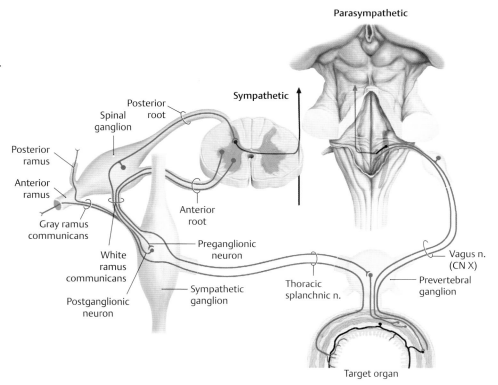

Review Questions: Introduction

1. Which of the following is associated with membranous bone formation?
   A. Primary ossification center
   B. Epiphyses
   C. Direct ossification of mesenchymal templates
   D. Long bones of the limbs
   E. Diaphysis

2. A portal system is associated with
   A. venous shunts that divert blood toward the heart
   B. the pulmonary circulation
   C. arterial–venous anastomoses
   D. capillary beds in the liver
   E. lymphatic capillaries

3. In the anatomic position the
   A. eyes are directed forward
   B. palms are directed forward
   C. body is erect with arms at the sides
   D. feet are directed forward
   E. All of the above

4. Which of the following is true of splanchnic nerves?
   A. They synapse in ganglia near their target organ.
   B. They innervate viscera of the abdomen.
   C. They may carry sympathetic fibers.
   D. They may carry parasympathetic fibers.
   E. All of the above

5. A 43-year-old high school teacher complained to her physician of abdominal bloating and pelvic pain. Radiographic studies showed a large tumor involving her right ovary. Although the patient was scheduled for surgery to remove the tumor, the physician was concerned about spread of the cancer along lymphatic channels. What is the lymphatic drainage pattern of pelvic viscera?
   A. Ipsilateral drainage to the right and left lymphatic ducts
   B. Contralateral drainage to the right and left lymphatic ducts
   C. Bilateral drainage to the right and left lymphatic ducts
   D. All pelvic viscera drain to the right lymphatic duct.
   E. All pelvic viscera drain to the left lymphatic duct.

Answers and Explanations

1. **C** In the process of membranous ossification, embryonic mesenchymal templates are replaced by bone (Section 1.5).
   A A primary ossification center, usually in the shaft of the long bones, is the site at which endochondral ossification begins.
   B Epiphyses, located on either end of the long bones, are the secondary ossification centers for endochondral ossification.
   D Long bones of the limbs undergo endochondral bone formation, in which a cartilaginous template forms from the embryonic mesenchyme before being replaced by bone.
   E A diaphysis is the shaft of a long bone, which undergoes endochondral ossification.

2. **A** The body's largest portal system diverts blood from capillary beds in the gastrointestinal tract to secondary capillary beds in the liver before returning it to systemic veins (Section 1.7).
   B A portal system is a venous system within the systemic (general body) circulation, but not within the pulmonary (lung) circulation.
   C A portal system diverts blood from one capillary network to another, unlike arterial–venous anastomoses, which divert blood away from capillary beds.
   D Lymphatic capillaries are restricted to the lymphatic system and are not involved with portal venous systems.

3. **E** The anatomic position is the standard position of the body used in medical references. The body is upright, facing the observer, with arms at the side and the head, eyes, palms, and feet directed forward (Section 1.1).
   A Eyes are directed forward, and other positions are correct as well (E).
   B Palms are directed forward, and other positions are correct as well (E).
   C Body is erect with arms at side, and other positions are correct as well (E).
   D Feet are directed forward, and other positions are correct as well (E).

4. **E** All of the above (Section 1.9c).
   A Splanchnic nerves synapse near their target organ either in prevertebral ganglia or in small ganglia on the viscera. B through D are correct also (E).
   B Splanchnic nerves are autonomic nerves that innervate viscera in the thorax, abdomen, and pelvis. A, C, and D are correct also (E).
   C Sympathetic fibers arise from the T1–L2 spinal cord to form thoracic, lumbar, and sacral splanchnic nerves. A, B, and D are correct also (E).
   D Parasympathetic fibers arise from the S2–S4 spinal cord and form pelvic splanchnic nerves. A through C are correct also (E).

5. **E** The left lymphatic duct receives lymph from the entire body below the diaphgram, as well as from the left side of the thorax, head, and neck and the left upper limb (Section 1.8). The right lymphatic duct receives lymph only from the right side of the thorax, head, and neck and the right upper limb.
   A Viscera from the right and left sides of the pelvis drain to the left lymphatic duct.
   B All pelvic viscera drain to the left lymphatic duct.
   C All pelvic viscera drain to the left lymphatic duct.
   D Only the right upper quadrant of the body drains to the right lymphatic duct.

2 Back

The back includes the vertebral column, the spinal cord and spinal nerves, and the overlying muscles and skin.

2.1a General Features

— The vertebral column
  • encloses and protects the spinal cord,
  • supports the head and trunk,
  • provides an attachment for the limbs, and
  • transfers the weight of the body to the lower limbs.
— The vertebral column, which extends from the skull to the coccyx, comprises 33 vertebrae and the intervening intervertebral disks, which are divided among five regions (**Fig. 2.1**):
  • 7 cervical vertebrae
  • 12 thoracic vertebrae
  • 5 lumbar vertebrae
  • 5 fused sacral vertebrae
  • 4 (3–5) fused coccygeal vertebrae

Osteoporosis

The spine is the primary target for degenerative diseases of the skeleton, such as osteoporosis, in which the rate of reabsorption by osteoclasts exceeds that of bone formation by osteoblasts. The resulting loss of bone mass predisposes the individual to compression fractures of the spine.

— Within each region, individual vertebrae are identified by number, a designation often referred to as a **vertebral level** (such as T8 vertebral level).
— Vertebrae increase in size from the cervical to the lumbar regions and decrease in size from the top of the sacrum to the coccyx.
— The **kyphotic curvatures** of the thoracic and sacral regions of the vertebral column, known as primary curvatures, are curved posteriorly and are present in the fetus. The **lordotic curvatures** of the cervical and lumbar regions, curved anteriorly, are secondary curvatures that develop postnatally.

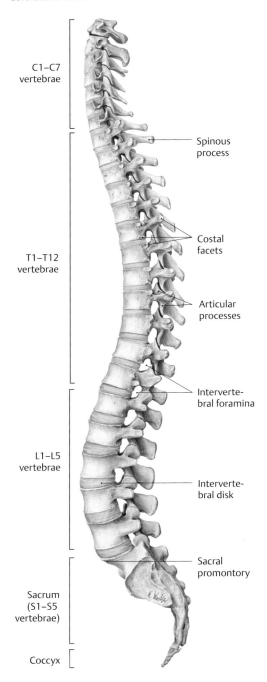

Fig. 2.1 ▶ **Vertebral column**
Left lateral view.

C1–C7 vertebrae

T1–T12 vertebrae

L1–L5 vertebrae

Sacrum (S1–S5 vertebrae)

Coccyx

Spinous process

Costal facets

Articular processes

Intervertebral foramina

Intervertebral disk

Sacral promontory

Abnormal curvatures of the vertebral column: kyphosis, lordosis, and scoliosis

Kyphosis ("hunchback"), an excessive anterior curvature of the thoracic spine, is often seen in elderly women. Although it may be congenital or posture related, it is usually secondary to degenerative changes (collapse) of the vertebral bodies. Lordosis ("swayback"), an excessive posterior curvature of the lumbar spine, frequently develops as a temporary side effect during pregnancy, but in nonpregnant individuals it may have pathologic or even weight-related causes. Scoliosis is a lateral curvature of the spine and may be congenital or neuromuscular, caused by diseases such as cerebral palsy and muscular dystrophy.

— A **vertebral canal** passes through the center of the vertebral column and encloses the spinal cord, the spinal meninges (membranes surrounding the spinal cord), and the roots of the spinal nerves, and associated vasculature (see Sections 2.3b, d).
— **Intervertebral foramina**, openings between vertebrae, allow the passage of spinal nerves.
— **Spinal cord segments** emit paired spinal nerves, and both the segment and the spinal nerve pair are identified by region and number (such as L4). Spinal cord segments do not necessarily lie adjacent to vertebra of the same number.

2.2 The Vertebral Column

2.2a Regional Characteristics of Vertebrae

Most vertebrae share a typical form (**Fig. 2.2**), although specific features vary by region.
— Most vertebrae have the following:
  • An anterior vertebral body
  • A posterior vertebral arch formed by paired pedicles and paired laminae (the pedicles attach to the vertebral body, and the paired laminae join to form a spinous process)
  • Paired transverse processes that project laterally from the vertebral arch
  • Superior and inferior articular processes that articulate with the vertebrae above and below
  • A vertebral foramen encircled by the vertebral body and vertebral arch (the combined vertebral foramina of all vertebrae form the vertebral canal)
— Cervical vertebrae, the smallest of all of the vertebrae, support the head and form the posterior skeleton of the neck (**Fig. 2.3**). The seven cervical vertebrae are characterized as typical or atypical.

Fig. 2.2 ▸ Structural elements of a vertebra
Left posterosuperior view. With the exception of the atlas (C1) and axis (C2), all vertebrae consist of the same structural elements.

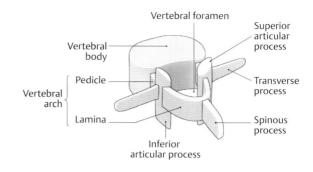

Spina bifida

Spina bifida is a congenital defect associated with the incomplete fusion of the vertebral arches (usually L5 and S1). In the mild form, spina bifida occulta, the defect is small and asymptomatic and is often marked only by a patch of hair, birthmark, or dimple over the affected vertebrae. Severe forms such as spina bifida cystica are caused by incomplete closure of the embryonic neural tube, resulting in incomplete development of the spinal cord, meninges, and overlying vertebrae. Severe cases are associated with neurologic deficits and herniation of the spinal cord and meninges through the vertebral arch defect.

Fig. 2.3 ▸ Cervical spine
Bones of the cervical spine, left lateral view.

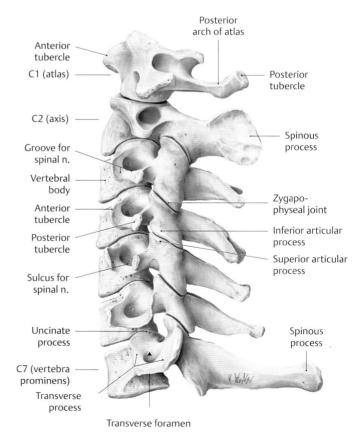

- Typical cervical vertebrae (**Fig. 2.4A**)
  - C3–C6 have a small body, a large vertebral foramen, and often bifid (two-pronged) spinous processes.
- Atypical cervical vertebrae
  - C1, the **atlas**, lacks a vertebral body and spinous process (**Fig. 2.4B**). It has anterior and posterior vertebral arches that are connected on each side by **lateral masses**. C1 articulates with the occipital bone of the skull and C2.
  - C2, the **axis**, has a peglike **dens** projecting superiorly from its body that articulates with the anterior arch of C1 (**Fig. 2.4C**).
  - C7, the **vertebra prominens**, has a long, palpable spinous process.
- All cervical vertebrae have paired **transverse foramina**, openings formed by the anterior and posterior tubercles of each transverse process.

— Paired **vertebral arteries** ascend in the neck through the transverse foramina of C1–C6, pass through a groove on the posterior arch of C1, and enter the skull through a large opening, the **foramen magnum**.

— Thoracic vertebrae (**Fig. 2.5A** and **B**) have
- long spinous processes that project inferiorly,
- heart-shaped vertebral bodies,
- **superior** and **inferior articular facets** that are oriented in the coronal plane, and
- **costal facets** that articulate with the ribs.

— Lumbar vertebrae (**Fig. 2.6A** and **B**), the largest vertebrae, have
- large bodies,
- short, broad spinous processes, and
- an **interarticular part** (pars interarticularis), part of the lamina between the superior and inferior articular facets, that forms the neck of the "Scottie dog" seen on oblique views of lumbar spine radiographs. It is a common site of vertebral fractures (**Fig. 2.7, Table 2.1**).

▌ Spondylolysis and spondylolisthesis

Spondylolysis is a fracture across the interarticular part of the lamina, usually at L5, and appears as a "collar" on the Scottie dog seen on lumbar radiographs. When the defect is bilateral, the vertebral body may separate from its vertebral arch and shift anteriorly relative to the vertebra below it, a condition known as spondylolisthesis. Mild cases can be asymptomatic, but more severe cases compress the spinal nerves and cause pain in the lower limbs and back.

Fig. 2.4 ▶ **Cervical vertebrae**

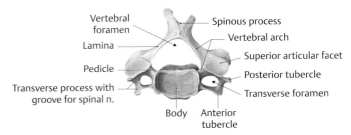

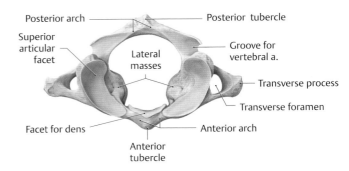

A Typical cervical vertebra (C4), superior view.

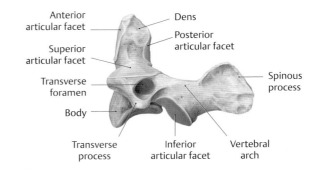

B Atlas (C1), superior view.

C Axis (C2), left lateral view.

Fig. 2.5 ▸ **Thoracic spine**

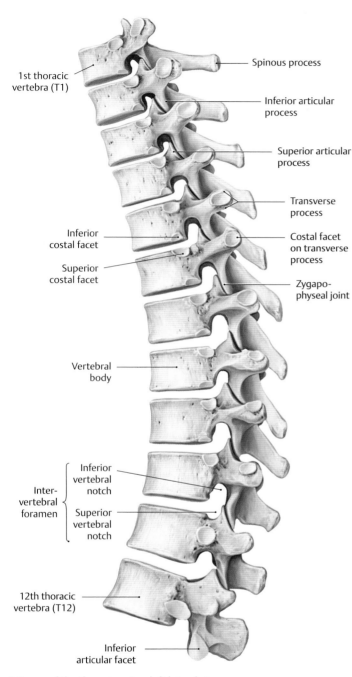

1st thoracic vertebra (T1)

Spinous process

Inferior articular process

Superior articular process

Transverse process

Inferior costal facet

Superior costal facet

Costal facet on transverse process

Zygapophyseal joint

Vertebral body

Inferior vertebral notch

Intervertebral foramen

Superior vertebral notch

12th thoracic vertebra (T12)

Inferior articular facet

A Bones of the thoracic spine, left lateral view.

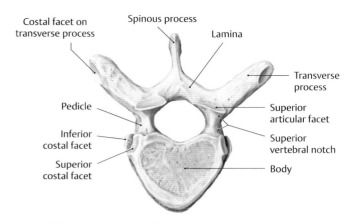

Costal facet on transverse process

Spinous process

Lamina

Transverse process

Pedicle

Inferior costal facet

Superior costal facet

Superior articular facet

Superior vertebral notch

Body

B Typical thoracic vertebra (T6), superior view.

Fig. 2.6 ▸ **Lumbar spine**

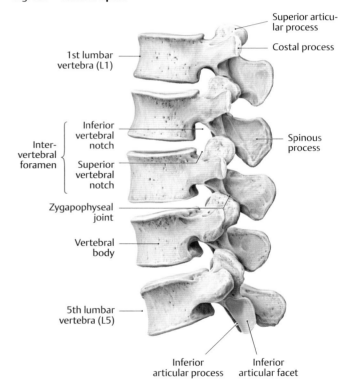

1st lumbar vertebra (L1)

Superior articular process

Costal process

Intervertebral foramen

Inferior vertebral notch

Superior vertebral notch

Spinous process

Zygapophyseal joint

Vertebral body

5th lumbar vertebra (L5)

Inferior articular process

Inferior articular facet

A Bones of the lumbar spine, left lateral view.

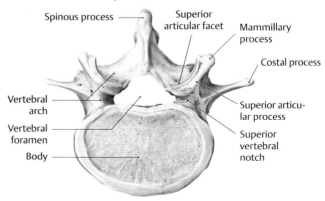

Spinous process

Superior articular facet

Mammillary process

Costal process

Vertebral arch

Vertebral foramen

Body

Superior articular process

Superior vertebral notch

B Typical lumbar vertebra (L4), superior view.

— The five sacral vertebrae are fused into a single bone, the **sacrum** (**Fig. 2.8A, B,** and **C**), which forms the posterosuperior wall of the pelvis and articulates laterally with the hip bones. The sacrum contains

  • the **sacral canal**, a continuation of the vertebral canal, which is open inferiorly at the **sacral hiatus;**
  • the **median sacral crest**, the fused spinous processes of the sacral vertebrae;
  • paired **medial sacral crests** that end inferiorly as the **sacral cornua** on either side of the sacral hiatus;
  • four pairs of **anterior** and **posterior sacral foramina** for the passage of spinal nerve branches; and
  • the **promontory,** formed by the anterior lip of the S1 vertebral body.

— The small coccygeal vertebrae, usually four (but this can vary from three to five), fuse into a single triangularly shaped bone, the **coccyx,** which articulates with the sacrum at the **sacrococcygeal joint**.

Fig. 2.7 ▸ **Oblique view of the lumbar spine**

1. Body of vertebra
2. Intervertebral disk space
3. Ribs
4. Interarticular part
5. Intervertebral disk space
6. Lamina
7. Ipsilateral transverse process

8. Contralateral transverse process
9. Pedicle
10. Superior articular process
11. Intervertebral foramen
12. Inferior articular process
13. Spinous process

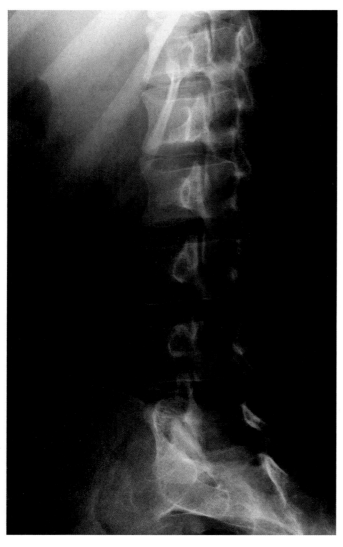

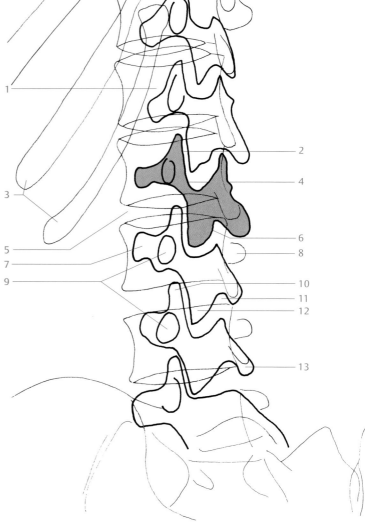

Fig. 2.8 ▶ **Sacrum and coccyx**

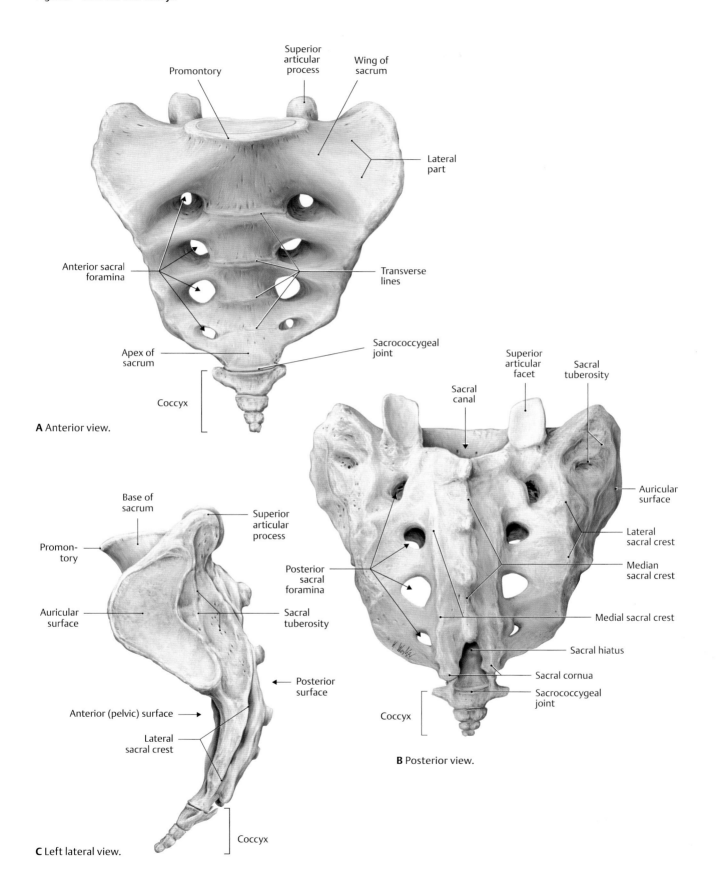

Promontory

Superior articular process

Wing of sacrum

Lateral part

Anterior sacral foramina

Transverse lines

Apex of sacrum

Sacrococcygeal joint

Coccyx

A Anterior view.

Base of sacrum

Superior articular process

Promontory

Auricular surface

Posterior sacral foramina

Sacral tuberosity

Posterior surface

Anterior (pelvic) surface

Lateral sacral crest

Coccyx

C Left lateral view.

Sacral canal

Superior articular facet

Sacral tuberosity

Auricular surface

Lateral sacral crest

Median sacral crest

Posterior sacral foramina

Medial sacral crest

Sacral hiatus

Sacral cornua

Sacrococcygeal joint

Coccyx

B Posterior view.

2.2b Joints of the Vertebral Column

Joints of the vertebral column include articulations between adjacent vertebral bodies and articulations between adjacent vertebral arches. Joints also form between the vertebral column and the skull (**Table 2.1**). Individual vertebral joints allow small local movements, but the combination of these movements over multiple vertebral levels accounts for the considerable flexibility of the vertebral column.

— **Craniovertebral joints** (**Fig. 2.9A** and **B**) are synovial joints between the skull and C1, and between C1 and C2:

- Paired **atlanto-occipital joints** between the occipital bone of the skull and the atlas (C1) allow flexion and extension of the head (as when nodding "yes").
- **Atlantoaxial joints**, which include one median and two lateral articulations between the atlas and axis (C1 and C2), allow rotation of the head (as when saying "no").

Injuries of the cervical spine

The laxity of the cervical spine makes it prone to hyperextension injuries, such as "whiplash," the excessive and often violent backward movement of the head, resulting in fractures of the dens of the axis and traumatic spondylolisthesis (see Spondylolysis and Spondylolisthesis on page 22). Patient prognosis is largely dependent on the spinal level of the injuries.

Fig. 2.9 ▶ **Craniovertebral joints**

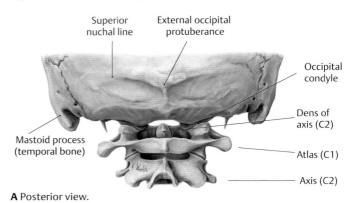

A Posterior view.

B Atlas and axis, posterosuperior view.

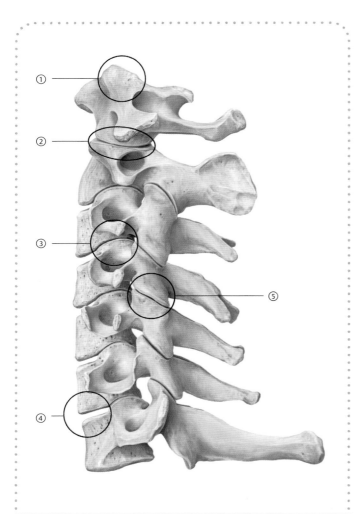

Table 2.1 ▶ Joints of the Vertebral Column		
Craniovertebral joints		
①	Atlanto-occipital joints	Occiput–C1
②	Atlantoaxial joints	C1–C2
Joints of the vertebral bodies		
③	Uncovertebral joints	C3–C7
④	Intervertebral joints	C2–S1
Joints of the vertebral arch		
⑤	Zygapophyseal joints	C1–S1

— **Uncovertebral joints** form between the **uncinate processes** (lateral lips on the superior edges of the vertebral bodies) of C3–C7 vertebrae and the vertebral bodies immediately superior to them.

   • These joints, which are not present at birth, form during childhood, probably as a result of a fissure in the cartilage of the intervertebral disk that then assumes a jointlike character.

— **Intervertebral joints** form between **intervertebral (IV) disks** and the articular surfaces of vertebral bodies. There are no IV disks between C1 and C2.

   • The IV disks act as shock absorbers and are composed of an outer fibrous ring, the **anulus fibrosus**, and a gelatinous core, the **nucleus pulposus** (**Fig. 2.10**).
   • The height of the IV disk relative to the height of the vertebral body determines the degree of mobility of the joint; mobility is greatest in the cervical and lumbar regions.
   • The differences between anterior and posterior heights of the cervical and lumbar disks contribute to the lordotic curvatures.

Fig. 2.10 ▶ **Intervertebral disk**
Fourth lumbar vertebra, superior view.

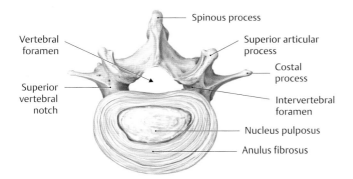

Spinous process

Vertebral foramen

Superior articular process

Costal process

Superior vertebral notch

Intervertebral foramen

Nucleus pulposus

Anulus fibrosus

Herniation of intervertebral disks

As elasticity of the anulus fibrosus declines with age, compressive forces can cause the nucleus pulposus to protrude through weakened areas. If the fibrous ring of the anulus ruptures posteriorly, the herniated material may compress the contents of the dural sac, but posterolateral herniations that compress spinal nerves are most common, particularly at the L4–L5 or L5–S1 level. In the lumbar region, where spinal nerves exit the vertebral canal above the IV disk, the hernia is likely to compress the spinal nerve inferior to that level (e.g., a herniation of the L4–L5 disk will impact the L5 spinal nerve), and pain is felt along the corresponding dermatome.

— **Zygapophyseal joints**, also known as **facet joints**, are synovial joints that join the superior and inferior articular facets of adjacent vertebrae. The orientation of these joints differs between regions and influences the degree and direction of movement of the vertebral column.

   • In the cervical region, the joints are mostly in the horizontal plane and allow movement in most directions.
   • In the thorax, the joints largely lie in the coronal plane, limiting movement to lateral flexion.
   • In the lumbar region, the joints are in the sagittal plane, facilitating flexion and extension.

Age-related changes in vertebrae

With advancing age, a decrease in bone density and aging of the IV disks can lead to an increase in compressive forces on the vertebral joints. Subsequent degenerative changes can include the depletion of articular cartilage and the formation of osteophytes (bony spurs). Osteophyte formation at the periphery of the vertebral bodies where they join the IV disks is known as spondylosis. Similar degenerative changes of the zygapophyseal joints indicate osteoarthritis, common in the cervical and lumbar spine but also manifested in the joints of the hand, hip, and knee.

2.2c Vertebral Ligaments

Vertebral ligaments support the joints of the vertebral column.

— Ligaments that support the cranial vertebral joints include (**Fig. 2.11A** and **B**)

- the **atlanto-occipital membranes**, which connect the occipital bone of the skull to the anterior and posterior arches of the atlas (C1);
- the **alar ligaments**, which secure the dens of C2 to the skull; and
- the **cruciform ligament**, formed by longitudinal fascicles (fibers) and a transverse ligament, which secures the dens against the anterior arch of the atlas.

Fig. 2.11 ▸ **Dissection of the craniovertebral joint ligaments** Posterior view.

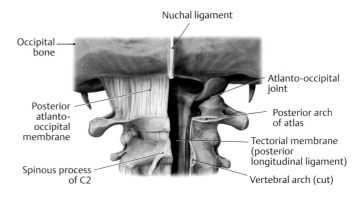

Nuchal ligament

Occipital bone

Atlanto-occipital joint

Posterior atlanto-occipital membrane

Posterior arch of atlas

Tectorial membrane (posterior longitudinal ligament)

Spinous process of C2

Vertebral arch (cut)

A Posterior longitudinal ligament. *Removed:* Spinal cord; vertebral canal windowed.

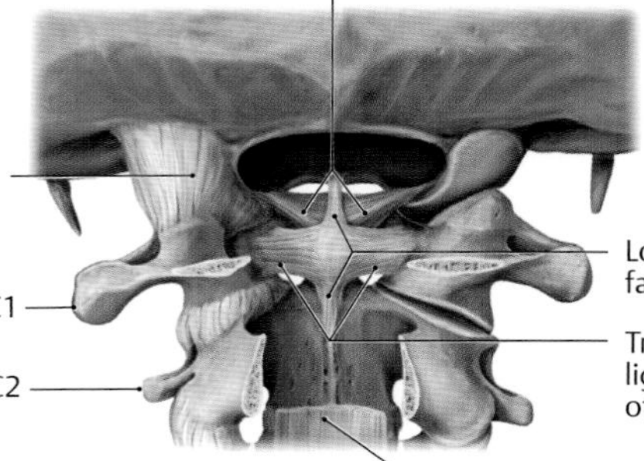

Alar ligaments

Atlanto-occipital capsule

C1

C2

Longitudinal fascicles*

Transverse ligament of atlas*

Posterior longitudinal ligament

B Cruciform ligament of atlas (*).
Removed: Tectorial membrane.

Fig. 2.12 ▸ **Ligaments of the vertebral column: Thoracolumbar junction**
Left lateral view of T11–L3, with T11–T12 sectioned in the midsagittal plane.

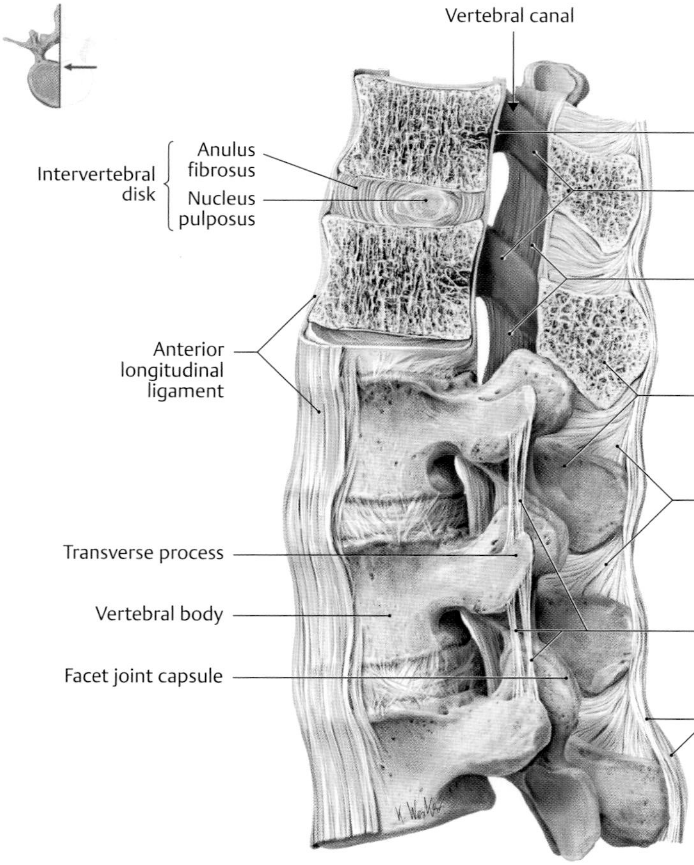

Vertebral canal

Anulus fibrosus

Intervertebral disk

Nucleus pulposus

Posterior longitudinal ligament

Vertebral arch

Ligamenta flava

Anterior longitudinal ligament

Spinous processes

Interspinous ligaments

Transverse process

Vertebral body

Intertransverse ligaments

Facet joint capsule

Supraspinous ligament

— Two longitudinal ligaments join all of the vertebral bodies (**Figs. 2.12** and **2.13**):

1. the **anterior longitudinal ligament**, a broad fibrous band extending from the occipital bone of the skull to the sacrum, attaches to the anterior and lateral surfaces of the vertebral bodies and IV disks and prevents hyperextension.
2. the **posterior longitudinal ligament**, a thin fibrous band extending from C2 to the sacrum along the anterior aspect of the vertebral canal, attaches primarily to the IV disks and offers weak resistance to hyperflexion. Superiorly, this ligament extends into the skull as the **tectorial membrane** (see **Fig. 2.11A**).

— Ligaments that join the vertebral arches (**Fig. 2.14**) include the following:
- the paired **ligamenta flava**, which join the laminae of adjacent vertebrae on the posterior wall of the vertebral canal. They limit flexion and provide postural support of the vertebral column (see also **Fig. 2.12**).
- the **supraspinous ligament**, which connects the posterior ridge of the spinous processes
- the **nuchal ligament**, a finlike expansion of the supraspinous ligament in the neck that extends from the occipital bone to the spinous process of C7

— Additional vertebral ligaments connect elements of the vertebral arches and spinous processes (see **Fig. 2.12**).

Fig. 2.14 ▶ **Ligaments of the cervical spine**
Midsagittal section, left lateral view. The nuchal ligament is the broadened, sagittally oriented part of the supraspinous ligament that extends from the vertebra prominens (C7) to the external occipital protuberance.

Fig. 2.13 ▶ **Posterior longitudinal ligament**
Posterior view of opened vertebral canal at level of L2–L5. *Removed:* L2–L4 vertebral arches at pedicular level.

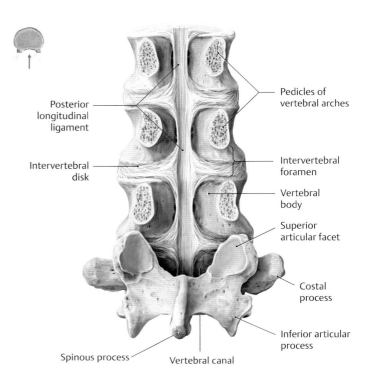

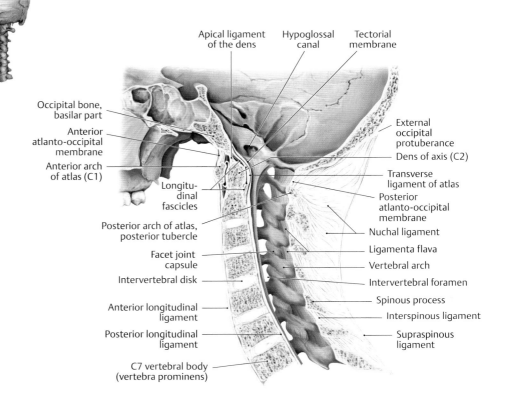

29

2.2d Neurovasculature of the Vertebral Column

— The following arteries supply the vertebrae, vertebral ligaments, meninges, and spinal cord (**Fig. 2.15**):
  • The segmental arteries, paired branches of the descending aorta such as the **posterior intercostal** and **lumbar arteries**, that arise in the thoracic and lumbar regions
  • Branches of the **subclavian artery** in the neck, including the vertebral and **ascending cervical arteries**
  • The **iliolumbar**, **medial**, and **lateral sacral arteries** in the pelvis
— The **vertebral venous** (Batson) **plexus** surrounds the vertebral bodies and drains the spinal cord, meninges, and vertebrae (**Figs. 2.16A** and **B**).

  • **Anterior** and **posterior external plexuses** surround the vertebrae, and **anterior** and **posterior internal plexuses** lie within the epidural space in the vertebral canal.
  • Both the internal and external plexuses drain into **intervertebral veins**, which in turn drain to **vertebral veins** of the neck (see **Fig. 2.20A**; see also **Fig. 17.20**) and segmental veins (paired tributaries of the inferior vena cava and azygos system) in the thoracic, lumbar, and sacral regions.
  • The veins of the vertebral venous plexus have few valves, which allows free venous communication between the skull, neck, thorax, abdomen, and pelvis.

Fig. 2.15 ▶ **Arteries of the trunk**
Right lateral view.

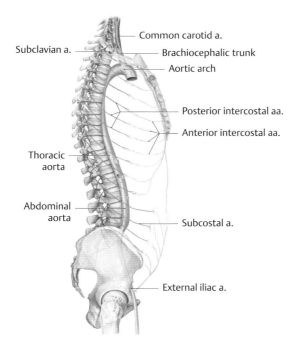

Fig. 2.16 ▶ **Vertebral venous plexus**
The intervertebral and basivertebral veins connect the internal and external venous plexuses, which drain into the azygos system.

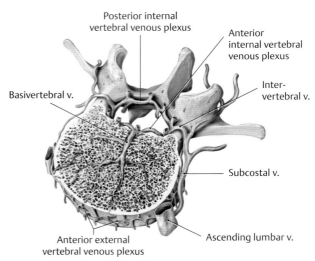

A Vertebral venous plexuses, superior view.

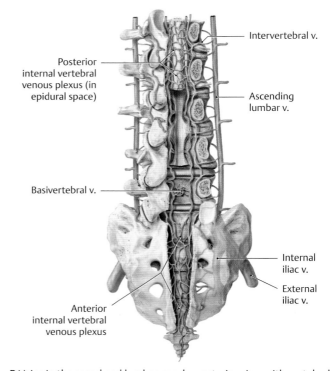

B Veins in the sacral and lumbar canals, posterior view with vertebral canal windowed.

Metastasis and the vertebral venous plexus

The vertebral venous plexus links the venous drainages of viscera in the thorax, abdomen, and pelvis and the venous sinuses of the brain. These communications have been identified as a likely route of metastases of carcinoma of the prostate (commonly), breast, and lung (less commonly) to the central nervous system and bone.

— Lymphatic drainage from the vertebrae and vertebral ligaments generally follows the arteries that supply each region and end in cervical, thoracic, lumbar, and sacral lymph nodes.
— Spinal nerves at each level innervate the vertebrae, vertebral joints, and spinal meninges through dorsal rami and meningeal branches of the anterior rami. A sympathetic branch also arises from the thoracic sympathetic ganglia.

2.3 The Spinal Cord and Spinal Nerves

The spinal cord is the part of the central nervous system that relays information between the brain and the body. The spinal cord, along

Fig. 2.17 ▶ **Spinal cord in situ** Posterior view with vertebral canal windowed.

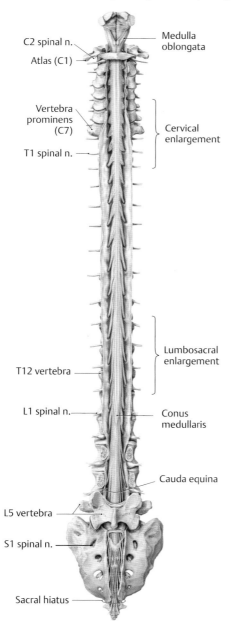

with its spinal nerves, surrounding membranes (the **meninges**), and associated vasculature, is enclosed within the vertebral canal.

2.3a Spinal Cord

— The spinal cord, continuous with the **medulla oblongata** of the brain (see **Fig. 18.8A**) superiorly, exits the skull base through the **foramen magnum** of the occipital bone. It descends within the vertebral canal and terminates as the **conus medullaris** adjacent to the L1 vertebra (**Fig. 2.17**; see also **Fig. 17.6**).
— During development the longitudinal growth of the vertebral column exceeds that of the spinal cord. At birth the conus medullaris is at the level of the L3 vertebra, but in the adult it lies adjacent to the L1/L2 intervertebral disk.
— Because the adult spinal cord is considerably shorter than the vertebral column, occupying only the superior two thirds of the vertebral canal, most spinal cord segments do not lie adjacent to the vertebral level of the same number (**Fig. 2.18**).
— The spinal cord consists of 31 segments, each of which innervates a specific area of the trunk or limbs. Each spinal cord segment has paired **spinal nerves** that contain both sensory and motor neurons.

Fig. 2.18 ▶ **Spinal cord segments and vertebral levels** The spinal cord is divided into four major regions: cervical, thoracic, lumbar, and sacral. Spinal cord segments are numbered by the exit points of their associated spinal nerves.

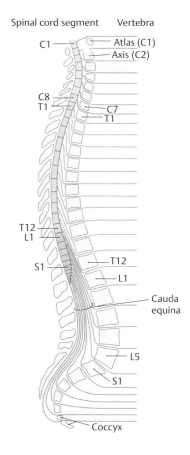

— Two swellings occur in the regions of the spinal cord that innervate the limbs:
  • The **cervical enlargement** at C4–T1 is related to the brachial plexus, a plexus of nerves that innervate the upper limb.
  • The **lumbosacral enlargement** at T11–S1 is related to the lumbar and sacral plexuses, nerve plexuses that innervate the abdominal wall and lower limb.

2.3b Meninges of the Spinal Cord

The spinal **meninges** are membranes that surround the spinal cord and nerve roots and that contain the **cerebrospinal fluid** (a fluid that cushions and nourishes the brain and spinal cord) (**Figs. 2.19** and **2.20A** and **B**; see also Section 18.2b).

— The three layers of spinal meninges are continuous with the meninges that surround the brain:
  1. **Dura mater**, a tough outer layer that forms the **dural sac** enclosing the spinal cord and extending along the nerve roots to the intervertebral foramina. The dural sac begins at the foramen magnum of the skull and ends at the level of S2.
  2. **Arachnoid mater**, a delicate middle layer that is connected to the underlying membrane by **arachnoid trabeculae** (strands of connective tissue).
  3. **Pia mater**, a thin layer that adheres to the surface of the spinal cord. **Denticulate ligaments**, transverse extensions of the pia mater, attach to the dura mater and suspend the spinal cord within the dural sac.

— The **filum terminale**, a thin cord of pia mater, extends from the conus medullaris to the apex of the dural sac. There it is surrounded by spinal dura mater and extends to the end of the vertebral canal, where it anchors both membranes to the coccyx.

— Three spaces separate the layers of meninges.
  • The **epidural space** lies between the bony wall of the vertebral canal and the dura mater. It contains fat and the vertebral venous plexus.
  • The **subdural space**, a potential space between the dura and arachnoid layers, contains a thin film of lubricating fluid.
  • The **subarachnoid space** lies deep to the arachnoid layer and contains the cerebrospinal fluid. The **lumbar cistern** is an enlargement of the subarachnoid space within the dural sac inferior to the conus medullaris.

Lumbar puncture, spinal anesthesia, and epidural anesthesia

A lumbar puncture, used to extract cerebrospinal fluid from the spinal subarachnoid space, is administered by inserting a needle between the spinous process of L3 and L4 (sometimes between L4 and L5). The needle pierces the ligamentum flavum and wall of the dural sac before entering the lumbar cistern. The injection of a local anesthetic for spinal anesthesia is also administered in this manner. A similar approach may be used for epidural anesthesia, to anesthetize emerging spinal nerves, but the anesthetic is injected into the epidural space without entering the dural sac. A caudal approach through the sacral hiatus also allows access to the epidural space.

Fig. 2.19 ▶ **Spinal cord and its meningeal layers**
Posterior view. The dura mater is opened, and the arachnoid mater is sectioned.

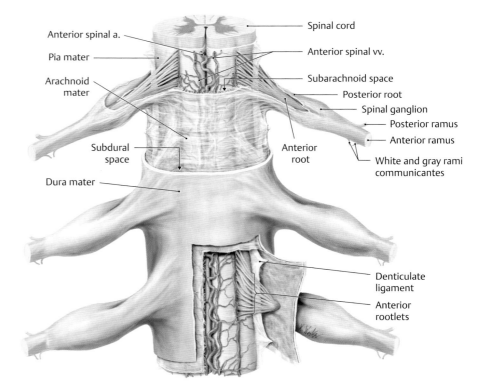

Anterior spinal a.
Pia mater
Arachnoid mater
Subdural space
Dura mater
Spinal cord
Anterior spinal vv.
Subarachnoid space
Posterior root
Spinal ganglion
Posterior ramus
Anterior ramus
White and gray rami communicantes
Anterior root
Denticulate ligament
Anterior rootlets

Fig. 2.20 ▶ **Spinal cord in situ: Transverse section**
Superior view.

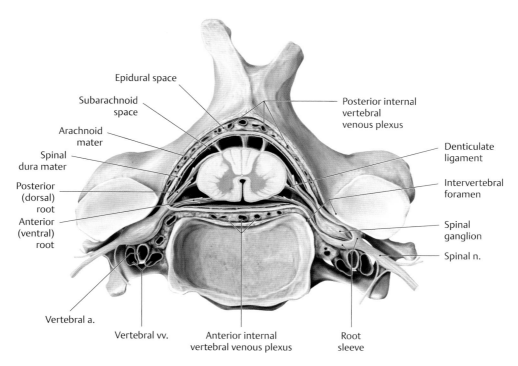

Epidural space

Subarachnoid space

Arachnoid mater

Spinal dura mater

Posterior (dorsal) root

Anterior (ventral) root

Posterior internal vertebral venous plexus

Denticulate ligament

Intervertebral foramen

Spinal ganglion

Spinal n.

Root sleeve

Anterior internal vertebral venous plexus

Vertebral vv.

Vertebral a.

A Spinal cord at level of C4 vertebra.

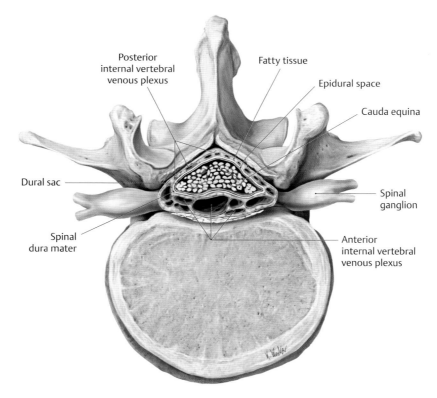

Posterior internal vertebral venous plexus

Fatty tissue

Epidural space

Cauda equina

Dural sac

Spinal ganglion

Spinal dura mater

Anterior internal vertebral venous plexus

B Cauda equina at level of L2 vertebra.

2.3c Blood Supply to the Spinal Cord (Fig. 2.21A and B)

— Longitudinal spinal arteries supply the superior part of the spinal cord.

- A single **anterior spinal artery** arises from the two vertebral arteries (branches of the subclavian arteries) and supplies the anterior two thirds of the spinal cord.
- Paired **posterior spinal arteries** arise from the vertebral arteries (or one of their branches, the posterior cerebellar artery) and supply the posterior third of the spinal cord.

— **Anterior** and **posterior segmental medullary arteries** are large, irregularly spaced vessels that communicate with the spinal arteries.

- They arise from branches of the subclavian artery and segmental arteries in the thoracic and lumbar region.
- The medullary arteries enter the vertebral canal through the intervertebral foramina and are found mainly at the cervical and lumbar enlargements.

Fig. 2.21 ▶ Arteries of the spinal cord
The unpaired anterior and paired posterior spinal arteries typically arise from the vertebral arteries. As they descend within the vertebral canal, the spinal arteries are reinforced by anterior and posterior segmental medullary arteries. Depending on the spinal level, these reinforcing branches may arise from the vertebral, ascending or deep cervical, posterior intercostal, lumbar, or lateral sacral arteries.

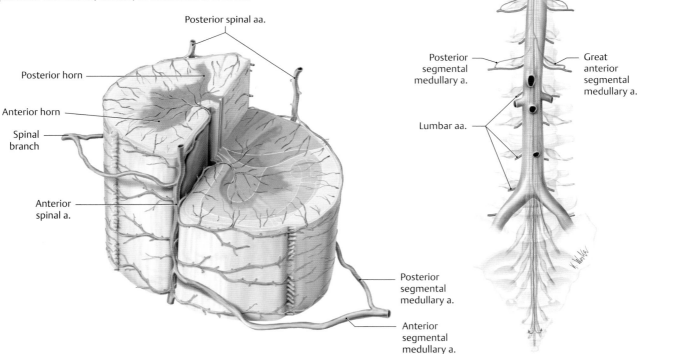

A Spinal and segmental medullary arteries.

B Arterial supply system.

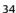

34

- The **great anterior segmental medullary artery** (of Adamkiewicz), a single large, usually left-sided vessel, can provide an important contribution to the circulation of the lower two thirds of the spinal cord.

  • It arises as a branch of a lower thoracic or lumbar segmental artery.
  • It enters the vertebral canal through an intervertebral foramen in the lower thorax or upper lumbar region.

- The **anterior** and **posterior radicular arteries** are small arteries that supply the roots of the spinal nerves and the superficial **gray matter** of the spinal cord. They do not communicate with the spinal arteries.

- Veins of the spinal cord, which are more numerous than the arteries, have the same distribution, anastomose freely with one another, and drain into the internal vertebral plexus (**Fig. 2.22**).

Fig. 2.22 ▶ **Veins of the spinal cord**
The interior of the spinal cord drains via venous plexuses into an anterior and a posterior spinal vein. The radicular and spinal veins connect the veins of the spinal cord with the internal vertebral venous plexus. The intervertebral and basivertebral veins connect the internal and external vertebral venous plexuses, which drain into the azygos system.

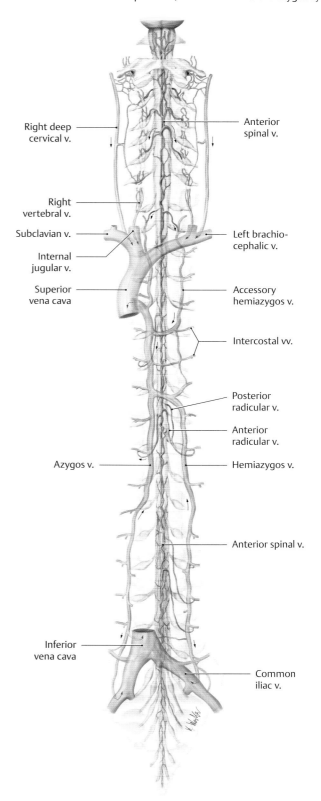

Right deep cervical v.

Right vertebral v.

Subclavian v.

Internal jugular v.

Superior vena cava

Azygos v.

Inferior vena cava

Anterior spinal v.

Left brachiocephalic v.

Accessory hemiazygos v.

Intercostal vv.

Posterior radicular v.

Anterior radicular v.

Hemiazygos v.

Anterior spinal v.

Common iliac v.

2.3d Spinal Nerves

Spinal nerves transmit information between peripheral body tissues and the spinal cord. A single pair of spinal nerves arises from each spinal cord segment.

— There are 31 pairs of spinal nerves: 8 cervical, 12 thoracic, 5 lumbar, 5 sacral, and 1 coccygeal.
— Spinal nerves are mixed (sensory and motor) nerves, which arise bilaterally from each spinal cord segment (**Fig. 2.23**). They are formed by the merging of
  • anterior roots containing motor (efferent) fibers and
  • posterior roots containing sensory (afferent) fibers.
— Spinal nerves are somatic nerves but most also carry visceral nerve fibers.
  • Spinal nerves T1–L2 carry sympathetic fibers that synapse in the ganglia of the sympathetic trunk or in preaortic ganglia.
  • Spinal nerves S2–S4 carry parasympathetic fibers that contribute to the visceral nerve plexuses of the pelvis.
— Each spinal nerve divides into an **anterior ramus** and a **posterior ramus**. Anterior rami innervate the anterolateral trunk wall and the limbs; posterior rami innervate the skin and muscles of the back and posterior scalp.

— Spinal nerves from each spinal cord segment pass through the intervertebral foramina at the corresponding vertebral level.
  • Cervical nerves C1–C7 exit the vertebral canal superior to the vertebra of the same number (e.g., C4 spinal nerve exits between C3 and C4 vertebrae).
  • C8 spinal nerve exits below the C7 vertebra (between the C7 and T1 vertebrae).
  • Spinal nerves T1–Co1 exit the canal inferior to the corresponding vertebra.
— Because the spinal cord is shorter than the vertebral column, nerve roots from the lower spinal cord (L2–Co1) must descend below the conus medullaris within the lumbar cistern of the dural sac before exiting through the respective intervertebral foramina. This loose group of nerve roots is called the **cauda equina** (see **Figs. 2.18** and **2.20B**).
— Anterior rami of thoracic spinal nerves become **intercostal nerves**, which run in the spaces between ribs of the thoracic wall. Anterior rami of the cervical, lumbar, and sacral regions (with contributions from T1) form plexuses (**Fig. 2.24A** and **B**):
  • Cervical plexus (C1–C4)
  • Brachial plexus (C5–T1)
  • Lumbar plexus (L1–L4)
  • Sacral plexus (L4–S3)
— The cutaneous (sensory) branches of the pair of spinal nerves derived from a spinal cord segment supply specific areas of skin called **dermatomes** (**Fig. 2.25**). The muscles that are innervated by the motor branches of each pair of spinal nerves are called **myotomes**.

Fig. 2.23 ► **Spinal cord segment**
Anterior view. The spinal cord consists of 31 segments innervating a specific area in the trunk or limbs, Afferent (sensory) posterior rootlets and efferent (motor) anterior rootlets form the posterior and anterior roots, respectively. The two roots fuse to form a mixed spinal nerve, which then divides into various branches.

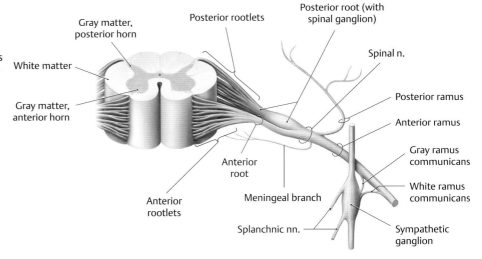

Gray matter, posterior horn
Posterior rootlets
Posterior root (with spinal ganglion)
Spinal n.
White matter
Posterior ramus
Gray matter, anterior horn
Anterior ramus
Gray ramus communicans
Anterior root
White ramus communicans
Anterior rootlets
Meningeal branch
Splanchnic nn.
Sympathetic ganglion

Fig. 2.24 ▶ **Nerves of the trunk wall**

Spinal Cord Segment	Anterior Branches (anterior rami)	Posterior Branches (dorsal rami)
C1		Suboccipital nerve
C2	Cervical plexus	Greater occipital nerve
C3		Third occipital nerve
C4		
C5		
C6	Branchial plexus	
C7		
C8		
T1		
T2		
T3		
T4		
T5		
T6	Intercostal nerves	
T7		
T8		
T9		Posterior rami
T10		
T11		
T12		
T13		
L1		
L2		
L3	Lumbar plexus	
L4		
L5		
S1		
S2		
S3	Sacral plexus	
S4		
S5	Coccygeal plexus	
Co1		
Co2		

A Anterior and posterior branches of the spinal nerves.

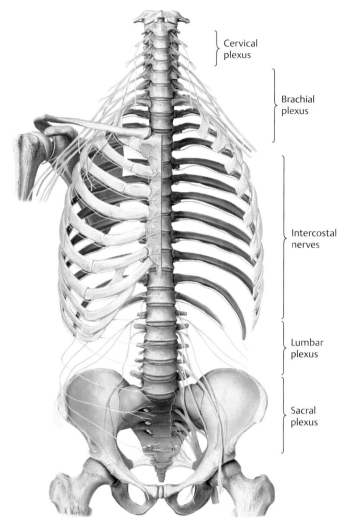

B Nerves of the trunk wall, anterior view. *Removed:* Anterior part of the left half of the thoracic cage.

Fig. 2.25 ▶ **Dermatomes of the head, trunk, and limbs**
Each spinal cord segment innervates a particular skin area (dermatome).

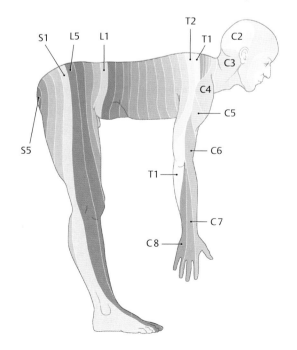

2.4 Muscles of the Back and Suboccipital Region (**Table 2.2**)

— **Extrinsic muscles**, the most superficial muscles that overlie the back, stabilize and move the upper limb. (See Chapter 14 for a discussion of the muscles of the upper limb.)

- Extrinsic muscles include the trapezius, latissimus dorsi, levator scapulae, and rhomboid major and minor.

— **Intrinsic muscles**, which attach to vertebrae or ribs, move and support the vertebral column.

- They are arranged in superficial, intermediate, and deep layers (**Figs. 2.26** and **2.27A** and **B**).
- The superficial layer includes the **splenius** muscle group that covers the deeper neck muscles laterally and posteriorly (**Fig. 2.26**). These muscles extend and rotate the head and neck. They extend superolaterally from the spinous processes of cervical and upper thoracic vertebrae to the occipital bone and transverse processes of C1 and C2
- The intermidiate layer includes the **erector spinae** muscle group that extends from the midline of the back to the angle of the ribs laterally. These large muscles are the main

extensors and stabilizers of the thoracic and lumbar vertebral column. They include

- the **iliocostalis**, the most lateral column that arises from the **thoracolumbar fascia**, the sacrum, iliac crest, and ribs and extends superolaterally to the ribs and to cervical and lumbar vertebrae.
- the **longissimus**, the middle column that arises from the sacrum, iliac crest, spinous processes of lumbar vertebrae, and transverse processes of thoracic and cervical vertebrae. It inserts superiorly on the temporal bone of the skull, to cervical, thoraric and lumbar vertebrae and to the ribs.
- the **spinalis**, the most medical column that extends between the spinous processes of cervical and thoracic vertebrae

Fig. 2.26 ► **Superficial and intermediate muscles of the back** Posterior view. *Removed:* Thoracolumbar fascia (left).

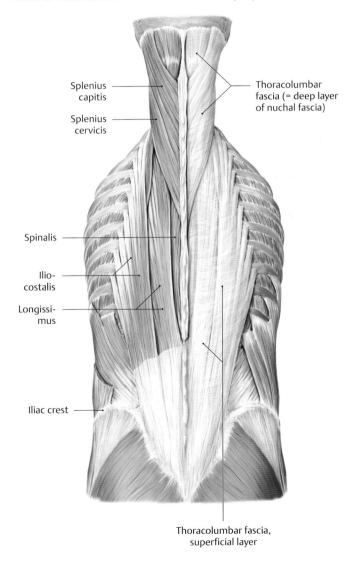

Table 2.2 ► **Muscles of the Back and Suboccipital Region**		
Muscle Group	**Innervation**	**Action**
Intrinsic muscles of the back		
Superficial layer Splenius capitis Splenius cervicis	Posterior rami of cervical spinal nerves	Extend, rotate, and laterally flex the head and cervical spine
Intermediate layer (erector spinae) Spinalis Longissimus Iliocostalis	Posterior rami of spinal nerves	Extend and laterally flex the spine
Deep layer Transversospinalis group Rotatores (brevis and longus) Multifidus Semispinalis Deep segmental group Interspinales Intertransversarii Levatores costarum	Posterior rami of spinal nerves	Extend, rotate, and laterally flex the head and spine
Muscles of the suboccipital region		
Rectus capitus posterior major Rectus capitus posterior minor Obliquus capitus superior Obliquus capitis inferior	Suboccipital n. (C1)	Extend and rotate the head

- The deep layer includes short muscles at multiple vertebral levels that produce small movements along the entire vertebral column (**Fig. 2.27A** and **B**). They are divided into **transversospinalis** muscle group and a **deep segmental** muscle group. The transversospinalis muscles extend between the transverse and spinous processes of the vertebrae, They include:
  - ○ the **semispinalis** muscles, the most superficial this group

- ○ the **multifidis**, most prominent in the lumbar region
- ○ the **rotatores**, the deepest muscles of the transversospinalis group, best developed in the thoraric region

- The deep segmental muscles are minor muscles of the back. They include the **interspinales** and **intertransversarii** that connect adjacent vertebrae, and the **levatores costarum** that connect vertebrae to ribs.

Fig. 2.27 ► **Deep intrinsic back muscles**
Posterior view.

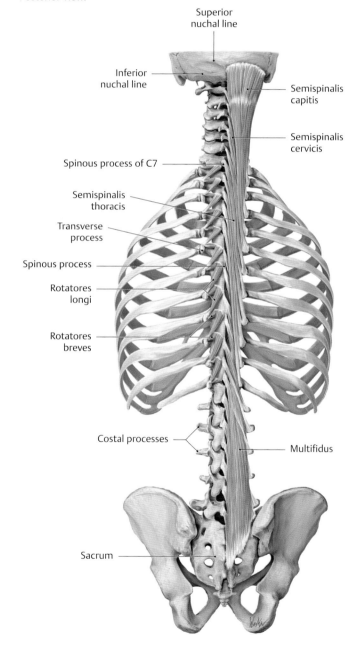

Superior nuchal line
Inferior nuchal line
Semispinalis capitis
Semispinalis cervicis
Spinous process of C7
Semispinalis thoracis
Transverse process
Spinous process
Rotatores longi
Rotatores breves
Costal processes
Multifidus
Sacrum

A Transversospinalis muscles: Rotatores, multifidus, and semispinalis.

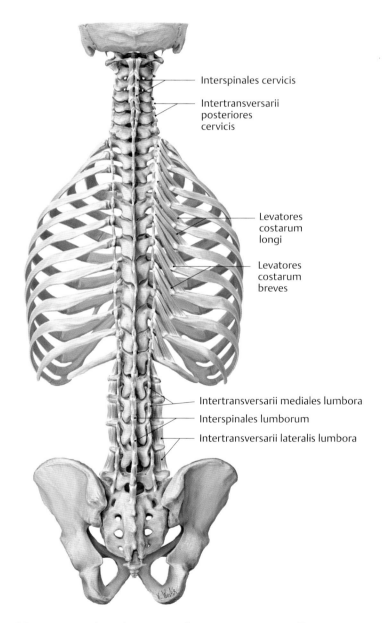

Interspinales cervicis
Intertransversarii posteriores cervicis
Levatores costarum longi
Levatores costarum breves
Intertransversarii mediales lumbora
Interspinales lumborum
Intertransversarii lateralis lumbora

B Deep segmental muscles: Interspinales, intertransversarii, and levatores costarum.

- A deep fascia that encloses the intrinsic muscles runs laterally from the posterior midline to the cervical and lumbar transverse processes and to the ribs. This **thoracolumbar fascia** continues into the neck as the deep layer of the **nuchal fascia**, the posterior extension of the **cervical fascia** (see Section 21.1).

— Muscles of the posterior neck occupy the small **suboccipital compartment** (**Fig. 2.28**) that is inferior to the base of the skull and deep to the trapezius and intrinsic back muscles that extend into the neck. The suboccipital muscles arise from C1 or C2 and extend upward to insert on the occipital bone or transverse process of C1. All assist in the positioning of the head and are innervated by the suboccipital nerve, the posterior ramus of C1. They include the **rectus capitis posterior major, rectus capitis posterior minor, obliquus capitis inferior,** and **obliquus capitis superior.**

— Posterior intercostal and lumbar arteries (branches of the descending aorta and subclavian artery) supply the skin and muscles of the back. The veins of the back accompany the arteries and are tributaries of the azygos system.

— Posterior rami of intercostal and lumbar nerves supply the skin and intrinsic muscles of the back (**Figs. 2.29** and **2.30**).

Fig. 2.29 ▶ **Cutaneous innervation of the back**
Dermatomes: Segmental (radicular) cutaneous innervation of the back. *Note:* The posterior ramus of C1 is purely motor; there is consequently no C1 dermatome.

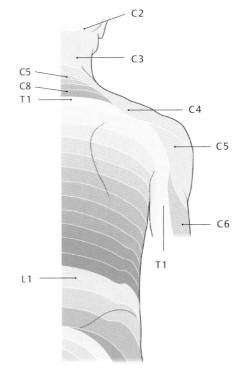

Fig. 2.28 ▶ **Short nuchal and craniovertebral joint muscles**
Suboccipital muscles, posterior view.

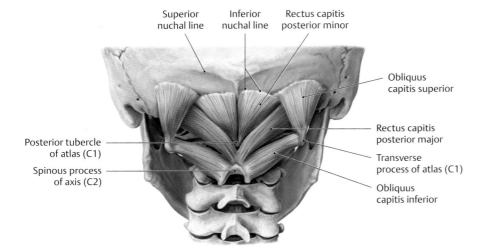

Fig. 2.30 ► **Nerves of the back**
Cross section through the vertebral column and spinal cord with
surrounding musculature, superior view.

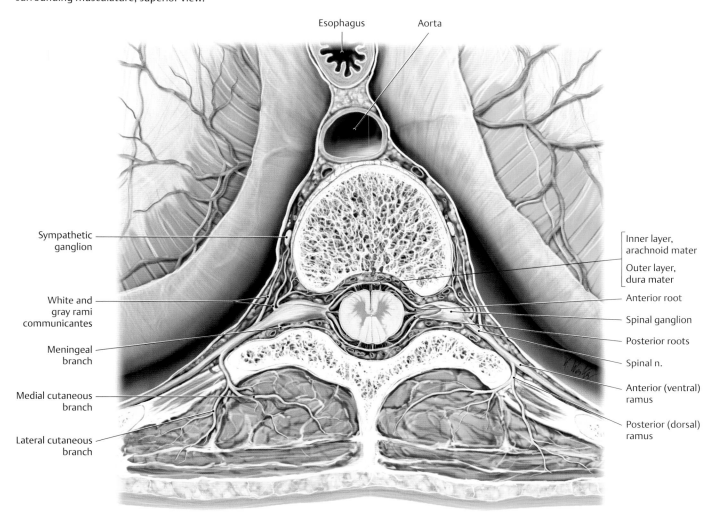

Esophagus   Aorta

Sympathetic
ganglion

Inner layer,
arachnoid mater

Outer layer,
dura mater

Anterior root

Spinal ganglion

White and
gray rami
communicantes

Posterior roots

Spinal n.

Meningeal
branch

Anterior (ventral)
ramus

Medial cutaneous
branch

Posterior (dorsal)
ramus

Lateral cutaneous
branch

Review Questions: Back

1. During the surgical repair of an aortic aneurysm in a 62-year-old patient, the left T10 intercostal artery that supplied the great anterior segmental artery (of Adamkiewicz) was inadvertently ligated. A likely consequence of this would be a disruption of the blood supply to
   A. the cervical enlargement of the spinal cord
   B. the lumbosacral enlargement of the spinal cord
   C. the lower thoracic vertebrae
   D. the deep intrinsic muscles of the back
   E. the posterior one-third of the spinal cord

2. A 57-year-old woman who runs a 4-mile route three times a week complained to her primary care physician of low back pain and an irritating paresthesia (tingling) along the inner aspect of her right leg. Electromyographic studies identified a lesion of her L4 spinal nerve on the right side.
   The L4 spinal nerve
   A. carries only sensory fibers
   B. contributes to both the lumbar and sacral nerve plexuses
   C. contains sympathetic nerve fibers that innervate pelvic viscera
   D. exits the intervertebral foramen between the L3 and L4 vertebrae
   E. innervates intrinsic muscles and skin of the back via its anterior ramus

3. The filum terminale is best described as
   A. an extension of the arachnoid mater that connects to the pia mater
   B. a transverse ligament that suspends the spinal cord within the dural sac
   C. an extension of the pia mater that descends within the lumbar cistern
   D. a ligament that connects the spinous processes of the vertebrae
   E. an extension of the pia mater that anchors the conus medullaris to the L2 vertebra

4. The nerves that descend within the lumbar cistern of the dural sac are called
   A. lumbar plexus
   B. sacral plexus
   C. cauda equina
   D. posterior rami
   E. sacral spinal nerves

5. An 87-year-old patient sees his primary care physician with a complaint of mental confusion and back pain. Although the physician considers that these symptoms may be a normal consequence of his age, examination reveals that he has advanced prostate cancer that has spread to his brain and vertebral column. The probable route of metastasis is identified as the vertebral venous plexus, which
   A. drains the vertebrae and intervertebral disks but does not drain the spinal cord
   B. lies within the subarachnoid space
   C. consists of veins with multiple valves along their length
   D. consists of paired longitudinal veins within the vertebral canal
   E. is a valveless system of veins

6. A 47-year-old construction worker presented to his physician with debilitating pain in his lower back and lower limb. Radiographic studies showed a herniated intervertebral disk at the L4–L5 vertebral level. Which of the following is true?
   A. The herniated disk most likely signals a weakness of the anterior longitudinal ligament.
   B. A posterior herniation of this disk could result in compression of the adjacent spinal cord.
   C. Pain from this hernia would most likely be felt along the L4 dermatome.
   D. The herniation is the result of a loss of elasticity of the anulus fibrosus, which allowed protrusion of the nucleus pulposus.
   E. None of the above

7. The splenius muscle group
   A. lies deep to the trapezius
   B. is enclosed by the thoracolumbar fascia
   C. extends the cervical spine and head
   D. is innervated by posterior rami of cervical spinal nerves
   E. All of the above

8. Ninety-two-year-old Sadie Parker remains mentally alert and physically active but has lost several inches in height, and her posture is stooped forward. Her geriatrician explains that this exaggerated curvature is due to degeneration of the bodies of two of her thoracic vertebrae and often occurs in older women as a result of decreased bone density. The curvature exhibited by this patient is known as
   A. scoliosis
   B. spondylolysis
   C. lordosis
   D. kyphosis
   E. spondylosis

9. The spinal cord terminates caudally as the
   A. denticulate ligament
   B. filum terminale
   C. conus medullaris
   D. lumbar cistern
   E. sacral hiatus

10. Which of the following ligaments would prevent hyperextension of the vertebral column?
   A. Anterior longitudinal ligament
   B. Posterior longitudinal ligament
   C. Ligamentum flavum
   D. Alar ligament
   E. Cruciform ligament

11. Which of the following vertebral characteristics is paired with the correct vertebral region?
   A. Promontory—sacral
   B. Vertebral prominens—thoracic
   C. Dens—thoracic
   D. Transverse foramen—lumbar
   E. Costal facet—cervical

Answers and Explanations

1. **B** The great anterior segmental artery (of Adamkiewicz) supplies the inferior two-thirds of the spinal cord, which includes the region of the lumbosacral enlargement (T11–S1) (Section 2.3c).
A The great anterior segmental artery (of Adamkiewicz) supplies the inferior two-thirds of the spinal cord, which does not include the region of the cervical enlargement (C4–T1).
C Vertebrae are supplied by segmental arteries of the descending aorta, as well as by branches of the subclavian arteries and arteries of the pelvis.
D Intrinsic muscles of the back get their blood supply from posterior branches of the intercostal and lumbar arteries.
E The posterior spinal arteries that usually arise from the vertebral arteries in the neck supply the posterior third of the spinal cord.

2. **B** The lumbar plexus includes anterior rami of spinal nerves L1–L4, and the sacral plexus includes anterior rami of spinal nerves L4–S4 (Section 2.3d).
A All spinal nerves carry both sensory and motor fibers
C Sympathetic fibers are carried only in spinal nerves between T1 and L2.
D Except for nerves in the cervical region, spinal nerves exit below the vertebra of the corresponding number; thus, L4 exits between the L4 and L5 vertebrae.
E Intrinsic muscles and skin of the back are innervated by posterior rami of spinal nerves.

3. **C** The filum terminale is a filament of pia mater that runs within the lumbar cistern with the cauda equina, from the conus medullaris to the end of the dural sac. Inferior to the dural sac, it is surrounded by spinal dura mater and extends to the coccyx (Section 2.3b).
A The arachnoid trabeculae connect the arachnoid mater to the pia mater.
B Denticulate ligaments suspend the spinal cord within the dural sac.
D The supraspinous ligament connects the spinous processes of all thoracic, lumbar, and sacral vertebrae. In the cervical region it expands as the nuchal ligament, a finlike ligament that attaches superiorly to the occipital bone.
E The end of the spinal cord, the conus medullaris, lies adjacent to the L2 vertebra but is not attached to it.

4. **C** Because the spinal cord is shorter than the vertebral column, spinal nerves L2–Co1 descend as a group (cauda equina) within the dural sac before exiting at the appropriate intervertebral foramen (Section 2.3d).
A The lumbar plexus forms outside the vertebral canal on the posterior abdominal wall and contains only anterior rami of lumbar spinal nerves (L1–L4).
B The sacral plexus forms outside the vertebral canal on the posterior wall of the pelvis and contains only anterior rami of L4–S4 spinal nerves.
D The nerves of the cauda equina are spinal nerves, which contain both anterior and posterior rami.
E The cauda equina contains both lumbar and sacral spinal nerves.

5. **E** The vertebral venous plexus is a valveless system that allows communication between the caval and azygos systems, which drain the trunk, and the venous sinuses of the brain (Section 2.2d).
A The vertebral venous plexus drains the vertebrae, meninges, and spinal cord.
B The internal vertebral venous plexus lies in the epidural space. The external plexus surrounds the outside of the vertebral column.
C The vertebral venous plexus is a valveless system that allows communication between the caval and azygos systems, which drain the trunk, and the venous sinuses of the brain.
D The venous plexus consists of interconnecting veins that form an internal plexus within the vertebral canal and an external plexus that surrounds the vertebrae.

6. **D** Loss in elasticity of the fibrous ring, which may occur with aging, allows herniation of the nucleus pulposus (Section 2.2b).
A The anterior longitudinal ligament supports the vertebral bodies and disks anteriorly. The posterior longitudinal ligament supports the disks posteriorly where herniation normally occurs.
B The spinal cord ends at L2 and is not present in this part of the vertebral canal.
C The L4 spinal nerve exits the intervertebral foramen superior to the intervertebral disk and is usually unaffected by the herniation. The hernia would compress the next inferior spinal nerve, L5, and pain would be felt along that dermatome.
E Not applicable

7. **E** All of the above (Section 2.4)

A The splenius muscles are superficial intrinsic back muscles that lie deep to the trapezius, an extrinsic muscle of the upper back. B through D are also correct (E).

B All intrinsic back muscles, including the splenius group, are enclosed by the deep fascia of the back, the thoracolumbar fascia. A, C, and D are also correct (E).

C Splenius muscles extend the cervical spine and head when working bilaterally. Unilaterally, they flex and rotate the head to the same side. A, B, and D are also correct (E).

D The splenius muscles are innervated by the posterior rami of C1–C6 spinal nerves. A through C are also correct (E).

8. **D** Kyphosis is an abnormal posterior curvature of the thoracic spine often seen in older women (Section 2.1a).

A Scoliosis is a lateral curvature of the spine.

B Spondylolysis refers to a fracture or defect across the interarticular part of the lamina of the lumbar vertebrae.

C Lordosis is an exaggerated anterior curvature of the lumbar spine often seen in pregnant women.

E Spondylosis is a degeneration of the intervertebral disk and corresponding vertebral body that results in osteophyte formation.

9. **C** The spinal cord terminates caudally as the conus medullaris. This usually corresponds to the L1–L2 vertebral level in an adult (Section 2.3a).

A Denticulate ligaments are transverse extensions of the pia mater that attach to dura mater and suspend the spinal cord within the dural sac.

B Pia mater terminates caudally as the filum terminale.

D The lumbar cistern is part of the subarachnoid space that lies between the conus medullaris and the inferior end of the dural sac.

E The sacral hiatus is the inferior opening of the sacral canal, which is a continuation of the vertebral canal.

10. **A** The anterior longitudinal ligament attaches the anterior and lateral surfaces of the vertebral bodies and intervertebral disks and prevents hyperextension (Section 2.2c).

B The posterior longitudinal ligament attaches primarily to the intervertebral disks and produces weak resistance to hyperflexion.

C The ligamenta flava join the laminae of adjacent vertebrae. They limit flexion and provide postural support of the vertebral column.

D The alar ligaments secure the dens of C2 to the skull.

E The cruciform ligament, formed by longitudinal fibers and a transverse ligament, secure the dens against the anterior arch of the atlas.

11. **A** The anterior lip of S1 forms the promontory of the sacrum (Section 2.2a).

B The vertebral prominens is the C7 vertebra, named for its long palpable spinous process.

C Only the C2 vertebra has a dens, the peglike process that articulates with C1.

D Only cervical vertebrae have transverse foramina.

E Only thoracic vertebrae have costal facets where they articulate with the ribs.

3   Overview of the Thorax

The thorax is the region of the trunk between the neck and abdomen. The thoracic cavity, surrounded by a bony cage, which protects the thoracic contents, is open to the neck but separated from the abdomen by a muscular diaphragm. The viscera of the thorax include the primary organs of the respiratory and cardiovascular systems, as well as components of the gastrointestinal, endocrine, and lymphatic systems.

3.1   General Features

— The thorax is divided into two lateral compartments, the **pulmonary cavities**, which contain the lungs and pleural sac, and a central compartment, the **mediastinum**, which contains the heart, pericardial sac, trachea and bronchi, esophagus, thymus, and neurovasculature (**Table 3.1**).
— A **pericardial sac** surrounds the heart, and a **pleural sac** surrounds each lung. These closed membranous sacs contain a thin layer of serous fluid that ensures frictionless movement, which is crucial to the function of these organs.
— The lungs are the organs of respiration. They communicate with the **tracheobronchial tree** (the passages for air between the lungs and outside environment) and the heart through the **hilum**, an indentation on the medial surface of each lung.
— The heart is a four-chambered muscular organ that functions as a dual pump that propels blood through the body. Each pump is made up of two chambers: a thin-walled **atrium** and a thick-walled **ventricle**.
— During a cardiac cycle, the right pump receives deoxygenated blood from the **systemic circulation** (circulation of blood through all regions of the body except the lungs) and directs it to the **pulmonary circulation** in the lungs. The left pump receives oxygenated blood from the pulmonary circulation and returns it to the systemic circulation for the distribution of oxygen and nutrients (**Fig. 3.1**).
— Coordinated contraction of atria and ventricles, known as the **cardiac cycle**, is self-moderated by specialized tissue within the cardiac muscle that makes up the heart's **conduction system**.

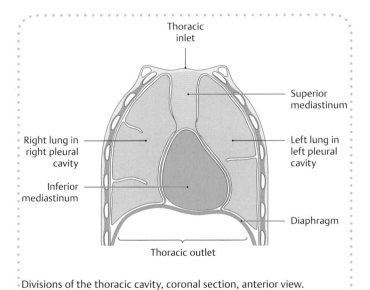

Divisions of the thoracic cavity, coronal section, anterior view.

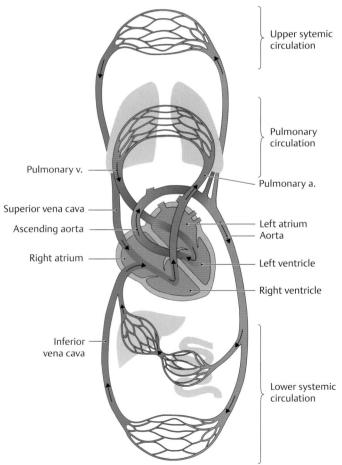

Fig. 3.1 ▶ **Systemic and pulmonary circulation**
Red, oxygenated blood; blue, deoxygenated blood.

Table 3.1 ▶ Major Structures of the Thoracic Cavity			
Mediastinum	Superior mediastinum		Thymus, great vessels, trachea, esophagus, and thoracic duct
	Inferior mediastinum	Anterior	Thymus
		Middle	Heart, pericardium, and roots of great vessels
		Posterior	Thoracic aorta, thoracic duct, esophagus, and azygos venous system
Pulmonary cavities	Right pulmonary cavity		Right lung, pleura
	Left pulmonary cavity		Left lung, pleura

3.2 Neurovasculature of the Thorax

The "great vessels," which include the pulmonary arteries and veins, the aorta, the superior vena cava, and the inferior vena cava, direct blood into and out of the heart and lungs. Their branches and further details of their anatomy, along with more detailed descriptions of lymphatic drainage and nerves of the thorax, are discussed in Chapters 5 and 6 on the mediastinum and pulmonary cavities.

3.2a   Arteries of the Thorax

— The **pulmonary trunk** directs deoxygenated blood from the right side of the heart into the pulmonary circulation. It arises from the right ventricle on the anterior surface of the heart, passes superiorly and posteriorly, and, under the arch of the aorta, divides into **right** and **left pulmonary arteries** (**Fig. 3.2**).
— One pulmonary artery enters each lung, where it branches into generations of smaller vessels that accompany the respiratory passages. The pulmonary arteries transport deoxygenated blood to the small respiratory units in the lungs.

Fig. 3.2 ▶ **Pulmonary arteries and veins**
Distribution of the pulmonary arteries and veins, anterior view.

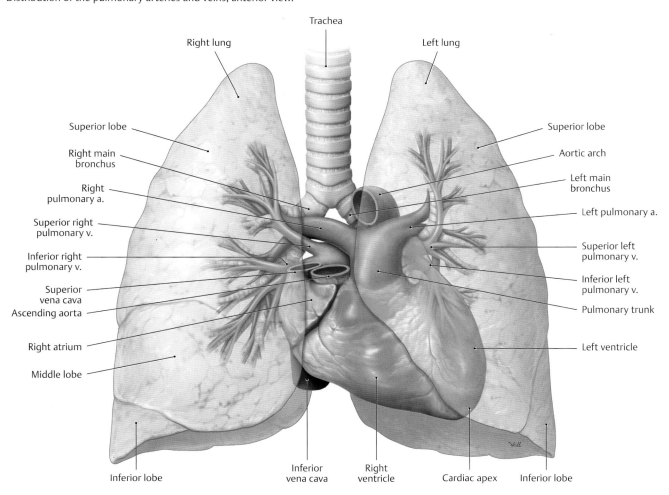

— The **thoracic aorta** arises from the left side of the heart and carries oxygenated blood that is distributed to the systemic circulation. It is divided into three sections:

- The **ascending aorta** arises from the left ventricle of the heart and ascends to the level of the fourth thoracic vertebra. The right and left coronary arteries are its only branches.
- The **aortic arch** (radiographically, the "aortic knob") ascends anterior to the right pulmonary artery and the bifurcation of the trachea (where the trachea splits into right and left bronchi). It courses posteriorly and to the left, arching over the structures entering the left lung, and then turns inferiorly to descend to the left of the trachea and esophagus. It terminates on the left side of the T4 vertebral body. Three large branches arise from the arch (**Fig. 3.3A**):

  ○ The **brachiocephalic trunk**, which ascends posterior to the right sternoclavicular joint, where it bifurcates into the **right common carotid** and **right subclavian arteries**
  ○ The **left common carotid artery**, which enters the neck posterior to the left sternoclavicular joint
  ○ The **left subclavian artery**, which arises from the distal segment of the arch and enters the neck posterior to the left sternoclavicular joint

- The **descending aorta**, a continuation of the aortic arch, descends within the posterior mediastinum, where it passes posterior to the root of the left lung and anterior and to the left of the thoracic vertebral bodies. It passes into the abdomen through the diaphragm at T12. Its thoracic branches are (**Fig. 3.3B**)

  ○ the **posterior intercostal arteries,** which run anteriorly within the 3rd through the 11th intercostal spaces (between the ribs), where they anastomose with the anterior intercostal arteries; and
  ○ the visceral branches to the esophagus, trachea, bronchi, and pericardium.

Fig. 3.3 ▶ **Thoracic aorta**

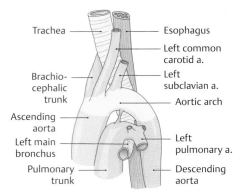

A Parts of the aortic arch, left lateral view. *Note:* The aortic arch begins and ends at the level of the sternal angle (T4–T5).

Fig. 3.3 ▶ **Thoracic aorta** (*continued*)

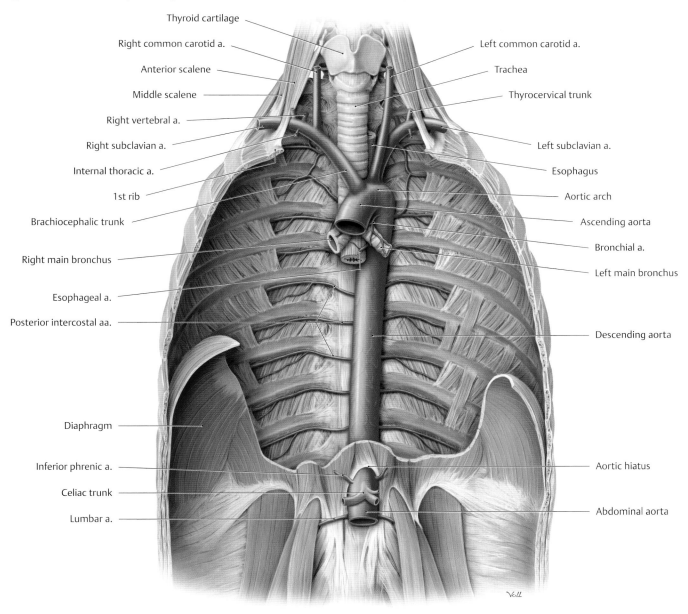

Thyroid cartilage

Right common carotid a.

Anterior scalene

Middle scalene

Right vertebral a.

Right subclavian a.

Internal thoracic a.

1st rib

Brachiocephalic trunk

Right main bronchus

Esophageal a.

Posterior intercostal aa.

Diaphragm

Inferior phrenic a.

Celiac trunk

Lumbar a.

Left common carotid a.

Trachea

Thyrocervical trunk

Left subclavian a.

Esophagus

Aortic arch

Ascending aorta

Bronchial a.

Left main bronchus

Descending aorta

Aortic hiatus

Abdominal aorta

B Thoracic aorta in situ, anterior view. *Removed*: Heart, lungs, and portions of diaphragm.

— The **internal thoracic artery** arises from the subclavian artery in the neck and descends deep to the ribs, just lateral to the sternum. Its branches supply the thoracic and abdominal walls (**Fig. 3.4**):

- The **anterior intercostal arteries**, which run within the intercostal spaces
- The **musculophrenic artery**, a terminal branch of the internal thoracic artery, which arises at the level of the sixth costal cartilage and follows the lower margin of the ribcage laterally
- The **superior epigastric artery**, a terminal branch of the internal thoracic artery, which runs inferiorly to supply muscles of the anterior abdominal wall

Fig. 3.4 ▶ **Arteries of the thoracic wall**
Anterior view.

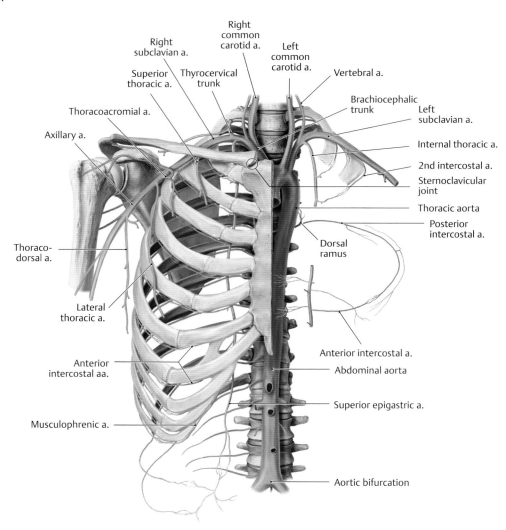

3.2b   Veins of the Thorax (Fig. 3.5)

— **Internal thoracic veins**, which receive the anterior intercostal veins, accompany the internal thoracic arteries and drain into the brachiocephalic veins of the superior mediastinum.
— The **right** and **left brachiocephalic veins**, which drain the head, neck, and upper limb, form behind the clavicle by the convergence of the internal jugular and subclavian veins. The left brachiocephalic vein, which is longer than the right, crosses the midline just anterior to the branches of the aortic arch and converges with the right vein to form the superior vena cava.

— The **superior vena cava**, which returns deoxygenated blood from the upper body to the heart, forms on the right side, posterior to the costal cartilage of the first rib by the junction of the brachiocephalic veins. It descends behind and to the right side of the aorta and drains into the superior pole of the right atrium.

Superior vena cava syndrome

The superior vena cava syndrome is an obstruction of the superior vena cava (SVC), which in the majority of cases is caused by mediastinal tumors such as metastatic lung carcinoma (the upper lobe of the right lung lies next to the SVC), lymphoma, breast cancer, or thyroid cancer. Noncancerous causes include thromboses (blood clots) that obstruct the lumen and infections that produce scarring. The onset of symptoms is usually gradual and includes dyspnea (shortness of breath) and swelling of the face, neck, and arms.

Fig. 3.5 ▶ **Veins of the thoracic wall**
Anterior view with rib cage opened. *Removed*: Clavicle.

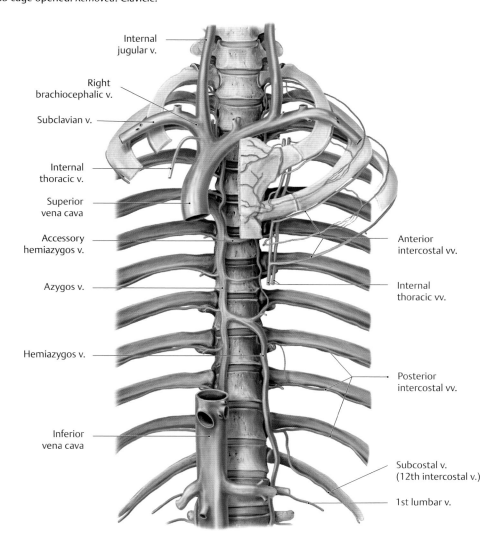

— The **inferior vena cava**, which returns deoxygenated blood to the heart from the abdomen, pelvis, and lower limbs, enters the right atrium after passing through the diaphragm from the abdomen. Only a small portion, therefore, is located within the thorax.

— The **pulmonary veins**, two on each side (often three on the left side), carry oxygenated blood from the lungs to the left side of the heart (see **Fig. 3.2**).

— The **azygos system** drains veins of the thoracic and anterolateral abdominal walls (**Fig. 3.6**; see also **Fig. 3.5**).

  • The **azygos vein** ascends along the right side of the thoracic vertebral bodies as it drains the **posterior intercostal veins** of the thoracic wall on that side. It arches over the hilum of the right lung to empty into the superior vena cava.

• The **accessory hemiazygos** and **hemiazygos veins** run along the left side of the thoracic vertebrae and drain the thoracic wall on the left side. They cross the midline independently (or they may join to form a single vessel) to drain into the azygos vein on the right side.

• The azygos and hemiazygos veins are the continuations of the **ascending lumbar veins** in the abdomen, which communicate with the inferior vena cava. Thus the azygos system links the drainages of the superior and inferior vena cavae and provides a collateral (alternate) pathway for blood back to the heart.

• Mediastinal, esophageal, and bronchial veins in the thorax, and the vertebral venous plexus (see Section 2.2d) are also tributaries of the azygos system.

Fig. 3.6 ▸ **Azygos system**
Anterior view.

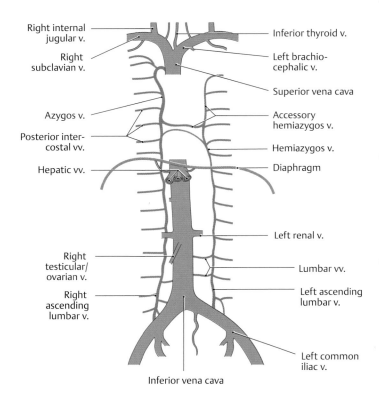

Right internal jugular v.
Right subclavian v.
Azygos v.
Posterior inter-costal vv.
Hepatic vv.
Right testicular/ovarian v.
Right ascending lumbar v.
Inferior thyroid v.
Left brachio-cephalic v.
Superior vena cava
Accessory hemiazygos v.
Hemiazygos v.
Diaphragm
Left renal v.
Lumbar vv.
Left ascending lumbar v.
Left common iliac v.
Inferior vena cava

3.2c Lymphatics of the Thorax (see Fig. 1.20)

— The **thoracic duct**, the main lymphatic vessel of the body,

  • drains the abdomen, pelvis, and lower limbs, and the left side of the thorax, head, neck, and left upper limb;

  • enters the thorax from its origin in the abdomen and passes superiorly in the midline of the posterior mediastinum; and

  • terminates at the junction of the left subclavian and left internal jugular veins (jugulosubclavian junction or "venous angle") in the neck.

— The **right lymphatic duct**, which has a variable form,

  • drains lymph from the right side of the thorax, head, and neck, and the right upper limb; and

  • usually terminates at the junction of the right subclavian and right interval jugular veins (the jugulosubclavian junction).

— Lymph from most thoracic structures drains through chains of lymph nodes that empty into **bronchomediastinal trunks** in the mediastinum (**Figs. 3.7** and **3.8**). This includes

  • parasternal and intercostal lymph nodes of the thoracic wall and superior surface of the diaphragm;

  • bronchopulmonary and intrapulmonary lymph nodes of the lungs and bronchi; and

  • tracheobronchial, paratracheal, and paraesophageal lymph nodes of the heart, pericardium, trachea, and esophagus.

— The bronchomediastinal trunks may empty into the thoracic and right lymphatic ducts, but, more commonly, they empty directly into the subclavian veins in the neck.

Fig. 3.7 ▶ **Lymphatic trunks in the thorax**
Anterior view of opened thorax.

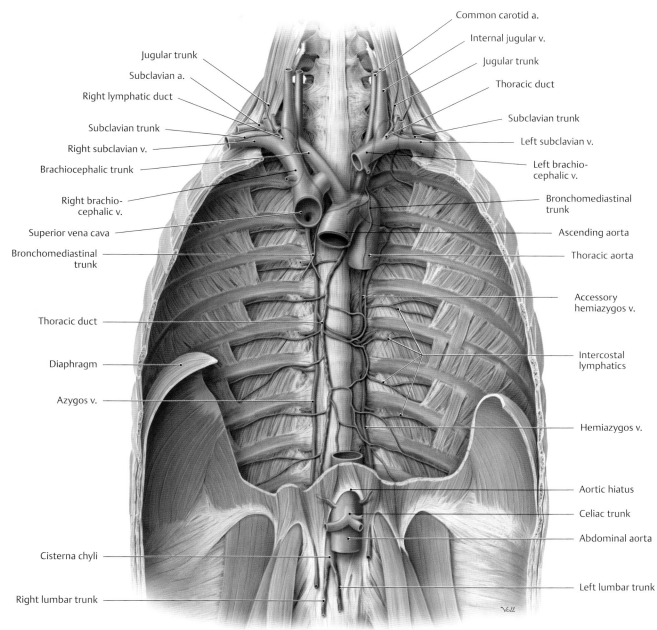

Fig. 3.8 ▶ **Thoracic lymph nodes**
Transverse section at the level of the tracheal bifurcation (at approximately T4), viewed from below. Topographically, the thoracic lymph nodes can be divided into three broad groups:

— Lymph nodes in the thoracic wall (pink)
— Lymph nodes in the lung and at the divisions of the bronchial tree (blue)
— Lymph nodes associated with the trachea, esophagus, and pericardium (green)

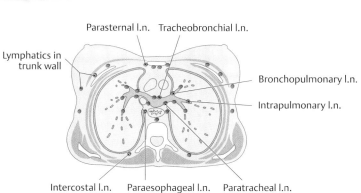

3.2d Nerves of the Thorax (Figs. 3.9, 3.10)

— Pairs of **posterior intercostal nerves** arise from the anterior (ventral) rami of T1–T11 and pass along the inferior edge of the ribs on their deep surface.

   V
   A
   N

• The nerves innervate the muscles between the ribs, overlying muscles and skin of the thoracic wall and the breast.

— **Phrenic nerves** arise in the neck from anterior rami of C3, 4, and 5 ("keeps the diaphragm alive") and descend into the thorax.

• On the right, the nerve runs along the superior vena cava; on the left, it crosses lateral to the aortic arch.

• Both nerves pass anterior to the hila of the lungs as they descend to the diaphragm between the pericardial and pleural sacs.

• The phrenic nerves innervate the pericardium, the medial part of the pleura, and the diaphragm.

— The **thoracic sympathetic trunks** run along either side of the thoracic vertebral column.

Fig. 3.10 ► **Nerves of the posterior mediastinum**
Anterior view.

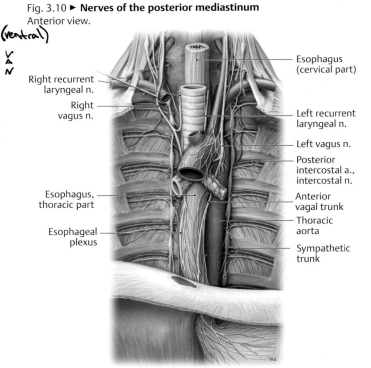

Right recurrent laryngeal n.
Right vagus n.
Esophagus, thoracic part
Esophageal plexus
Esophagus (cervical part)
Left recurrent laryngeal n.
Left vagus n.
Posterior intercostal a., intercostal n.
Anterior vagal trunk
Thoracic aorta
Sympathetic trunk

Fig. 3.9 ► **Nerves of the thorax**
Anterior view of opened thorax.

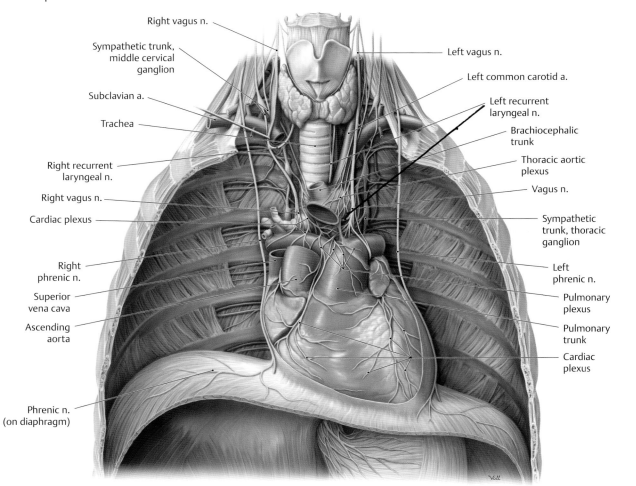

Right vagus n.
Sympathetic trunk, middle cervical ganglion
Subclavian a.
Trachea
Right recurrent laryngeal n.
Right vagus n.
Cardiac plexus
Right phrenic n.
Superior vena cava
Ascending aorta
Phrenic n. (on diaphragm)
Left vagus n.
Left common carotid a.
Left recurrent laryngeal n.
Brachiocephalic trunk
Thoracic aortic plexus
Vagus n.
Sympathetic trunk, thoracic ganglion
Left phrenic n.
Pulmonary plexus
Pulmonary trunk
Cardiac plexus

- Sympathetic (paravertebral) ganglia at each spinal level communicate with spinal nerves through white and gray rami communicans.
- The T1 ganglion may combine with the ganglion at C8 to form a large star-shaped stellate ganglion.
- Splanchnic nerves, derived from the sympathetic trunk, pass medially to contribute to the autonomic plexuses of the thorax, which innervate thoracic viscera.

— Nerves derived from the thoracic sympathetic trunk, called the **greater** (T5 to T9 or T10), **lesser** (T10–T11), and **least splanchnic nerves** course inferomedially along the thoracic vertebral bodies into the abdomen. They contain preganglionic fibers that synapse in prevertebral ganglia of abdominal autonomic nerve plexuses.

— The **vagus nerves** (CN X) descend from the neck into the thorax.

- The right vagus courses behind the superior vena cava, medial to the arch of the azygos vein; the left vagus runs lateral to the aortic arch.
- Both vagus nerves pass posterior to the hilum of the lung before merging on the wall of the esophagus.
- The vagus nerves contribute parasympathetic fibers to the cardiac, pulmonary, and esophageal plexuses.

— The **left recurrent laryngeal nerve**, a branch of the left vagus nerve, passes under the aortic arch, posterior to the **ligamentum arteriosum** (see Section 5.6), and turns superiorly to ascend in the neck in the groove between the trachea and esophagus.

- The right recurrent laryngeal nerve, a branch of the right vagus, recurs around the subclavian artery in the neck and is not a thoracic structure.

— The **esophageal plexus** surrounds the lower esophagus.

- It is composed of preganglionic parasympathetic fibers from the right and left vagus nerves and postganglionic fibers from the thoracic sympathetic trunk.
- **Anterior** and **posterior vagal trunks** arise from the plexus and pass into the abdomen, anterior and posterior to the esophagus.

— The **cardiac plexus** (**Fig. 3.11**; see also **Fig. 3.9**), which is located above the heart in the concavity of the arch of the aorta, continues along the coronary arteries and over the bifurcations of the trachea and pulmonary trunk. It innervates the conducting system of the heart and contains

- preganglionic sympathetic fibers from T1 to T5 and postganglionic sympathetic fibers from cardiopulmonary branches of the cervical and thoracic sympathetic trunk;
- preganglionic parasympathetic fibers from cardiac branches of the vagus nerve that arise in the cervical region and contributions from the recurrent laryngeal nerves; and
- visceral sensory fibers that travel with sympathetic and parasympathetic nerves.

— The **pulmonary plexus** is a continuation of the cardiac plexus onto the bifurcation of the trachea and the bronchi that penetrate the hilum of each lung.

- It regulates the constriction and dilation of the pulmonary vessels and respiratory passages.
- It transmits sensation from the lung and visceral, or inner, layer of the pleural sac that is adherent to the surface of the lung.

Fig. 3.11 ► **Autonomic innervation of the heart** Schematic.

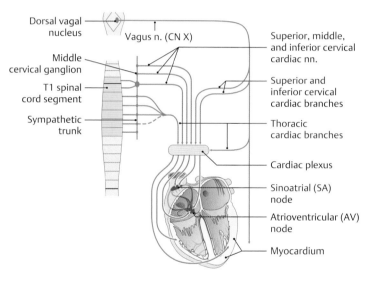

4 Thoracic Wall

A bony and muscular cage, which communicates superiorly with the neck and inferiorly with the abdomen, encloses and protects the thoracic contents. A superficial layer of extrinsic muscles overlies the thoracic cage, although these muscles act primarily on the upper limb. The breast, a derivative of the epidermis (outermost layer of skin), is a prominent superficial structure of the thoracic wall.

4.1 The Breast

4.1a General Features

The breast is made up of the **mammary gland**, a modified sweat gland, and its supporting fat and fibrous tissue (**Fig. 4.1A, B, C, and D**). Breasts remain rudimentary in males but are prominent structures of the female pectoral region.

— Female breasts extend from the lateral border of the sternum to the midaxillary line and overlie the 2nd through 6th ribs.
— The breast is embedded in the subcutaneous layer of the skin overlying the deep fascia of the pectoralis major and serratus anterior muscles.
— The **retromammary space** is a plane of loose connective tissue that separates the breast from underlying fascia of the pectoralis major muscle and allows movement of the breasts on the thoracic wall.
— The highest prominence of the breast, the **nipple**, is located at the center of the areola. Circularly arranged smooth muscle fibers cause erection of the nipple in response to cold or tactile stimulation. In men and young women, the nipple is at the T4 vertebral level, but in older women this location varies considerably.
— The **areola**, the pigmented skin surrounding the nipple, contains sebaceous glands whose oily secretions lubricate the area during nursing.
— An **axillary tail**, or small finger of glandular tissue, may extend into the axilla (armpit) along the lower edge of the pectoralis muscle.
— The volume of fat, not the volume of glandular tissue, largely determines the differences in breast size among women.

4.1b Mammary Gland

The mammary gland has two components:

— The **parenchyma**, or milk-producing part of the gland (see **Fig. 4.1B**)
  • The parenchyma consists of lobes divided into 15 to 20 lobules, which contain grapelike clusters of **alveoli**, hollow balls lined by secretory cells.
  • **Lactiferous ducts** in the parenchyma drain each lobule and open at the nipple. Deep to the areola, each duct has a small, dilated portion called the **lactiferous sinus** where, in lactating females, a small amount of milk is stored.
— The **stroma**, or fibrous framework, of the gland that separates the lobules and supports the lobes
  • Stroma is attached to the overlying dermis of the skin by **suspensory (Cooper) ligaments**, which are particularly strong on the superior surface of the breast.

4.1c Neurovasculature of the Breast

— Anterior intercostal branches and medial mammary branches (from perforating branches) of the internal thoracic artery, **lateral thoracic** and **thoracodorsal branches** of the axillary artery, and the 2nd, 3rd, and 4th posterior intercostal arteries supply the breast (see **Fig. 3.4**).
— Venous blood drains primarily to the axillary vein but also to the internal thoracic vein.

Fig. 4.1 ▶ **Structures of the breast**

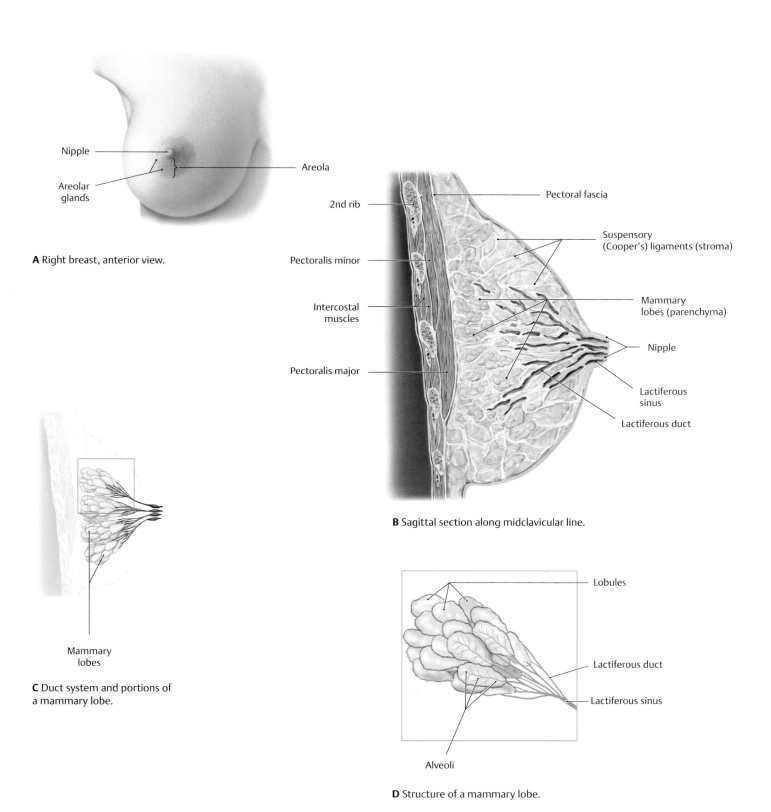

A Right breast, anterior view.

B Sagittal section along midclavicular line.

C Duct system and portions of a mammary lobe.

D Structure of a mammary lobe.

— Most lymph (> 75%) from the breast drains (particularly from the lateral quadrant) to axillary lymph nodes (**Fig. 4.2**); from there it travels to nodes around the clavicle and the ipsilateral lymphatic duct.

  • Some lymph may drain to deep pectoral nodes, where it joins the bronchomediastinal drainage in the mediastinum.
  • Medial portions of the breast may drain to parasternal nodes and to the contralateral breast; inferior segments may drain to abdominal nodes.

— The anterior and lateral cutaneous branches of the 4th, 5th, and 6th intercostal nerves innervate the breast.

Fig. 4.2 ► **Lymphatic drainage of the female breast**
Axillary, parasternal, and cervical lymph nodes. Right thoracic and axillary region with the arm abducted, anterior view.

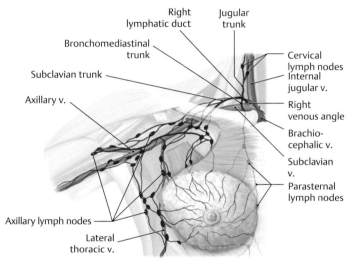

Carcinoma of the breast

The most common type of breast cancer, invasive ductal carcinoma, arises from the lining of the lactiferous ducts. Typically, it metastasizes through lymphatic channels, most abundantly to axillary nodes, but it may also travel to supraclavicular nodes, the contralateral breast, and the abdomen. Obstruction of the lymphatic drainage causes edema, and fibrosis (shortening) of the suspensory ligaments can cause a pitted appearance of the skin. Through venous communication with the azygos system and vertebral venous plexus, breast cancer can metastasize to the vertebrae, cranium, and brain. Elevation of the breast with contraction of the pectoralis major muscle suggests invasion of the pectoralis fascia and retromammary space.

4.2 The Thoracic Skeleton

The thoracic skeleton protects the thoracic viscera and provides attachment for the upper limb. The thoracic cage includes the sternum, 12 pairs of ribs, and the 12 thoracic vertebrae (**Fig. 4.3**; see also Section 2.2).

4.2a The Sternum

The **sternum** is a flat, elongated bone that has three parts:

1. The **manubrium**, which articulates laterally with the costal cartilages (cartilage that attaches the ribs to the sternum) of the 1st and 2nd ribs. A deep **jugular notch** separates the right and left sternoclavicular joints (see **Fig. 1.7A**), where the manubrium articulates with the clavicles.
2. The **body**, which is fused superiorly with the manubrium at the **manubriosternal joint**. Laterally, the body articulates with costal cartilages of the 2nd to 7th ribs.
3. The **xiphoid process**, the lowest part of the sternum, which joins superiorly with the body of the sternum at the xiphisternal joint.

  • The **sternal angle** is an important surface landmark on the anterior thoracic wall that provides orientation to the internal anatomy of the thorax. It is a palpable ridge that marks the fusion of the manubrium and body of the sternum. A horizontal plane through the sternal angle intersects
    ○ the articulation between the sternum and the costal cartilages of the 2nd ribs,
    ○ the division of the mediastinum into superior and inferior regions,
    ○ the origin and termination of the aortic arch,
    ○ the bifurcation of the trachea, and
    ○ the T4–T5 intervertebral disk.

Fig. 4.3 ► **Thoracic skeleton**
Anterior view.

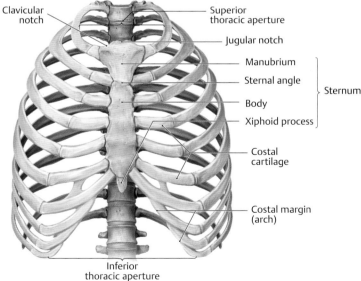

4.2b   The Ribs

— The ribs are numbered 1 to 12 from superior to inferior, and each rib articulates with a thoracic vertebra of the same number.
— The ribs hang obliquely downward from their articulation with the vertebral column. Their anterior ends may be two to five vertebral levels lower than their posterior attachment (**Fig. 4.4**).
— Ribs 1 to10 articulate anteriorly with a cartilaginous segment called the **costal cartilage**.
— The ribs are classified according to their articulation with the sternum (see **Fig. 4.4**):
  • **True ribs** (1 to 7) articulate directly with the sternum via individual costal cartilages.
  • **False ribs** (8 to 10) articulate indirectly with the sternum through costal cartilages that are connected to the cartilage superior to it.
  • **Floating ribs** (11 and 12) have no connection to the sternum.
— Most ribs articulate at three joints (**Fig. 4.5**):
  1. **Costochondral joints** between the bony segments of ribs 1 to 10 and their respective **costal cartilages**
  2. **Sternocostal joints** between the sternum and costal cartilages of ribs 1 to 7 on each side
  3. **Costovertebral joints** between the ribs and vertebrae. These joints may contain multiple articulations.
     ◦ The **costal tubercle** of each rib articulates with the costal facet on its accompanying vertebra (see **Fig. 2.5A**).
     ◦ The **heads** of ribs 2 to 10 articulate with the vertebra of the same number and with the vertebra superior to them. Ribs 1, 11, and 12 articulate only with their own vertebra.

Fig. 4.4 ▶ **Types of ribs**
Left lateral view.

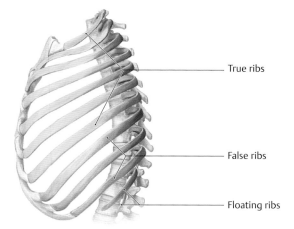

True ribs

False ribs

Floating ribs

Fig. 4.5 ▶ **Structure of a thoracic segment**
Superior view of 6th rib pair.

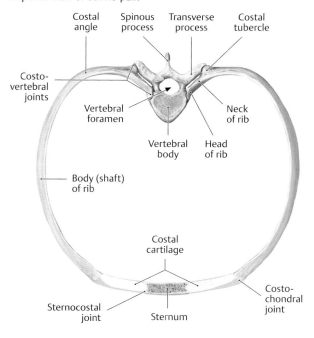

Costal angle
Spinous process
Transverse process
Costal tubercle
Costo-vertebral joints
Vertebral foramen
Neck of rib
Vertebral body
Head of rib
Body (shaft) of rib
Costal cartilage
Sternocostal joint
Sternum
Costo-chondral joint

4.2c   Thoracic Apertures

— The thoracic cage has superior and inferior openings (see **Fig. 4.3**):
  • The **superior thoracic aperture (thoracic inlet)**, which is bounded by the T1 vertebra, the 1st ribs, and the manubrium of the sternum. The thorax communicates with the neck through this opening.
  • The **inferior thoracic aperture (thoracic outlet)**, which is bounded by the T12 vertebra, 11th and 12th ribs, the **costal margin** (lower border of the thoracic cage), and the xiphoid process. A muscular diaphragm closes this aperture, separating the thoracic cavity from the abdominal cavity (see Section 4.3b).

Table 4.1 ▶ Muscles of the Thoracic Wall

Muscle		Origin	Insertion	Innervation	Action
Scalene mm.	Anterior scalene	C3–C6 (transverse processes, anterior tubercles)	1st rib (anterior scalene tubercles)	C3–C6	Raise the upper ribs during inspiration
	Middle scalene	C3–C7 (transverse processes, posterior tubercles)	1st rib (posterior to groove for subclavian a.)		
	Posterior scalene	C5–C7 (transverse processes, posterior tubercles)	2nd rib (outer surface)		
Intercostal mm.	External intercostal mm.	Lower margin of rib to upper margin of next lower rib (courses obliquely forward and downward from costal tubercle to chondro-osseous junction)		1st to 11th intercostal nn.	Raise the ribs during inspiration
	Internal intercostal mm.	Lower margin of rib to upper margin of next lower rib (courses obliquely forward and upward from costal angle to sternum)			Lower the ribs during expiration
	Innermost intercostal mm.				
Subcostal mm.		Lower margin of lower ribs to inner surface of ribs two to three ribs below		Adjacent lower intercostal nn.	Lower the ribs during expiration
Transversus thoracis		Sternum and xiphoid process (inner surface)	2nd to 6th ribs (costal cartilage, inner surface)	2nd to 6th intercostal nn.	Weakly lower the ribs during expiration

Fig. 4.6 ▶ **Muscles of the thoracic wall**
Anterior view with thoracic cage opened to expose posterior surface of anterior wall.

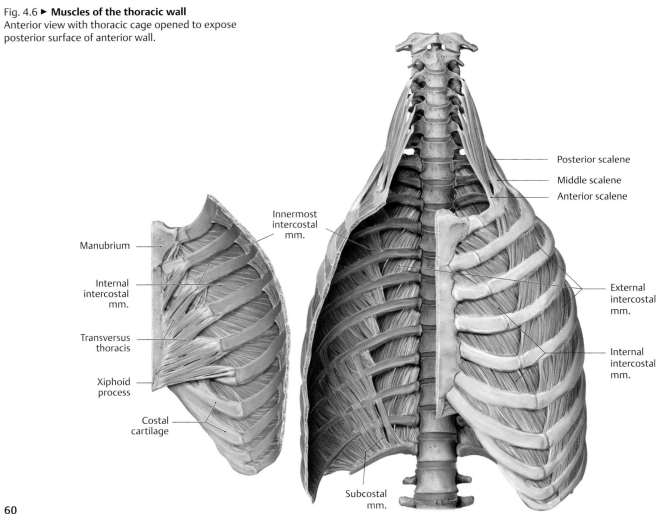

4.3 Muscles of the Thorax (**Fig. 4.6, Table 4.1**)

4.3a Muscles of the Thoracic Wall

— Extrinsic muscles of the upper limb, including the **pectoralis major, pectoralis minor**, and **serratus anterior**, cover the thorax. Although they mainly move or stabilize the upper limb, these muscles also assist in movements of the ribs during deep inspiration. (See Chapter 13, Overview of the Upper Limb.)

— The **anterior scalene, middle scalene** and **posterior scalene muscles** originate on the transverse processes of the cervical vertebrae and insert onto the 1st and 2nd ribs. They assist the intrinsic thoracic muscles during inspiration and are considered extrinsic muscles of respiration.

— Intrinsic muscles of the thoracic wall are the chief muscles that move the ribs during respiration.

• The **intercostal muscles** occupy the intercostal spaces between the ribs. They extend from the inferior border of one rib to the superior border of the next inferior rib. The intercostal muscles move the ribs primarily during forced repiration. During quiet respiration, they stabilize the thoracic wall. They include

◦ the **external intercostal muscles**, with fibers directed inferoanteriorly, which make up the most superficial layer

◦ the **internal intercostal** and **innermost intercostal muscles**, which occupy the middle and deepest layers of the thoracic wall, respectively, with their fibers directed inferosuperiorly

• The **subcostal muscles** are most prominent along the lower thoracic wall, where they cross the inner surface of one or two intercostal spaces.

• The **transversus thoracic muscles** consist of four of five thin slips that extend superiorly and laterally from the posterior surface of the sternum to the ribs.

4.3b The Thoracic Diaphragm

The **thoracic diaphragm** (or simply, the **diaphragm**), a musculotendinous sheet that separates the thorax from the abdomen, is the principal muscle of respiration. The diaphragm forms the floor of the thorax, the roof of the abdomen, and a portion of the posterior abdominal wall (**Fig. 4.7A** and **B**).

— The skeletal muscle fibers of the diaphragm originate along the costal margin, the vertebral bodies of L1–L3, the **medial** and **lateral arcuate ligaments**, and the xiphoid process. They insert on the diaphragm's **central tendon**.

Fig. 4.7 ▶ Diaphragm
The diaphragm, which separates the thorax from the abdomen, has two asymmetric domes and three apertures (for the aorta, vena cava, and esophagus).

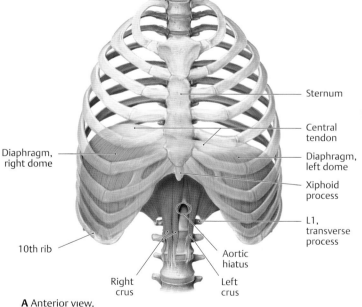

A Anterior view.

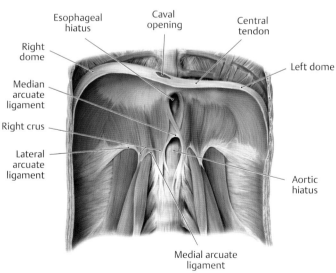

B Coronal section with diaphragm in intermediate position.

— Right and left **crura**, extensions of the posterior diaphragm, attach to the bodies of the lumbar vertebrae, with the right crus extending slightly lower than the left crus.
— The domes on the right and left sides of the diaphragm are asymmetric; the right hemidiaphragm is generally higher than the left.
— During full expiration the diaphragm is 4 to 6 cm higher than during full inspiration. During expiration it ascends to the level of the 4th or 5th rib on the right and slightly lower on the left, although this varies with respiration, posture, and body type.
— The diaphragm has three openings to allow the passage of structures between the thorax and abdomen (**Fig. 4.8**):

1. The **caval aperture** (hiatus), which is a passage for the inferior vena cava through the central tendon at the T8 vertebral level
2. The **esophageal aperture** (hiatus), which is an opening at the T10 vertebral level for the esophagus, the anterior and posterior vagal trunks, and left gastric artery and vein. It is usually formed by the right crus of the diaphragm (occasionally by the right and left crura) that, when contracted, forms a sphincter around the esophagus.
3. The **aortic aperture (hiatus)**, which is a passageway for the aorta between the right and left crura as it passes behind the diaphragm at T12. The thoracic duct, and often the azygos and hemiazygos veins, also passes through this aperture.

— The inferior phrenic arteries, branches of the abdominal aorta (or celiac trunk), are the primary blood supply to the diaphragm. The superior phrenic, pericardiacophrenic, and musculophrenic arteries make additional contributions (**Fig. 4.9**).
— Venous blood drains to the azygos system through posterior intercostal and superior phrenic veins.
— The phrenic nerve (C3–C5) provides all of the motor and most of the sensory innervation to the diaphragm. The subcostal and lower intercostal nerves supply sensory innervation to the periphery of the diaphragm (**Fig. 4.10**).

Fig. 4.8 ▶ **Diaphragmatic apertures**
Left lateral view.

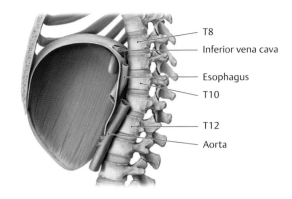

T8
Inferior vena cava
Esophagus
T10
T12
Aorta

Fig. 4.9 ▶ Neurovasculature of the diaphragm
Anterior view of opened thoracic cage.

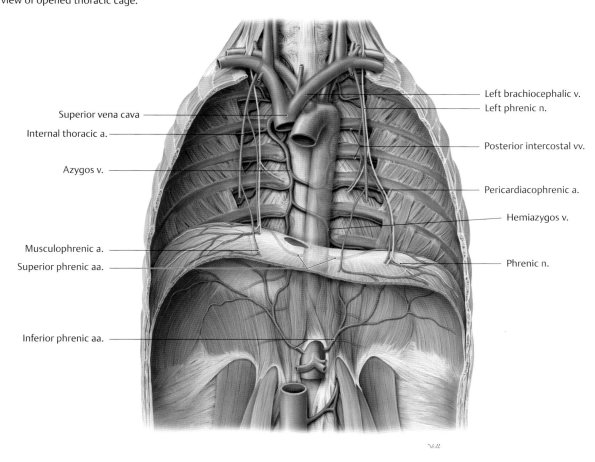

Left brachiocephalic v.

Left phrenic n.

Superior vena cava

Internal thoracic a.

Posterior intercostal vv.

Azygos v.

Pericardiacophrenic a.

Hemiazygos v.

Musculophrenic a.

Superior phrenic aa.

Phrenic n.

Inferior phrenic aa.

Fig. 4.10 ▶ Innervation of the diaphragm
Anterior view. The phrenic nerve lies on the lateral surface of the fibrous pericardium together with the pericardiacophrenic arteries and veins.
Note: The phrenic nerve also innervates the pericardium.

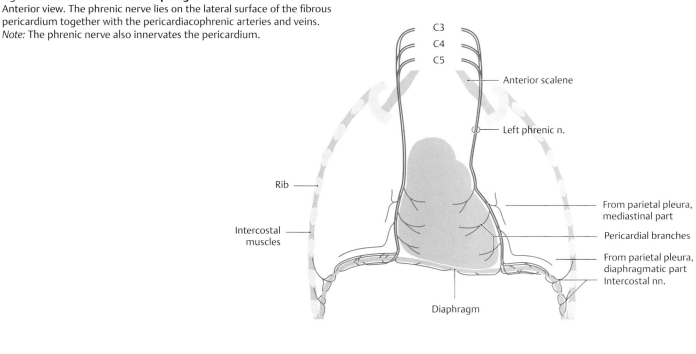

C3
C4
C5

Anterior scalene

Left phrenic n.

Rib

From parietal pleura, mediastinal part

Pericardial branches

Intercostal muscles

From parietal pleura, diaphragmatic part

Intercostal nn.

Diaphragm

—— Efferent fibers   —— Afferent fibers

4.4 Neurovasculature of the Thoracic Wall (Fig. 4.11)

— Anterior intercostal arteries (branches of the internal thoracic artery) and posterior intercostal arteries (branches of the thoracic aorta and subclavian artery) supply the muscles and skin of the thoracic wall (see **Fig. 3.4**).
— Intercostal veins drain primarily to the azygos system but also into the brachiocephalic and internal thoracic veins, which join the superior vena cava (see **Fig. 3.5**).

— The **thoracoepigastric vein** is a superficial vein that drains the subcutaneous tissue of the anterolateral thoracic and abdominal walls. It drains superiorly to the axillary vein of the upper limb and inferiorly to the superficial epigastric vein (**Fig. 4.12**).

Fig. 4.11 ▶ **Intercostal structures in cross section**
Transverse setion, anterosuperior view.

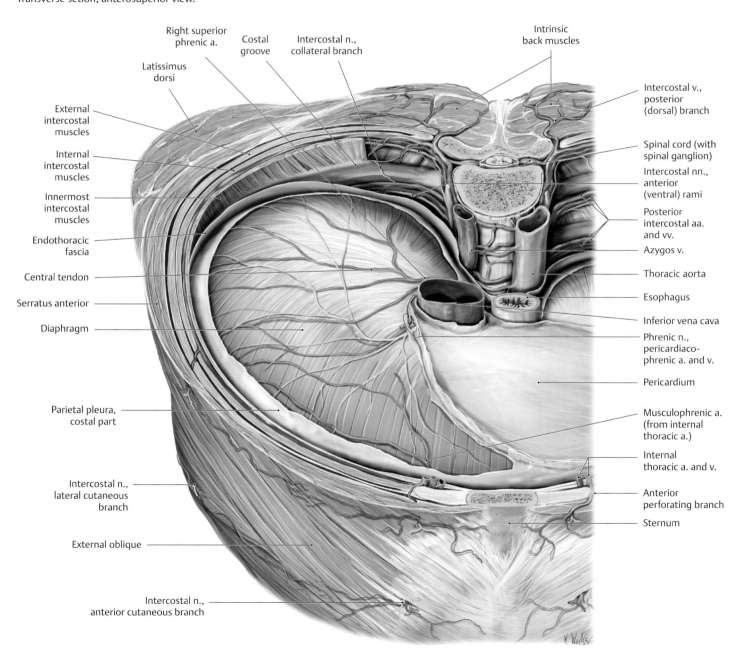

— The thoracic wall is drained by three major groups of lymph nodes:

- The **parasternal nodes,** which are scattered along the internal thoracic artery. They receive lymph from the breast, anterior thoracic wall, liver, and upper deep surface of the anterior abdominal wall.
- The **intercostal nodes,** which are located in the intercostal spaces near the heads and necks of the ribs. They drain the posterolateral part of the chest and mammary glands.
- The **diaphragmatic nodes,** which are located on the superior surface of the diaphragm. They drain the central tendon of the diaphragm, the fibrous pericardium, and the superior surface of the liver.

— Intercostal nerves T1–T11 innervate the muscles of the thoracic wall. In the midaxillary line these nerves give off a lateral cutaneous branch that supplies the superficial muscles and skin of the thorax (**Fig. 4.13A and B**).

— Intercostal nerves and vessels are protected within the **costal groove** on the deep inferior edge of the ribs (see **Fig. 4.11**). Within this bundle of neurovascular structures, the nerve runs inferior to its accompanying vessels.

— The 7th through 11th intercostal nerves continue anteriorly from the intercostal space to innervate the anterior abdominal wall.

— Landmark dermatomes on the thoracic wall include T4 at the nipple and T6 over the xiphoid process.

Fig. 4.12 ▶ **Superficial veins**
Anterior view. The thoracoepigastric veins are a potential superficial collateral venous drainage route in the event of superior or inferior vena cava obstruction.

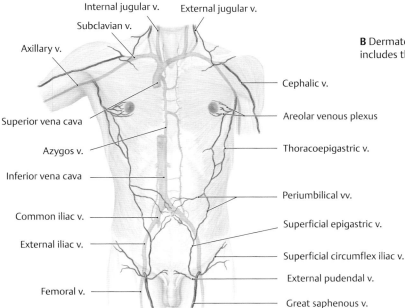

Fig. 4.13 ▶ **Cutaneous innervation of the thoracic wall**
Anterior view.

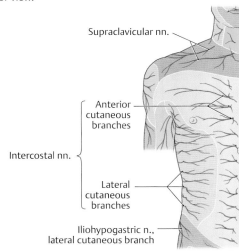

A Sensory nerves of the anterior thoracic wall.

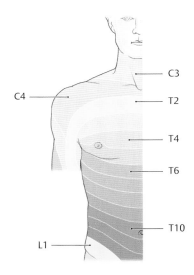

B Dermatomes of the anterior thoracic wall. *Landmarks:* T4 generally includes the nipple; T6 innervates the skin over the xiphoid.

65

5 Mediastinum

The **mediastinum** is the region within the thorax between the right and left pulmonary cavities (see **Table 3.10**). The sternum and the costal cartilages of ribs 1 through 7 form its anterior boundary, and the thoracic vertebrae form its posterior boundary. The mediastinum contains the heart, great vessels, and pericardium, as well as the esophagus, trachea, thymus, and associated neurovasculature (**Fig. 5.1A** and **B**).

Fig. 5.1 ▸ **Mediastinum**

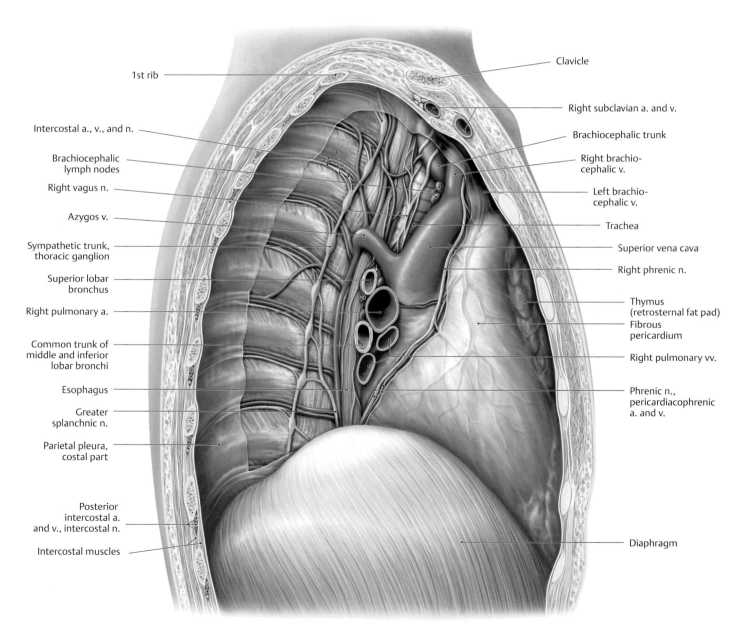

A Parasagittal section, right lateral view. Note the many structures passing between the superior and inferior (middle and posterior) mediastinum.

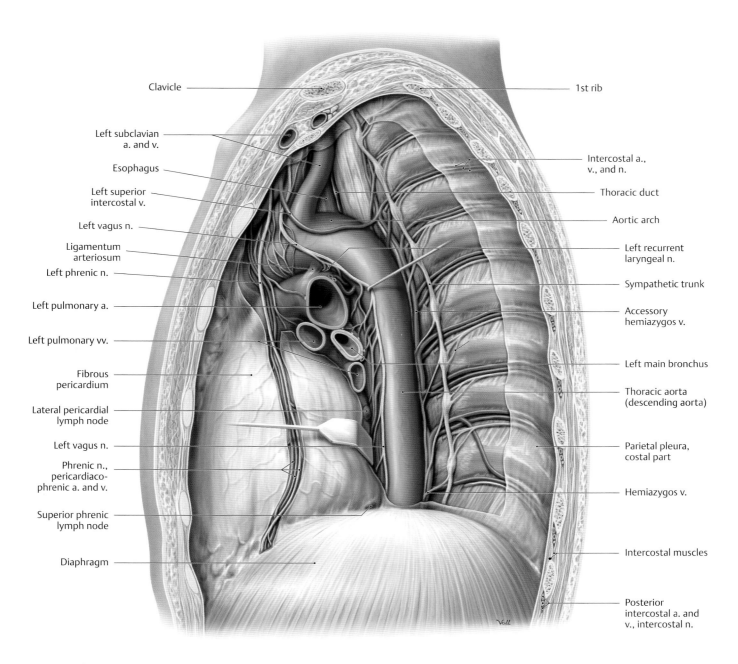

Clavicle

1st rib

Left subclavian
a. and v.

Intercostal a.,
v., and n.

Esophagus

Thoracic duct

Left superior
intercostal v.

Aortic arch

Left vagus n.

Left recurrent
laryngeal n.

Ligamentum
arteriosum

Sympathetic trunk

Left phrenic n.

Accessory
hemiazygos v.

Left pulmonary a.

Left pulmonary vv.

Left main bronchus

Fibrous
pericardium

Thoracic aorta
(descending aorta)

Lateral pericardial
lymph node

Left vagus n.

Parietal pleura,
costal part

Phrenic n.,
pericardiaco-
phrenic a. and v.

Hemiazygos v.

Superior phrenic
lymph node

Intercostal muscles

Diaphragm

Posterior
intercostal a. and
v., intercostal n.

B Parasagittal section, left lateral view. *Removed:* Left lung and parietal pleura. *Revealed:* Posterior mediastinal structures.

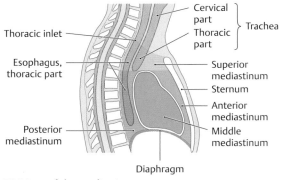

Divisions of the mediastinum.

Table 5.1 ▶ Contents of the Mediastinum				
	Superior ○ mediastinum	**Inferior mediastinum**		
		Anterior ○	**Middle ○**	**Posterior ○**
Organs	• Thymus • Trachea • Esophagus	• Thymus	• Heart • Pericardium	• Esophagus
Arteries	• Aortic arch • Brachiocephalic trunk • Left common carotid a. • Left subclavian a.	• Smaller vessels	• Ascending aorta • Pulmonary trunk and branches • Pericardiaco-phrenic aa.	• Thoracic aorta and branches
Veins and lymph vessels	• Superior vena cava • Brachiocephalic vv. • Thoracic duct	• Smaller vessels, lymphatics, and lymph nodes	• Superior vena cava • Azygos v. • Pulmonary vv. • Pericardiaco-phrenic vv.	• Azygos v. • Hemiazygos v. • Thoracic duct
Nerves	• Vagus nn. • Left recurrent laryngeal n. • Cardiac nn. • Phrenic nn.	• None	• Phrenic nn.	• Vagus nn.

5.1 Regions of the Mediastinum (**Table 5.1**)

— A horizontal plane passing through the sternal angle (at T4–T5 intervertebral disk) divides the region into a **superior mediastinum**, bounded above by the superior thoracic aperture, and an **inferior mediastinum** limited inferiorly by the thoracic diaphragm.

— The inferior mediastinum is further divided into

  • the **anterior mediastinum**, a narrow space posterior to the sternum and anterior to the pericardium;
  • the **middle mediastinum**, the largest section of the inferior mediastinum, which contains the pericardium, heart and major vessels; and
  • the **posterior mediastinum**, a small area posterior to the pericardium and anterior to the 5th through 12th thoracic vertebrae.

5.2 The Pericardium and Pericardial Cavity

5.2a Pericardium

The **pericardium**, a double fibroserous membrane, forms the **pericardial sac** that surrounds the heart and the origins of the great vessels (**Figs. 5.2, 5.3,** and **5.4**).

— The pericardium is composed of two layers: an outer fibrous layer and an inner serous layer.

  1. The outer fibrous **pericardium** is composed of tough inelastic connective tissue. It is attached inferiorly to the diaphragm and is continuous superiorly with the tunica adventitia (outer layer) of the great vessels.
  2. The thin **serous pericardium** consists of a parietal part and a visceral part.

    ○ The **parietal layer** (part) **of serous pericardium** lines the inner surface of the parietal pericardium.
    ○ The **visceral layer** (part) **of serous pericardium** firmly adheres to the outer surface of the heart as the **epicardium**. This layer is continuous with the parietal layer of the serous pericardium at the root of the great vessels.

— **Pericardiacophrenic arteries**, branches of the internal thoracic arteries, provide the main blood supply to the pericardium. Veins that accompany the arteries drain into the superior vena cava.

— The vagus (CN X) and phrenic nerves (C3–C5) and branches from the sympathetic trunks innervate the pericardium.

— Pericardial pain is often referred via the phrenic nerve to the skin of the ipsilateral supraclavicular region (dermatomes C3–C5).

Fig. 5.2 ▶ Pericardium
Anterior view of opened thorax. *Removed:* Thymus. *Reflected:*
Flaps of the fibrous pericardium.

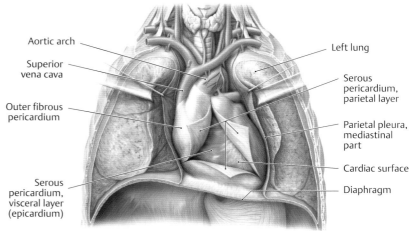

Aortic arch
Superior vena cava
Outer fibrous pericardium
Serous pericardium, visceral layer (epicardium)
Left lung
Serous pericardium, parietal layer
Parietal pleura, mediastinal part
Cardiac surface
Diaphragm

Fig. 5.3 ▶ Serous pericardial reflections
Sagittal section through the mediastinum. Note the continuity of the parietal serous and visceral serous pericardia.

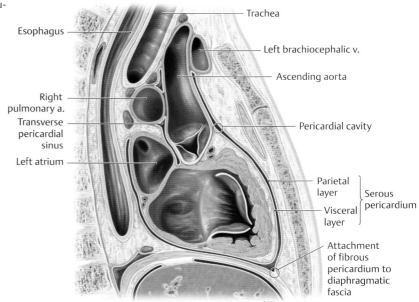

Esophagus
Right pulmonary a.
Transverse pericardial sinus
Left atrium
Trachea
Left brachiocephalic v.
Ascending aorta
Pericardial cavity
Parietal layer
Visceral layer
Serous pericardium
Attachment of fibrous pericardium to diaphragmatic fascia

Pericarditis

Pericarditis is an inflammation of the pericardium, which causes sharp, retrosternal or epigastric pain and a characteristic pericardial friction rub (a sound like the rustle of silk) that's heard on auscultation. This is caused by friction from the roughened layers of the inflamed pericardium rubbing together. Pericarditis can lead to pericardial effusion (fluid in the pericardial cavity) or cardiac tamponade (abnormal accumulation of fluid in the pericardial cavity that prevents venous return to the heart) and may be accompanied by dyspnea (shortness of breath) and peripheral edema (swelling).

Fig. 5.4 ▶ **Heart in situ**
Anterior view of the opened thorax. *Removed:* Thymus and anterior pericardium. *Revealed:* Heart.

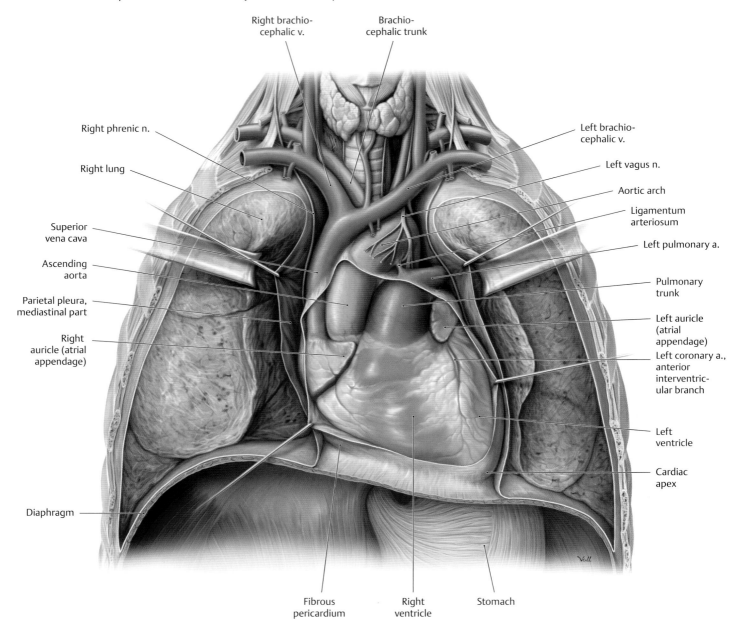

Right brachio-cephalic v.

Brachio-cephalic trunk

Right phrenic n.

Right lung

Superior vena cava

Ascending aorta

Parietal pleura, mediastinal part

Right auricle (atrial appendage)

Diaphragm

Fibrous pericardium

Right ventricle

Stomach

Left brachio-cephalic v.

Left vagus n.

Aortic arch

Ligamentum arteriosum

Left pulmonary a.

Pulmonary trunk

Left auricle (atrial appendage)

Left coronary a., anterior interventricular branch

Left ventricle

Cardiac apex

5.2b The Pericardial Cavity

The **pericardial cavity** is the space within the pericardial sac between the parietal and visceral layers of the serous pericardium (see **Fig. 5.3**).

— The pericardial cavity is filled with a thin layer of serous fluid that allows for frictionless movement of the heart.
— Two pericardial recesses form where the serous pericardium reflects around the roots of the great vessels (**Figs. 5.5** and **5.6**).

1. The **transverse pericardial sinus** is a passage between the inflow channels (superior vena cava and pulmonary veins) and the outflow channels (aorta and pulmonary trunk) of the heart.
2. The **oblique pericardial sinus** is a recess of the pericardial cavity posterior to the heart between the right and left pulmonary veins.

Fig. 5.5 ▶ Posterior pericardial cavity
Anterior view. The heart has been elevated to partially visualize the posterior pericardial cavity and the oblique pericardial sinus.

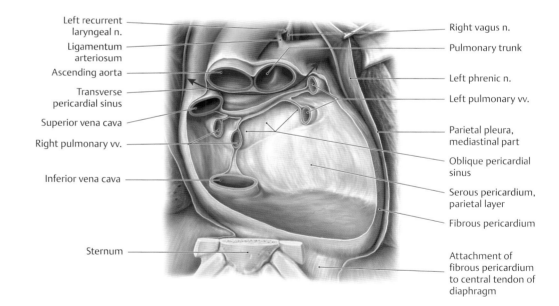

Left vagus n.

Superior vena cava

Pericardiacophrenic a. and v., left phrenic n.

Ascending aorta

Pulmonary trunk

Left auricle (atrial appendage)

Left pulmonary vv.

Heart, diaphragmatic surface

Oblique pericardial sinus

Right pulmonary v.

Coronary sinus

Inferior vena cava

Fig. 5.6 ▶ Pericardial recesses
Posterior pericardium, anterior view. *Removed:* Anterior pericardium and heart. *Revealed:* The posterior pericardium and the oblique pericardial sinus. The double-headed arrow illustrates the course of the transverse pericardial sinus, the passage between the reflections of the serous layer of the pericardium around the arterial and venous great vessels of the heart.

Left recurrent laryngeal n.

Right vagus n.

Ligamentum arteriosum

Pulmonary trunk

Ascending aorta

Left phrenic n.

Transverse pericardial sinus

Left pulmonary vv.

Superior vena cava

Right pulmonary vv.

Parietal pleura, mediastinal part

Inferior vena cava

Oblique pericardial sinus

Serous pericardium, parietal layer

Fibrous pericardium

Sternum

Attachment of fibrous pericardium to central tendon of diaphragm

---

Cardiac tamponade

Cardiac tamponade is a life-threatening condition in which fluid collects in the pericardial space. The increased intrapericardial pressure restricts the filling of the heart during diastole and reduces cardiac output but increases the heart rate. Inhibition of venous return to the heart causes peripheral edema, hepatomegaly (enlarged liver), and increased venous pressure (often noted by distension of the internal jugular vein). Pericardiocentesis, aspiration of the fluid from the pericardial space, can relieve the tamponade.

Surgical significance of the transverse pericardial sinus

During cardiac surgery, the surgeon is able to isolate (and clamp) the heart's outflow tracts, the aorta and pulmonary trunk, from its inflow tracts, the superior vena cava and pulmonary veins, by passing the clamps through the transverse pericardial sinus.

Fig. 5.7 ▶ **Surfaces of the heart**
The heart has three surfaces: anterior (sternocostal), posterior (base), and inferior (diaphragmatic).

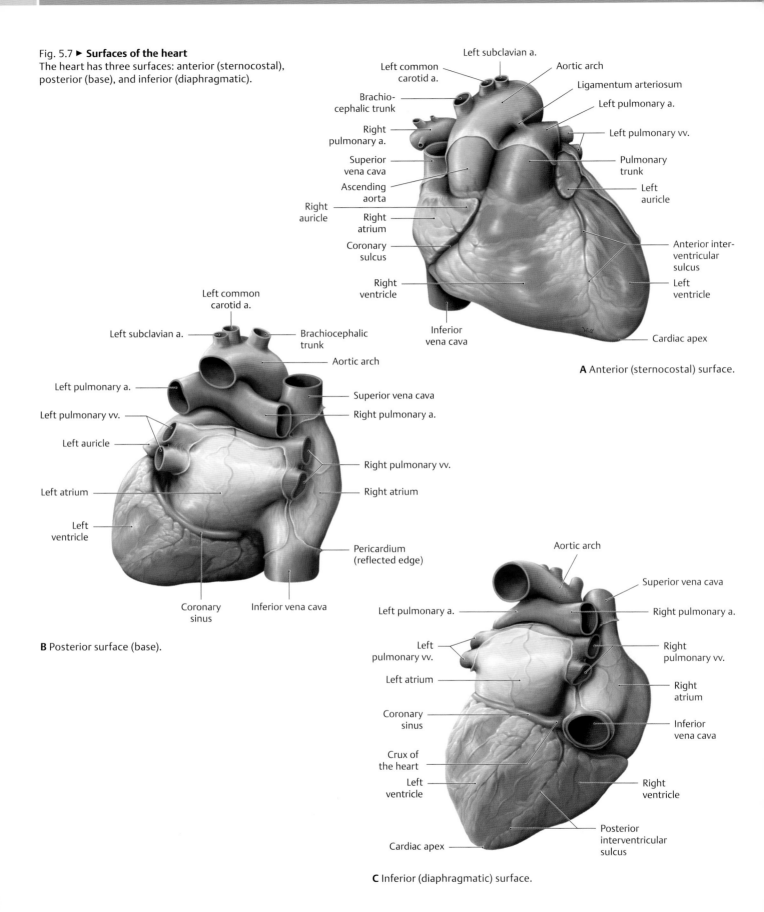

Left subclavian a.
Left common carotid a.
Aortic arch
Brachio-cephalic trunk
Ligamentum arteriosum
Left pulmonary a.
Right pulmonary a.
Left pulmonary vv.
Superior vena cava
Pulmonary trunk
Ascending aorta
Left auricle
Right auricle
Right atrium
Coronary sulcus
Anterior inter-ventricular sulcus
Right ventricle
Left ventricle
Inferior vena cava
Cardiac apex

A Anterior (sternocostal) surface.

Left common carotid a.
Left subclavian a.
Brachiocephalic trunk
Aortic arch
Left pulmonary a.
Superior vena cava
Left pulmonary vv.
Right pulmonary a.
Left auricle
Right pulmonary vv.
Left atrium
Right atrium
Left ventricle
Pericardium (reflected edge)
Coronary sinus
Inferior vena cava

B Posterior surface (base).

Aortic arch
Superior vena cava
Left pulmonary a.
Right pulmonary a.
Left pulmonary vv.
Right pulmonary vv.
Left atrium
Right atrium
Coronary sinus
Inferior vena cava
Crux of the heart
Left ventricle
Right ventricle
Posterior interventricular sulcus
Cardiac apex

C Inferior (diaphragmatic) surface.

5.3 The Heart

5.3a General Features

— The heart is a hollow muscular organ located in the middle mediastinum within the pericardial sac. It rests on the central tendon of the diaphragm and is flanked on either side by the right and left pulmonary cavities.

— The heart has a conical shape. The **base**, anchored by the great vessels, is on its superior and posterior surfaces. The **apex**, located approximately at the 5th intercostal space, projects anteriorly, inferiorly, and to the left and moves freely within the pericardial sac.

— Internally, the heart is divided into four chambers: the right and left atria and the right and left ventricles (see Sections 5.3b and c).

  • The right and left atria, separated by an **interatrial septum**, are the inflow chambers of the heart, receiving blood from the systemic circulation on the right and pulmonary circulation on the left.

  • The right and left ventricles, separated by an **interventricular septum**, are the outflow chambers of the heart. Blood flows from the right ventricle into the pulmonary circulation and from the left into the systemic circulation.

— Two small appendages, the **right** and **left auricles**, are extensions of the atria and are visible externally.

— The surfaces of the heart are (**Fig. 5.7A, B,** and **C**)

  • the **sternocostal surface** on the anterior side of the heart, formed mostly by the right ventricle with portions of the right atrium and left ventricle;

  • the base on the posterior and superior sides of the heart, formed by the left atrium and a portion of the right atrium; and

  • the **diaphragmatic surface** on the inferior side of the heart, formed by the left and right ventricles.

— The borders of the heart define the cardiac shadow that is seen on radiographic images (**Table 5.2**; **Fig. 5.8A** and **B**).

— Three grooves on the external surface of the heart can be used to determine the position of the chambers.

  1. The **coronary sulcus** encircles the heart between the atria and ventricles. Because the heart has an oblique orientation, the sulcus is nearly vertical.

  2. The **anterior interventricular sulcus** is a longitudinal groove that marks the position of the interventricular septum on the anterior surface.

  3. The **posterior interventricular sulcus** is a longitudinal groove that marks the position of the interventricular septum on the diaphragmatic surface.

— The **crux of the heart is** a point on the posterior surface of the heart where the coronary (atrioventicular) and interventricular sulci meet. It marks the junction of the four chambers of the heart.

— The wall of the heart consists of three layers:

  1. The **epicardium**, the thin outermost layer, formed by the visceral layer of the serous pericardium

  2. The **myocardium**, the thick layer of cardiac muscle, thickest in the walls of the ventricles

Table 5.2 ▶ Borders of the Heart	
Border	**Defining structures**
Right cardiac border	Right atrium
	Superior vena cava
Apex	Left ventricle
Left cardiac border	Aortic arch ("aortic knob")
	Pulmonary trunk
	Left atrium
	Left ventricle
Inferior cardiac border	Left ventricle
	Right ventricle

Fig. 5.8 ▶ **Radiographic appearance of the heart**

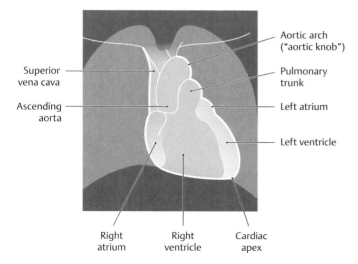

Superior vena cava
Ascending aorta
Aortic arch ("aortic knob")
Pulmonary trunk
Left atrium
Left ventricle
Right atrium
Right ventricle
Cardiac apex

A Schematic of posteroanterior chest radiograph in **B**.

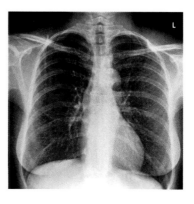

B Posteroanterior chest radiograph.

3. The **endocardium**, the thin internal layer, which lines the chambers and valves of the heart

— A **cardiac skeleton** of dense fibrous connective tissue forms four **fibrous anuli** (rings) and intervening **trigones** that separate the chambers of the heart, provide anchoring points for cardiac muscle fibers and cardiac valves, and insulate electrical impulses of the heart's conduction system (**Fig. 5.9**).

Fig. 5.9 ▶ **Cardiac skeleton**
Superior view. Red dotted circles are attachment sites of papillary muscles on valves.

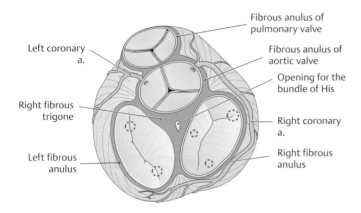

5.3b The Atria (Fig. 5.10A, B, and C)

The **atria** are the thin-walled inflow chambers of the heart.

— The right atrium receives the superior and inferior venae cavae from the systemic circulation and the cardiac veins from the heart. The left atrium receives the pulmonary veins from the lungs.

— Each atrium is associated with an auricle, a small pouch that expands the capacity of the atrium and whose roughened walls contain pectinate muscles.

— A depression on the right ride of the interatrial septum, the **oval fossa** (fossa ovalis), is a remnant of the **oval foramen** (foramen ovale), an opening through which blood was shunted from the right to left atria in the prenatal circulation.

— The right atrium is divided into two parts by a muscular ridge, the **terminal crest** (crista terminalis). The ridge is evident on the outside of the heart as the **terminal sulcus**. The two parts of the right atrium are

1. the **venous sinus** (sinus venarum), a smooth-walled region on the posterior wall that contains the openings of the superior vena cava, inferior vena cava, coronary sinus, and anterior cardiac veins; and

2. the **atrium proper**, the anterior muscular portion that, like the right auricle, contains pectinate muscles.

— The left atrium is smaller but thicker walled than the right atrium and receives the four to five pulmonary veins from the lungs. The atrial walls are smooth, with the pectinate muscles confined to the left auricle.

5.3c The Ventricles

The ventricles are thick-walled chambers that connect to the outflow channels of the heart: the right ventricle to the pulmonary artery and the left ventricle to the aorta (see **Fig. 5.10A, B,** and **C**).

— The walls of the ventricles are marked with a meshwork of thick muscular ridges known as **trabeculae carneae**.

— Most of the interventricular septum is muscular, but there is a small membranous part at the superior end that is a common site of septal defects.

— The right ventricle is the smaller and thinner walled of the two ventricles. A muscular ridge, the **supraventricular crest**, separates it into two parts:

1. The **right ventricle proper,** the inflow portion of the ventricle that receives blood from the right atrium

   ○ An **anterior** and a **posterior papillary muscle** arise from its floor, and a **septal papillary muscle** arises from the interventricular septum.

   ○ A muscular **septomarginal trabecula** (moderator band) extends from the septum to the base of the anterior papillary muscle and carries a part of the electrical conduction system (the right branch of the antrioventricular bundle) that facilitates the coordinated contraction of the papillary muscle.

2. The **conus arteriosus** (infundibulum), the smooth-walled outflow channel through which blood flows into the pulmonary trunk

— The left ventricle, which includes the apex of the heart, is the thickest-walled chamber of the heart. Similar to the right ventricle, the left is divided into inflow and outflow portions:

1. The **left ventricle proper**, which receives blood from the left atrium. A large anterior and small posterior papillary muscle arise from its floor

2. The **aortic vestibule**, the smooth-walled outflow channel through which blood flows into the aorta

Ventricular septal defect

Ventricular septal defects (VSDs), the most common of congenital heart defects, usually involve the membranous part of the interventricular septum and are associated with Down syndrome, tetralogy of Fallot, and Turner syndrome. VSDs may also occur traumatically from rupture of the membranous septum following a myocardial infarction. When the VSD is large, the resulting left-to-right shunt increases blood flow through the pulmonary circulation, causing pulmonary hypertension and cardiac failure.

Tetralogy of Fallot

Tetralogy of Fallot is a rare combination of four congenital cardiac defects: pulmonary stenosis, overriding aorta, ventricular septal defect (VSD), and right ventricular hypertrophy. Symptoms include cyanosis, dyspnea (shortness of breath), fainting, finger clubbing, fatigue, and prolonged crying in infants.

Fig. 5.10 ▶ **Chambers of the heart**

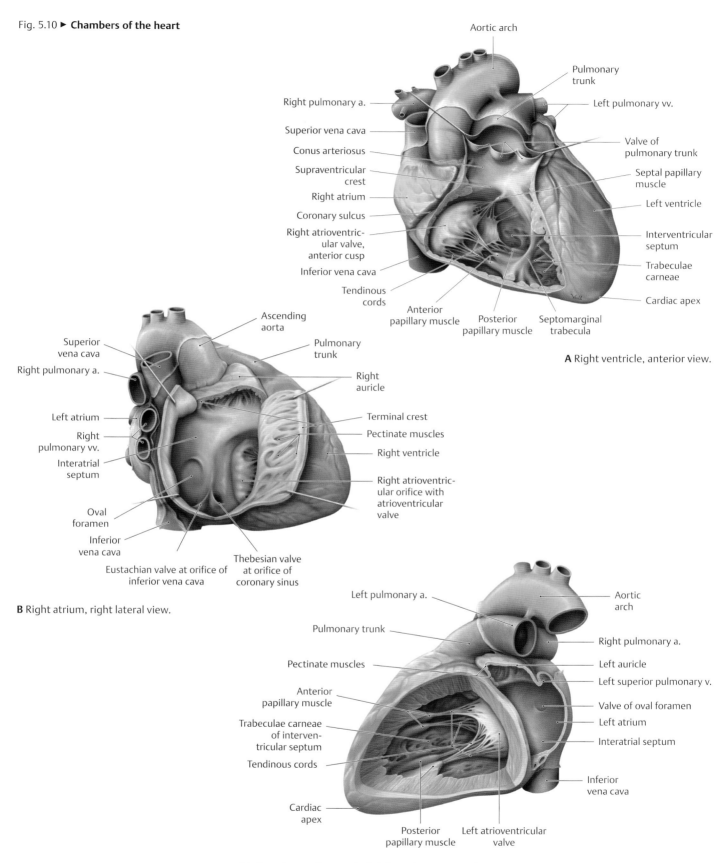

A Right ventricle, anterior view.

B Right atrium, right lateral view.

C Left atrium and ventricle, left lateral view. Note the irregular trabeculae carneae characteristic of the ventricular wall.

Fig. 5.11 ► **Cardiac valves**

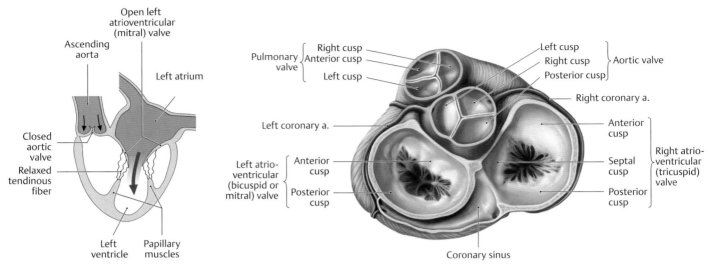

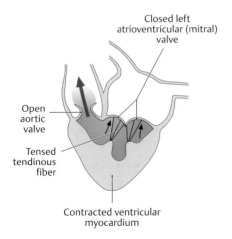

A Blood flow through the left side of the heart during ventricular diastole (relaxation of the ventricles), anterior view. *Closed:* Semilunar valves. *Open:* Atrioventricular valves.

B Superior view of cardiac valves during ventricular diastole. *Closed:* Semilunar valves. *Open:* Atrioventricular valves. *Removed:* Atria and great arteries.

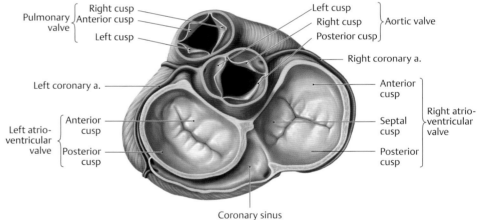

C Blood flow through the left side of the heart during ventricular systole (contraction of the ventricles). *Closed:* Atrioventricular valves. *Open:* Semilunar valves.

D Superior view of cardiac valves during ventricular systole. *Closed:* Atrioventricular valves. *Open:* Semilunar valves. *Removed:* Atria and great arteries.

5.3d Valves of the Heart

There are two types of cardiac valves: atrioventricular and semilunar (**Fig. 5.11A, B, C,** and **D**).

1. **Atrioventricular valves** separate the atria from the ventricles and prevent regurgitation of blood into the atria during contraction of the ventricles (see **Fig. 5.10**).

   - The atrioventricular valves are made up of cusps, thin leaflets with free inner margins and outer margins that are attached to the fibrous rings of the cardiac skeleton.
   - Slender threads called **tendinous cords** (chordae tendinae) attach the free edges of the valve leaflets to the papillary muscles in the ventricles. These cords maintain closure of the valves and prevent regurgitation of blood during ventricular contraction. Each cusp attaches to tendinous cords from more than one papillary muscle.
   - The atrioventricular valves include
     - the **tricuspid valve**, which separates the right atrium from the right ventricle and is composed of anterior, posterior, and septal cusps; and
     - the **bicuspid** (or **mitral**) **valve**, which separates the left atrium from the left ventricle and is composed of anterior and posterior cusps. The anterior cusp is immediately adjacent to, and continuous with, the wall of the aorta.

Mitral valve prolapse

Mitral valve prolapse is a condition in which one or both leaflets of the mitral valve prolapse (evert) into the left atrium, allowing regurgitation of blood through the mitral valve during systole. This condition is usually asymptomatic but is noted by a midsystolic click (valve prolapsing) and murmur (regurgitation).

2. **Semilunar valves** prevent outflow from the ventricles as the chambers fill and backflow of blood into the ventricles after it has been expelled.

- Each valve is composed of three semilunar cusps with free inner margins and attached outer margins. A **sinus**, or pocket, is created between each cusp and the vessel wall. The thickened free margin of the cusp, the **lunule**, is the point of contact of the cusps. A **nodule** marks the center of the lunule.
- The semilunar valves include the following:
  - The **pulmonary semilunar valve** (**pulmonary valve**, is located in the pulmonary trunk at the top of the conus arteriosus, where it moderates blood flow through the right ventricular outflow channel. Its cusps are in the anterior, right, and left positions.
  - The **aortic semilunar valve** (**aortic valve**) is located within the aorta immediately adjacent to the mitral valve, where it moderates blood flow through the left ventricular outflow channel. Its cusps are in the posterior, right, and left positions. The coronary arteries arise from the sinuses above the right and left cusps.

Aortic valve stenosis

Stenosis of the aortic valve is the most common valve abnormality. Calcifications of the valve leaflets narrow the outflow tract and lead to overload of the left ventricle, resulting in left ventricular hypertrophy.

5.3e Heart Sounds and Auscultation Sites

When the heart valves close, they produce characteristic sounds described as "lub dub."

— Closure of the tricuspid and mitral valves during contraction of the ventricles produces the first sound ("lub").
— Closure of the pulmonary and aortic valves as the ventricles relax produces the second sound ("dub").
— The sounds, carried by the blood as it flows into the next vessel or chamber, are best distinguished at **auscultation sites** downstream from the valves (**Table 5.3**).

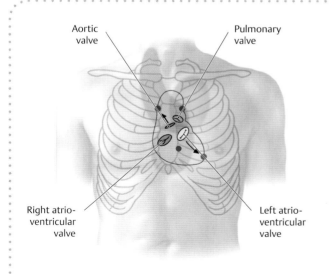

Table 5.3 ▶ **Position and Auscultation Sites of Cardiac Valves**		
Valve	**Anatomical projection**	**Auscultation site**
Aortic valve	Left sternal border (at level of 3rd rib)	Right 2nd intercostal space (at sternal margin)
Pulmonary valve	Left sternal border (at level of 3rd costal cartilage)	Left 2nd intercostal space (at sternal margin)
Left atrioventricular valve	Left 4th/5th costal cartilage	Left 5th intercostal space (at midclavicular line) or cardiac apex
Right atrioventricular valve	Sternum (at level of 3rd costal cartilage)	Right 5th intercostal space (at sternal margin)

Auscultation sites of the cardiac valves, indicated by dark colored circles. Valvular heart disease causes turbulent blood flow through a valve; this produces a murmur that may be detected in the colored region around the valve.

5.3f Conduction System of the Heart (Fig. 5.12A, B, and C)

The conduction system of the heart generates and transmits impulses that modulate the contraction of the cardiac muscle. It consists of nodes, which initiate the impulses, and conducting fibers, which distribute the impulses to cardiac muscle to effect a coordinated contraction of the heart chambers.

— The **sinoatrial** (SA) **node**, the pacemaker of the heart, initiates and coordinates the timing of the contraction of the heart chambers.

  • At a frequency of 60 to 70 beats per minute, the SA node transmits impulses to both atria and to the atrioventricular node.

• It is subepicardial, located on the external surface of the heart, just within the myocardium of the right atrium at the junction with the superior vena cava.

• A branch of the right coronary artery usually supplies the SA node.

— The **atrioventricular** (AV) **node** is stimulated by the SA node and transmits impulses to the AV bundle.

  • It is subendocardial, located at the base of the interatrial septum above the septal cusp of the tricuspid valve.

  • The AV nodal artery, a branch of the right coronary artery, arises near the origin of the posterior interventricular artery at the crux of the heart.

Fig. 5.12 ▶ **Cardiac conduction system**

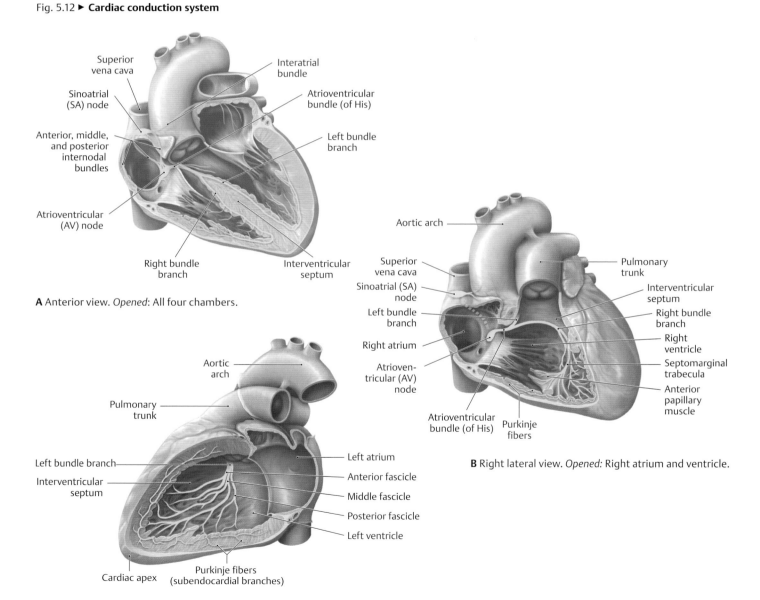

A Anterior view. *Opened*: All four chambers.

B Right lateral view. *Opened:* Right atrium and ventricle.

C Left lateral view. *Opened:* Left atrium and ventricle.

— The **atrioventricular** (AV) **bundle** (of His) arises from cells of the AV node and transmits impulses to the walls of the ventricles.

- It runs first along the membranous part of the interventricular septum and then divides into **right** and **left bundle branches** that descend to the apex on either side of the muscular part of the septum.
- The bundle branches end as **Purkinje fibers**, modified cardiac fibers, which ascend within the muscular walls of the ventricles.

Atrioventricular heart block

Atrioventricular (AV) heart block is a partial or complete blockage of the conduction of electrical impulses between the atria and ventricles. This causes bradycardia (slow heartbeat) and arrhythmias (irregular heartbeat) and ultimately prevents the heart from effectively contracting and delivering blood to the body. Although heart block may be congenital, it is frequently the result of damage to the heart muscle after myocardial infarction (MI).

5.3g The Cardiac Cycle

The heart's conduction system moderates the cardiac cycle, the coordinated **systole** (contraction) and **diastole** (relaxation) of the atria and ventricles. **Figure 5.13A, B, C,** and **D** summarizes the sequence of events of the cycle.

1. In the initial phase of diastole, the atria and ventricles are relaxed, and the AV and semilunar valves are closed.
2. In late diastole, the atria fill, the AV valves open, and blood flows passively into the ventricles.
3. Stimulation from the SA node initiates the contraction of the atria, forcing the remaining atrial blood volume into the ventricles.
4. As pressure in the ventricles rises above that in the atria, the AV valves close.
5. Stimulation from the AV node and the AV bundles initiates contraction of the ventricles (ventricular systole).
6. Rising intraventricular pressure forces the semilunar valves to open. Blood is ejected from the right ventricle into the pulmonary trunk and from the left ventricle into the aorta.
7. Relaxation of the ventricles (ventricular diastole) causes backward flow in the pulmonary trunk and aorta and closure of the pulmonary and aortic valves.

Fig. 5.13 ► **The cardiac cycle**

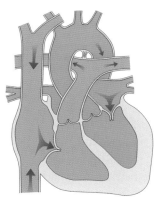
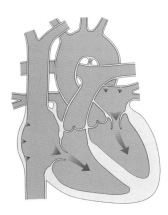

A and **B** Ventricular diastole.

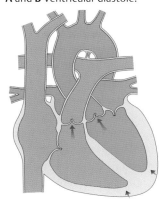
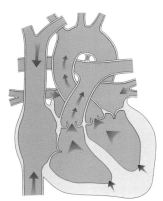

C and **D** Ventricular systole.

5.4 Neurovasculature of the Heart

5.4a Coronary Arteries (Fig. 5.14A and B; Table 5.4)

The **right** and **left coronary arteries** arise from the ascending aorta just superior to the right and left cusps of the aortic valve. In the initial phase of ventricular diastole, the local surge in aortic pressure caused by the backflow closes the aortic valve and drives blood into the coronary arteries. Blood flow in the arteries is greatest during diastole because of the compression of arteries within the myocardium during systole.

— The right and left coronary arteries supply the myocardium and epicardium of the heart.

- The **right coronary artery** descends within the coronary sulcus around the right side of the heart. Its major branches and their distribution are
    - the **SA nodal artery**, which supplies the right atrium and the SA node;
    - the **right marginal branch**, which supplies the apex and part of the right ventricle;
    - the **posterior interventricular branch**, which supplies the right and left ventricles and posterior third of the interventricular septum and anastomoses with the interventricular branch of the left coronary artery near the apex on the diaphragmatic surface; and
    - the **AV nodal artery**, which supplies the AV node.

- The **left coronary artery**, typically larger than the right coronary artery, arises from the aorta posterior to the pulmonary trunk. After a short but variable course, it divides into two large branches, the **anterior interventricular** (left anterior descending) **artery**, which descends in the anterior interventricular sulcus, and the **circumflex artery**, which runs around the left side of the heart in the coronary sulcus. Their branches and distributions include
    - the anterior interventricular artery, which supplies the anterior aspects of the right and left ventricles and the anterior two-thirds of the interventricular septum, including the AV bundle of the conducting system; and
    - the circumflex artery, which supplies the left atrium and, via its **left marginal branch**, the left ventricle. In ~40% of the population, an **SA nodal branch** arises to supply the SA node.

— Variation in the coronary circulation is common but the descriptive language is misleading. The term "dominance" refers not to the artery that supplies the greater volume of cardiac tissue (that is almost always the left coronary artery), but to the artery that gives rise to the posterior interventricular branch.

- A right dominant circulation occurs in about two-thirds of the population. The posterior interventricular branch arises from the right coronary artery and supplies the posterior third of the interventricular septum.
- Approximately 15% of people exhibit left dominance in which the posterior interventricular artery is a branch of the circumflex artery. In these cases, the entire interventricular septum and the AV node are supplied by the left coronary artery.
- Approximately 15% of people have a shared dominance in which branches from both coronary arteries run in the interventricular groove and jointly supply the interventricular septum.

Angina

Angina (angina pectoris), a sudden, crushing substernal pain, is a result of myocardial ischemia (insufficient blood supply) caused by a narrowing of the coronary arteries. Exercise following a heavy meal, stress, or even cold weather can trigger an episode. Although angina pain may be severe, it is relieved by a short rest and does not result in infarction of cardiac muscle.

Coronary artery disease

Coronary artery disease results in ischemia of the myocardium and is a leading cause of death in the United States. In atherosclerosis of the coronary arteries, lipid deposits build up on the inner wall of the vessel and gradually narrow the lumen. In acute disease a fragment of plaque breaks off and completely obstructs the vessel. This creates a necrotic (dead) area of myocardium known as a myocardial infarction. Chronic disease is characterized by a gradual narrowing of the vessels. Over time a collateral circulation develops that circumvents the narrowed segment and may prevent, or limit, damage from other ischemic events.

Coronary artery bypass graft

Coronary artery bypass graft (CABG) is a surgical procedure performed to bypass atherosclerotic narrowings of the coronary arteries that are the cause of anginal pain. If left untreated these narrowings can eventually occlude the vessel and lead to myocardial infarction (MI). The internal thoracic artery and the great saphenous vein are most commonly used as the bypass vessel.

5.4b Coronary Veins (see Fig. 5.14A and B)

— The **coronary sinus**, which receives most of the venous return from the heart, runs in the posterior coronary sulcus between the left atrium and ventricle. The **thebesian valve** guards the orifice of the coronary sinus where it drains into the right atrium near the opening of the inferior vena cava (see **Fig. 5.10B**).
— The large veins of the heart are tributaries of the coronary sinus.

- The **great cardiac vein** travels with the anterior interventricular artery and drains the left atrium and both ventricles.
- The **posterior left ventricular** vein drains the diaphragmatic surface of the left ventricle.
- The **posterior interventricular (middle cardiac) vein** runs in the posterior interventricular groove with the posterior interventricular artery and drains the posterior part of the interventricular septum.
- The **small cardiac vein**, which drains the posterior right atrium and the right ventricle, accompanies the right coronary artery in the atrioventricular groove.

— **Anterior cardiac veins** drain the anterior surface of the right ventricle and open directly into the right atrium.

Table 5.4 ▶ Branches of the Coronary Arteries	
Left coronary artery	**Right coronary artery**
Circumflex a. • Atrial branch • Left marginal a. • Posterior left ventricular a.	Branch to sinoatrial node
	Conus branch
	Atrial branch
	Right marginal a.
Anterior interventricular a. (left anterior descending a.) • Conus branch • Lateral branch • Interventricular septal branches	Posterior interventricular (descending) a. • Interventricular septal branches
	Branch to atrioventricular node
	Right posterolateral a.

Fig. 5.14 ▶ **Coronary arteries and cardiac veins**

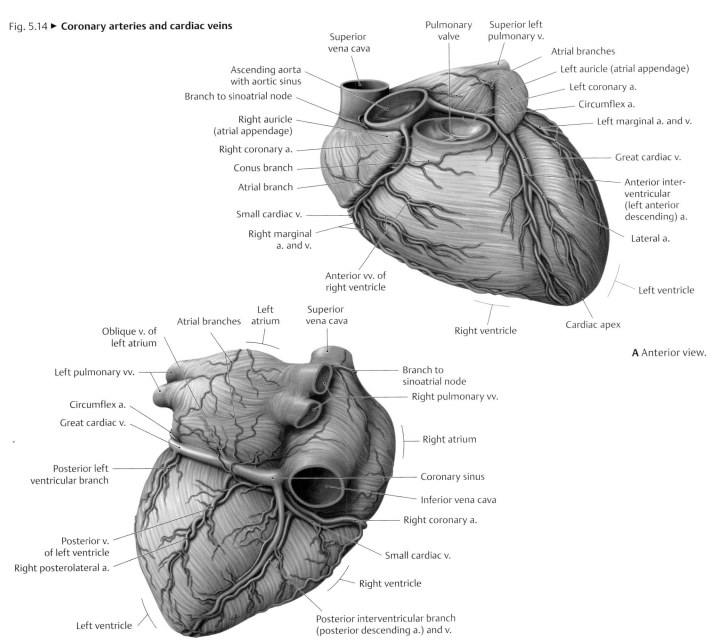

A Anterior view.

B Posteroinferior view. *Note:* The right and left coronary arteries typically anastomose posteriorly at the left atrium and ventricle.

5.4c   Lymphatic Drainage of the Heart

— Lymphatic vessels of the heart have a crossed drainage pattern. Lymph from the left atrium and ventricle drains via a left coronary trunk to inferior tracheobronchial nodes. Efferents from these nodes usually drain to the right venous junction via the bronchomediastinal trunk. Lymph from the right ventricle and atrium drains via a right coronary trunk that runs along the ascending aorta to brachiocephalic nodes near the left venous junction (**Fig. 5.15A** and **B**).

— The pericardium usually drains to the right and left venous junctions via superior phrenic nodes and bronchomediastinal trunks, but it may also drain superiorly to the brachiocephalic nodes.

Fig. 5.15 ▶ **Lymphatic drainage of the heart**
A unique "crossed" drainage pattern exists in the heart: lymph from the left atrium and ventricle drains to the right venous junction, whereas lymph from the right atrium and ventricle drains to the left venous junction.

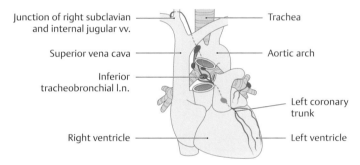

A Lymphatic drainage of the left chambers, anterior view.

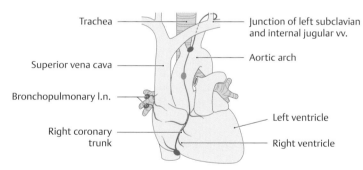

B Lymphatic drainage of the right chambers, anterior view.

5.4d   Innervation of the Heart

The autonomic nerves of the cardiac plexus innervate the conduction system of the heart; they therefore regulate the heart rate but do not initiate the heartbeat.

— Sympathetic innervation increases the rate and force of contractions by increasing the response of the SA and AV nodes. It also allows dilation of the coronary arteries.

— Parasympathetic innervation decreases the rate of contractions and causes vasoconstriction of the coronary arteries.

— Visceral sensory fibers innervating the baroreceptors (receptors that measure blood pressure) and chemoreceptors (receptors that measure blood CO_2) in the heart and aortic arch travel with the parasympathetic fibers of the vagus nerve.

— Visceral sensory fibers carrying pain sensation travel with sympathetic fibers to the T1–T5 spinal cord.

5.5   Prenatal and Neonatal Circulation

5.5a   Prenatal Circulation

Fetal shunts that direct the flow of blood through the liver, heart, and lungs create a prenatal circulation that differs from that of the adult. The numbered steps in **Fig. 5.16** illustrate the blood flow in the fetal circulation.

1. Fetal blood supplied with oxygen and nutrients in the placenta courses through the umbilical vein toward the liver of the fetus.

2. Although a portion of the blood is distributed to the liver, over half bypasses the liver and is redirected through a shunt, the **ductus venosus**, which empties directly into the inferior vena cava. This blood mixes with smaller amounts from the liver and lower parts of the body before entering the right atrium of the heart.

3. The **eustachian valve** (see **Fig. 5.10B**) at the orifice of the inferior vena cava directs this well-oxygenated mixture across the right atrium into the left atrium through the oval foramen on the interatrial septum. The higher systolic pressure in the right atrium relative to that in the left creates this right-to-left shunt.

From the left atrium, the flow continues into the left ventricle, the aorta, and the systemic circulation of the head and neck. Thus the most highly oxygenated and nutrient-rich blood from the placenta is directed into the coronary, carotid, and subclavian arteries to supply the upper body, especially the heart and developing brain.

4. Oxygen-depleted blood entering the right atrium from the superior vena cava is directed downward through the tricuspid valve into the right ventricle and out through the pulmonary trunk.

Because the high vascular resistance in the lungs prevents much blood from entering the pulmonary arteries, most is diverted to the descending aorta through the **ductus arteriosus**, a connection between the left pulmonary artery and the aortic arch.

5. The blood entering the aorta from the ductus arteriosus mixes with some blood from the aortic arch. This partially oxygenated blood flows into the descending aorta and is distributed to the lower body, or back to the placenta by way of the paired umbilical arteries.

Fig. 5.16 ▶ **Prenatal circulation**
After Fritsch and Kühnel.

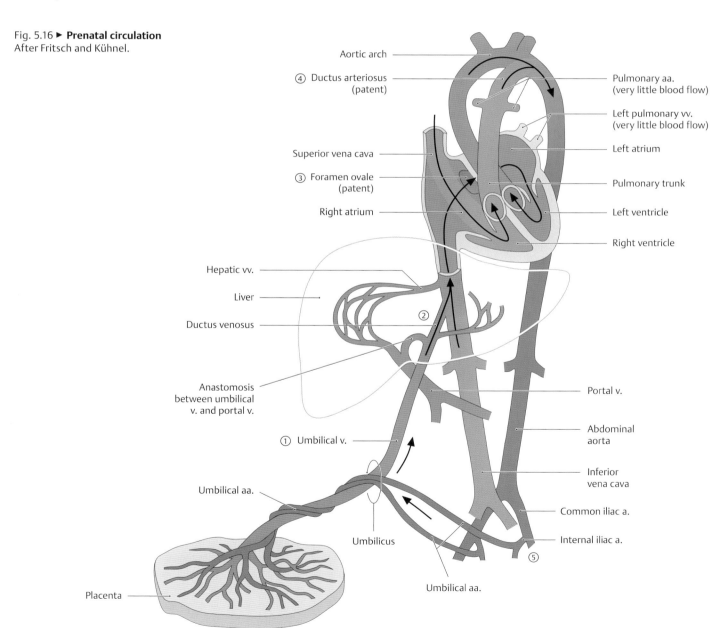

5.5b Cardiovascular Changes at Birth

At birth, a series of changes occurs in the cardiovascular system (**Fig. 5.17; Table 5.5**).

1. Pressure in the right atrium decreases as a result of
   a. ligation of the umbilical vein, which cuts off blood flow from the placenta; and
   b. the onset of pulmonary respiration, which dramatically decreases the pulmonary blood pressure and increases blood flow to the lungs.
3. As a result of increased flow through the lungs, there is a decreased blood flow through the ductus arteriosus, which constricts within 10 to 15 hours of birth. In the adult, the remnant of this structure is the **ligamentum arteriosum**.
4. Blood returning to the heart through the pulmonary veins increases pressure in the left atrium.
5. Increased pressure in the left atrium, coupled with a corresponding decrease in pressure in the right atrium, causes a functional closure of the foramen ovale within hours of birth. Complete closure of the oval foramen usually occurs after several months, forming the **oval fossa** (fossa ovalis) in the adult heart.

6. Functional closure of the umbilical arteries, umbilical vein, and ductus venosus occurs within minutes of birth, although the obliteration of the lumen in each vessel may take several months. The remnants of these vessels in the adult are ligamentous structures.

Table 5.5 ▶ **Derivatives of Fetal Circulatory Structures**

Fetal structure	Adult remnant
Ductus arteriosus	Ligamentum arteriosum
Oval foramen	Oval fossa
Ductus venosus	Ligamentum venosum
Umbilical v.	Round ligament of the liver (ligamentum teres)
Umbilical a.	Medial umbilical ligament

Fig. 5.17 ▶ **Postnatal circulation**
After Fritsch and Kühnel.

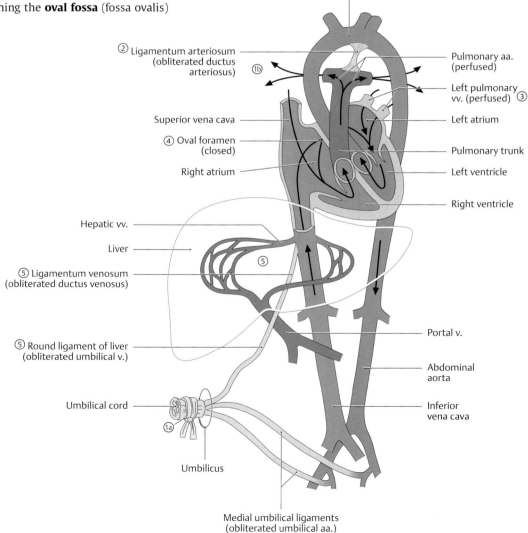

Atrial septal defect

Atrial septal defects (ASDs) are among the most common congenital cardiac anomalies and are particularly associated with Down syndrome. Most ASDs result from a failure of the oval foramen to close at birth, but they may also result from incomplete development of the septal components. ASDs result in left-to-right shunting and an increase in blood volume through the pulmonary circulation. Small ASDs are often asymptomatic, but larger ASDs will cause hypertrophy of the right atrium, right ventricle, and pulmonary arteries due to the fluid overload.

Patent ductus arteriosus

The opening of the pulmonary circulation at birth causes the ductus arteriosus to constrict, probably in response to an increase in local oxygen tension. If the ductus remains open, as a patent ductus arteriosus (PDA), deoxygenated blood continues to enter the descending aorta. There may be no symptoms if the defect is small, but larger defects may cause failure to thrive, dyspnea (shortness of breath), fatigue, tachycardia (increased heart rate), and cyanosis. Because prostaglandins maintain patency of the ductus during fetal life, premature infants whose ductus does not constrict spontaneously at birth may be treated with prostaglandin inhibitors.

Coarctation of the aorta

Coarctation, or stenosis, of the aorta usually occurs in proximity to the ligamentum arteriosum, where it limits (or obstructs) the normal blood flow from the aortic arch through the descending aorta. When the narrowing is distal to the ligamentum, an effective collateral circulation links the proximal and distal aortic segments via the internal thoracic arteries and their intercostal branches. The intercostal arteries may become large and tortuous enough to form notches along the lower margins of the ribs.

5.6 Thymus

The thymus is a gland of the immune system, responsible for maturation of T-lymphocytes (**Fig. 5.18**).

— In childhood, the thymus presents as a large bilobed organ that overlies the heart and great vessels in the superior and anterior mediastinum.

— At puberty, high levels of circulating sex hormones cause the gland to atrophy.

Fig. 5.18 ▶ **Thymus**
Anterior view of opened thorax.

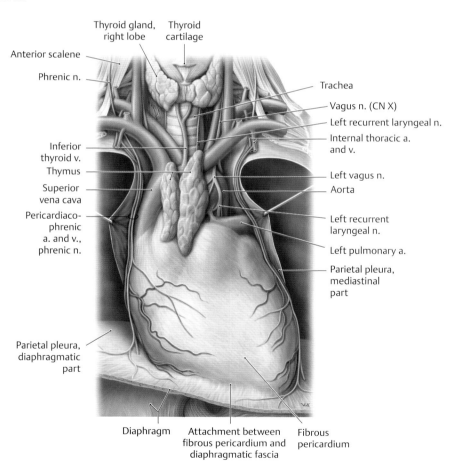

5.7 Esophagus

The esophagus, the thoracic segment of the gastrointestinal tract, is a narrow, but highly distensible, muscular tube. It connects the pharynx in the neck to the stomach in the abdomen (**Fig. 5.19**).

— The esophagus descends anterior to the thoracic vertebral bodies in the posterior mediastinum. Superiorly, it lies posterior to the trachea; inferiorly, it lies posterior to the left atrium of the heart.

— In the upper thorax, the esophagus descends on the right side of the aorta. Before passing through the esophageal aperture of the diaphragm, the esophagus passes first anterior to, and then to the left of, the aorta.

— The upper esophagus is composed mostly of striated muscle arranged in inner circular and outer longitudinal layers. Striated muscle is gradually replaced by smooth muscle fibers inferiorly.

— Three constrictions narrow the lumen of the esophagus (**Fig. 5.20**):

1. The upper **esophageal constriction**, created by the cricopharyngeus muscle (part of the inferior constrictor muscle of the pharynx), which surrounds the upper esophageal opening in the neck

2. The **middle esophageal constriction**, created by the aortic arch and left main bronchus

3. The **lower esophageal constriction**, or **cardiac sphincter**, created by circular muscles of the distal esophagus, folds in the mucosa formed by a submucosal venous plexus, and the muscular esophageal aperture of the diaphragm

— The blood supply to the upper, middle, and lower esophagus arises from vessels in the neck (inferior thyroid), thorax (esophageal branches of the descending aorta), and abdomen (left gastric and left inferior phrenic), respectively.

Fig. 5.19 ► **Esophagus in situ**
Anterior view.

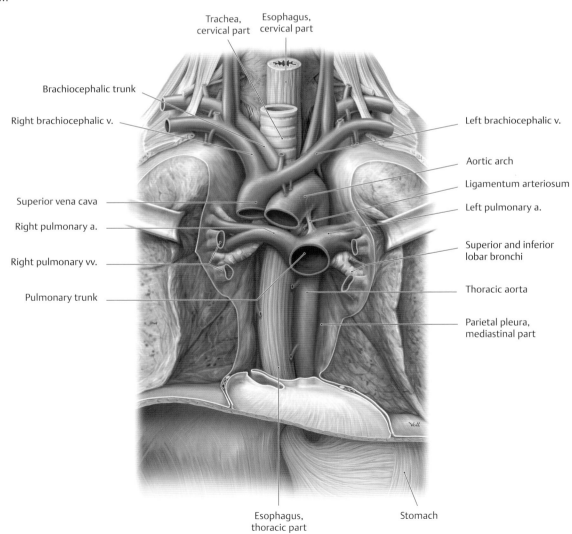

Trachea, cervical part

Esophagus, cervical part

Brachiocephalic trunk

Right brachiocephalic v.

Left brachiocephalic v.

Aortic arch

Ligamentum arteriosum

Superior vena cava

Left pulmonary a.

Right pulmonary a.

Right pulmonary vv.

Superior and inferior lobar bronchi

Thoracic aorta

Pulmonary trunk

Parietal pleura, mediastinal part

Esophagus, thoracic part

Stomach

Fig. 5.20 ▶ **Esophagus: Location and constrictions**
Esophageal constrictions, right lateral view.

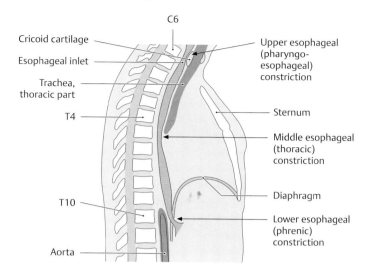

- Cricoid cartilage
- Esophageal inlet
- Trachea, thoracic part
- T4
- T10
- Aorta
- C6
- Upper esophageal (pharyngo-esophageal) constriction
- Sternum
- Middle esophageal (thoracic) constriction
- Diaphragm
- Lower esophageal (phrenic) constriction

— The veins of upper and middle esophageal segments drain into the azygos system. Veins of the lower esophageal segment drain inferiorly along inferior phrenic veins into the hepatic portal system (the venous drainage for organs of the abdominal gastrointestinal tract).

— The **esophageal plexus**, formed by the right and left vagus nerves with contributions from the greater splanchnic, nerves, innervates the esophagus.

Achalasia

Achalasia is a deficiency of inhibitory neurons in the lower part of the esophagus. These neurons are responsible for overriding the normal resting tonic contraction of the smooth muscle cells in the lower esophageal sphincter. Their deficiency results in failure of the sphincter to relax during swallowing. As food accumulates above the sphincter, there is an increased risk of aspiration pneumonia.

5.8 Trachea and Bronchi

The trachea, located in the superior mediastinum, is the proximal part of the **tracheobronchial tree**, a passageway for air between the lungs and the external environment. The distal part of this passageway, the **bronchial tree**, extends into the lungs and is discussed with the pulmonary cavities in Chapter 6.

— As the trachea descends through the superior mediastinum, slightly to the right of the midline, it lies anterior to the esophagus and posterior to the great vessels.

— C-shaped cartilaginous rings form the skeleton of the trachea and prevent collapse of the lumen. A muscular membrane connects the ends of the rings posteriorly (**Fig. 5.21A and B**).

— The **carina**, a wedge-shaped cartilage, marks the bifurcation of the trachea into a **right** and **left bronchus** at the T4–T5 vertebral level.

— Of the two main bronchi, the right is shorter, wider, and more vertical than the left, and therefore is more prone to obstruction by foreign objects.

— Descending branches of the inferior thyroid artery in the neck (see **Fig. 21.21C**), as well as bronchial arteries that arise from the descending aorta (see **Fig. 3.3B**), supply the trachea. Venous blood drains to the inferior thyroid veins.

— Thoracic splanchnic nerves and parasympathetic fibers from the vagus (CN X) nerve innervate the trachea via the pulmonary plexus.

Fig. 5.21 ▶ **Trachea**

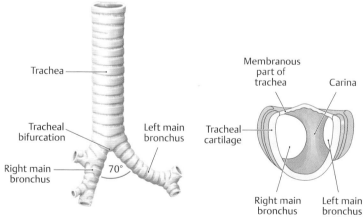

- Trachea
- Tracheal bifurcation
- Right main bronchus
- Left main bronchus
- 70°
- Membranous part of trachea
- Carina
- Tracheal cartilage
- Right main bronchus
- Left main bronchus

A Anterior view.

B Tracheal bifurcation, superior view.

6 Pulmonary Cavities

The right and left pulmonary cavities, which flank the mediastinum laterally and anteriorly, extend superiorly above the costal cartilages of the first rib and inferiorly to the thoracic diaphragm (see **Table 3.1**). Each pulmonary cavity contains a lung and bronchial tree and a pleural sac.

6.1 The Pleura and Pleural Cavity

6.1a The Pleura

The **pleura** is a fibroserous membrane that surrounds each lung and lines the pulmonary cavities (**Fig. 6.1**).

— The pleura is composed of two layers:

- The **parietal pleura**, which is a continuous layer that lines the inner wall of the thoracic cavity, the superior surface of the diaphragm, and the mediastinum. Its parts are named according to location: cervical, costal, diaphragmatic, and mediastinal (**Fig. 6.2**).

Fig. 6.2 ▶ **Parts of the parietal pleura**
Anterior view. *Opened:* Right pleural cavity.

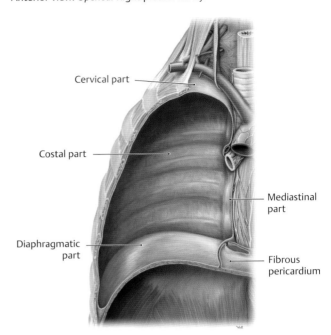

Cervical part

Costal part

Diaphragmatic part

Mediastinal part

Fibrous pericardium

Fig. 6.1 ▶ **Lungs in situ**
Anterior view. *Removed:* Anterior thoracic wall and costal part of the parietal pleura.

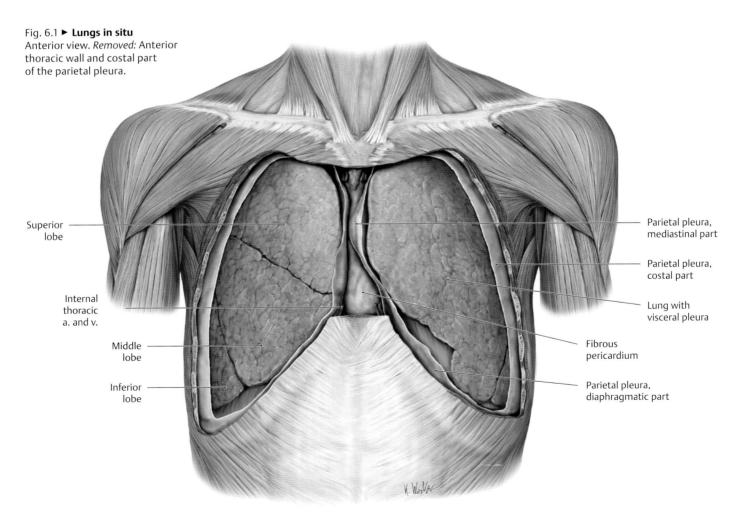

Superior lobe

Internal thoracic a. and v.

Middle lobe

Inferior lobe

Parietal pleura, mediastinal part

Parietal pleura, costal part

Lung with visceral pleura

Fibrous pericardium

Parietal pleura, diaphragmatic part

— The **visceral pleura**, which covers the surface of the lung and extends into its fissures.

— The visceral and parietal layers are continuous with one another at the hilum of the lung (see Section 6.2a). Together they form the inner and outer walls of a closed pleural sac that contains a **pleural cavity** (**Fig. 6.3**).

— The **pulmonary ligament** is a double-layered fold of visceral and parietal pleura that extends vertically from the hilum to the diaphragm along the mediastinal border of each lung (see **Fig. 6.5B** and **D**).

The blood supply and innervation of the pleura are derived from nerves and vessels that supply adjacent structures. Visceral pleura shares the neurovasculature of the lungs and bronchi; parietal pleura shares the neurovasculature of the thoracic wall.

Pleuritis

Inflammation of the pleura, or pleuritis, creates friction between the visceral and parietal layers that produces a sharp, stabbing pain as the layers glide over one another during respiration. The inflammation may also produce adhesions between the two layers.

6.1b   The Pleural Cavity

The **pleural cavity**, the cavity within the pleural sac, is the potential space between the visceral and parietal layers of pleura (see **Fig. 6.3**).

Fig. 6.4 ▶ **Costomediastinal and costodiaphragmatic recesses**
On the left side of the thorax, an examiner's fingertips are placed in the costomediastinal and costodiaphragmatic recesses. These recesses are formed by the acute reflection of the costal part of the parietal pleura onto the fibrous pericardium (costomediastinal) or diaphragm (costodiaphragmatic).

Fig. 6.3 ▶ **Pleura and pleural cavity**
Schematic.

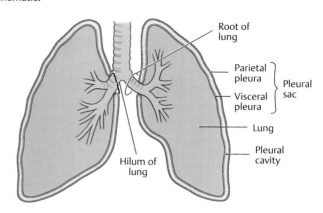

— The pleural cavity contains a thin layer of serous fluid, which lubricates the adjacent pleural surfaces, facilitates the movement of the lung, and maintains surface tension that is crucial to respiration.

— On most surfaces, the two pleural layers approximate one another, but the lung and its visceral pleura are somewhat smaller than the outer wall of the pleural cavity and its lining of parietal pleura. Two recesses that form as a result of this discrepancy accommodate the expansion of the lungs during inspiration (**Fig. 6.4**):

• The **costodiaphragmatic recess** forms where the diaphragmatic pleura reflects from the perimeter of the diaphragm to meet the costal pleura on the thoracic wall.

• The **costomediastinal recess** forms between the pericardial sac and the sternum, where the mediastinal pleura reflects to meet the costal pleura.

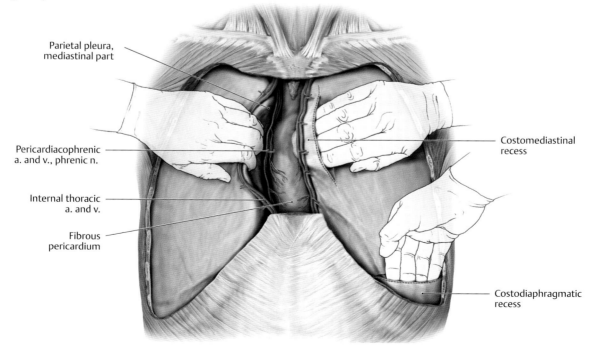

Pneumothorax

Pneumothorax is a condition in which air enters the pleural space. It may result from a tear in the chest wall and parietal pleura (such as from a stab wound) or a tear of the visceral pleura (such as from a rupture of a pulmonary lesion). Air in the pleural space decreases the negative pressure that normally keeps the lungs inflated and leads to a partial or complete lung collapse.

Tension pneumothorax

Tension pneumothorax is a life-threatening condition in which air accumulates in the pleural space and becomes trapped because the injured tissue acts as a one-way valve. This causes complete collapse of the lung on the affected side and a shifting of the heart to the opposite side, thus compromising venous return and cardiac output. This mediastinal shift also compresses the opposite lung and impairs its ventilatory capacity.

Pleural effusion

Pleural effusion is a condition in which there is excess fluid in the pleural space. Effusions are designated by their protein concentration into transudates (< 30 g/L protein) and exudates (> 30 g/L protein). Transudates are usually caused by congestive heart failure or fluid overload (causing increased venous pressure). Less commonly they are caused by liver failure or renal disease. Exudates may leak from the pleural capillaries in inflammatory states, pneumonia, tuberculosis (TB), or lung cancer. Symptoms include dyspnea (shortness of breath), cough, and dull chest pain. Pleural effusions are treated by draining the fluid through a procedure known as thoracentesis (see call-out box below).

Chylothorax

Chylothorax is a type of pleural effusion (fluid in the pleural space) in which chyle leaks from the thoracic duct or one of the main lymphatic vessels and accumulates in the pleural space.

Thoracentesis

Thoracentesis (chest drain) is a procedure in which a needle is inserted into the pleural cavity to drain fluid, blood, or pus. In an upright patient the fluid accumulates in the costodiaphragmatic recesses. In order to access these recesses without damaging the inferior border of the lung, the diaphragm, the liver, or the spleen, the needle is usually inserted at the posterior axillary line in the 7th intercostal space or in the mid-axillary line at the 7th or 8th intercostal space. The needle is inserted above the rib to avoid the intercostal neurovascular bundle that runs in the costal groove along the lower margin of the rib.

6.2 The Lungs

6.2a General Features (Fig. 6.5A, B, C, and D, Table 6.1)

— Each lung has costal, mediastinal, and diaphragmatic surfaces.
— The **apex** of each lung projects into the neck above the first costal cartilage; the **base** of each lung rests on the diaphragm.
— The **root** of the lung, which connects the lung to the mediastinum, contains the pulmonary vessels, nerves, and bronchi. The root enters the lung at the **hilum**, an indentation on the mediastinal surface (see **Fig. 6.3**).
— Fissures, lined by visceral pleura, divide each lung into lobes: three lobes on the right and two lobes on the left.
— Thin connective tissue septa (intersegmental septa) that are continuous with the visceral pleura subdivide lobes of the lungs into discrete pyramidal-shaped units called **bronchopulmonary segments** (**Fig. 6.6A, B, C, D,** and **E**).

Table 6.1 ▶ Structure of the Lungs	Right lung	Left lung
Lobes	Superior, middle, inferior	Superior, inferior
Fissures	Oblique, horizontal	Oblique
Bronchopulmonary Segments	10	8–10
Unique Features	Larger and heavier than the left, but shorter and wider due to higher right hemidiaphragm	Superior lobe characterized by the lingula and a deep cardiac notch

- Each bronchopulmonary segment is an anatomically and functionally independent respiratory unit. This independence allows the surgical resection of individual segments.
- There are 10 bronchopulmonary segments in the right lung and 8 to 10 segments in the left lung.

Carcinoma of the lung

Carcinoma of the lung accounts for ~20% of all cancers and is mainly caused by cigarette smoking. It arises first in the lining of the bronchi and metastasizes quickly to bronchopulmonary lymph nodes and subsequently to other node groups, including supraclavicular nodes. It can also spread via the blood to the lungs, brain, bone, and suprarenal glands. Lung cancer can invade adjacent structures such as the phrenic nerve, resulting in paralysis of a hemidiaphragm, or the recurrent laryngeal nerve, resulting in hoarseness due to paralysis of the vocal cord.

6.2b Right Lung

— Because the dome of the diaphragm is higher on the right side, the right lung is shorter and wider than the left lung.
— Horizontal and oblique fissures divide the right lung into superior, middle, and inferior lobes (see **Fig. 6.5A** and **B**).
— The root of the lung passes under the arch of the aorta, posterior to the right atrium, and under the arch of the azygos vein (see **Figs. 3.2** and **5.1A**).
— The right bronchus and its branches are the most posterior structures within the root of the lung. The pulmonary artery passes anterior to the bronchus, and the pulmonary veins lie anterior and inferior to the artery.

6.2c Left Lung

— An oblique fissure divides the left lung into superior and inferior lobes (see **Fig. 6.5C** and **D**).
— A deep indentation along the anterior border of the superior lobe called the **cardiac notch** accommodates the leftward projection of the apex of the heart.
— The **lingula**, a thin tongue of lung tissue from the superior lobe, forms the inferior border of the cardiac notch and moves into and out of the costomediastinal recess during respiration.
— The aortic arch crosses over the left bronchus, and the descending aorta passes behind the root of the lung (see **Fig. 5.1B**).
— The left pulmonary artery arches over the left bronchus to become the most superior structure in the root of the lung. Pulmonary veins pass anterior and inferior to the bronchus.

Fig. 6.5 ▶ **Gross anatomy of the lungs**

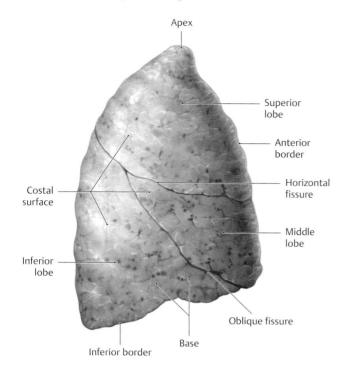

Apex

Superior
lobe

Anterior
border

Horizontal
fissure

Costal
surface

Middle
lobe

Inferior
lobe

Oblique fissure

Inferior border

Base

A Right lung, lateral view.

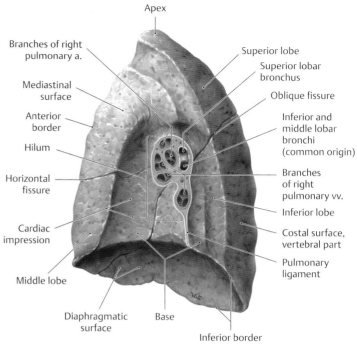

Apex

Branches of right
pulmonary a.

Superior lobe

Superior lobar
bronchus

Mediastinal
surface

Oblique fissure

Anterior
border

Inferior and
middle lobar
bronchi
(common origin)

Hilum

Horizontal
fissure

Branches
of right
pulmonary vv.

Inferior lobe

Cardiac
impression

Costal surface,
vertebral part

Pulmonary
ligament

Middle lobe

Diaphragmatic
surface

Base

Inferior border

B Right lung, medial view.

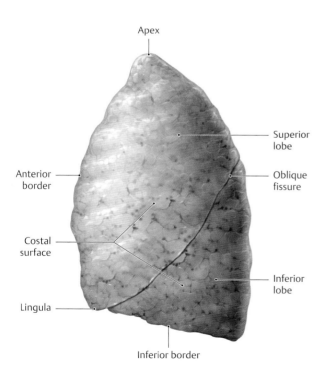

Apex

Superior
lobe

Anterior
border

Oblique
fissure

Costal
surface

Inferior
lobe

Lingula

Inferior border

C Left lung, lateral view.

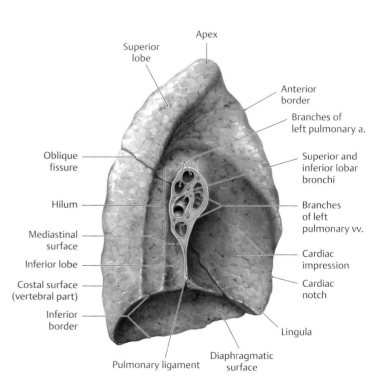

Apex

Superior
lobe

Anterior
border

Branches of
left pulmonary a.

Oblique
fissure

Superior and
inferior lobar
bronchi

Hilum

Branches
of left
pulmonary vv.

Mediastinal
surface

Cardiac
impression

Inferior lobe

Cardiac
notch

Costal surface
(vertebral part)

Inferior
border

Lingula

Pulmonary ligament

Diaphragmatic
surface

D Left lung, medial view.

Fig. 6.6 ► **Segmentation of the lungs**

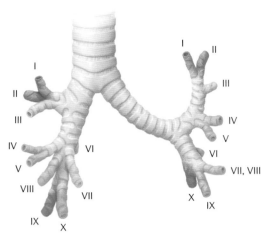

A Trachea with segmental bronchi, anterior view.

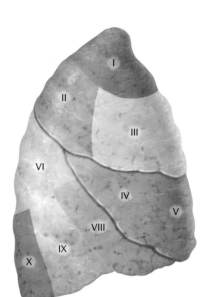

B Right lung, lateral view.

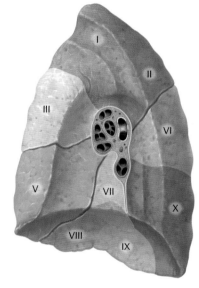

C Right lung, medial view.

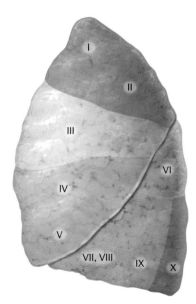

D Left lung, lateral view.

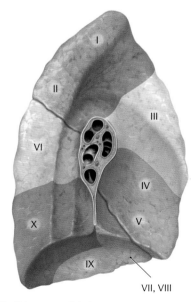

E Left lung, medial view.

6.3 The Tracheobronchial Tree

The tracheobronchial tree consists of the trachea and the bronchi in the mediastinum, and the bronchial tree (generations of branches formed by successive bifurcations) within the lungs. (The trachea is discussed in Section 5.8.) The tracheobronchial tree has conducting and respiratory components.

— The trachea and its larger proximal branches form the conducting component, a passageway for air exchange between the lung and the external environment (**Figs. 6.7** and **6.8A**). All except the most distal of these branches have cartilaginous rings or plates in their walls. The branches include

- the **right** and **left main** (primary) **bronchi**, formed by the bifurcation of the trachea in the superior mediastinum. One main bronchus enters the root of each lung.
- the **lobar** (secondary) **bronchi**, which branch from the main bronchi. One lobar bronchus enters each lobe of the respective lung (three on the right and two on the left).

- the **segmental** (tertiary) **bronchi**, which branch from the lobar bronchi. One segmental bronchus enters each bronchopulmonary segment.
- the **conducting bronchioles**, a network of airways without cartilage that are formed as the segmental bronchi subdivide and decrease in size.
- the **terminal bronchioles**, the last branches of the conducting bronchioles and the final part of the conducting airway.

— The respiratory component (seen only histologically), made up of passages distal to the terminal bronchioles, is involved in air conduction as well as in gas exchange (**Fig. 6.8B**).

- The structures in this part of the bronchial tree include the **respiratory bronchioles**, **alveolar sacs**, and **alveoli**.
- The single-celled walls of the alveoli are designed for efficient gas exchange.

Fig. 6.7 ► **Trachea**
Anterior view. The numbers I to IX of the segmental bronchi correspond with bronchopulmonary segments shown in **Fig. 6.6B** to **D**.

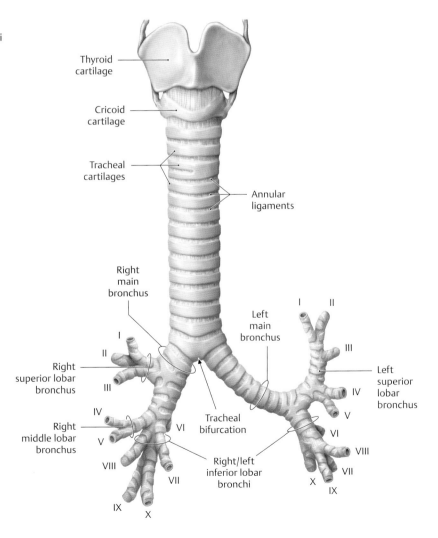

Fig. 6.8 ▶ **Bronchial tree**

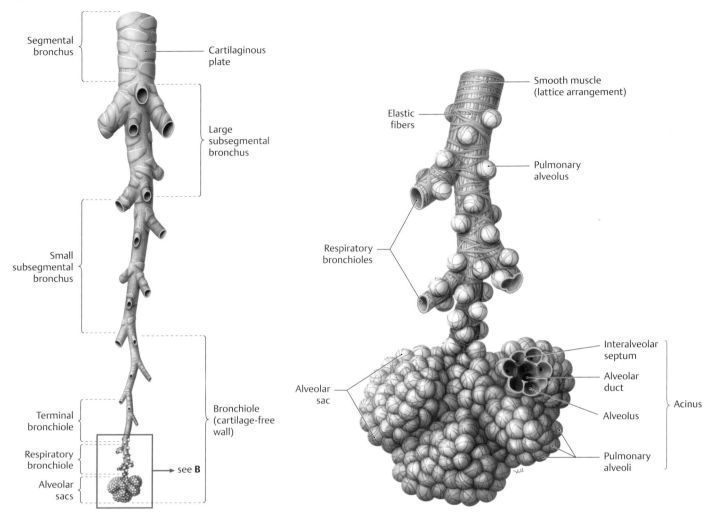

A Divisions of the bronchial tree.

B Respiratory portion of the bronchial tree.

▊ Atelectasis

Atelectasis is the partial or complete collapse of alveoli within the lung and can result from mucus in the airways following surgery (most common), cystic fibrosis, asthma, or obstruction of the airways by a foreign object (e.g., a tumor or blood clot). When severe, it can lead to respiratory failure.

▊ Neonatal respiratory distress syndrome

Neonatal respiratory distress syndrome (neonatal RDS), common in preterm infants, results from a deficiency of surfactant, which leads to alveolar collapse (atelectasis). The use of synthetic surfactant and administration of continuous positive airway pressure (CPAP) can help maintain airway patency in these infants.

▊ Chronic obstructive pulmonary disease

Chronic obstructive bronchitis and emphysema, both caused by cigarette smoking, contribute in varying degrees to chronic obstructive pulmonary disease (COPD). Inflammation from chronic bronchitis leads to thickened bronchial tubes, excess mucus production, and a narrowed airway. Emphysema destroys alveolar walls, thereby reducing the capacity for gas exchange, and, as small airways collapse during expiration, air is trapped in the lungs. This chronic hyperinflation of the lungs and the increased work of expiration create a typical barrel chest appearance (increased antero-posterior diameter).

6.4 Mechanics of Respiration

Respiration, the exchange of oxygen and carbon dioxide, requires a continuous flow of air between the lungs and external environment and is accomplished through the rhythmic change in thoracic volume and corresponding expansion (during **inspiration**) and contraction (during **expiration**) of the lungs (**Figs. 6.9, 6.10,** and **6.11**).

— Inspiration requires an expansion of the pulmonary cavities and decrease in intrapleural pressure.

- During quiet respiration, the diaphragm, the chief respiratory muscle, contracts and flattens, increasing the vertical dimension of the cavity.
- Forced inspiration engages other respiratory muscles (primarily the intercostals, scalene, and posterior serratus) that elevate the ribs and sternum and expand the cavities horizontally.

- As the cavities expand, the pleural sac is pulled outward, causing an increase in lung volume and a decrease in intrapleural pressure. When the pressure drops below atmospheric pressure (negative pressure), air is pulled into the respiratory passageways.

— Expiration requires a contraction of the pulmonary cavities and increase in intrapleural pressure.

- Quiet expiration is a passive process. With relaxation of the diaphragm, there is a decrease in thoracic volume and a corresponding contraction of the lungs. As the intrapleural pressure increases, air is expelled.
- Forced expiration requires the contraction of anterior abdominal and intercostal muscles to decrease thoracic volume.

Fig. 6.9 ▶ **Respiratory changes in thoracic volume**
Inspiratory position (red); expiratory position (blue).

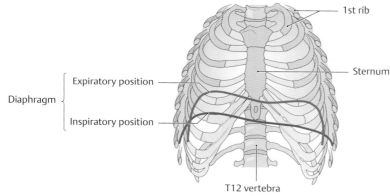

1st rib

Expiratory position

Diaphragm

Inspiratory position

Sternum

T12 vertebra

Fig. 6.10 ▶ **Respiratory changes in lung volume**

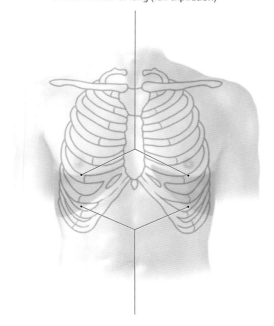

Inferior border of lung (full expiration)

Inferior border of lung (full inspiration)

Fig. 6.11 ▶ **Movements of the lung and bronchial tree**
As the volume of the lung changes with the volume of the thoracic cavity, the entire bronchial tree moves within the lung. These structural movements are more pronounced in portions of the bronchial tree distant from the pulmonary hilum.

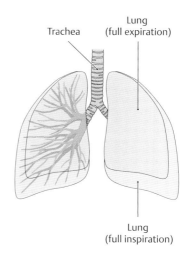

Trachea

Lung
(full expiration)

Lung
(full inspiration)

6.5 Neurovasculature of the Lungs and Bronchial Tree

6.5a Arteries of the Lungs and Bronchial Tree

- The **pulmonary arteries**, branches of the pulmonary trunk, transport deoxygenated blood to the capillary network surrounding the respiratory alveoli (**Fig. 6.12**). Within the lungs, branches of the arteries follow the branches of the bronchial tree as they ramify within the lobes and bronchopulmonary segments.
- **Bronchial arteries**, branches of the thoracic aorta, supply the bronchial tree, the connective tissue of the lungs, and the visceral pleura. Typically one branch to the right lung and two to the left lung, these bronchial arteries travel along the posterior aspect of the main bronchi and eventually anastomose with distal branches of the pulmonary arteries.

Fig. 6.12 ▶ **Pulmonary vasculature**
Pulmonary arteries (shown in blue) carry *deoxygenated* blood and follow the bronchial tree. Pulmonary veins (red) are the only veins in the body carrying *oxygenated* blood, which they receive from the alveolar capillaries at the periphery of the lobule.

Pulmonary embolism

Pulmonary embolism (PE) is the obstruction of a pulmonary artery or its branches by fat emboli, air bubbles, or, most commonly, thromboses (blood clots) that have traveled up from the deep veins of the legs. Large obstructions can impede blood flow into the lung and consequently cause cor pulmonale, right-sided heart failure. Large obstructions are often fatal, but smaller obstructions may affect only a single bronchopulmonary segment and result in a pulmonary infarction.

6.5b Veins of the Lungs and Bronchial Tree

- **Pulmonary veins** arise from the capillary beds surrounding the alveoli (see **Fig. 6.12**). Arising first as small veins that travel within the intersegmental septa carrying oxygenated blood, they receive veins from adjacent bronchopulmonary segments as well as from the visceral pleura. These veins join to form two pulmonary veins within each lung, which traverse the hilum and enter the left atrium of the heart.
- **Bronchial veins**, one from each lung, drain only the proximal portion of the root and terminate in the azygos and accessory hemiazygos (or superior intercostals) veins.

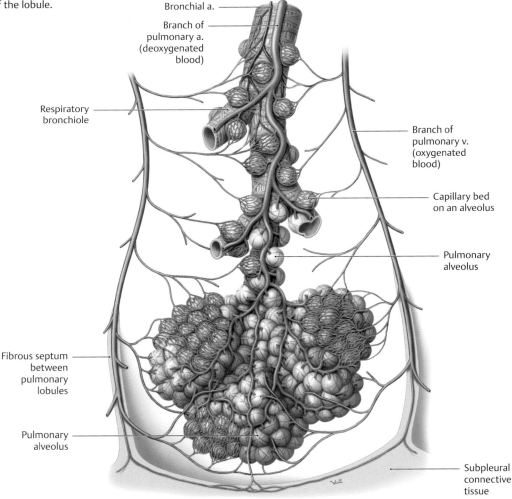

Bronchial a.

Branch of pulmonary a. (deoxygenated blood)

Respiratory bronchiole

Branch of pulmonary v. (oxygenated blood)

Capillary bed on an alveolus

Pulmonary alveolus

Fibrous septum between pulmonary lobules

Pulmonary alveolus

Subpleural connective tissue

6.5c Lymphatics of the Lungs and Bronchial Tree

— The **superficial lymphatic plexus** of the lungs, deep to the visceral pleura, drains the pleura and the lung tissue.
— The **deep lymphatic plexus**, within the walls of the bronchi, drains structures associated with the lung root.
— Whereas the superficial and deep plexuses eventually drain to the superior and inferior (carinal) **tracheobronchial nodes**, the deep plexus drains initially to the **bronchopulmonary** nodes along the lobar bronchi (**Fig. 6.13**).
— Lymph from tracheobronchial nodes drains to **paratracheal nodes** and then to the **bronchomediastinal trunks** on either side, which terminate in the junction of the subclavian and jugular veins (jugulosubclavian venous junctions).
— The superior, middle, and inferior lobes of the right lung and the superior lobe of the left lung normally drain along ipsilateral channels. Some lymph from the inferior lobe of the left lung, however, drains to the right tracheobronchial nodes, and from there it continues to follow right-sided channels.

6.5d Nerves of the Lungs and Bronchial Tree

— The **pulmonary plexus**, an autonomic nerve plexus that lies anterior and posterior to the root of the lung, innervates the lung, bronchial tree, and visceral pleura (**Table 6.2**).
— Visceral afferent fibers carrying pain from the bronchi and visceral pleura travel with sympathetic splanchnic nerves.
— Visceral afferent fibers from receptors related to cough and stretch reflexes, and receptors for blood pressure and blood gas levels travel with the vagus (parasympathetic) nerve.
— The parietal pleura is innervated by somatic nerves of the thoracic wall, and it is extremely sensitive to pain. Intercostal nerves innervate the costal surface, and phrenic nerves (C3–C5) innervate the mediastinal and diaphragmatic surfaces.
— Irritation of the parietal pleura in the areas supplied by the phrenic nerve is referred to the dermatomes C3–C5 on the neck and shoulder.

Table 6.2 ▶ Autonomic Innervation of the Lungs and Bronchial Tree		
Target structures	**Sympathetic**	**Parasympathetic**
Bronchial muscles	Inhibitory (bronchodilation)	Motor (bronchoconstriction)
Pulmonary vessels	Motor (vasoconstriction)	Inhibitory (bronchodilation)
Secretory cells of alveoli	Secretomotor	Inhibitory

Fig. 6.13 ▶ **Lymphatic drainage of the pleural cavity**
Peribronchial network, coronal section.

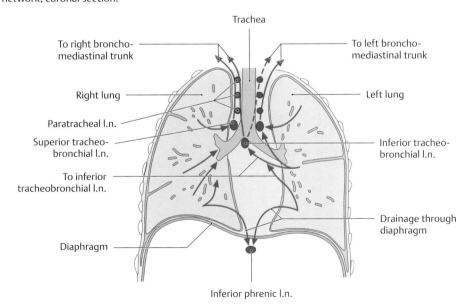

Review Questions: Thorax

1. Which of the following nerves contribute to the phrenic nerve?
   A. Anterior rami of C3–C5 spinal nerves
   B. Anterior rami of C5–T1 spinal nerves
   C. Sympathetic fibers from C3–C5 spinal cord segments
   D. Sympathetic fibers from T1–T4 spinal cord segments
   E. Cardiac nerves from the cervical sympathetic trunk

2. Which of the following is true of bronchopulmonary segments?
   A. Each is served by one terminal bronchiole.
   B. There are three in the right lung and two in the left lung.
   C. Each is supplied by one bronchial artery.
   D. Each is an anatomically and functionally distinct respiratory unit of the lung.
   E. They have single-celled walls designed for efficient gas exchange.

3. Which of the following structures is/are found in the right atrium?
   A. Chordae tendineae
   B. Oval fossa
   C. Mitral valve
   D. Papillary muscles
   E. Trabeculae carneae

4. The sternal angle (of Louis) marks the location of the
   A. second costal cartilage
   B. T4–T5 intervertebral disk
   C. origin of the aortic arch
   D. bifurcation of the trachea
   E. All of the above

5. You are studying the CT images of your patient who is being treated for lung cancer. You focus on the scan that shows the carina where you note several enlarged lymph nodes. What other structure is most likely visible in this CT image?
   A. Left atrium
   B. Brachiocephalic artery
   C. Sternal angle
   D. Tricuspid valve
   E. Right pulmonary vein

6. Within hours of arriving home after a 10-hour bus ride, a 77-year-old grandmother was rushed to the emergency room with shortness of breath, sweating, and nausea. Although she died shortly after being admitted, her workup in the emergency room revealed a pulmonary embolus in her left pulmonary artery. What other findings would you expect in this patient?
   A. Collapse of the left lung
   B. Acute dilation of the right ventricle
   C. A shift of mediastinal structures to the right side
   D. Hypertrophy of the left ventricle
   E. Dilation of the left atrium

7. A malignancy involving the lateral breast would *most* likely metastasize first to which of the following groups of nodes?
   A. Parasternal nodes
   B. Abdominal nodes
   C. Deep pectoral nodes
   D. Axillary nodes
   E. Nodes of the contralateral breast

8. The mother of a three-month-old infant was concerned because her child had little energy and did not seem to be thriving. As a young pediatrician, you examine the child and suspect the presence of a congenital cardiac defect, most likely a patent ductus arteriosus. What other symptoms would accompany this diagnosis?
   A. Increased blood flow in the pulmonary circulation
   B. Distension of the right atrium
   C. Decreased oxygen in the systemic circulation
   D. Notching of the ribs created by dilated intercostal arteries
   E. Left-to-right shunting between the atria

9. What is the surface landmark on the chest that approximates the position of the apex of the heart?
   A. Sternal angle
   B. Left 3rd intercostal space
   C. Left 5th intercostal space
   D. Right 5th intercostal space
   E. Xiphoid process of the sternum

10. Dr. P. was performing a cardiac bypass on his 53-year-old male patient whose anterior interventricular artery (also known as left anterior descending artery, LAD) was narrowed near its origin. Although Dr. P. frequently used a saphenous vein graft for this procedure, he chose to use the left internal thoracic artery instead. Leaving its origin intact, he cut its distal connections and anastomosed it to the LAD beyond the narrowed segment. This successfully restored flow to the anterior part of the heart. What path does the blood take through this diverted route?
    A. Aortic arch to left subclavian artery to internal thoracic artery
    B. Aortic arch to brachiocephalic artery to internal thoracic artery
    C. Aortic arch to internal thoracic artery
    D. Aortic arch to left subclavian artery to pericardiacophrenic artery to internal thoracic artery
    E. Aortic arch to axillary artery to internal thoracic artery

11. Your grandfather, who admits to some dizziness and minor chest palpitations during the past week, is finally admitted to the emergency department for chest pain and shortness of breath. Imaging reveals a major blockage of his right coronary artery near the crux of the heart just proximal to the origin of the posterior interventricular artery. Which part of the heart would be affected by the ischemia that results from this blockage?
    A. Sinoatrial (SA) node
    B. Atrioventricular (AV) node
    C. Anterior two-thirds of the interventricular septum
    D. Left atrium
    E. Right ventricle

12. Janet Jones, who had a recent history of a myocardial infarction (MI), complained to her cardiologist of a sharp, stabbing pain behind her sternum that radiated to her shoulder and was accompanied by shortness of breath, particularly when she was lying down. Her physician noted a pericardial friction rub and treated her for pericarditis, an inflammation of her pericardium caused by the recent MI.
    Pain from her pericardium was transmitted by the
    A. phrenic nerves
    B. cardiac plexus
    C. pulmonary plexus
    D. intercostal nerves
    E. None of the above

13. The right lymphatic duct drains the lymph from
    A. the entire right side of the body
    B. the right side of the thorax, right upper limb, and right side of the head and neck
    C. only the right side of the thorax
    D. only the right side of the head and neck and right upper limb
    E. the right side of the thorax, the abdomen, and the right lower and the right upper limbs

14. Which of the following features are paired with the correct lung?
    A. Lingula—right lung
    B. Horizontal fissure—left lung
    C. Cardiac notch—left lung
    D. Two lobar bronchi—right lung
    E. Shorter and wider than the contralateral lung—left lung

15. Several weeks after suffering a severe myocardial infarction, JR was rushed to the emergency department but died shortly afterward. It was discovered at autopsy that the muscle anchoring one leaflet of his mitral valve had ruptured, probably as a consequence of his earlier heart attack. Which was the affected muscle?
    A. Papillary muscle
    B. Trabeculae carneae
    C. Pectinate muscle
    D. Terminal crest
    E. Septomarginal trabecula (moderator band)

16. What is the origin of the posterior intercostal arteries?
    A. Aorta
    B. Internal thoracic artery
    C. Lateral thoracic artery
    D. Subclavian artery
    E. Superior epigastric artery

17. A patient with a history of asthma presents to the emergency department with shortness of breath and wheezing. Drugs and oxygen are administered, but her condition worsens. She is transferred to the intensive care unit and put on a ventilator. Twenty-four hours after admission, she dies from complications of asthma. On autopsy it is found that she has severe inflammation, an increase in smooth muscle, and other pathologic changes around a part of the respiratory tree that does not contain cartilage. Which part of the airway was most likely affected in this patient?
    A. Trachea
    B. Main (primary) bronchi
    C. Lobar (secondary) bronchi
    D. Segmental (tertiary) bronchi
    E. Bronchioles

18. During the physical examination of a 28-year-old construction worker, you mention that his heart sounds strong and healthy. He asks you to explain what creates the heart sounds. You tell him that the first heart sound (the "lub") is produced by the
    A. closure of the tricuspid and pulmonary valves
    B. closure of the atrioventricular valves
    C. opening of the semilunar valves
    D. contraction of the ventricles
    E. turbulent flow through the valves

19. All of the following structures are in contact with thoracic vertebral bodies except
    A. Azygos vein
    B. Trachea
    C. Sympathetic trunk
    D. Thoracic duct
    E. Right posterior intercostal artery

20. What is/are the primary muscle(s) used in quiet respiration?
    A. Intercostal muscles
    B. Scalene muscles
    C. Diaphragm
    D. Pectoralis major
    E. Anterior abdominal muscles

21. Which of the following valves is most audible at the right 2nd intercostal space just lateral to the sternum?
    A. Aortic valve
    B. Left atrioventricular valve
    C. Pulmonary valve
    D. Right atrioventricular valve
    E. Valve for the coronary sinus

22. During auscultation of the heart, which of the following relationships is *most* likely to be correct in a normal adult?
    A. The left 4th intercostal space at the midaxillary line is the site
       for ausculation of the mitral valve.
    B. The left 2nd intercostal space at the sternal border is the site
       for ausculation of the aortic valve.
    C. The right 3rd intercostal space at the sternal border is the site
       for ausculation of the pulmonary valve.
    D. The right 2nd intercostal space at the sternal border is the site
       for ausculation of the aortic valve.
    E. The right 4th intercostal space at the midclavicular line is the
       site for ausculation of the tricuspid valve.

23. Which of the following events occurs during either quiet or forced
expiration?
    A. Collapse of alveolar sacs
    B. Increase in lung volume
    C. Elevation of the ribs
    D. Increase in intrapleural pressure
    E. Temporary collapse of the segmental bronchi

24. During a routine physical exam of a young athlete who is training to compete in the Olympic trials, you scrutinize her cardiac
rhythm for abnormalities. Which of the following events normally
occur during ventricular diastole?
    A. Contraction of the ventricles
    B. Ejection of blood into the pulmonary trunk
    C. Opening of the semilunar valves
    D. Filling of the coronary arteries
    E. Closure of the atrrioventricular valves

Answers and Explanations

1. **A** The phrenic nerve is a somatic nerve containing C3–C5 anterior rami (Section 3.2d).
B The anterior rami of C5–T1 form the brachial plexus.
C There are no autonomic nerves that arise from the C3–C5 spinal cord.
D Sympathetic splanchnic nerves that arise from T1–T4 contribute to the cardiac and pulmonary plexuses.
E Cardiac branches from the cervical sympathetic trunk contribute to the cardiac plexus and are not related to the phrenic nerve.

2. **D** Bronchopulmonary segments function independently from other segments and are separated from them by thin septa (Section 6.2a).
A One segmental bronchi enters each bronchopulmonary segment and ramifies into many conducting bronchioles, which in turn divide into many terminal bronchioles.
B The right lung has 10 bronchopulmonary segments, and the left lung has 8 to 10 segments.
C Bronchial arteries supply the bronchi and connective tissue of the lungs, including the visceral pleura. Branches of the pulmonary arteries supply the bronchopulmonary segments.
E Alveoli, the smallest unit of the respiratory tree, have single-celled walls that facilitate gas exchange.

3. **B** The oval fossa on the interatrial septum is the remnant of the opening between the atria that allows right-to-left shunting in the fetal circulation (Section 5.3b).
A Chordae tendineae are found in the ventricles.
C The mitral valve separates the left atrium and ventricle.
D Papillary muscles are found only in the ventricles.
E Trabeculae carneae are muscular ridges in the walls of the ventricles.

4. **E** The sternal angle is a palpable bony prominence created at the junction of the body and manubrium of the sternum. It marks the transverse plane that passes through the 2nd costal cartilage, T4–T5 intervertebral disk, origin of the aortic arch, and bifurcation of the trachea (Section 4.2a).

5. **C** The carina, at the bifurcation of the trachea, lies approximately at the T4–T5 vertebral level, which is also the level of the sternal angle (Section 4.2d).
A The left atrium lies approximately at the level of T6–T7, below the carina at the bifurcation of the trachea.
B The brachiocephalic artery, the first branch of the aortic arch, lies approximately at the level of T3. The carina lies at the level of the sternal angle at T4–T5.
D The tricuspid valve lies at the level of the 5th costal cartilage. The carina lies at the level of the 2nd costal cartilage and the sternal angle.
E Pulmonary veins on both sides lie at the level of the left atrium, approximately at the level of T6–T7, well below the carina at T4–T5.

6. **B** Obstruction of the pulmonary artery impedes blood flow into the lung and causes pooling of blood in the right side of the heart. This causes acute dilation of the right atrium and right ventricle (Section 6.5a).
A Collapse of the lung is a symptom of a pneumothorax in which air enters the pleural cavity.
C The pressure of a tension pneumothorax can cause the heart to shift to the opposite side.
D Hypertrophy of the left ventricle is the result of a chronic condition that causes the myocardium to work harder in response to a fluid overload or an obstruction in the aortic outflow tract. A pulmonary embolism is usually an acute event that causes a fluid overload in the right ventricle but decreases venous return to the left ventricle.
E A pulmonary embolism reduces the volume of blood entering the lung from the right side of the heart and therefore results in a diminished venous return to the left side of the heart. The right atria and ventricle may be acutely dilated, but the left atria and ventricle are not.

7. **D** A malignancy involving the lateral breast would most likely metastasize via the axillary nodes and then on to nodes around the clavicle and the ipsilateral lymphatic duct (Section 4.1c).
A Medial portions of the breast may drain to the parasternal nodes. These nodes also receive lymph from the anterior abdominal wall above the umbilicus, the deeper parts of the anterior portion of the thoracic wall, and the superior surface of the liver.
B Nodes of the anterior abdominal wall receive lymph from the medial and inferior parts of the breast.
C Although some lymph from the breast may drain to deep pectoral nodes posterior to the pectoralis muscle, most lymph from the breast drains to axillary nodes.
E Lymphatic drainage from the medial breast may drain to the contralateral breast, but lymphatic drainage from the lateral breast most abundantly passes to the axillary nodes.

8. **C** A patent ductus arteriosus allows deoxygenated blood from the right side of the heart to mix with oxygenated blood in the descending aorta. This results in delivery of poorly oxygenated blood to peripheral tissues (Section 5.5b).
A A patent ductus arteriosus reduces flow through the pulmonary circulation by diverting blood to the descending aorta.
B Distension of the right atrium can result from fluid overload in the right side of the heart as might occur as a result of left-to-right shunting through a septal defect or stenosis of the pulmonary artery.
D Dilated intercostal arteries and rib notching are characteristics of coarctation of the aorta.
E Left-to-right shunting between the atria occurs as a result of a patent oval foramen.

9. **C** The apex lies at the level of the 5th intercostal space (Section 5.3a).
A The sternal angle is at the level of the 2nd costal cartilages.
B The 3rd intercostal space is above the level of the heart.
D The apex of the heart is found at the most inferior and left border of the heart, which lies to the left of the sternum.
E The xiphoid process lies in the midline, whereas the apex lies to the left side of the sternum.

10. **A** The internal thoracic artery is a branch of the subclavian artery, the third branch of the aortic arch (Section 3.2a).
B The internal thoracic artery arises from the subclavian artery.
C The internal thoracic artery does not arise directly from the aortic arch. It is a branch of the subclavian artery.
D The pericadiacophrenic arteries arise from the internal thoracic arteries to supply the pericardium and diaphragm. They do not contribute to the blood supply of the heart.
E The internal thoracic artery arises from the subclavian artery, not the axillary artery.

11. **B** The AV nodal artery, which branches from the right coronary artery near the origin of the posterior interventricular artery, usually supplies the AV node (Section 5.4a).
A The SA node is supplied by the SA nodal artery, a branch of the proximal part of the right coronary artery, or by the circumflex branch of the left coronary artery.
C The left anterior interventricular artery (LAD) supplies the anterior two-thirds of the interventricular septum.
D The circumflex branch of the left coronary artery supplies the left atrium.
E The marginal branch of the right coronary artery supplies most of the right ventricle. Its origin is well proximal to the crux of the heart and would not be affected by this blockage.

12. **A** The phrenic nerves (C3–C5) are the primary sensory nerves of the pericardium. Referred pain is often felt in the supraclavicular region, the C3–C5 dermatome (Section 5.2a).
B The cardiac plexus is a plexus of autonomic fibers that innervate the heart.
C The pulmonary plexus, an extension of the cardiac plexus, regulates the constriction and dilation of the pulmonary vessels and bronchial passages.
D Intercostal nerves innervate structures of the thoracic and abdominal walls.
E Not applicable

13. **B** The right lymphatic duct drains the lymph from the right side of the thorax, right upper limb, and right side of the head and neck (Section 3.2c).
A Lymph from all structures below the diaphragm drains to the left lymphatic duct (thoracic duct).
C The right side of the head and neck and right upper limb also drain to the right lymphatic duct.
D The right side of the thorax also drains to the right lymphatic duct.
E Lymph from the abdomen and both lower limbs drains to the thoracic duct (left lymphatic duct).

14. **C** The cardiac notch is a deep indentation along the anterior border of the superior lobe of the left lung (Section 6.2c).
A The lingula is a thin tongue of tissue that forms the lower border of the cardiac notch of the superior lobe of the left lung.
B The left lung has only an oblique fissure that separates the superior and inferior lobes.
D The right lung has three lobes supplied by three lobar bronchi.
E The right lung is shorter and wider than the left lung due to the presence of the liver below the right side of the diaphragm.

15. **A** The papillary muscles of the left ventricle attach to the tendinous cords of the mitral valve leaflets and prevent them from prolapsing during ventricular systole (Section 5.3d).
B Trabeculae carneae are the thick muscular ridges of the ventricular walls.
C Pectinate muscles are found in the right and left auricles.
D The terminal crest (crista terminalis) is a muscular ridge within the right atrium that separates its two parts, the venous sinus and the atrium proper.
E The interventricular septomarginal trabecula is a muscular band that connects the septum to the anterior papillary muscle of the right ventricle and carries the right branch of the atrioventricular bundle of the conducting system.

16. **A** The aorta supplies the posterior intercostal arteries (Section 4.4).
B The internal thoracic artery supplies the anterior intercostal arteries.
C The lateral thoracic artery originates from the axillary artery and supplies the pectoralis major and minor, and the serratus anterior muscles and the lateral mammary arteries.
D The subclavian artery supplies the internal thoracic, vertebral, and axillary arteries, as well as branches to the neck and shoulder.
E The superior epigastric artery is a branch of the internal thoracic artery. It supplies the lower anterior intercostal arteries and the anterior abdominal wall.

17. **E** The bronchioles have no cartilage but do contain a layer of smooth muscle that often hypertrophies (cells increase in size) in severe asthma (Section 6.3).
A The trachea contains C-shaped cartilage rings.
B The main bronchi contain C-shaped cartilage rings, similar to those in the trachea.
C Lobar bronchi contain plates of cartilage.
D Segmental bronchi contain plates of cartilage.

18. **B** Closure of tricuspid and mitral (atrioventricular) valves produces the first ("lub") sound (Section 5.3e).
A Closure of the tricuspid valve contributes to the first heart sound ("lub"); closure of the pulmonary valve contributes to the second heart sound ("dub").
C Opening of the semilunar valves does not produce discernible heart sounds.
D Contraction of the ventricles does not produce any sound, although it coincides with the closure of the atrioventricular valves, which produces the first heart sound.
E Turbulent flow through the valves, often associated with valvular stenosis and regurgitation, produces a murmur heard on auscultation.

19. **B** The trachea lies anterior to the esophagus along its entire length and is not in contact with the vertebral bodies (Sections 4.4 and 5.8).
A The azygos vein ascends along the anterior surface of the thoracic vertebrae.
C The sympathetic trunks lie along the lateral aspects of the thoracic vertebrae.
D The thoracic duct ascends along the vertebral bodies between the azygos and hemiazygos veins.
E The posterior intercostal arteries arise from the aorta and cross the vertebral bodies to run within the intercostal spaces on the right side.

20. **C** During quiet respiration the contraction and relaxation of the diaphragm change the volume of the pulmonary cavities and consequently the expansion and contraction of the lungs (Section 6.4).
A The intercostal muscles are used to elevate and lower the ribs during forced inspiration and forced expiration.
B Scalene muscles are extrinsic muscles of respiration that move the ribs during forced inspiration.
D The pectoralis major moves and stabilizes the upper limb but also assists movements of the ribs during deep inspiration.
E Anterior abdominal muscles contract during forced expiration.

21. **A** The aortic valve is most audible at the right 2nd intercostal space just lateral to the sternum (Section 5.3e).
B Sound from the left atrioventricular (AV) valve is most audible over the left 5th intercostal space on the midclavicular line.
C Sound from the pulmonary valve is most audible over the left 2nd intercostal space just lateral to the sternum.
D Sound from the right AV valve is most audible from the right lower aspect of the body of the sternum.
E There is usually no audible sound from the valve of the coronary sinus.

22. **D** The right 2nd intercostal space at the sternal border is the site for auscultation of the aortic valve (Section 5.3e).
A The left 5th intercostal space at the midclavicular line is the site for auscultation of the mitral valve.
B The left 2nd intercostal space at the sternal border is the site for auscultation of the aortic valve.
C The left 2nd intercostal space at the sternal border is the site for auscultation of the pulmonary valve.
E The left 5th intercostal space at the sternal border is the site for auscultation of the tricuspid valve.

23. **D** During expiration, the contraction of the pulmonary cavity causes an increase in intrapleural pressure, which forces air to be expelled from the lung (Section 6.4).
A Surfactant lining the walls of the alveoli prevents them from collapsing during expiration.
B During inspiration the thoracic cavity expands, pulling the pleural sac outward and causing an increase in lung volume.
C The elevation of the ribs increases the size of the thoracic cavity during inspiration.
E Incomplete cartilaginous rings in the walls of the bronchi prevent them from collapsing during expiration.

24. **D** At the beginning of ventricular diastole (relaxation of the ventricles), the semilunar valves close, and backflow in the aorta fills the coronary arteries (Section 5.3g).
A The ventricles contract during ventricular systole.
B Blood from the right ventricle is ejected into the pulmonary trunk during ventricular systole.
C The semilunar valves open during ventricular systole to allow blood to flow into the aorta and pulmonary trunk.
E During the initial phase of ventricular systole, as ventricular pressure increases, the atrioventricular valves close.

7 The Abdominal Wall and Inguinal Region

The abdomen, the region of the trunk between the thorax and the pelvis, contains the largest portion of the **abdominopelvic cavity**, a peritoneal-lined space that it shares with the pelvis. The abdomen houses the primary organs of the gastrointestinal and urinary systems, although some abdominal viscera (i.e., small intestine) typically overflow the boundaries of the abdomen to occupy pelvic spaces, and pelvic viscera, when distended (i.e., bladder and uterus), can extend superiorly into the abdomen (**Fig. 7.1**).

The abdominal wall, composed of skin, fascia, and muscles, is supported by its attachments to the ribs, lumbar vertebrae, and bony pelvis. It moves and stabilizes the trunk, supports the abdominal viscera, and creates intra-abdominal pressure that is crucial in digestion and respiration. The muscular abdominal wall provides little protection for underlying viscera, but much of the upper abdominal viscera lie under the dome of the diaphragm, where they are protected by the thoracic skeleton. The bony pelvis protects most viscera in the lower abdomen.

Fig. 7.1 ► **Peritoneal relationships**
Midsagittal section through male pelvis, viewed from the left side.
Peritoneal cavity. The peritoneum is shown in red.

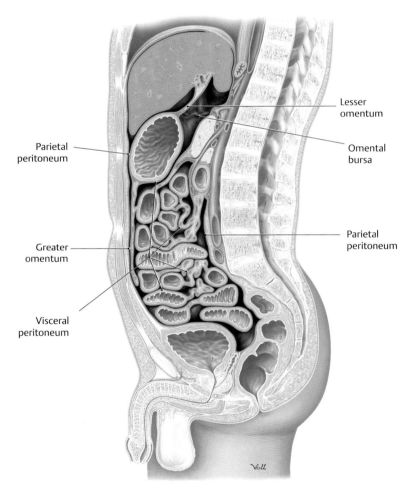

7.1 Regions and Planes of the Abdominal Wall

— In order to describe the location of abdominal viscera, we divide the abdomen into four quadrants or nine regions, using vertical reference lines and standard transverse planes (**Fig. 7.2A** and **B**).

— The **transpyloric plane**, a transverse plane measured halfway between the jugular notch and pubic crest, is a useful horizontal plane that provides orientation to the internal anatomy of the abdomen (**Fig. 7.3**; see also **Fig. 1.4**). The T12–L1 plane passes through (or very close to)

- the pylorus of the stomach,
- the ampulla of the duodenum,
- the celiac trunk,
- the superior mesenteric artery,
- the origin of the portal vein,
- the neck of the pancreas, and
- the left colic flexure of the large intestine.

Fig. 7.3 ▶ **Transpyloric plane (dashed red line) and its relationship to abdominal viscera**
Anterior view. RUQ, right upper quadrant; LUQ, left upper quadrant.

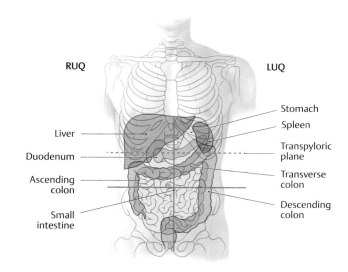

Fig. 7.2 ▶ **Criteria for dividing the abdomen into regions**

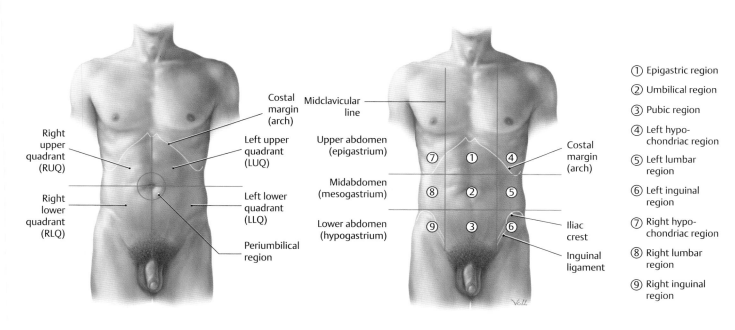

① Epigastric region
② Umbilical region
③ Pubic region
④ Left hypochondriac region
⑤ Left lumbar region
⑥ Left inguinal region
⑦ Right hypochondriac region
⑧ Right lumbar region
⑨ Right inguinal region

A The abdomen is divided into four quadrants by two perpendicular lines that intersect at the umbilicus.

B Coordinate system composed of two vertical and two horizontal lines divide the abdomen into nine regions, each located in either the upper, middle, or lower abdomen. The two vertical lines are the left and right midclavicular lines. One of the two horizontal lines passes through the lowest point of the 10th ribs and the other through the summit of the two iliac crests.

7.2 Structure of the Abdominal Wall

7.1a Superficial Fascial Layer (see **Fig. 7.5C**)

— **The superficial fascia** lies deep to the skin and superficial to the muscular layer. It has two components:

- The **superficial fatty layer (Camper's fascia)**, a subcutaneous layer of fat whose thickness varies among individuals and that is continuous with the superficial fascia of the thorax, back, and lower limb
- The **deep membranous layer (Scarpa's fascia)**, a tough fibrous sheet that lies deep to the superficial fatty layer, covers the lower anterior abdominal wall, and extends inferiorly into the perineum, where it is continuous with the **superficial perineal (Colles') fascia**.

7.1b Muscular Layer (Table 7.1)

— Three flat muscles make up most of the muscular layer of the lateral and anterior walls of the abdomen: the **external oblique**, **internal oblique**, and **transversus abdominis**. Their large aponeuroses constitute the most anterior part of the abdominal wall (**Fig. 7.4A, B,** and **C**).

- The thickened inferior edge of the external oblique aponeurosis forms the **inguinal ligament**, which attaches laterally to the **anterior superior iliac spine** and medially to the **pubic tubercle** of the pubis (see **Fig. 10.8A**). Some fibers of the medial end of the ligament reflect downward as the **lacunar ligament** to attach to the superior edge of the pubis (see **Table 7.2**).
- Inferiorly, the aponeuroses of the internal oblique and transversus abdominis muscles join to form the **conjoined tendon**, where they attach to the pubis.
- In the anterior midline, the aponeuroses of the three muscles overlap with the contralateral muscles, forming the **linea alba**, a tendinous raphe (junction) that extends from the xiphoid process to the pubis. The **umbilical ring**, a remnant of the opening for the umbilical cord, interrupts the raphe at its midpoint.

Fig. 7.4 ► **Muscles of the anterior abdominal wall**
Right side, anterior view.

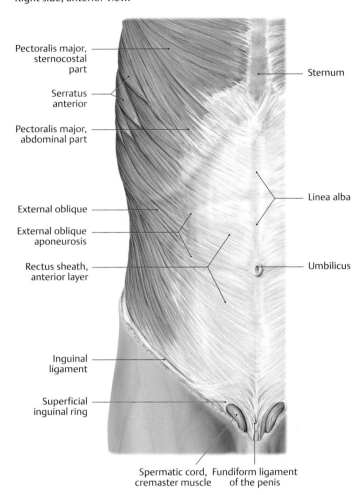

A Superficial abdominal wall muscles.

Table 7.1 ► Muscles of the Anterolateral and Posterior Abdominal Walls				
Muscle	**Origin**	**Insertion**	**Innervation**	**Action**
Anterolateral abdominal wall				
External oblique	5th to 12th ribs (outer surface)	Linea alba, pubic tubercle, anterior iliac crest	Intercostal nn. (T7–T12)	*Unilateral:* bends trunk to same side, rotates trunk to opposite side *Bilateral:* flexes trunk, compresses abdomen, stabilizes pelvis
Internal oblique	Thoracolumbar fascia(deep layer), iliac crest (intermediate line), anterior superior iliac spine, iliopsoas fascia	10th to 12 ribs (lower borders), linea alba (anterior and posterior layers)	Intercostal nn. (T7–T12), iliohypogastric n., ilioinguinal n.	*Unilateral:* bends trunk to same side, rotates trunk to opposite side *Bilateral:* flexes trunk, compresses abdomen, stabilizes pelvis
Transversus abdominis	7th to 12th costal cartilages (inner surfaces), thoracolumbar fascia (deep layer), iliac crest, anterior superior iliac spine (inner lip), iliopsoas fascia	Linea alba, pubic crest	Intercostal nn. (T7–T12), iliohypogastric n., ilioinguinal n.	*Unilateral:* rotates trunk to same side *Bilateral:* compresses abdomen

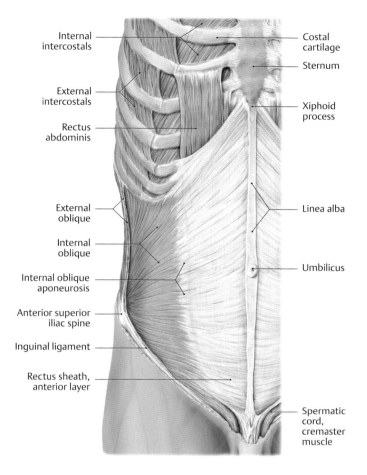

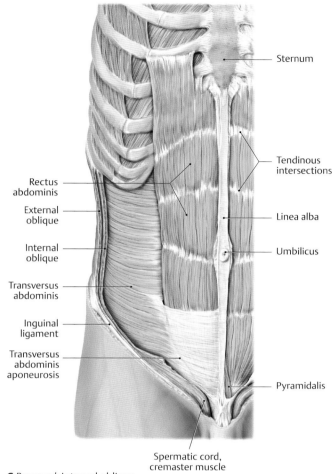

B *Removed:* External oblique, pectoralis major, and serratus anterior.

C *Removed:* Internal oblique.

Table 7.1 ► **Muscles of the Anterolateral and Posterior Abdominal Walls (*Continued*)**				
Muscle	**Origin**	**Insertion**	**Innervation**	**Action**
Rectus abdominis	*Lateral head:* Crest of pubis to pubic tubercle *Medial head:* Anterior region of pubic symphysis	Cartilages of 5th to 7th ribs, xiphoid process of sternum	Intercostal nn. (T5–T12)	Flexes trunk, compresses abdomen, stabilizes pelvis
Pyramidalis	Pubis (anterior to rectus abdominis)	Linea alba (runs within the rectus sheath)	Subcostal n.	Tenses linea alba
Posterior abdominal wall				
Psoas major — Superficial layer	T12-L4 vertebral bodies and associated intervertebral disks (lateral surfaces)	Femur (lesser trochanter), joint insertion with iliopsoas muscle	Lumbar plexus	Hip joint: flexion and external rotation Lumbar spine (with femur fixed): *Unilateral:* contraction bends trunk laterally *Bilateral:* contraction raises trunk from supine position
Psoas major — Deep layer	L1-L5 (costal processes)			
Psoas minor	T12, L1 vertebrae and intervertebral disk (lateral surfaces)	Pecten pubis, iliopubic ramus, iliac fascia; lowermost fibers may reach inguinal ligament	Lumbar plexus	
Iliacus	Iliac fossa		Femoral n.	Hip joint: Flexion and external rotation Lumbar spine (with femur fixed): *Unilateral:* contraction bends trunk laterally *Bilateral:* contraction raises trunk from supine position
Quadratus lumborum	Iliac crest and iliolumbar ligament (not shown)	12th rib, L1–L4 vertebrae (transverse processes)	T12, L1–L4 spinal nn.	*Unilateral:* bends trunk to same side *Bilateral:* bearing down and expiration, stabilizes 12th rib

Fig. 7.5 ► **Anterior abdominal wall and rectus sheath**

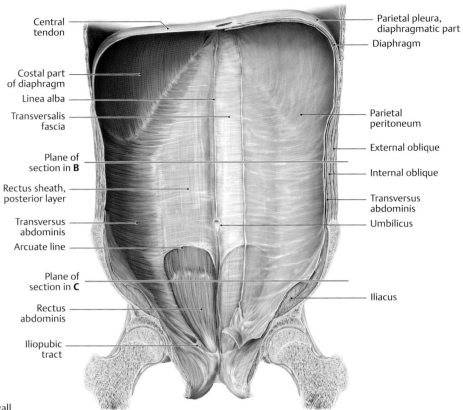

Central tendon

Costal part of diaphragm

Linea alba

Transversalis fascia

Plane of section in **B**

Rectus sheath, posterior layer

Transversus abdominis

Arcuate line

Plane of section in **C**

Rectus abdominis

Iliopubic tract

Parietal pleura, diaphragmatic part

Diaphragm

Parietal peritoneum

External oblique

Internal oblique

Transversus abdominis

Umbilicus

Iliacus

A Posterior (internal) view of anterior abdominal wall.

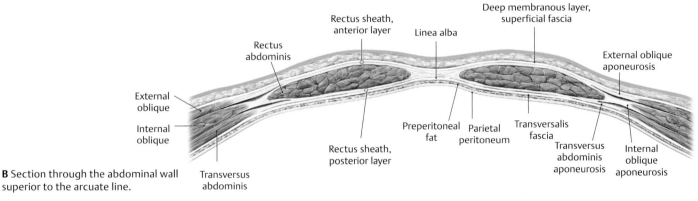

Rectus abdominis

Rectus sheath, anterior layer

Linea alba

Deep membranous layer, superficial fascia

External oblique aponeurosis

External oblique

Internal oblique

Transversus abdominis

Rectus sheath, posterior layer

Preperitoneal fat

Parietal peritoneum

Transversalis fascia

Transversus abdominis aponeurosis

Internal oblique aponeurosis

B Section through the abdominal wall superior to the arcuate line.

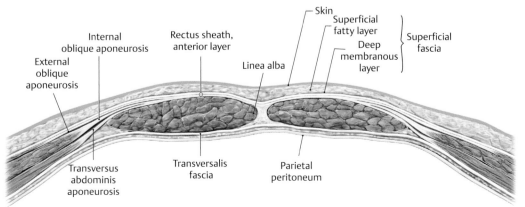

External oblique aponeurosis

Internal oblique aponeurosis

Rectus sheath, anterior layer

Linea alba

Skin

Superficial fatty layer

Deep membranous layer

Superficial fascia

Transversus abdominis aponeurosis

Transversalis fascia

Parietal peritoneum

C Section through the abdominal wall inferior to the arcuate line.

— A **rectus sheath** encloses the **rectus abdominis** and **pyramidalis muscles** on either side of the anterior midline (**Fig. 7.5A, B,** and **C**; see also **Fig. 7.4C**).

- The lateral edges of the sheath are visible externally as the **semilunar lines**.
- The sheath has anterior and posterior layers, formed by the aponeuroses of the anterolateral muscles as they split to pass around the rectus muscles.
- The **arcuate line** is the inferior end of the posterior layer of the rectus sheath. Inferior to this, the aponeuroses only pass anterior to the rectus muscles.

— Five muscles form most of the posterior abdominal wall: the **psoas major**, **psoas minor** (sometimes absent), **quadratus lumborum**, **iliacus**, and diaphragm (**Fig. 7.6**).

- The psoas major and iliacus muscles unite to form the **iliopsoas muscle**, which passes into the thigh and acts on the hip joint.
- The thoracic diaphragm forms part of the superior portion of the posterior abdominal wall.
- The transversus abdominis muscle contributes to the lateral part of the posterior abdominal wall.

— **Endoabdominal fascia** is a deep fascial layer that lines the internal surface of the abdominal wall muscles. It lies superficial to (outside of) the parietal peritoneum and in most places is separated from it by a layer of fat called **preperitoneal fat**.

- Each part of the endoabdominal fascia is named for the muscle it lines: **transversalis fascia** (see **Fig. 7.5B**), **diaphragmatic fascia**, **psoas fascia**.
- In the inguinal region (groin), a thickened line of the transversalis fascia, the **iliopubic tract**, attaches to the inner edge of the inguinal ligament, where it supports the posterior wall of the inguinal canal (see **Fig. 7.5A**).

Fig. 7.6 ▶ **Muscles of the posterior abdominal wall**
Coronal section with the diaphragm in the intermediate position, anterior view.

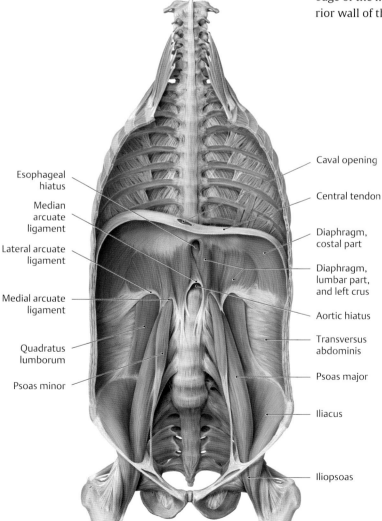

Esophageal hiatus

Median arcuate ligament

Lateral arcuate ligament

Medial arcuate ligament

Quadratus lumborum

Psoas minor

Caval opening

Central tendon

Diaphragm, costal part

Diaphragm, lumbar part, and left crus

Aortic hiatus

Transversus abdominis

Psoas major

Iliacus

Iliopsoas

7.1c Internal Surface of the Anterior Abdominal Wall (Fig. 7.7)

The internal surface of the anterior abdominal wall is lined with transversalis fascia and parietal peritoneum, with a variable amount of intervening preperitoneal fat.

— **Peritoneal folds** form where structures tent the peritoneum as they course between it and the transversalis fascia. The folds include

- the **median umbilical fold**, a single midline fold created by the **median umbilical ligament**, a remnant of the **urachus** (a fetal connection between the bladder and umbilicus);
- the **medial umbilical folds**, paired folds created by the **medial umbilical ligaments**, remnants of the umbilical arteries in the fetus; and
- the **lateral umbilical fold**, paired folds created by the **inferior epigastric vessels**.

— **Peritoneal fossae** are formed between the peritoneal folds and are potential sites of herniation (protrusion of viscera through a wall or tissue). The fossae include

- the **supravesical fossa** between the median and medial umbilical folds;
- the **medial inguinal fossa**, commonly known as the **inguinal triangle of Hesselbach** (Hesselbach's triangle) between the medial and lateral umbilical folds; and
- the **lateral umbilical fossa**, lateral to the lateral umbilical folds.

— The **falciform ligament** is a double-layered peritoneal reflection between the liver and the anterior abdominal wall that extends superiorly from the umbilicus to the roof of the abdominal cavity. It encloses the round ligament (remnant of the umbilical vein) and paraumbilical veins.

Fig. 7.7 ▶ **Internal surface anatomy of the anterior abdominal wall in the male**
Coronal section through the abdominal and pelvic cavity at the level of the hip joints, posterior view.

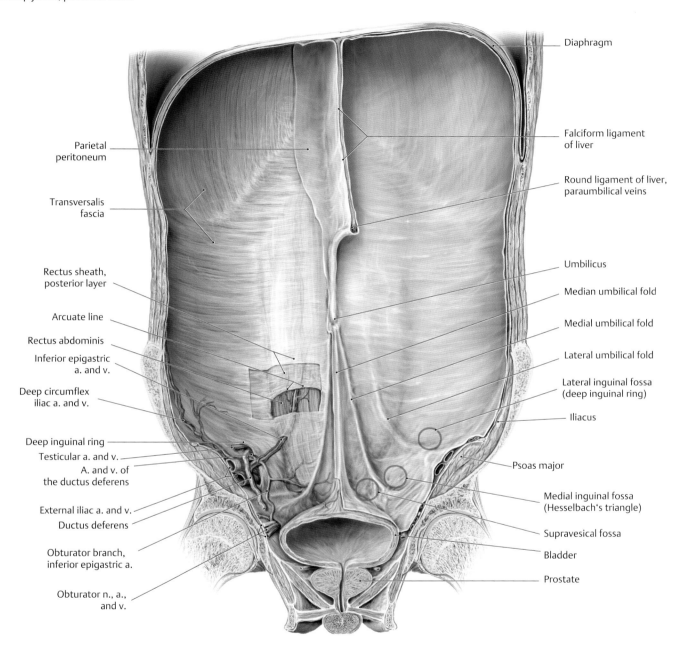

Parietal peritoneum

Transversalis fascia

Rectus sheath, posterior layer

Arcuate line

Rectus abdominis

Inferior epigastric a. and v.

Deep circumflex iliac a. and v.

Deep inguinal ring

Testicular a. and v.

A. and v. of the ductus deferens

External iliac a. and v.

Ductus deferens

Obturator branch, inferior epigastric a.

Obturator n., a., and v.

Diaphragm

Falciform ligament of liver

Round ligament of liver, paraumbilical veins

Umbilicus

Median umbilical fold

Medial umbilical fold

Lateral umbilical fold

Lateral inguinal fossa (deep inguinal ring)

Iliacus

Psoas major

Medial inguinal fossa (Hesselbach's triangle)

Supravesical fossa

Bladder

Prostate

7.2 Neurovasculature of the Abdominal Wall (**Fig. 7.8**)

7.2a Arteries of the Abdominal Wall

Arteries of the abdominal wall, which anastomose extensively with one another, arise from the internal thoracic artery, the abdominal aorta, the external iliac artery, and the femoral artery.

— The branches of each internal thoracic artery are

- the musculophrenic artery and
- the superior epigastric artery, which descends within the rectus sheath posterior to the rectus abdominis muscle, where it anastomoses with the inferior epigastric artery.

— The paired segmental branches of the abdominal aorta are

- the intercostal, subcostal, and lumbar arteries.

— The branches of the external iliac artery are

- the inferior epigastric artery and deep circumflex iliac artery.

— The branches of the femoral artery in the thigh that supply the abdominal wall are

- the **superficial epigastric artery** and
- the **superficial circumflex iliac artery**.

7.2b Veins of the Abdominal Wall

— The deep veins of the abdominal wall accompany the arteries of similar name and drain to the superior and inferior venae cavae via the brachiocephalic, azygos, hemiazygos, and common iliac veins.

— An extensive subcutaneous venous network drains superiorly to the internal thoracic and **lateral thoracic veins** of the thorax and inferiorly to the **inferior** and **superficial epigastric veins**.

— Obstruction of the superior or inferior vena cava may alter the venous flow across the abdominal wall, resulting in the development or enlargement of a superficial anastomosis between the axillary and femoral veins through the thoracoepigastric vein (see Section 4.4).

Fig. 7.8 ▶ **Neurovascular structures of the anterior trunk wall**
Anterior view. *Left side:* superficial dissection. *Right side:* deep dissection. *Removed:* pectoralis major and minor. *Partially removed:* external oblique, internal oblique, transversus abdominis, rectus abdominis, and intercostal muscles.

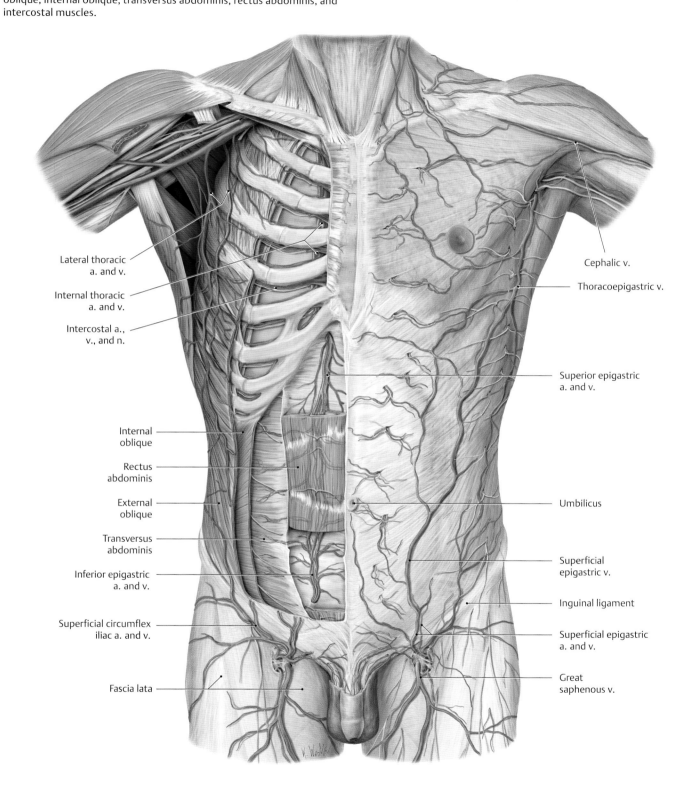

Lateral thoracic a. and v.

Internal thoracic a. and v.

Intercostal a., v., and n.

Internal oblique

Rectus abdominis

External oblique

Transversus abdominis

Inferior epigastric a. and v.

Superficial circumflex iliac a. and v.

Fascia lata

Cephalic v.

Thoracoepigastric v.

Superior epigastric a. and v.

Umbilicus

Superficial epigastric v.

Inguinal ligament

Superficial epigastric a. and v.

Great saphenous v.

7.2c Lymphatic Drainage of the Abdominal Wall

— Lymphatic drainage of the abdominal wall is divided into upper and lower regions by a curved line ("watershed") located between the umbilicus and costal margin (**Fig. 7.9**).

- From the upper region, lymph drains to axillary and parasternal nodes before draining to the right and left jugulo-subclavian junctions (venous angles).
- From the lower region, lymph drains inferiorly to ipsilateral superficial inguinal nodes. These drain to external iliac and common iliac nodes and eventually to the thoracic duct.

7.2d Nerves of the Abdominal Wall

— Nerves of the abdominal wall arise from thoracic and lumbar spinal nerves and include (**Fig. 7.10A and B**)

- the lower intercostal nerves (T7–T11) and the subcostal nerve (T12) of the thorax, and
- the iliohypogastric nerve of the lumbar plexus.

— Dermatomes of the abdominal wall follow the slope of the ribs. Landmark dermatomes that correspond to visible surface features of the abdominal wall include T10 at the umbilicus and L1 at the inguinal ligament and top of the pubis.

7.3 The Inguinal Region

The **inguinal region,** or groin, includes the inferolateral region of the anterior abdominal wall (**Fig. 7.11**).

Fig. 7.9 ▶ **Lymphatic pathways and regional lymph nodes of the anterior trunk wall**
Anterior view. Arrows indicate direction of lymph flow.

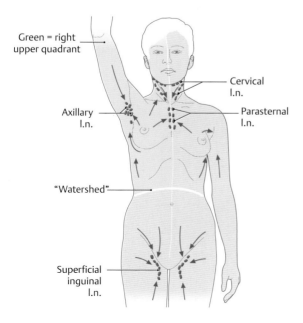

7.3a Inguinal Canal

The inguinal canal is an oblique passage through the abdominal wall that allows structures to pass between the abdominal and pelvic cavities and the perineum. Deficiencies in the anterolateral abdominal muscles, their aponeuroses, and their deep fascia create the inguinal canal (**Table 7.2**).

— The boundaries of the canal are

- the anterior wall, formed by the aponeurosis of the external oblique muscle;
- the posterior wall, formed by transversalis fascia and conjoined tendon;
- the floor, formed by the inguinal ligament; and
- the roof, formed by the arching fibers of the aponeuroses of the internal oblique and transversus abdominis muscles.

Fig. 7.10 ▶ **Cutaneous innervation of the anterior abdominal wall**

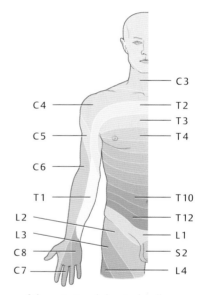

A Sensory nerves of the anterior abdominal wall.

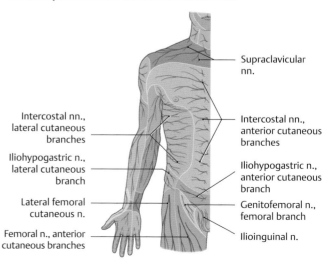

B Dermatomes of the anterior abdominal wall.

Fig. 7.11 ▶ Male inguinal region
Right side, anterior view.

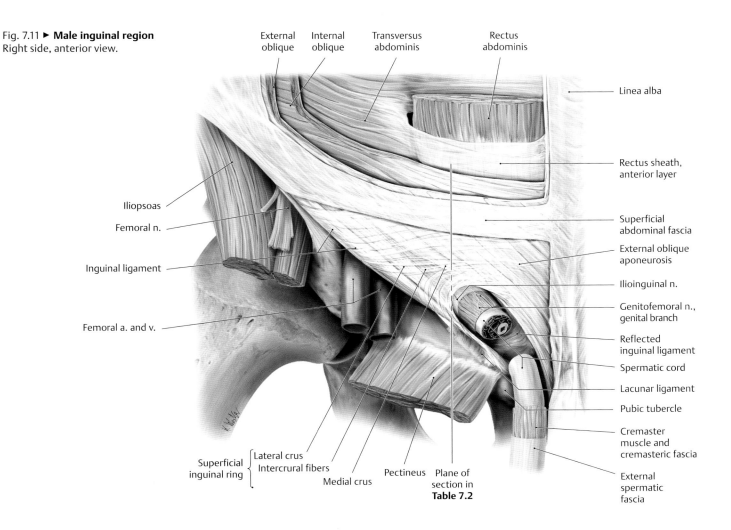

External oblique
Internal oblique
Transversus abdominis
Rectus abdominis
Linea alba
Rectus sheath, anterior layer
Superficial abdominal fascia
External oblique aponeurosis
Ilioinguinal n.
Genitofemoral n., genital branch
Reflected inguinal ligament
Spermatic cord
Lacunar ligament
Pubic tubercle
Cremaster muscle and cremasteric fascia
External spermatic fascia

Iliopsoas
Femoral n.
Inguinal ligament
Femoral a. and v.

Superficial inguinal ring
Lateral crus
Intercrural fibers
Medial crus
Pectineus
Plane of section in **Table 7.2**

Table 7.2 ▶ Structures of the Inguinal Canal		
Structures		**Formed by**
Wall	Anterior wall	① External oblique aponeurosis
	Roof	② Internal oblique muscles
		③ Transversus abdominis
	Posterior wall	④ Transversalis fascia
		⑤ Parietal peritoneum
	Floor	⑥ Inguinal ligament (densely interwoven fibers of the lower external oblique aponeurosis and adjacent fascia lata of thigh)
Openings	Superficial inguinal ring	Opening in external oblique aponeurosis; bounded by medial and lateral crus, intercrural fibers, and reflected inguinal ligament
	Deep inguinal ring	Outpouching of the transversalis fascia lateral to the lateral umbilical fold (inferior epigastric vessels)

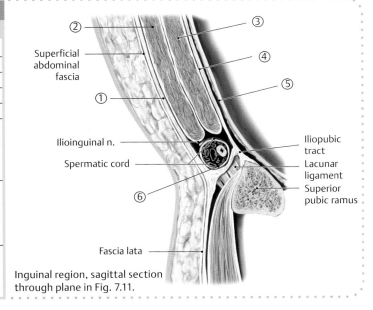

Superficial abdominal fascia
Ilioinguinal n.
Spermatic cord
Iliopubic tract
Lacunar ligament
Superior pubic ramus
Fascia lata

Inguinal region, sagittal section through plane in Fig. 7.11.

Inguinal hernia and hydrocele

Inguinal hernias account for the large majority of abdominal wall hernias, and of those, most occur in males. A hernia is the protrusion of a visceral structure into a space that it doesn't normally occupy. Inguinal hernias involve the protrusion of parietal peritoneum, peritoneal fat, or the small intestine. Of the two types of inguinal hernias, the indirect hernia is the result of a congenital defect and is common in young males, whereas the direct hernia results from a weakening of the abdominal wall and generally occurs in middle-aged males.

During development, a tongue of peritoneum, the processus vaginalis, evaginates into the inguinal canal and accompanies the testis in its descent into the scrotum. Before birth most of the processes obliterate, closing the communication between it and the peritoneal cavity. If the processus vaginalis fails to obliterate, abdominal contents can herniate (indirect hernia) through its opening at the deep inguinal ring (lateral to the inferior epigastric vessels) and extend into the scrotum (or labia in females). Herniated viscera travel within the spermatic cord and are covered by the layers of the cord.

Weakening of the anterior abdominal wall in the inguinal triangle (medial to the inferior epigastric vessels) can allow viscera to protrude through the medial end of the canal and through an enlarged superficial ring (direct hernia). The herniated viscera travel outside the spermatic cord and are covered only by peritoneum and transversalis fascia of the abdominal wall.

The opening into a persistent processus vaginalis may be small enough to prevent herniation but large enough to form a hydrocele, the accumulation of excess peritoneal fluid. The hydrocele can be confined to the scrotum (hydrocele of the testis) or to the cord (hydrocele of the cord). Confirmation is by transillumination of the scrotum, which allows detection of the excess fluid.

— The canal has two openings:

- At the medial end of the canal, fibers of the external oblique aponeurosis split to create an opening known as the **superficial inguinal ring**. This ring lies in the anterior wall of the inguinal triangle of Hesselbach.
- At the lateral end of the inguinal canal, immediately lateral to the origin of the inferior epigastric vessels, the transversalis

fascia evaginates into the canal and creates the **deep inguinal ring**. This ring lies in the lateral inguinal fossa (see **Fig. 7.7**).

— The contents of the inguinal canal include the **spermatic cord** in males and the **round ligament** of the uterus in females (**Fig. 7.12**; also see Section 11.2c).

7.3b The Spermatic Cord

The spermatic cord forms at the deep inguinal ring, traverses the inguinal canal, and exits through the superficial inguinal ring. It enters the scrotum and descends to the posterior surface of the testis (**Fig. 7.13**).

— The structures in the spermatic cord include

- the ductus deferens;
- the testicular artery and pampiniform plexus of veins, the artery of the ductus deferens, and the cremasteric artery;
- lymphatic vessels of the testis and spermatic cord; and
- sympathetic and parasympathetic fibers of the testicular plexus and the genital branch of the genitofemoral nerve.

— Derivatives of the muscles and fascia of the abdominal wall surround the contents of the spermatic cord as they pass through the inguinal canal. The layers formed by the muscles and fascia are the same as those surrounding the testis (**Table 7.3**):

- **Internal spermatic fascia** derived from the transversalis fascia
- **Cremaster muscle** and **cremasteric fascia** derived from the internal oblique muscle and fascia
- **External spermatic fascia** derived from the external oblique aponeurosis and fascia

Fig. 7.12 ► **Female inguinal region**
Right side, anterior view.

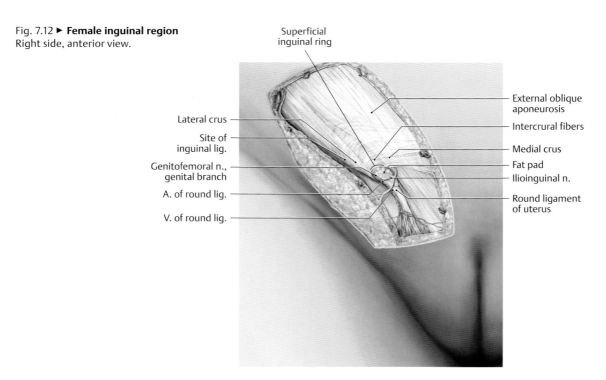

Superficial inguinal ring

Lateral crus

Site of inguinal lig.

Genitofemoral n., genital branch

A. of round lig.

V. of round lig.

External oblique aponeurosis

Intercrural fibers

Medial crus

Fat pad

Ilioinguinal n.

Round ligament of uterus

Fig. 7.13 ▶ Spermatic cord
Male pelvis, anterior view. *Opened:* Inguinal canal and coverings of the spermatic cord.

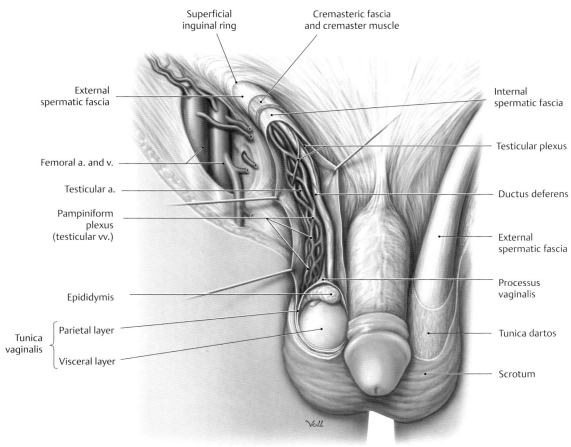

Superficial inguinal ring

Cremasteric fascia and cremaster muscle

External spermatic fascia

Internal spermatic fascia

Testicular plexus

Femoral a. and v.

Testicular a.

Ductus deferens

Pampiniform plexus (testicular vv.)

External spermatic fascia

Processus vaginalis

Epididymis

Tunica dartos

Tunica vaginalis { Parietal layer
Visceral layer

Scrotum

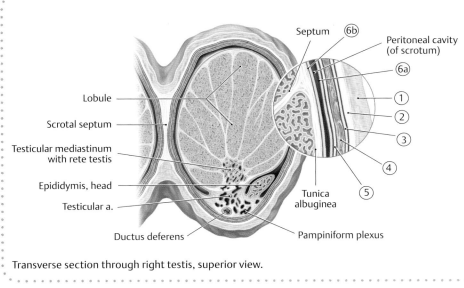

Septum

Peritoneal cavity (of scrotum)

6b

6a

Lobule

Scrotal septum

Testicular mediastinum with rete testis

Epididymis, head

Testicular a.

Tunica albuginea

1
2
3
4
5

Ductus deferens

Pampiniform plexus

Transverse section through right testis, superior view.

Table 7.3 ▶ Coverings of the Testis	
Covering of the Testis	**Abdominal Wall Derivative**
① Scrotal skin	Abdominal skin
② Tunica dartos	Dartos fascia and muscle
③ External spermatic fascia	External oblique fascia
④ Cremaster muscle and cremasteric fascia*	Internal oblique muscle and fascia
⑤ Internal spermatic fascia	Transversalis fascia
⑥a Tunica vaginalis, parietal layer	Peritoneum
⑥b Tunica vaginalis, visceral layer	

* The transversus abdominis has no contribution to the spermatic cord or covering of the testis.

7.3c   The Testes

The testes are paired ovoid reproductive organs, 4 to 5 cm long and 3 cm wide, located in separate compartments within the scrotum. They produce spermatozoa and secrete the male hormone testosterone (**Fig. 7.14A** and **B**; see also **Table 7.3**).

— An extension of the peritoneum known as the **tunica vaginalis** forms a closed sac that folds around the testis, surrounding it on all sides except on its posterior edge. The tunic has an outer parietal layer and an inner visceral layer that is adherent to the surface of the testis.

— Each testis is enveloped by the **tunica albuginea**, a tough capsule of connective tissue that thickens along the posterior border as the mediastinum of the testis and invaginates to divide the testis into over 200 lobules.

— Sperm are produced in the **seminiferous tubules**, highly coiled tubules within the lobules. They exit the testes through a ductal network, the **rete testis** in the mediastinum, and then pass through **efferent ductules** to the **epididymis**.

— The testicular artery, a branch of the abdominal aorta, supplies the testis. A rich collateral blood supply arises from anastomoses with the artery of the ductus deferens, the **cremasteric artery**, a branch of the inferior epigastric artery, and the **external pudendal artery** from the femoral artery (**Fig. 7.15**).

— The **pampiniform plexus** of veins drains the testis and converges to form the testicular vein. The testicular veins drain to the inferior vena cava on the right and to the renal vein on the left.

Fig. 7.14 ▶ **Testis and epididymis**
Left lateral view.

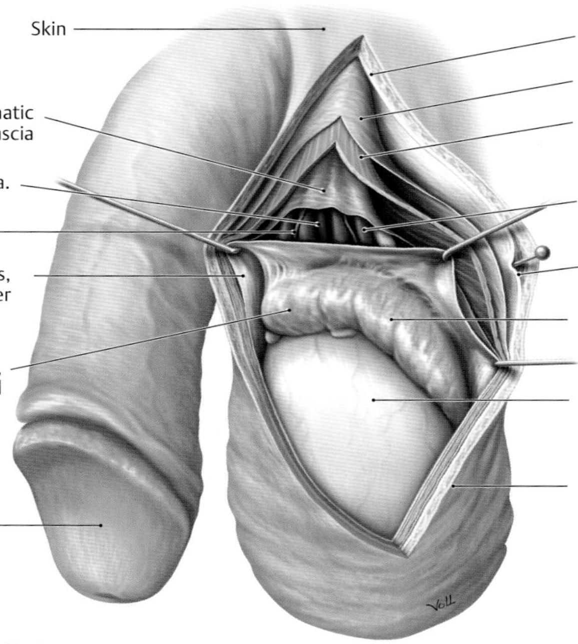

A Testis and epididymis in situ.

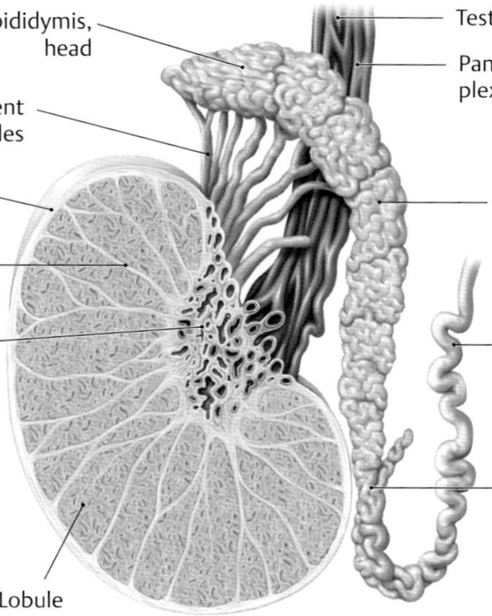

B Sagittal section.

Fig. 7.15 ▶ **Blood vessels of the testis**
Left lateral view.

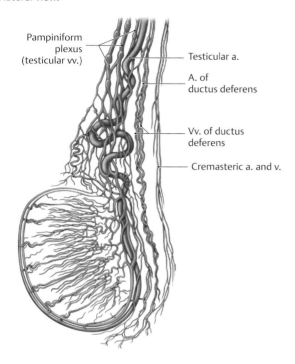

Pampiniform
plexus
(testicular vv.)

Testicular a.

A. of
ductus deferens

Vv. of ductus
deferens

Cremasteric a. and v.

Varicocele

The pampiniform plexus from each testis surrounds the testicular artery and converges to form a testicular vein. When the venous valves become incompetent, the plexus can become dilated and tortuous, forming a varicocele that is often reported to feel like "a bag of worms." Varicoceles are predominantly on the left side. This is generally attributed to the abrupt termination of the left testicular vein at the left renal vein, which may slow venous return.

— The lymph vessels of the testes drain directly to lateral aortic and preaortic lymph nodes.
— The **cremasteric reflex**, initiated by stroking of the inner thigh, contracts the cremaster muscle and elevates the testis. The ilioinguinal nerve provides the sensory limb; the genital branch of the genitofemoral nerve provides the motor limb.

Absent or reduced cremasteric reflex

An absent or reduced cremasteric reflex that is accompanied by sudden testicular pain, inflammation and elevation of one testis, nausea, and vomiting may indicate testicular torsion (twisting of a testis). Prompt surgery for testicular torsion (to untwist the affected testis and anchor both testes) may prevent loss of a testis.

— The testicular nerve plexus arises from the aortic plexus and travels along with the testicular artery. It contains sympathetic fibers from the T7 spinal cord level, as well as visceral afferent and vagal parasympathetic fibers.

Testicular cancer

Testicular cancer is the most common cancer in males between 15 and 34 years of age. The vast majority of these cancers are seminomas or germ cell tumors that arise in the germ cells that produce immature sperm. Symptoms include a lump in the affected testis (usually only one testis is affected), a feeling of heaviness in the scrotum, pain in the affected testis or scrotum, a sudden collection of fluid in the scrotum, and the development of excess breast tissue (gynecomastia). Testicular cancer commonly metastasizes via lymph nodes to the lungs or via the bloodstream, commonly to the liver, lungs, brain, and spine.

7.3d The Epididymis and Ductus Deferens

The epididymis and ductus deferens are parts of the male ductal system that transport sperm from the testis to the genital structures in the pelvis (see **Fig. 7.14A** and **B**).

— The epididymis, a highly coiled tubule where sperm are stored and mature, hugs the posterior surface of the testis. Its expanded head contains the lobules with the efferent ductules, its body is made up of a long convoluted duct, and its tail is continuous with the ductus deferens.
— The **ductus deferens** is a muscular tube that transmits sperm from the scrotum to the pelvis.
   • It begins at the tail of the epididymis and continues as part of the spermatic cord through the inguinal canal.
   • At the deep inguinal ring, the ductus deferens descends into the pelvis posterior to the bladder, where, near its termination, it enlarges as the **ampulla of the ductus deferens** (see **Fig. 11.2**).
   • The ampulla joins with the duct of the seminal gland (vesicle) to form the ejaculatory duct (see Section 11.1a).

8 The Peritoneal Cavity and Neurovasculature of the Abdomen

8.1 The Peritoneum and Peritoneal Cavity

The **peritoneum**, a thin, transparent serous membrane, lines the abdominopelvic cavity. Parietal and visceral layers of the peritoneum enclose the **peritoneal cavity**, which contains a thin film of serous fluid that facilitates the movement of the viscera during digestion and respiration (see **Fig. 7.1**).

8.1a Peritoneal Relations

— Structures in the abdomen are defined with respect to their relationship to the peritoneum (**Table 8.1**; **Figs. 8.1** and **8.2**).

- **Intraperitoneal** organs, almost completely enclosed by the visceral layer of the peritoneum, are suspended within the peritoneal cavity by **mesenteries**, double layers of peritoneum that attach to the body wall.

- **Extraperitoneal** structures lie posterior or inferior to the peritoneal cavity.

  o **Primarily retroperitoneal** structures lie posterior to the peritoneal cavity, are not suspended by a mesentery, and are usually covered by peritoneum only on their anterior surface.

  o **Secondarily retroperitoneal** structures were previously intraperitoneal structures that became fixed to the posterior abdominal wall when their mesentery fused with the parietal peritoneum of the posterior abdominal wall during development.

  o **Subperitoneal structures** include pelvic organs that lie below the peritoneum.

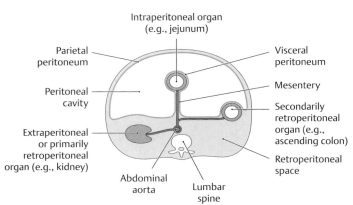

Fig. 8.2 ▶ **Peritoneal relations of the organs in the abdomen**
Transverse section through the abdomen showing the peritoneal relationships of abdominal organs. Viewed from above.

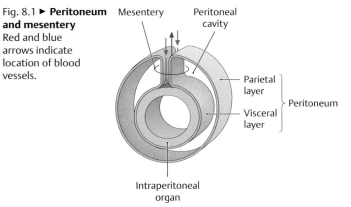

Fig. 8.1 ▶ **Peritoneum and mesentery**
Red and blue arrows indicate location of blood vessels.

Table 8.1 ▶ Organs of the Abdomen	
Location	**Organs**
Intraperitoneal organs: These organs have a mesentery and are completely covered by the peritoneum.	
Abdominal peritoneal cavity	• Stomach • Small intestine (jejunum, ileum, some of the superior part of the duodenum) • Spleen • Liver (with the exception of the bare area) • Gallbladder • Cecum with vermiform appendix (portions of variable size may be retroperitoneal) • Large intestine (transverse and sigmoid colons)
Extraperitoneal organs: These organs either have no mesentery or lost it during development.	
Retroperitoneum — Primarily retroperitoneal	• Kidneys • Suprarenal glands
Retroperitoneum — Secondarily retroperitoneal	• Duodenum (descending, horizontal, and ascending) • Pancreas • Ascending and descending colon

— Organs associated with the gastrointestinal tract are intraperitoneal or secondarily retroperitoneal. Organs of the urinary system are retroperitoneal.

8.1b Peritoneal Structures

Most of the abdominal viscera are somewhat mobile during digestion and respiration. Reflections of the peritoneum that connect organs to the body wall or to other organs prevent excessive movement (i.e., twisting), which can compromise normal function. These reflections form mesenteries, omenta, and peritoneal ligaments.

— A **mesentery** is a double layer of peritoneum that connects intraperitoneal organs to the posterior abdominal wall and transmits vessels and nerves (see **Fig. 8.1**). There are three major mesenteries in the abdomen (**Fig. 8.3**):

- The **mesentery of the small intestine**, or the "mesentery," is a fan-shaped apron of peritoneum that suspends the second and third parts (jejunum and ileum) of the small intestine.
- The **transverse mesocolon** suspends the transverse section of the large intestine.
- The **sigmoid mesocolon** suspends the sigmoid colon of the large intestine in the left lower quadrant.

Fig. 8.3 ▶ **Mesenteries of the peritoneal cavity**
Anterior view. *Reflected:* Greater omentum and transverse colon. *Removed:* Intraperitoneal small intestine.

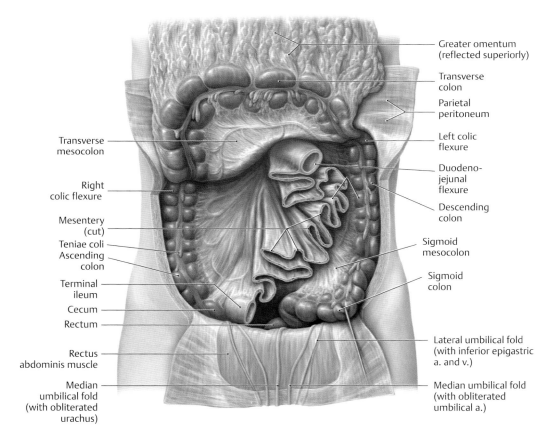

— An **omentum** is a double layer of peritoneum that connects the stomach and duodenum to another organ. There are two omenta (**Figs. 8.4** and **8.5**; see also **Fig. 9.1**):

• The **greater omentum**, a four-layered apron of peritoneum, originates as a double layer of peritoneum from the greater curvature of the stomach and proximal duodenum. It drapes inferiorly, anterior to the coils of small intestine, before looping upward to its distal attachment on the posterior abdominal wall.

   ◦ The **gastrocolic ligament** is a portion of the greater omentum that adheres to the transverse colon (**Fig. 8.6**).

Fig. 8.4 ► **Greater and lesser omenta**
Anterior view of the opened upper abdomen. Arrow indicates the omental foramen.

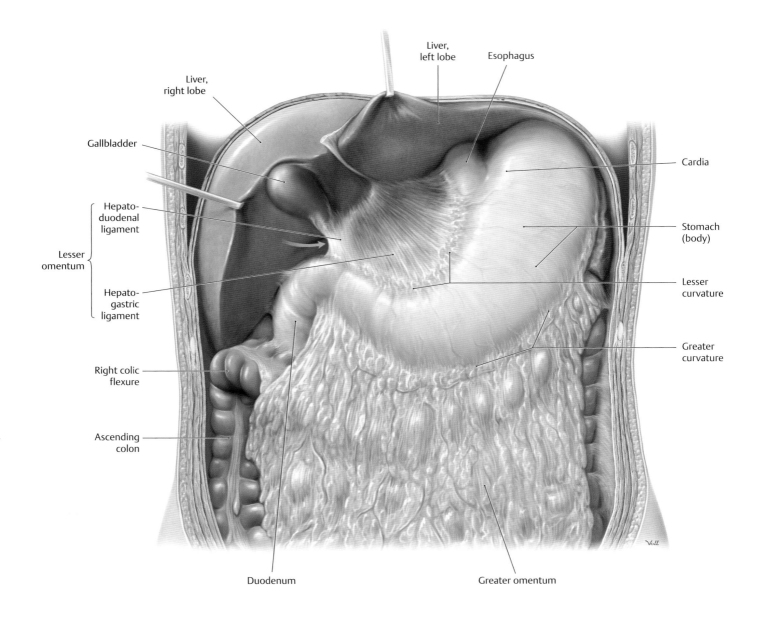

Fig. 8.5 ► **Peritoneal structures**

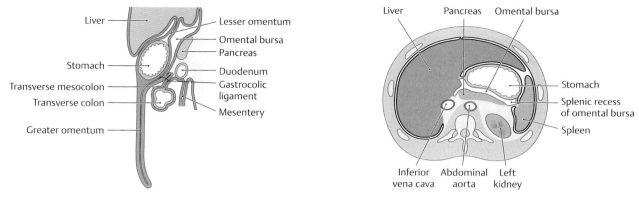

Liver
Lesser omentum
Omental bursa
Pancreas
Stomach
Duodenum
Transverse mesocolon
Gastrocolic ligament
Transverse colon
Mesentery
Greater omentum

A Sagittal section.

Liver
Pancreas
Omental bursa
Stomach
Splenic recess of omental bursa
Spleen
Inferior vena cava
Abdominal aorta
Left kidney

B Transverse section, interior view.

Fig. 8.6 ► **Omental bursa in situ**

Anterior view. *Divided:* Gastrocolic ligament. *Retracted:* Liver. *Reflected:* Stomach.

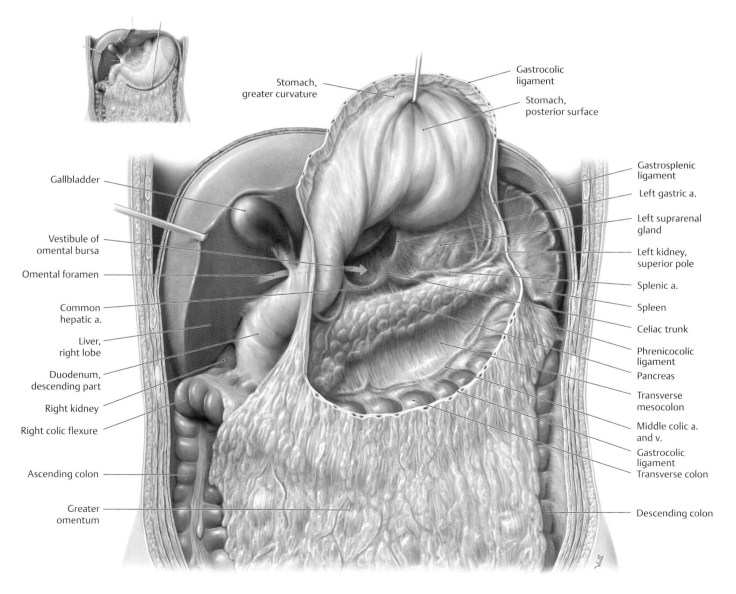

Stomach, greater curvature
Gastrocolic ligament
Stomach, posterior surface
Gallbladder
Gastrosplenic ligament
Left gastric a.
Left suprarenal gland
Vestibule of omental bursa
Left kidney, superior pole
Omental foramen
Splenic a.
Common hepatic a.
Spleen
Celiac trunk
Liver, right lobe
Phrenicocolic ligament
Duodenum, descending part
Pancreas
Right kidney
Transverse mesocolon
Right colic flexure
Middle colic a. and v.
Gastrocolic ligament
Ascending colon
Transverse colon
Greater omentum
Descending colon

∘ The **gastrosplenic ligament** is a lateral extension of the greater omentum that connects the stomach to the spleen and is traversed by branches of the splenic artery (**Fig. 8.7**).

- The **lesser omentum**, a double layer of peritoneum, extends from the liver to the stomach and proximal duodenum. It is formed by
  ∘ the **hepatogastric ligament**, between the liver and stomach, and
  ∘ the **hepatoduodenal ligament**, between the liver and duodenum, which encloses the structures of the **portal triad** (the portal vein, hepatic artery, and **bile duct**) in its free edge.

Fig. 8.7 ▶ **Posterior wall of the peritoneal cavity**
Anterior view. *Removed:* All intraperitoneal organs.

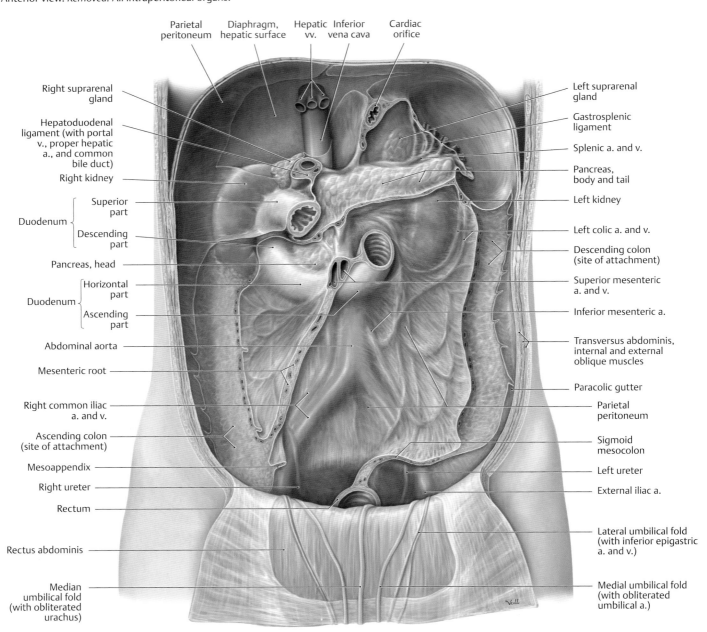

124

— **Peritoneal ligaments** are reflections of peritoneum that connect organs to each other or to the body wall. They support the organ in position and may convey their neurovasculature. Individual ligaments are discussed in Sections 9.2 to 9.4 with the specific abdominal organs.

8.1c Neurovasculature of the Peritoneum

The **neurovasculature** for the **parietal and visceral peritoneum** is derived from different sources.

— Parietal peritoneum derives its neurovasculature from vessels and nerves of the body wall. Its sensitivity to pain, pressure, and temperature is well localized (felt acutely) through somatic nerves of the overlying muscles and skin.
— Visceral peritoneum derives its neurovasculature from the underlying organs. Autonomic nerves mediate sensitivity to stretching and chemical irritation, but the visceral peritoneum lacks sensitivity to touch and temperature.
— Sensation is poorly localized and is usually referred to regions that reflect the embryological origins of the underlying organ.

  • Sensation from foregut structures is referred to the epigastric region.
  • Sensation from midgut structures is referred to the umbilical region.
  • Sensation from hindgut structures is referred to the pubic region.

8.1d Subdivisions of the Peritoneal Cavity

— The peritoneal cavity is divided into two spaces:

  • The **greater sac**, which includes the entire peritoneal cavity except that space defined as the lesser sac
  • The **omental bursa (lesser sac)**, which is a small extension of the peritoneal cavity that lies behind the stomach and lesser omentum (**Table 8.2**; see also **Figs. 8.5** and **8.6**). It communicates with the greater sac through a single opening, the **omental (epiploic) foramen** (**Table 8.3**).

— Attachments of the peritoneum to the body wall that form during development of the gastrointestinal tract further subdivide the greater sac. These attachments can influence the flow of fluid within the cavity (**Figs. 8.8** and **8.9**).

  • The **subphrenic recess** between the diaphragm and liver is limited by the coronary ligaments and separated into right and left spaces by the falciform ligament.
  • The **subhepatic space** lies between the liver and the transverse colon. A posterior extension of this space, the **hepatorenal recess** (hepatorenal pouch, Morison's pouch), lies between the visceral surface of the liver and the right kidney and suprarenal gland. The hepatorenal recess communicates with the right subphrenic recess.
  • The **supracolic** and **infracolic compartments** are defined by the attachment of the transverse mesocolon on the posterior abdominal wall—with the supracolic compartment above the attachment site and the infracolic compartment below it. The root of the mesentery of the small intestine further divides the infracolic compartment into right and left spaces.
  • The **paracolic gutters**, which lie adjacent to the ascending and descending colons, allow communication between the supracolic and infracolic compartments.

Fig. 8.8 ▶ **Drainage spaces within the peritoneal cavity**
Anterior view.

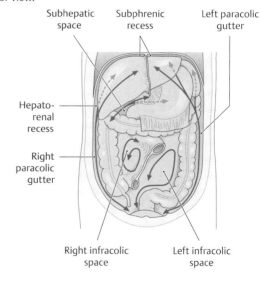

Subhepatic space   Subphrenic recess   Left paracolic gutter

Hepato-renal recess

Right paracolic gutter

Right infracolic space   Left infracolic space

Table 8.2 ▶ Boundaries of the Omental Bursa (Lesser Sac)		
Direction	**Boundary**	**Recess**
Anterior	Lesser omentum, gastrocolic ligament	—
Inferior	Transverse mesocolon	Inferior recess
Superior	Liver (with caudate lobe)	Superior recess
Posterior	Pancreas, aorta (abdominal part), celiac trunk, splenic a. and v., gastrosplenic fold, left suprarenal gland, left kidney (superior pole)	—
Right	Liver, duodenal bulb	—
Left	Spleen, gastrosplenic ligament	Splenic recess

Table 8.3 ▶ Boundaries of the Omental Foramen	
The communication between the greater and lesser sacs is the omental (epiploic) foramen (see arrow in **Figs. 8.4** and **8.6**).	
Direction	**Boundary**
Anterior	Hepatoduodenal ligament with the portal v., proper hepatic a., and bile duct
Inferior	Duodenum (superior part)
Posterior	Inferior vena cava, diaphragm (right crus)
Superior	Liver (caudate lobe)

Peritonitis and ascites

Bacterial contamination of the peritoneum following surgery or rupture of an inflamed organ (duodenum, gallbladder, appendix) results in peritonitis, inflammation of the peritoneum. It is accompanied by severe abdominal pain, tenderness, nausea, and fever and can be fatal when generalized throughout the peritoneal cavity. It often results in ascites, the accumulation of excess peritoneal fluid due to a change in concentration gradients that results in loss of capillary fluid. Ascites can also accompany other pathological conditions, such as metastatic liver cancer and portal hypertension. In these cases, many liters of acitic fluid can accumulate in the peritoneal cavity. The fluid is aspirated by paracentesis. The needle is carefully inserted into the abdominal wall so as to avoid the urinary bladder and inferior epigastric vessels.

Peritoneal infections and abscesses

The flow of fluid in the peritoneal cavity can spread intraperitoneal infections and determine the sites of peritoneal abscess formation. Fluid commonly collects in the right and left subphrenic recesses, although abscesses are more likely to form on the right side due to duodenal or appendyceal ruptures. Fluid in the supracolic compartment, such as subphrenic recesses and the omental bursa, can drain to the hepatorenal recess, the lowest part of the abdominal cavity in the supine patient. Therefore, this is a common site of pus accumulation and abscess formation. In the infracolic compartment, the paracolic gutters direct peritoneal fluid and infections toward the pelvis.

8.2 Neurovasculature of the Abdomen

8.2a Arteries of the Abdomen (Fig. 8.9)

— The **abdominal aorta** supplies abdominal viscera and most of the anterior abdominal wall.
  - It enters the abdomen at T12 through the aortic hiatus of the diaphragm and descends along the vertebral column to the left of the midline.
  - It terminates at the L4 vertebral level, where it bifurcates into two **common iliac arteries**.
  - A single **median sacral artery** arises near the bifurcation.

Abdominal aortic aneurysm

Abdominal aortic aneurysms (AAAs) most commonly occur between the renal arteries and the bifurcation of the aorta. When small they can remain asymptomatic, but large aneurysms can be palpated through the abdominal wall to the left of the midline. Ruptured AAAs present with severe abdominal pain that radiates to the abdomen or back. Mortality rates for ruptured aneurysms approach 90% due to overwhelming hemorrhage.

— **Table 8.4** lists major branches of the abdominal aorta.
  - Paired parietal (segmental) branches supply the structures of the posterior abdominal wall. These include the **inferior phrenic** and **lumbar arteries**.
  - Paired visceral branches supply organs of the retroperitoneum. These are the middle **suprarenal, testicular** or **ovarian**, and **renal arteries**.

Table 8.4 ▶ **Branches of the Abdominal Aorta**			
The abdominal aorta gives rise to three major unpaired trunks (bold) and the unpaired median sacral artery, as well as six paired branches.			
Branch from abdominal aorta	**Branches**		
Inferior phrenic aa. (paired)	Superior suprarenal aa.		
Celiac trunk	Left gastric a.		
	Splenic a.		
	Common hepatic a.	Proper hepatic a.	
		Right gastric a.	
		Gastroduodenal a.	
Middle suprarenal aa. (paired)			
Superior mesenteric a.			
Renal aa. (paired)	Inferior suprarenal aa.		
Lumbar aa. (1st through 4th, paired)			
Testicular/ovarian aa. (paired)			
Inferior mesenteric a.			
Common iliac aa. (paired)	External iliac a.		
	Internal iliac a.		
Median sacral a.			

Fig. 8.9 ► **Abdominal aorta**

Female abdomen, anterior view. *Removed:* Abdominal organs and peritoneum. The abdominal aorta is the distal continuation of the thoracic aorta. It enters the abdomen at the T12 level and bifurcates into the common iliac arteries at L4.

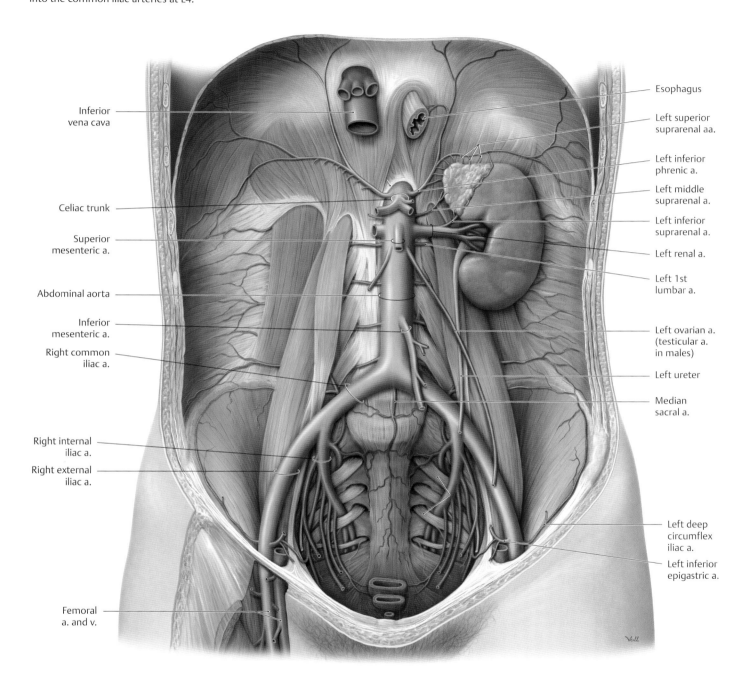

Inferior vena cava

Celiac trunk

Superior mesenteric a.

Abdominal aorta

Inferior mesenteric a.

Right common iliac a.

Right internal iliac a.

Right external iliac a.

Femoral a. and v.

Esophagus

Left superior suprarenal aa.

Left inferior phrenic a.

Left middle suprarenal a.

Left inferior suprarenal a.

Left renal a.

Left 1st lumbar a.

Left ovarian a. (testicular a. in males)

Left ureter

Median sacral a.

Left deep circumflex iliac a.

Left inferior epigastric a.

- Three unpaired visceral branches supply the intestines and accessory organs of the gastrointestinal tract:

    1. The **celiac trunk**, a short trunk that arises at T12/L1 and supplies the abdominal foregut. Its branches, the **splenic**, **left gastric**, and **common hepatic arteries**, anastomose extensively with each other (**Figs. 8.10** and **8.11**).

Fig. 8.10 ▶ **Celiac trunk: Stomach, liver, and gallbladder**
Anterior view. *Opened:* Lesser omentum. *Incised:* Greater omentum. The celiac trunk arises from the abdominal aorta at about the level of L1.

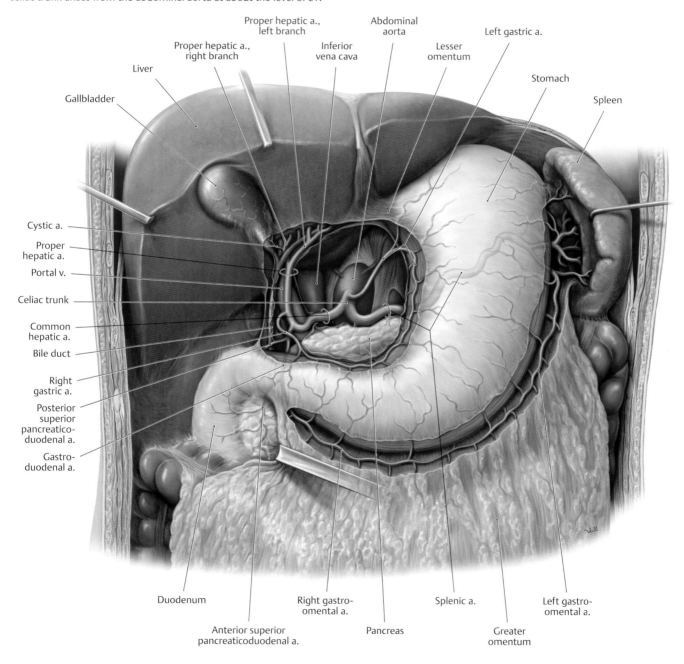

Fig. 8.11 ▸ **Celiac trunk: Pancreas, duodenum, and spleen**
Anterior view. *Removed:* Stomach (body) and lesser omentum.

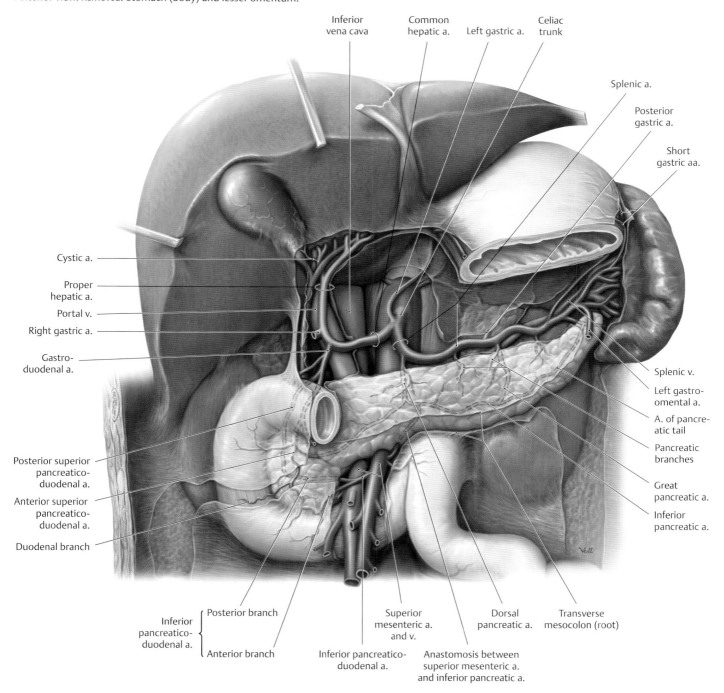

Inferior
vena cava

Common
hepatic a.

Left gastric a.

Celiac
trunk

Splenic a.

Posterior
gastric a.

Short
gastric aa.

Cystic a.

Proper
hepatic a.

Portal v.

Right gastric a.

Gastro-
duodenal a.

Splenic v.

Left gastro-
omental a.

A. of pancre-
atic tail

Pancreatic
branches

Great
pancreatic a.

Inferior
pancreatic a.

Posterior superior
pancreatico-
duodenal a.

Anterior superior
pancreatico-
duodenal a.

Duodenal branch

Inferior
pancreatico-
duodenal a.

Posterior branch

Anterior branch

Superior
mesenteric a.
and v.

Inferior pancreatico-
duodenal a.

Dorsal
pancreatic a.

Anastomosis between
superior mesenteric a.
and inferior pancreatic a.

Transverse
mesocolon (root)

2. The **superior mesenteric artery** (SMA), which arises at L1, posterior to the neck of the pancreas. It supplies mid-gut structures, and its major branches include the **inferior pancreaticoduodenal**, **middle colic**, **right colic**, and **ileocolic arteries**, as well as a series of **jejunal** and **ileal branches** (**Fig. 8.12**).

Fig. 8.12 ▶ **Superior mesenteric artery**
Anterior view. *Partially removed:* Stomach and peritoneum. *Note:* The middle colic artery has been truncated. The superior mesenteric artery arises from the aorta opposite L2.

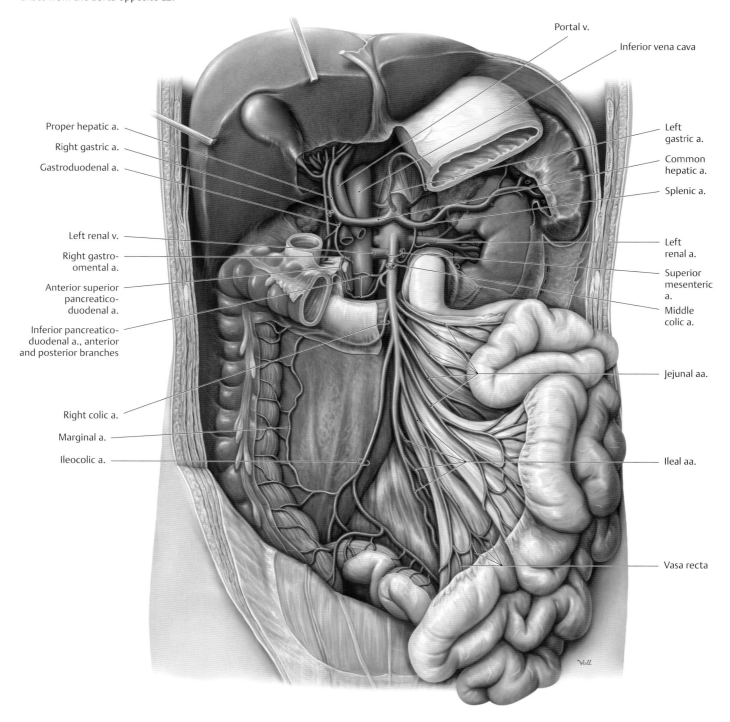

3. The **inferior mesenteric artery** (IMA), which arises at L3 and has the smallest caliber of the three visceral trunks. It supplies the hindgut through its **left colic**, **sigmoidal**, and **superior rectal** branches (**Fig. 8.13**).

- Common iliac arteries pass along the brim of the pelvis and terminate by bifurcating into two major branches (see **Fig. 8.9**):
  - The **internal iliac artery**, which descends into the pelvis
  - The **external iliac artery**, which gives off the **inferior epigastric** and **deep circumflex iliac arteries** before passing into the lower limb as the **femoral artery**.

Fig. 8.13 ▶ **Inferior mesenteric artery**
Anterior view. *Removed:* Jejunum and ileum. *Reflected:* Transverse colon. The inferior mesenteric artery arises from the aorta opposite L3.

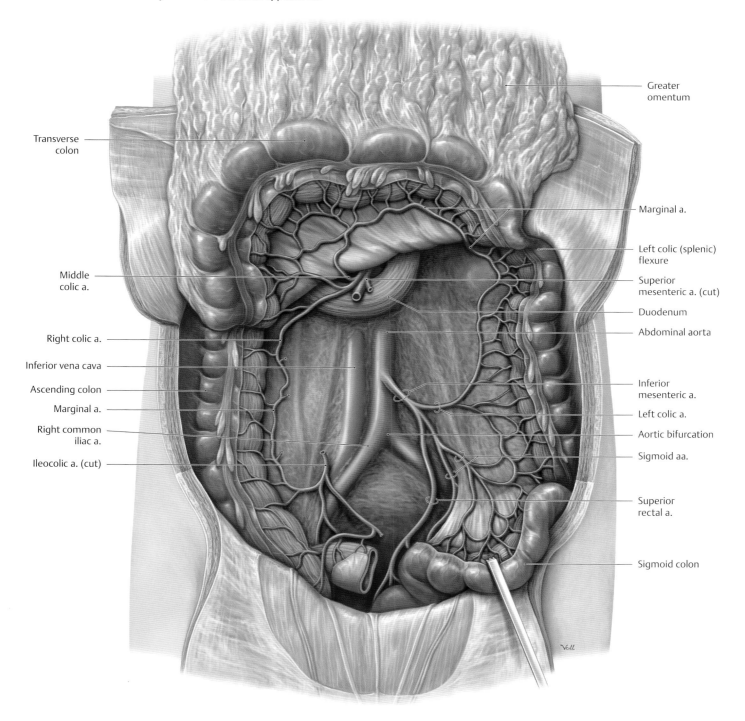

Transverse colon

Greater omentum

Marginal a.

Left colic (splenic) flexure

Middle colic a.

Superior mesenteric a. (cut)

Duodenum

Abdominal aorta

Right colic a.

Inferior vena cava

Ascending colon

Inferior mesenteric a.

Marginal a.

Left colic a.

Right common iliac a.

Aortic bifurcation

Sigmoid aa.

Ileocolic a. (cut)

Superior rectal a.

Sigmoid colon

— Important anastomoses connect the three unpaired visceral branches of the aorta and provide a collateral blood supply to the intestinal organs (**Fig. 8.14**).

- The celiac trunk and superior mesenteric artery anastomose in the head of the pancreas through the **pancreaticoduodenal arteries** and in the body and tail of the pancreas through **dorsal pancreatic** and **inferior pancreatic arteries**.
- The superior mesenteric and inferior mesenteric arteries anastomose near the junction of the transverse and descending colons through the middle and left colic arteries. The **marginal artery** runs along the mesenteric border of the large intestine and connects the ileocolic, right colic, middle colic, and left colic arteries (see **Fig. 8.13**).
- The inferior mesenteric artery anastomoses with arteries of the rectum through its **superior rectal artery** (see **Fig. 10.18**).

Fig. 8.14 ▶ **Abdominal arterial anastomoses**
Three major anastomoses provide overlap in the arterial supply to ensure adequate blood flow to abdominal areas: (1) between the celiac trunk and the superior mesenteric artery via the pancreaticoduodenal arteries; (2) between the superior and inferior mesenteric arteries via the middle and left colic arteries; and (3) between the inferior mesenteric and internal iliac arteries via the superior and middle or inferior rectal arteries

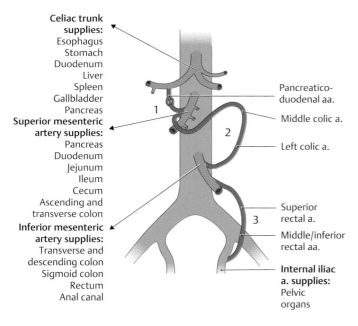

8.2b Veins of the Abdomen

— The **inferior vena cava** (IVC) receives blood from retroperitoneal and pelvic organs, walls of the abdomen and pelvis, and the lower limbs (**Fig. 8.15**).

- It originates at the L5 vertebral level where the **common iliac veins** merge.
- It ascends along the right side of the vertebral column, passes posterior to the liver, and pierces the central tendon of the diaphragm at the T8 vertebral level, where it enters the right atrium of the heart.

— **Table 8.5** lists the tributaries of the inferior vena cava.

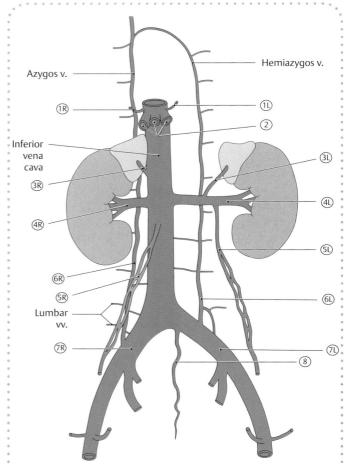

Table 8.5 ▶ **Tributaries of the Inferior Vena Cava**		
①R	①L	Inferior phrenic vv. (paired)
	②	Hepatic vv. (3)
③R	③L	Suprarenal vv. (the right vein is a direct tributary)
④R	④L	Renal vv. (paired)
⑤R	⑤L	Testicular/ovarian vv. (the right vein is a direct tributary)
⑥R	⑥L	Ascending lumbar vv. (paired)
⑦R	⑦L	Common iliac vv. (paired)
	⑧	Median sacral v.

- Paired common iliac veins drain the **external iliac** and **internal iliac veins.**
- Paired **inferior phrenic** and **lumbar veins** drain the posterior abdominal wall and diaphragm and accompany the arteries of similar name.
- Veins of the retroperitoneal organs include the **right** and **left renal veins**, the right **suprarenal vein**, and the right **testicular** or **ovarian** (gonadal) **vein**. The suprarenal and gonadal veins on the left side drain to the left renal vein.

- Typically three **hepatic veins** enter the IVC from the liver immediately below the diaphragm.
— Paired **ascending lumbar veins** communicate with the lumbar veins and are continuous with the azygos and hemiazygos veins of the thorax. These communications between the lumbar, ascending lumbar, azygos, and hemiazygos veins function as a collateral pathway between the inferior and superior venae cavae (see **Fig. 3.6**)

Fig. 8.15 ▶ **Inferior vena cava**
Anterior view. *Removed:* All organs except the kidneys and suprarenal glands.

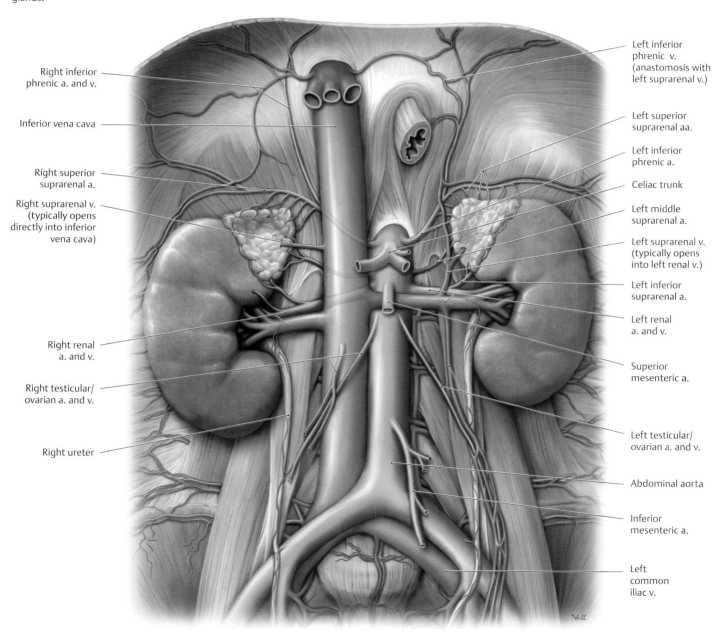

— The **hepatic portal vein** (usually known as the **portal vein**), part of the **hepatic portal system**, shunts nutrient-rich venous blood from the capillary beds of the gastrointestinal tract and its associated organs to sinusoids of the liver (**Figs. 8.16** and **8.17**). This blood eventually enters the inferior vena cava through the hepatic veins.

— Tributaries of the portal vein include the following:

- The **splenic vein**, which drains the spleen, and the **superior mesenteric vein**, which drains the small intestine and most of the large intestine. These two veins unite behind the neck of the pancreas to form the hepatic portal vein.

- The **inferior mesenteric vein**, which drains the hindgut portion of the gastrointestinal tract. It usually joins the splenic vein but may empty directly into the portal vein.

- Veins from the lower esophagus, stomach, pancreas, duodenum, and gallbladder

— Normal connections between the systemic (caval) venous system and portal venous system, called **portosystemic pathways**, can become abnormally dilated when there is an obstruction of the portal or systemic circulations (i.e., cirrhosis of the liver or pregnancy). These dilations are most prominent in (**Fig. 8.18**)

1. **esophageal veins**,
2. **periumbilical veins** through the superior and inferior epigastric veins of the abdominal wall,
3. **colic veins** in the retroperitoneum, and
4. **rectal veins** of the rectum and anal canal.

Fig. 8.16 ▶ **Portal vein: In situ**
Anterior view. *Partially removed:* Stomach, pancreas, and peritoneum.

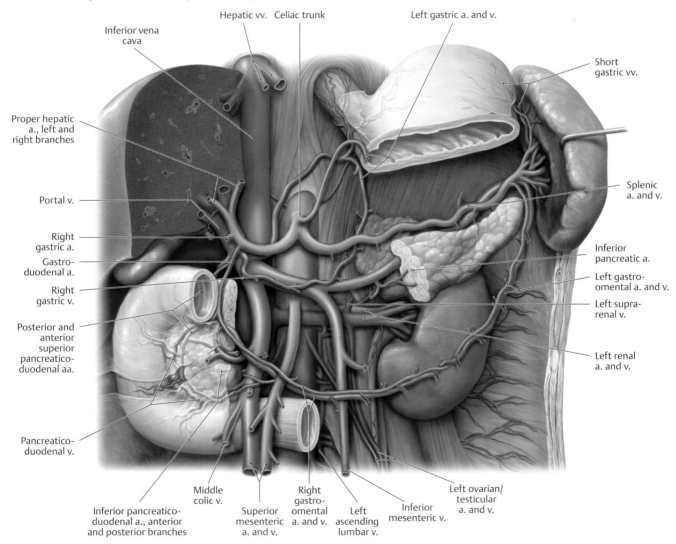

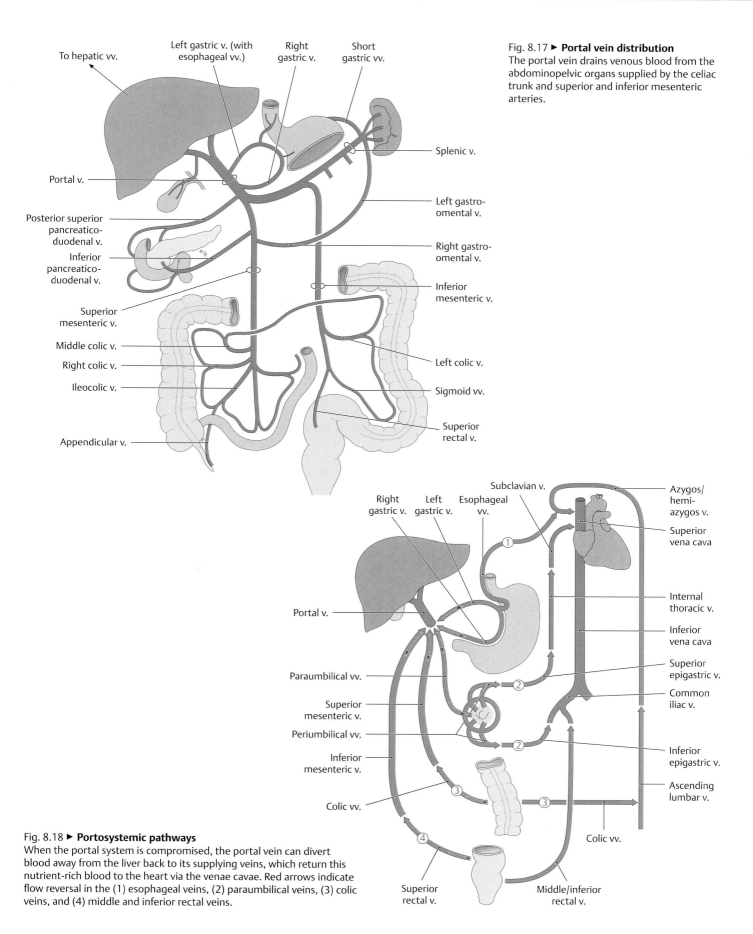

To hepatic vv.

Left gastric v. (with esophageal vv.)

Right gastric v.

Short gastric vv.

Portal v.

Posterior superior pancreatico-duodenal v.

Inferior pancreatico-duodenal v.

Superior mesenteric v.

Middle colic v.

Right colic v.

Ileocolic v.

Appendicular v.

Splenic v.

Left gastro-omental v.

Right gastro-omental v.

Inferior mesenteric v.

Left colic v.

Sigmoid vv.

Superior rectal v.

Fig. 8.17 ▶ Portal vein distribution
The portal vein drains venous blood from the abdominopelvic organs supplied by the celiac trunk and superior and inferior mesenteric arteries.

Subclavian v.

Right gastric v.

Left gastric v.

Esophageal vv.

Azygos/hemi-azygos v.

Superior vena cava

Portal v.

Paraumbilical vv.

Superior mesenteric v.

Periumbilical vv.

Inferior mesenteric v.

Colic vv.

Superior rectal v.

Middle/inferior rectal v.

Internal thoracic v.

Inferior vena cava

Superior epigastric v.

Common iliac v.

Inferior epigastric v.

Ascending lumbar v.

Colic vv.

Fig. 8.18 ▶ Portosystemic pathways
When the portal system is compromised, the portal vein can divert blood away from the liver back to its supplying veins, which return this nutrient-rich blood to the heart via the venae cavae. Red arrows indicate flow reversal in the (1) esophageal veins, (2) paraumbilical veins, (3) colic veins, and (4) middle and inferior rectal veins.

Portal hypertension and surgical portocaval shunts

Portal hypertension occurs secondary to liver disease (e.g., cirrhosis) or thrombosis of the portal vein. Increased resistance to the flow of blood in the portal system forces portal blood through portocaval anastomoses to the systemic circulation. Symptoms of portal hypertension include ascites, caput medusa (enlargement of periumbilical veins on the anterior abdominal wall), varices of the rectal veins (hemorrhoids), and esophageal varices. Symptoms may be relieved by surgically creating a portocaval shunt between the portal and systemic circulations (portal vein to the inferior vena cava or splenic vein to the left renal vein).

Esophageal varices

Submucosal veins of the esophagus drain superiorly to the systemic system (through the azygos veins) and inferiorly to the portal system. When flow through the portal vein is obstructed (as in portal hypertension), these portosystemic anastomoses allow blood in the lower esophagus to drain to the systemic veins. The esophageal varices, enlarged veins that result from this increased flow, can rupture, causing severe hemorrhaging.

8.2c Lymphatic Drainage of the Abdomen

Lymph vessels from the abdominal walls and viscera usually accompany the arteries that supply those regions and ultimately drain to the chyle cistern (if present) or the thoracic duct.

— The cisterna chyli (chyle cistern) is an elongated, lobulated, thin-walled dilation that, when present, gives rise to the thoracic duct. It lies to the right of the T12 vertebral body and receives the **lumbar** and **intestinal trunks** (see **Fig. 1.20**).

— Groups of lumbar lymph nodes drain all of the abdominal viscera (except a small hepatic segment) and most of the abdominal wall (**Fig. 8.19**; **Table 8.6**).

• **Preaortic nodes**, which lie anterior to the abdominal aorta, receive lymph from the gastrointestinal tract (as far as the midrectum) and associated organs. Nodes surrounding the base of the major arteries form preterminal groups, such as the **superior** and **inferior mesenteric nodes**. These drain to **celiac nodes**, which drain to intestinal lymph trunks.

• **Lateral aortic nodes** (right and left lumbar nodes) lie along the medial border of the psoas muscles, the crura of the diaphragm, and along the inferior vena cava. They drain the abdominal and pelvic walls and the viscera of the retroperitoneum, including the ovaries and testes, and receive lymph from the common iliac nodes, which drain the pelvic viscera and the lower limb. Drainage from these lateral aortic nodes forms a lumbar trunk on each side.

• **Retroaortic nodes** that lie behind the aorta are considered peripheral nodes of the lateral aortic group and have no specific area of drainage.

• **Common iliac nodes** drain organs of the pelvis and the lower limbs.

Fig. 8.19 ▶ Lymphatic drainage of the internal organs of the abdomen and pelvis

See **Table 8.6** for numbering. Lymph drainage from the abdomen, pelvis, and lower limb ultimately passes through the lumbar lymph nodes (clinically: aortic nodes). The lumbar lymph nodes consist of the right (caval) and left lateral aortic nodes, the preaortic nodes, and the retroaortic nodes. Efferent lymph vessels from the lumbar and preaortic nodes form the lumbar and intestinal trunks, respectively. The lumbar and intestinal trunks terminate in the cisterna chyli.

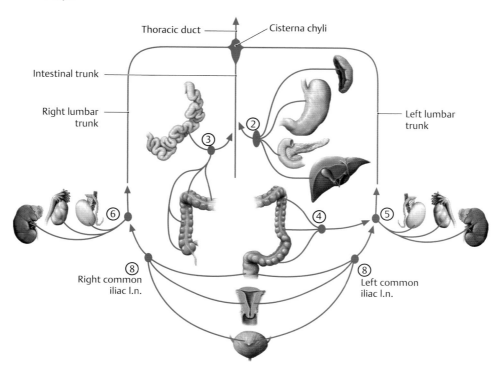

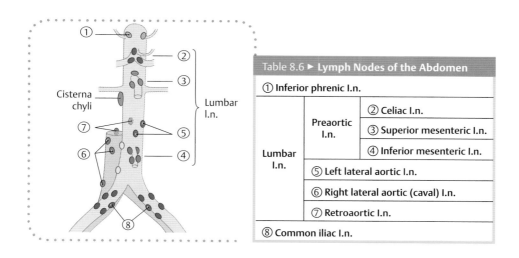

Table 8.6 ▶ Lymph Nodes of the Abdomen			
① Inferior phrenic l.n.			
Lumbar l.n.	Preaortic l.n.	② Celiac l.n.	
		③ Superior mesenteric l.n.	
		④ Inferior mesenteric l.n.	
	⑤ Left lateral aortic l.n.		
	⑥ Right lateral aortic (caval) l.n.		
	⑦ Retroaortic l.n.		
⑧ Common iliac l.n.			

Fig. 8.20 ▶ **Nerves of the lumbar plexus**
Anterior view.

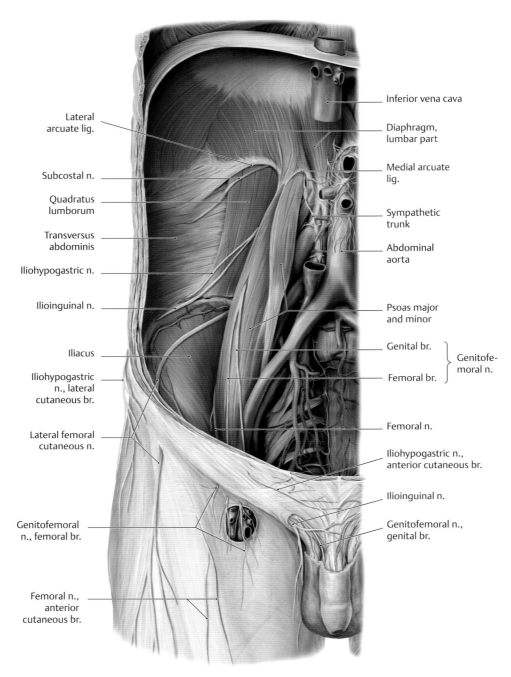

Lateral
arcuate lig.

Subcostal n.

Quadratus
lumborum

Transversus
abdominis

Iliohypogastric n.

Ilioinguinal n.

Iliacus

Iliohypogastric
n., lateral
cutaneous br.

Lateral femoral
cutaneous n.

Genitofemoral
n., femoral br.

Femoral n.,
anterior
cutaneous br.

Inferior vena cava

Diaphragm,
lumbar part

Medial arcuate
lig.

Sympathetic
trunk

Abdominal
aorta

Psoas major
and minor

Genital br. ⎫
⎬ Genitofe-
Femoral br. ⎭ moral n.

Femoral n.

Iliohypogastric n.,
anterior cutaneous br.

Ilioinguinal n.

Genitofemoral n.,
genital br.

A Lumbar plexus in situ.

8.2d Nerves of the Abdomen

— Lower intercostal nerves (T7–T11) and the **subcostal nerve** (T12) continue anteroinferiorly from their position on the thoracic wall to innervate most of the muscles and skin of the anterolateral abdominal wall.

— The nerves of the **lumbar plexus**, a somatic nerve plexus formed by the anterior rami of spinal nerves T12–L4, emerge from the psoas major muscle on the posterior abdominal wall (**Fig. 8.20A and B**). Most nerves of this plexus innervate the lower limb (see Section 15.4d and **Table 15.1**). Branches that innervate the abdominal wall and inguinal region include the

- **iliohypogastric** and **ilioinguinal nerves** (L1), which innervate the skin and muscles of the inferior anterior abdominal wall and the skin over the inguinal and pubic regions;
- **genitofemoral nerve** (L1–L2), whose genital branch innervates the cremaster muscle surrounding the spermatic cord and the skin over the scrotum and labia; and
- short muscular branches (T12–L4) that innervate the muscles of the posterior abdominal wall.

— **Lumbar sympathetic trunks**, the continuations of the sympathetic trunks in the thorax, descend along the lateral aspect of the lumbar vertebral bodies and give off three to four **lumbar splanchnic nerves**, which join the autonomic plexuses of the abdomen.

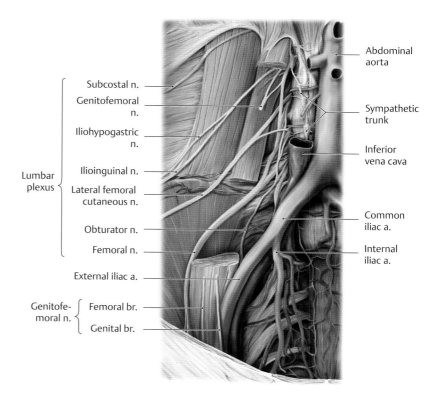

B Lumbar plexus dissection. *Windowed:* psoas major.

— Autonomic plexuses form along the aorta and travel with the major abdominal arteries to innervate the abdominal viscera (**Fig. 8.21** and **Table 8.7; Fig. 8.22** and **Table 8.8**). The plexuses contain

- preganglionic sympathetic nerves that synapse in the ganglia associated with the plexuses. (Note that the sympathetic nerves innervating the adrenal medulla are an exception and do not synapse in these ganglia.) The preganglionic sympathetic nerves arise from
  - thoracic splanchnic nerves (T5–T12) and
  - lumbar splanchnic nerves (T11–L2).
- preganglionic parasympathetic nerves, which pass through the plexuses and synapse in ganglia near their target organ. They arise from
  - the vagus nerves (CN X), which enter the abdomen as anterior and posterior vagal trunks from the esophageal plexus. They supply most of the abdominal viscera, including the digestive tract, except for its most distal segment (the descending colon to the anal canal).
  - **pelvic splanchnic nerves** (S2–S4), which ascend from the pelvis to innervate the descending and sigmoid colons in the abdomen. They also innervate viscera of the pelvis.

Table 8.7 ▶ **Autonomic Plexuses in the Abdomen and Pelvis**

Ganglia	Subplexus	Distribution	
Celiac plexus			
Celiac ganglia	Hepatic plexus	• Liver, gallbladder	
	Gastric plexus	• Stomach	
	Splenic plexus	• Spleen	
	Pancreatic plexus	• Pancreas	
Superior mesenteric plexus			
Superior mesenteric ganglia	—	• Pancreas (head) • Duodenum • Jejunum • Ileum	• Cecum • Colon (to left colic flexure) • Ovary
Suprarenal and renal plexus			
Aorticorenal ganglion	Ureteral plexus	• Suprarenal gland • Kidney • Proximal ureter	
Ovarian/testicular plexus			
—	—	• Ovary/testis	
Inferior mesenteric plexus			
—	Left colic plexus	• Left colic flexure	
	Superior rectal plexus	• Descending and sigmoid colon • Upper rectum	
Superior hypogastric plexus			
—	Hypogastric nn.	• Pelvic viscera	
Inferior hypogastric plexus			
Pelvic ganglia	Middle and inferior rectal plexus	• Middle and lower rectum	
	Prostatic plexus	• Prostate • Seminal vesicle • Bulbourethral gland	• Ejaculatory duct • Penis • Urethra
	Deferential plexus	• Ductus deferens • Epididymis	
	Uterovaginal plexus	• Uterus • Uterine tube	• Vagina • Ovary
	Vesical plexus	• Urinary bladder	
	Ureteral plexus	• Ureter (ascending from pelvis)	

Fig. 8.21 ► **Autonomic plexuses in the abdomen and pelvis**
Anterior view of the male abdomen. *Removed:* Peritoneum and majority
of the stomach.

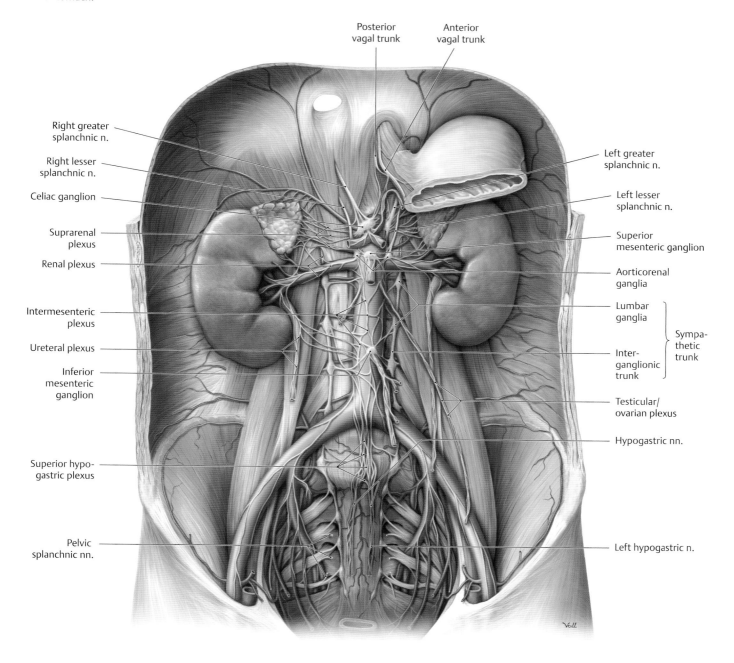

Posterior vagal trunk

Anterior vagal trunk

Right greater splanchnic n.

Right lesser splanchnic n.

Celiac ganglion

Suprarenal plexus

Renal plexus

Intermesenteric plexus

Ureteral plexus

Inferior mesenteric ganglion

Superior hypogastric plexus

Pelvic splanchnic nn.

Left greater splanchnic n.

Left lesser splanchnic n.

Superior mesenteric ganglion

Aorticorenal ganglia

Lumbar ganglia

Interganglionic trunk

Sympathetic trunk

Testicular/ovarian plexus

Hypogastric nn.

Left hypogastric n.

Fig. 8.22 ▶ **Sympathetic and parasympathetic nervous systems in the abdomen and pelvis**

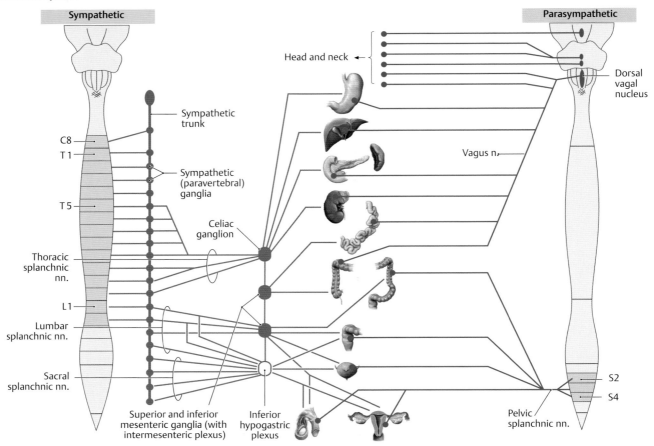

Sympathetic		Parasympathetic

Head and neck ◄

Dorsal vagal nucleus

Sympathetic trunk

C8
T 1

Sympathetic (paravertebral) ganglia

Vagus n.

T 5

Celiac ganglion

Thoracic splanchnic nn.

L 1

Lumbar splanchnic nn.

Sacral splanchnic nn.

S2
S4

Superior and inferior mesenteric ganglia (with intermesenteric plexus)

Inferior hypogastric plexus

Pelvic splanchnic nn.

A Sympathetic nervous system.

B Parasympathetic nervous system.

Table 8.8 ▶ Effects of the Autonomic Nervous System in the Abdomen and Pelvis

Organ (Organ System)		Sympathetic effect	Parasympathetic effect
Gastrointestinal tract	Longitudinal and circular muscle fibers	Decreases motility	Increases motility
	Sphincter muscles	Contraction	Relaxation
	Glands	Decreases secretions	Increases secretions
Splenic capsule		Contraction	No effect
Liver		Increases glycogenolysis/gluconeogenesis	
Pancreas	Endocrine pancreas	Decreases insulin secretion	
	Exocrine pancreas	Decreases secretion	Increases secretion
Urinary bladder	Detrusor muscle	Relaxation	Contraction
	Functional bladder sphincter	Contraction	Inhibits contraction
Seminal vesicle and ductus deferens		Contraction (ejaculation)	No effect
Uterus		Contraction or relaxation, depending on hormonal status	
Arteries		Vasoconstriction	Vasodilation of the arteries of the penis and clitoris (erection)
Suprarenal glands (medulla)		Release of adrenaline	No effect
Urinary tract	Kidney	Vasoconstriction (decreases urine formation)	Vasodilation

9 Abdominal Viscera

The peritoneal cavity of the abdomen contains the primary and accessory organs of the gastrointestinal tract. The primary organs are the stomach, small intestine, and large intestine; the accessory organs are the liver, gallbladder, pancreas, and spleen. The kidneys, proximal ureters, and suprarenal glands are found outside the peritoneal cavity within the retroperitoneum on the posterior abdominal wall (**Fig. 9.1**).

Fig. 9.1 ► **Organs of the abdomen and pelvis**
Midsagittal section through male pelvis, viewed from the left side.

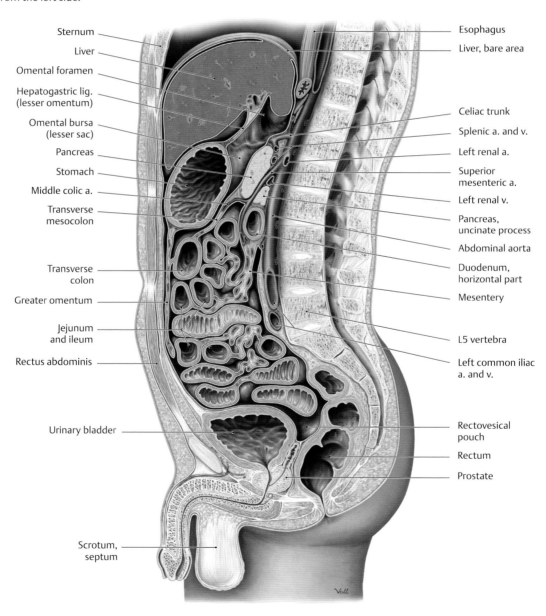

Sternum
Liver
Omental foramen
Hepatogastric lig. (lesser omentum)
Omental bursa (lesser sac)
Pancreas
Stomach
Middle colic a.
Transverse mesocolon
Transverse colon
Greater omentum
Jejunum and ileum
Rectus abdominis
Urinary bladder
Scrotum, septum

Esophagus
Liver, bare area
Celiac trunk
Splenic a. and v.
Left renal a.
Superior mesenteric a.
Left renal v.
Pancreas, uncinate process
Abdominal aorta
Duodenum, horizontal part
Mesentery
L5 vertebra
Left common iliac a. and v.
Rectovesical pouch
Rectum
Prostate

9.1 Divisions of the Gastrointestinal Tract

The three divisions of the embryonic gastrointestinal tract are retained in the adult system and reflected in its blood supply and innervation. These divisions are

— the **foregut**, which consists of the distal esophagus, the stomach, the proximal half of the duodenum, the liver, the gallbladder, and the superior part of the pancreas;
— the **midgut**, which includes the distal half of the duodenum, the jejunum, ileum, cecum, and appendix, and the ascending and proximal two thirds of the transverse colon; and
— the **hindgut**, which includes the distal third of the transverse colon, the descending and sigmoid colons, the rectum, and the upper part of the anal canal.

Rotation of the midgut tube

Development of the midgut is characterized by rapid elongation of the gut and its mesentery, resulting in the formation of the primary intestinal loop. The loop is attached to the yolk sac by the omphaloenteric duct (yolk stalk) and to the posterior abdominal wall by the superior mesenteric artery. As a result of this rapid elongation and expansion of the liver, the abdominal cavity becomes too small to contain all the intestinal loops, and they physiologically herniate into the proximal part of the umbilical cord. Coincident with growth in length, the primary intestinal loop rotates 270 degrees counterclockwise (if viewed from the front) around the axis established by the attachment of the superior mesenteric artery. Rotation occurs during herniation (approximately 90 degrees) and during the return of the intestinal loops into the abdominal cavity (remaining 180 degrees), which is thought to occur when the relative size of the liver and kidney decreases. Malrotation of the midgut can result in congenital abnormalities such as volvulus (twisting) of the intestine.

Localization of pain from foregut, midgut, and hindgut derivatives

Pain from gastrointestinal organs follows pathways determined by embryological origin. Pain from foregut structures is localized to the epigastric region, pain from structures of the midgut localizes in the periumbilical region, and pain arising from structures of the hindgut localizes in the hypogastric region.

9.2 Organs of the Gastrointestinal Tract

9.2a Stomach

The **stomach**, a hollow reservoir that stores, churns, and initiates digestion of food, communicates with the esophagus proximally and the duodenum of the small intestine distally (**Fig. 9.2A and B**; see also **Fig. 8.5**).

— It is normally J-shaped and lies in the left upper quadrant, although its shape and position vary among individuals and can change depending on its contents.

— The stomach has four parts:
  1. The **cardia**, which surrounds the opening to the esophagus
  2. The **fundus**, the superior portion that rises above and to the left of the opening between the esophagus and stomach (**cardiac orifice**)
  3. The **body**, the large expanded portion below the fundus
  4. The **pyloric part**, which is the outflow channel made up of the wide **pyloric antrum**, a narrow **pyloric canal**, and the **pyloris** or sphincteric region, which contains a muscular **pyloric sphincter** that surrounds the pyloric orifice into the first part of the duodenum.

— The stomach has a lesser curvature and a greater curvature.
  • The **lesser curvature** makes up the superior concave border. An **angular notch** (or incisure) along the curvature marks the junction of the body and pyloric part.
  • The **greater curvature** makes up the inferior convex border.

— The inner surface of the stomach is highly distensible; in adults, the stomach can accommodate 2 to 3 liters. **Rugae** (longitudinal folds) of the gastric mucosa, formed during contraction of the stomach, are most prominent in the pyloric part and along the greater curvature. Gastric filling causes the mucosal folds to disappear.

— The layers of peritoneum on the stomach's anterior and posterior surfaces unite along the lesser curvature to form the lesser omentum; along the greater curvature they unite to form the greater omentum (see **Figs. 9.1** and **8.6**).

— Anteriorly, the stomach is in contact with the abdominal wall, the diaphragm, and the left lobe of the liver. Posteriorly, it forms the anterior wall of the omental bursa.

— When the body is supine, the stomach rests on the pancreas, the spleen, the left kidney, the left suprarenal gland, and the transverse colon and its mesentery.

— Right and left gastric arteries, **right** and **left gastro-omental arteries**, and **short gastric arteries** (all derived from branches of the celiac trunk) supply the stomach (see **Fig. 8.10**).

— Veins that accompany the arteries of the stomach drain to the hepatic portal venous system.

— Lymph vessels drain to gastric and gastro-omental nodes, which drain to the celiac lymph nodes.

Fig. 9.2 ▶ **Stomach**
Anterior view.

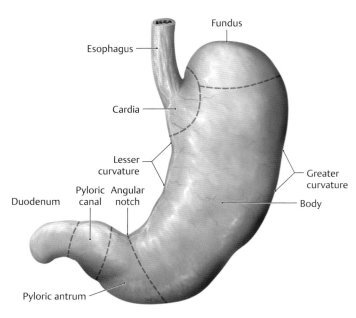

A Anterior wall.

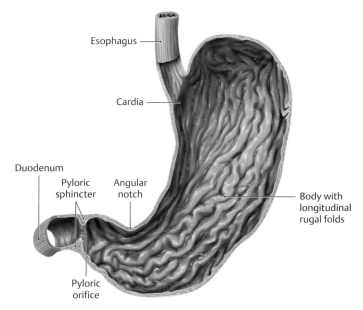

B Interior. *Removed:* Anterior wall.

■ **Gastric ulcers**

Gastric ulcers are open lesions of the mucosa that are believed to be initiated by increased acid secretion and exacerbated by the presence of the
bacterium *Helicobacter pylori*. Gastric ulcers can cause hemorrhaging if
they erode into gastric arteries. Posteriorly located ulcers can erode into
the pancreas and splenic artery, causing severe hemorrhaging. Patients
with chronic ulcers may undergo a vagotomy, the surgical sectioning of
the vagus nerve, which may curtail the production of gastric acid.

— The celiac nerve plexus innervates the stomach.

 • Sympathetic nerves promote vasoconstriction and inhibit
 peristalsis (**Fig. 9.3A** and **B**).
 • Parasympathetic nerves stimulate gastric secretion.

Fig. 9.3 ► **Autonomic innervation of the intraperitoneal organs**

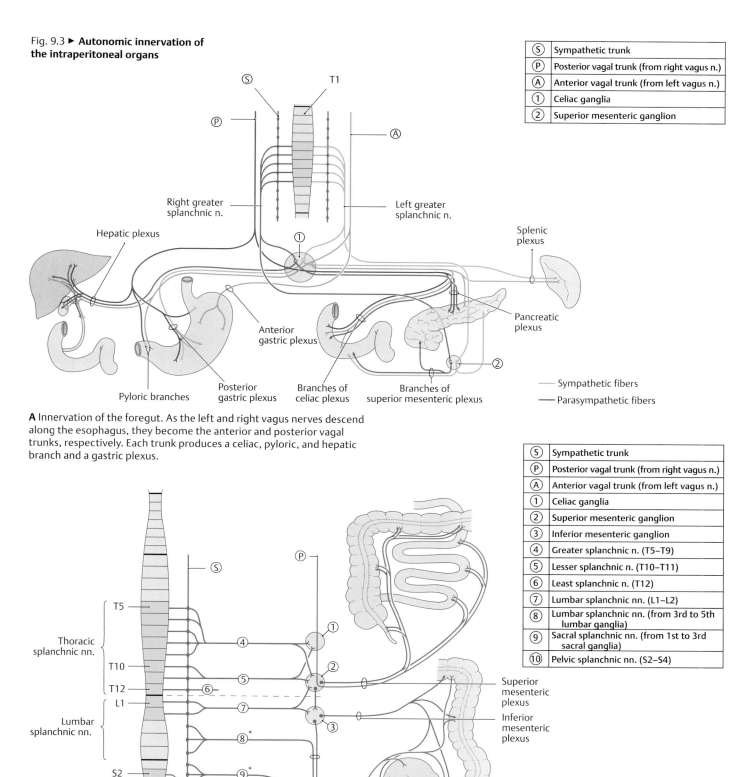

	S	Sympathetic trunk
	P	Posterior vagal trunk (from right vagus n.)
	A	Anterior vagal trunk (from left vagus n.)
	1	Celiac ganglia
	2	Superior mesenteric ganglion

A Innervation of the foregut. As the left and right vagus nerves descend along the esophagus, they become the anterior and posterior vagal trunks, respectively. Each trunk produces a celiac, pyloric, and hepatic branch and a gastric plexus.

	S	Sympathetic trunk
	P	Posterior vagal trunk (from right vagus n.)
	A	Anterior vagal trunk (from left vagus n.)
	1	Celiac ganglia
	2	Superior mesenteric ganglion
	3	Inferior mesenteric ganglion
	4	Greater splanchnic n. (T5–T9)
	5	Lesser splanchnic n. (T10–T11)
	6	Least splanchnic n. (T12)
	7	Lumbar splanchnic nn. (L1–L2)
	8	Lumbar splanchnic nn. (from 3rd to 5th lumbar ganglia)
	9	Sacral splanchnic nn. (from 1st to 3rd sacral ganglia)
	10	Pelvic splanchnic nn. (S2–S4)

*Synapse in the lumbar sympathetic ganglia.

B Innervation of the midgut and hindgut.

9.2b Small Intestine

The **small intestine** extends from the pyloric orifice of the stomach to the ileocecal orifice at the ileocecal junction and is the primary site of digestion and absorption of digested products. It is made up of three sections, the **duodenum**, which is mostly retroperitoneal, and the **jejunum** and **ileum,** which are suspended by the mesentery of the small intestine.

— The duodenum, the first and shortest section, is in a C-shaped curve around the head of the pancreas and has four parts (**Figs. 9.4** and **9.5**):

1. The **superior** (first) **part** is at the level of the L1 vertebra.

   ○ The proximal 2 cm segment, called the **duodenal bulb** or ampulla, is suspended from a mesentery.

2. The **descending** (second) **part** extends along the right side of the L1–L3 vertebral bodies.

   ○ This is the site of the junction of the foregut and midgut.
   ○ The **hepatopancreatic duct**, formed by the common bile duct and main pancreatic duct, enters the duodenum through the **major duodenal papilla** on the posteromedial wall. Superior to that, the **accessory pancreatic duct** enters through the **minor duodenal papilla**.

3. The **horizontal** (third) **part** crosses to the left, anterior to the inferior vena cava, the aorta, and the L3 vertebra, along the inferior border of the pancreas.

   ○ The root of the mesentery of the small intestine (mesenteric root) and superior mesenteric vessels cross anteriorly (see **Fig. 8.5**).

4. The **ascending** (fourth) **part** ascends along the left side of the aorta to the level of the L2 vertebra at the inferior border of the pancreas.

   ○ It joins the jejunum at the duodenojejunal flexure, which is suspended from the posterior abdominal wall by the **suspensory ligament** (of Treitz).

Fig. 9.4 ▶ **Parts of the duodenum**
Anterior view.

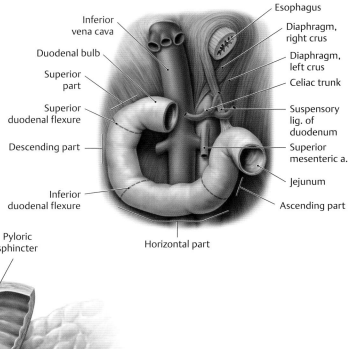

Fig. 9.5 ▶ **Duodenum**
Anterior view with the anterior wall opened.

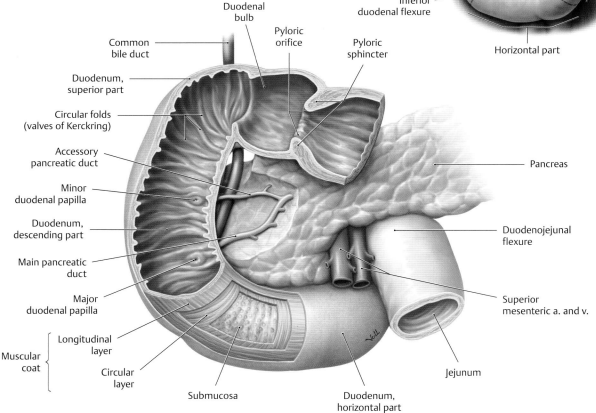

Duodenal (peptic) ulcers

Duodenal ulcers usually occur within a few centimeters of the pylorus on its posterior wall. Perforation of the duodenum can lead to peritonitis and ulceration of adjacent organs. Severe hemorrhaging results if the ulcer erodes through the gastroduodenal artery, which runs along the posterior side of the duodenum.

— The jejunum, the proximal two fifths of the intraperitoneal portion of the small intestine, is suspended by the small bowel mesentery and is located predominantly in the left upper quadrant (**Fig. 9.6**; see also **Fig. 8.4**).

- It is thicker walled and larger in diameter than the ileum.
- Tall, closely packed **circular folds** (**plicae circulares**) line its inner surface, increasing its surface area (**Fig. 9.7**).
- Widely spaced arterial arcades within its mesentery give rise to long, straight arteries, the **vasa recta** (see **Fig. 8.12**).

— The ileum, which makes up the distal three fifths of the intraperitoneal portion of the small intestine, is also suspended by the mesentery of the small intestine. The ileum extends from the end of the jejunum to its junction with the cecum (**ileocecal junction**) and resides in the lower left quadrant and the greater pelvis (see **Fig. 9.6**).

- It is longer in length than the jejunum.
- Lymphoid nodules (**Peyer's patches**) bulge outward from the connective tissue layer underlying the epithelium (lamina propria).
- Circular folds (plicae circulares) are low and sparse.
- The ileum has more fat, denser arterial arcades, and shorter vasa recta in its mesentery than the jejunum.

Ileal diverticulum

Ileal diverticulum (also known as Meckel's diverticulum), the most common congenital abnormality of the bowel, is an outpouching of the ileum that is a remnant of the omphalomesenteric duct (yolk stalk) that fails to resorb. The diverticulum may be unattached distally or connect to the umbilicus via a fibrous cord or fistula. They are present in ~2% of the population, are located ~2 feet proximal to the ileocecal junction, and often contain two or more types of mucosa. The diverticulum can contain gastric, pancreatic, jejunal, or colonic tissue. An ileal diverticulum is usually asymptomatic but when inflamed may mimic acute appendicitis.

— The blood supply, lymphatic drainage, and innervation of the parts of the small intestine reflect their development from the embryonic foregut and midgut.

- The section that extends from the pyloric sphincter to below the major duodenal papilla (foregut) is supplied by the **superior pancreaticoduodenal** branch of the **gastroduodenal artery** (supplied through the celiac trunk) (see **Fig. 8.12**).
- The midgut (distal part of the descending duodenum, the jejunum, and the ileum) is supplied by the **inferior pancreaticoduodenal, jejunal,** and **ileal arteries,** branches of the superior mesenteric artery.
- Veins of similar names accompany the arteries and terminate in the hepatic portal system.
- Lymph vessels from the small intestine follow the course of the arteries and drain into the celiac and superior mesenteric nodes.
- The celiac (to foregut) and superior mesenteric (to midgut) plexuses innervate the small intestine (see **Fig. 9.3A** and **B**).
  - Sympathetic innervation inhibits intestinal mobility, secretion, and vasodilation.
  - Parasympathetic innervation restores normal digestive activity following sympathetic stimulation.
  - Visceral sensory fibers transmit feelings of distension (often perceived as cramping), but the intestine is insensitive to most pain stimuli.

Inflammatory bowel disease

There are two types of inflammatory bowel disease (IBD): Crohn's disease and ulcerative colitis. Crohn's disease is a chronic inflammatory disease that can affect the entire GI tract but most commonly affects the terminal ileum and colon. It causes ulcers, fistulas (abnormal communications), and granulomata, producing symptoms such as fever, diarrhea, weight loss, and abdominal pain. Ulcerative colitis is a recurrent inflammatory disease of the colon and rectum that produces bloody diarrhea, weight loss, fever, and abdominal pain. These diseases are treated with drugs that reduce the inflammatory response.

Fig. 9.6 ▶ Jejunum and ileum in situ
Anterior view. *Reflected:* Transverse colon and greater omentum.

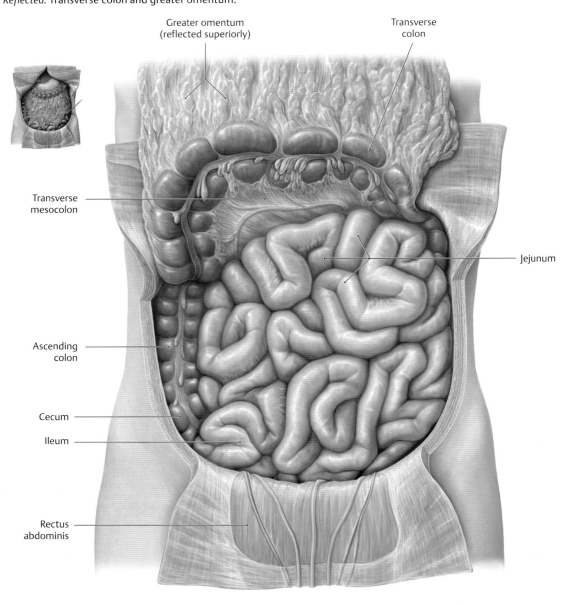

Greater omentum
(reflected superiorly)

Transverse
colon

Transverse
mesocolon

Jejunum

Ascending
colon

Cecum

Ileum

Rectus
abdominis

Fig. 9.7 ▶ Wall structure of the small intestine
Macroscopic views of the longitudinally opened small intestine.

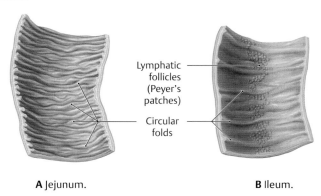

Lymphatic
follicles
(Peyer's
patches)

Circular
folds

A Jejunum.

B Ileum.

9.2c   Large Intestine

The **large intestine** extends from the cecum to the anal canal (**Fig. 9.8**). It converts liquid feces to a semisolid state through the absorption of water, electrolytes, and salts. It also stores and lubricates fecal matter. Although it consists of five parts, only the **cecum**, **appendix**, and **colon** reside in the abdomen. The **rectum** and **anal canal** are described in Chapter 11 with the pelvic viscera.

— The cecum is a blind pouch located in the right lower quadrant.

  • It is attached proximally in an end-to-side fashion to the terminal ileum and is continuous distally with the ascending colon.

  • It lacks a mesentery but is surrounded by peritoneum and therefore is fairly mobile.

— The (vermiform) appendix is a blind muscular diverticulum (outpouching) that opens into the posteromedial wall of the cecum below the **ileocecal orifice**.

  • Its walls contain large masses of lymphoid tissue.

  • Its mesoappendix (mesentery) suspends it from the ileum.

  • Its position is highly variable, but it is often retrocecal (posterior to the cecum).

— The colon has four parts that frame the abdominal viscera (see also **Fig. 8.4**).

  1. The **ascending colon** ascends from the cecum in the right lower quadrant to the **right colic** (hepatic) **flexure** under the liver.

  2. The **transverse colon** crosses the abdomen from the right colic flexure to the left upper quadrant, where it terminates at the **left colic** (splenic) **flexure**.

  3. The **descending colon** descends along the left side of the abdomen to the left lower quadrant.

  4. The **sigmoid colon** crosses the iliac fossa to join the rectum in the pelvis.

— The appendix, transverse colon, and sigmoid colon are intraperitoneal. Each is suspended by its respective **mesocolon** (mesentery). The left colic flexure is attached to the diaphragm by the **phenicocolic ligament**.

— The ascending and descending colons are secondarily retroperitoneal and therefore lack mesenteries.

— External features of the colon distinguish it from the small intestine:

  • **Teniae coli**, three longitudinal bands formed by the outer muscular layer

  • **Haustra**, outpouchings of the intestinal wall visible between the teniae coli

  • **Epiploic appendices**, small sacs of fat aligned along the teniae

— The blood supply, lymphatic drainage, and innervation of the parts of the large intestine reflect their development from the embryonic midgut and hindgut.

  • The ileocolic, right colic, and middle colic branches of the superior mesenteric artery supply the cecum, ascending colon, and proximal two thirds of the transverse colon (midgut) (see **Fig. 8.13**).

  • The left colic and sigmoidal branches of the inferior mesenteric artery supply the distal third of the transverse colon, and the descending and sigmoid colons (hindgut). A superior rectal branch supplies the upper rectum in the pelvis.

  • The marginal artery runs along the mesenteric border of the large intestine, anastomosing branches of the superior mesenteric artery with those of the inferior mesenteric artery. In turn, the superior rectal artery anastomoses with middle rectal and inferior rectal branches in the pelvis.

  • Veins of the colon follow the arteries and drain into the hepatic portal system.

  • Lymph vessels follow arterial pathways to drain into superior mesenteric or inferior mesenteric nodes.

  • The superior mesenteric (midgut) and inferior mesenteric (hindgut) nerve plexuses innervate the large intestine (see **Fig. 9.3B**).

Fig. 9.8 ▶ **Large intestine**
Anterior view.

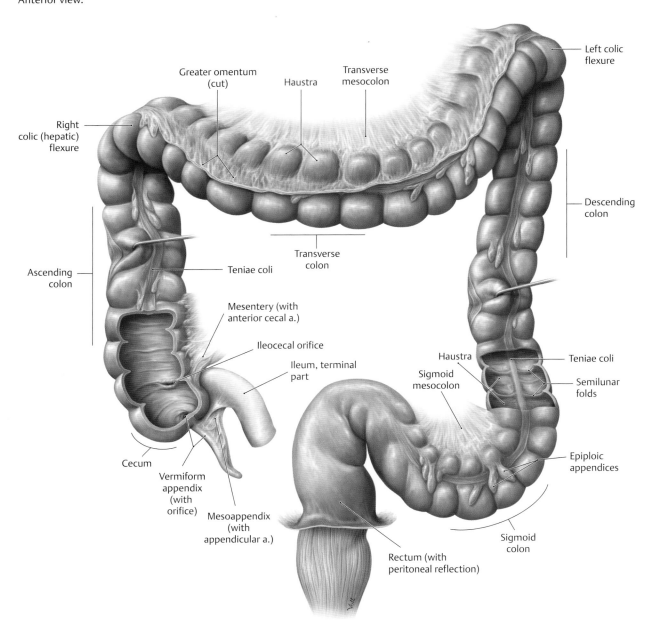

Right colic (hepatic) flexure

Greater omentum (cut)

Haustra

Transverse mesocolon

Left colic flexure

Ascending colon

Teniae coli

Transverse colon

Descending colon

Mesentery (with anterior cecal a.)

Ileocecal orifice

Ileum, terminal part

Haustra

Sigmoid mesocolon

Teniae coli

Semilunar folds

Cecum

Vermiform appendix (with orifice)

Mesoappendix (with appendicular a.)

Rectum (with peritoneal reflection)

Epiploic appendices

Sigmoid colon

Appendicitis

Inflammation of the appendix is felt initially as vague pain in the peri-umbilical region, transmitted via visceral fibers from the T10 spinal cord segment. As the inflammation irritates the overlying parietal peritoneum, acute pain is felt in the lower right quadrant and can be elicited by pressure near McBurney's point (located one third of the distance along a line between the anterior superior iliac spine and the umbilicus). Although the attached part of the appendix usually lies deep to this point, its free end is variable and may lie posterior to the cecum (retrocecal) or drape over the pelvic brim.

Volvulus of the sigmoid colon

Rotation and twisting of the sigmoid colon on its mesentery can lead to ob-struction of the descending and sigmoid colons. Constipation, the primary symptom, may progress to fecal impaction where the bowel becomes obstructed by hardened feces. This may be accompanied by abdominal pain, distension, and vomiting. The volvulus can become ischemic (have a reduced blood supply) and necrotic (tissue death) if not treated. Surgery is required to untwist the affected segment and resect any necrotic bowel.

9.3 Accessory Organs of the Gastrointestinal Tract

9.3a Liver

The **liver** is located in the right upper quadrant under the right hemidiaphragm and extends inferiorly to the costal margin (**Fig. 9.9**). It has a primary role in carbohydrate, protein, and fat metabolism. It also produces and secretes bile and bile pigments; detoxifies substances absorbed by the gastrointestinal tract; and stores vitamins and minerals, such as iron. In the fetus, the liver is the site of hematopoiesis (red blood cell production).

— Externally, ligaments and fissures divide the liver into four anatomic (topographic) lobes: the **right**, **left**, **caudate**, and **quadrate lobes** (**Fig. 9.10A, B,** and **C**).

— The liver's diaphragmatic surface conforms to the shape of the diaphragm and is marked by the **bare area**, which lacks peritoneum and is in direct contact with the diaphragm.

— The liver's visceral (inferior) surface has three prominent fissures:

1. The left sagittal fissure accommodates

   ○ the **round ligament** (ligamentum teres) of the liver anteriorly between the left and quadrate lobes. The round ligament is a remnant of the fetal umbilical vein.

   ○ the **ligamentum venosum** posteriorly between the left and caudate lobes. The ligamentum venosum is a remnant of the fetal ductus venosus.

2. The right sagittal fissure accommodates

   ○ the gallbladder anteriorly between the right and quadrate lobes and

   ○ the inferior vena cava posteriorly between the right and caudate lobes.

3. The transverse fissure accommodates

   ○ the **porta hepatis,** or hilum of the liver. Structures of the **portal triad** [proper hepatic artery, portal vein, and (common) **bile duct**] enter or exit here.

— The liver is intraperitoneal, covered by peritoneum except at the bare area, gallbladder fossa, and porta hepatis. Peritoneal reflections include

• the **coronary** and **triangular ligaments**, single-layered reflections between the liver and diaphragm that surround the bare area;

• the falciform ligament, a double layer of peritoneum, which attaches the liver to the anterior abdominal wall and contains the round ligament in its free edge; and

• the hepatogastric and hepatoduodenal ligaments (both parts of the lesser omentum), which attach the liver to the stomach and proximal duodenum (see **Fig. 8.5**).

— A subperitoneal fibrous capsule, **Glisson's capsule**, covers the surface of the liver.

Fig. 9.9 ▶ **Liver in situ**
Anterior view.

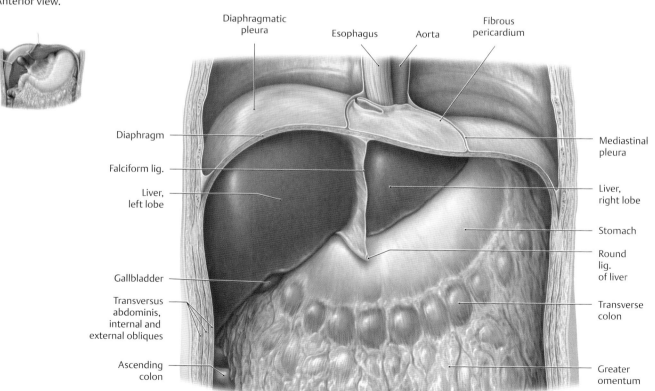

Diaphragmatic pleura — Esophagus — Aorta — Fibrous pericardium

Diaphragm

Falciform lig.

Liver, left lobe

Gallbladder

Transversus abdominis, internal and external obliques

Ascending colon

Mediastinal pleura

Liver, right lobe

Stomach

Round lig. of liver

Transverse colon

Greater omentum

Fig. 9.10 ▸ **Surfaces of the liver**
The liver is divided by its ligaments into four lobes: right, left, caudate, and quadrate.

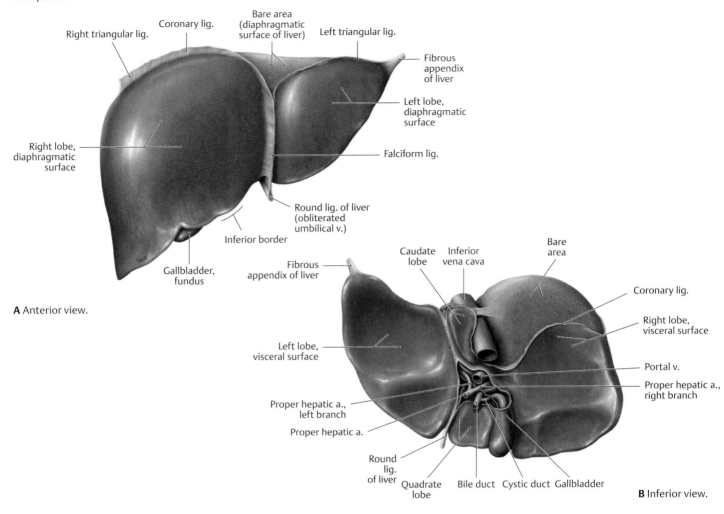

A Anterior view.

B Inferior view.

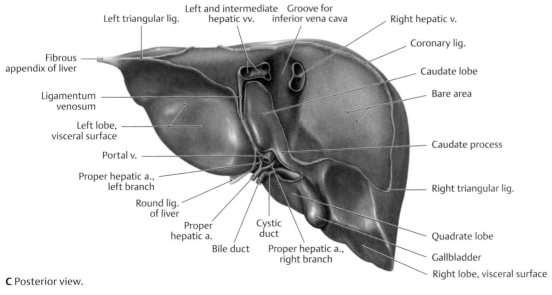

C Posterior view.

— Internally, branching of the intrahepatic blood vessels divides the liver into eight functional segments (designated as I through VIII) (**Fig. 9.11**, **Table 9.1**). This segmental arrangement of the blood supply facilitates the resection of individual diseased segments.

— The liver has a dual blood supply: the portal vein and the proper hepatic artery (see **Fig. 8.11**). Both vessels divide to form primary and secondary branches that supply the liver segments.

- The portal vein, carrying nutrient-rich blood from the digestive tract, provides 75 to 80% of the blood volume to the liver.
- The proper hepatic artery, supplied by the celiac trunk via the common hepatic artery, contributes 20 to 25% of the blood volume to the liver.

— Right, left, and intermediate (middle) hepatic veins run intersegmentally, draining adjacent segments, and open into the inferior vena cava immediately below the diaphragm.

— The liver has superficial and deep lymphatic drainages.

- The superficial lymphatic plexus, found within the fibrous capsule, drains the anterior liver surfaces to hepatic nodes (and eventually into the celiac nodes) and drains the posterior surfaces toward the bare area, which flow into phrenic or posterior mediastinal nodes.
- The deep plexus, which accompanies vessels within the liver segments, drains most of the liver, flowing first into the hepatic nodes in the porta hepatis and lesser omentum, before draining to the celiac nodes.

— The hepatic nerve plexus, a division of the celiac plexus, travels along the vessels of the portal triad to innervate the liver (see **Fig. 9.3A**).

■ Cirrhosis of the liver

Cirrhosis, most commonly caused by chronic alcoholism, is characterized by a progressive fibrosis of hepatic tissue around the intrahepatic vessels and biliary ducts that impedes blood flow. The liver becomes hard and nodular in appearance. Symptoms include ascites, splenomegaly, peripheral edema, esophageal varices, and other signs of portal hypertension.

Fig. 9.11 ► **Segmentation of the liver**
Anterior view. Branches of the hepatic artery, portal vein, and hepatic ducts divide the liver into hepatic segments.

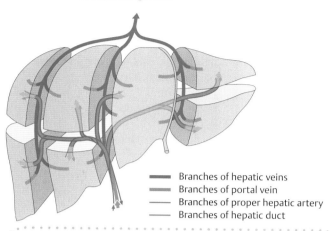

━━ Branches of hepatic veins
━━ Branches of portal vein
── Branches of proper hepatic artery
── Branches of hepatic duct

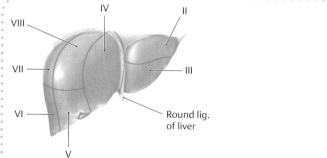

A Liver, diaphragmatic surface, anterior view.

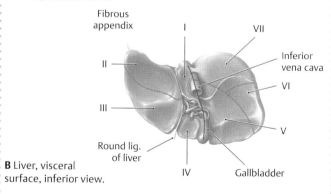

B Liver, visceral surface, inferior view.

Table 9.1 ► **Hepatic Segments**			
Part	**Division**	**Segment**	
Left part	Posterior part	I	Caudate lobe
	Left lateral division	II	Left posterolateral
		III	Left anterolateral
	Left medial division	IV	Left medial
Right part	Right medial division	V	Right anteromedial
		VI	Right anterolateral
	Right lateral division	VII	Right posterolateral
		VIII	Right posteromedial

9.3b Gallbladder and Extrahepatic Biliary System

The gallbladder is a pear-shaped sac that lies in a fossa on the visceral surface of the liver (**Fig. 9.12**). It stores the bile produced and secreted by the liver and concentrates it by absorbing salts and water. Hormonal or neural stimulation causes the gallbladder to release bile into the **extrahepatic biliary ducts**.

Fig. 9.12 ▶ **Biliary tract in situ**
Anterior view. *Removed:* Stomach, small intestine, transverse colon, and large portions of the liver. The gallbladder is intraperitoneal, covered by visceral peritoneum where it is not attached to the liver.

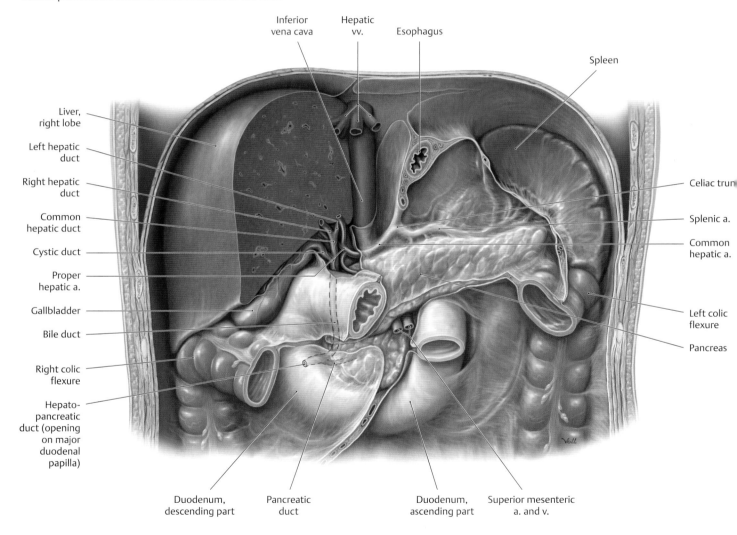

— The gallbladder has four parts (**Fig. 9.13**):

1. The **fundus**, the expanded distal end that is in contact with the anterior abdominal wall
2. The **body**, the main portion
3. The **infundibulum** between the body and neck
4. The **neck**, the narrow distal segment that joins with the cystic duct

— The extrahepatic biliary system of ducts transports bile from the liver and gallbladder to the duodenum. It consists of

- the **common hepatic duct** formed by the junction of the right and left hepatic ducts, which drain the liver;
- the **cystic duct**, which drains the gallbladder and communicates with the common hepatic duct from the liver (a **spiral valve** in the neck of the gallbladder keeps the cystic duct open); and
- the **bile duct**, formed by the junction of the common hepatic duct and cystic duct, which drains bile into the second part of the duodenum.

— The bile duct passes posterior to the first part of the duodenum and posterior to, or through, the head of the pancreas. It ends at the **hepatopancreatic ampulla** (of Vater), a dilation of the distal end of the duct, where it joins with the **main pancreatic duct** of the pancreas.

— A muscular **sphincter** (of Oddi) surrounds the hepatopancreatic ampulla as it traverses the medial wall of the duodenum through the major duodenal papilla and opens into the descending part of the duodenum (**Fig. 9.14**).
— The **cystic artery**, usually a branch of the right hepatic artery, supplies the gallbladder (see **Fig. 8.11**).
— Venous blood from the gallbladder drains into hepatic veins in the liver, which drain into the inferior vena cava.
— The hepatic plexus innervates the gallbladder (see **Fig. 9.3A**).

- Sympathetic stimulation inhibits bile secretion.
- Parasympathetic stimulation causes the gallbladder to contract and release bile.

Fig. 9.14 ▶ **Biliary sphincter system**
Sphincters of the pancreatic and bile ducts.

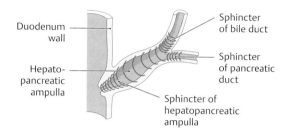

Fig. 9.13 ▶ **Extrahepatic bile ducts**
Anterior view. *Opened:* Gallbladder and duodenum.

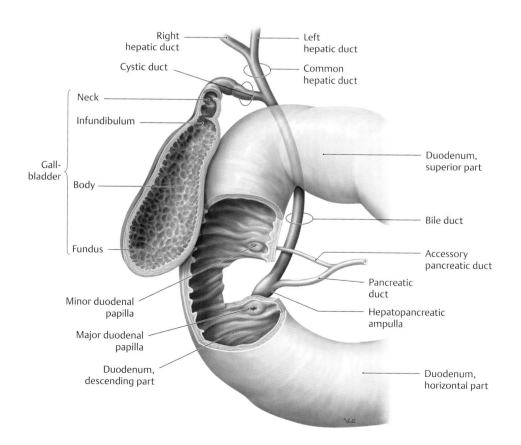

Gallstones

Gallstones are concretions of cholesterol crystals that lodge within the biliary tree. They most commonly occur in females over the age of 40. Gallstones can remain asymptomatic, but when they obstruct the hepatopancreatic ampulla, the narrowest part of the biliary tract, they impede the flow of bile and pancreatic secretions to the duodenum. This may cause bile to enter the pancreas, leading to pancreatitis. Gallstones that obstruct the cystic duct cause biliary colic, characterized by severe waves of pain, cholecystitis, and jaundice. Stones that accumulate in the fundus of a diseased gallbladder (also known as Hartmann's pouch) may ulcerate through the wall of the fundus into the transverse colon. These can pass naturally via the rectum, or they may pass into the duodenum and travel through the small intestine, where they are held up at the ileocecal valve, producing an intestinal obstruction (gallstone ileus). Pain arising from gallstones begins in the epigastric region and right hypochondriac region. Pain may also be referred to the posterior thoracic wall or right shoulder due to irritation of the diaphragm.

Cholecystectomy and the cystohepatic triangle (of Calot)

Cholecystectomy (removal of the gallbladder) is usually performed in patients with severe biliary colic. It is important during cholecystectomy to identify the cystohepatic triangle (of Calot) whose borders are defined by the cystic duct (inferiorly), the common hepatic duct (medially), and the inferior surface of the liver (superiorly) and dissect it carefully as the cystic artery arises from the right hepatic artery within the cystohepatic triangle.

Implications of the shared emptying of the bile duct and pancreatic duct

The common bile duct and the pancreatic duct both empty into the major duodenal papilla. This has important clinical implications (e.g., a tumor at the head of the pancreas may obstruct the common bile duct, causing biliary reflux into the liver and jaundice). Similarly, a gallstone that lodges in the common bile duct may obstruct the terminal part of the pancreatic duct, causing acute pancreatitis.

9.3c Pancreas

The **pancreas** is a lobulated gland that has dual functions. As an exocrine gland it synthesizes digestive enzymes, and as an endocrine gland it produces and secretes the hormones insulin and glucagon.

- It is secondarily retroperitoneal and lies on the posterior wall of the omental bursa.
- It crosses the midline with its head within the "C" of the duodenum and its tail touching the splenic hilum (see **Fig. 9.12**).
- The four parts of the pancreas are the **head** and **uncinate process**, the **neck**, the **body**, and the **tail** (**Fig. 9.15**).
- The **main pancreatic duct** (of Wirsung) traverses the length of the gland to join with the common bile duct at the hepatopancreatic ampulla. Together they drain into the descending part of the duodenum at the **major duodenal papilla** (see **Fig. 9.13**).
- When present, an **accessory pancreatic duct** (of Santorini) may drain to the descending part of the duodenum at the **minor duodenal papilla**, 2 cm proximal to the drainage site of the main pancreatic duct.

Fig. 9.15 ▶ **Pancreas**
Anterior view with dissection of the pancreatic duct.

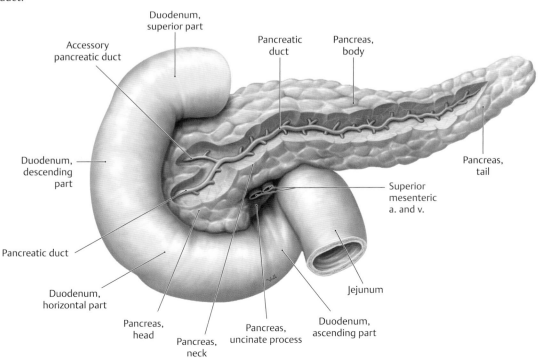

— Because of its central location in the upper abdomen, the pancreas is related topographically to many of the major abdominal vascular structures (**Fig. 9.16**; see also **Fig. 8.16**):

- The head lies anterior to the right renal vessels, left renal vein, and inferior vena cava.
- The neck and body cross anterior to the abdominal aorta, superior mesenteric vessels, and portal vein. The celiac trunk arises from the aorta immediately superior to this.
- The tail crosses anterior to the left kidney and extends to the hilum of the spleen. The splenic artery runs along its superior border, and the splenic vein courses behind it.

— Branches of the celiac trunk and superior mesenteric artery supply the pancreas (see **Fig. 8.11**).

- Pancreaticoduodenal branches of the gastroduodenal artery (from the celiac trunk) and superior mesenteric artery supply the head.
- Branches of the splenic artery supply the neck, body, and tail.

— Venous blood drains into the splenic and superior mesenteric veins, which merge to form the hepatic portal system (see **Fig. 8.16**).

— Lymphatic drainage is as varied as its blood supply but generally follows arterial pathways, ultimately draining into celiac and superior mesenteric nodes.

— The celiac and superior mesenteric plexuses innervate the pancreas (see **Fig. 9.3A** and **B**).

Carcinoma of the pancreas

Relations of the pancreas are of clinical significance in patients with pancreatic cancer. It metastasizes extensively to deep nodes and adjacent organs. Tumors of the head are most common and can obstruct the drainage of the bile and pancreatic ducts, resulting in obstructive jaundice. Tumors of the neck and body can obstruct the portal vein or inferior vena cava.

9.3d Spleen

The **spleen** is an intraperitoneal organ located in the hypochondriac region of the left upper quadrant (**Figs. 9.17, 9.18,** and **9.19**). It functions as a lymphoid gland and as a filter for old or abnormal red blood cells.

Fig. 9.16 ▶ **Pancreas and spleen**
Transverse section through L1 vertebra, inferior view.

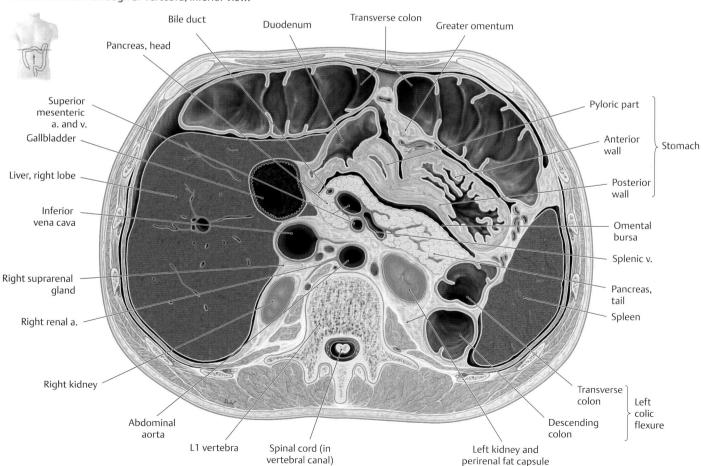

— Nestled under the dome of the diaphragm, the spleen does not normally project below the costal margin and therefore is not palpable on examination.
— The convex surface admits the splenic vessels and nerves at the **splenic hilum**.
— The spleen is connected to adjacent organs by peritoneal ligaments.

- The **splenorenal ligament**, which contains the branches of the splenic vessels and the tail of the pancreas, connects the spleen to the kidney.

- The **gastrosplenic ligament**, which contains the short gastric and left gastro-omental vessels, connects the spleen to the stomach.
- The **splenocolic ligament** connects the spleen to the left colic flexure.
- The **phrenicosplenic ligament** connects the spleen to the diaphragm.

— Although it is sheltered by the 9th, 10th, and 11th ribs, the spleen is particularly vulnerable to lacerations from fractured ribs, and because of its dense vascularity, it bleeds profusely.

Fig. 9.17 ▶ Pancreas and spleen: Location
Anterior view. RUQ, right upper quadrant; LUQ, left upper quadrant.

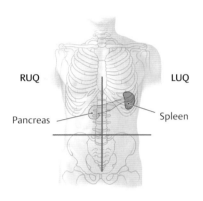

Fig. 9.18 ▶ Spleen
Visceral surface.

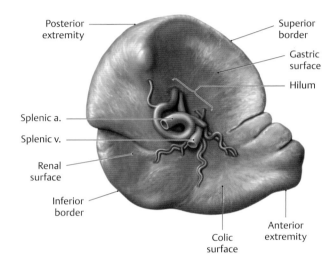

Fig. 9.19 ▶ The spleen in situ: peritoneal relationships
Anterior view into the left upper quadrant (LUQ) with the stomach removed.

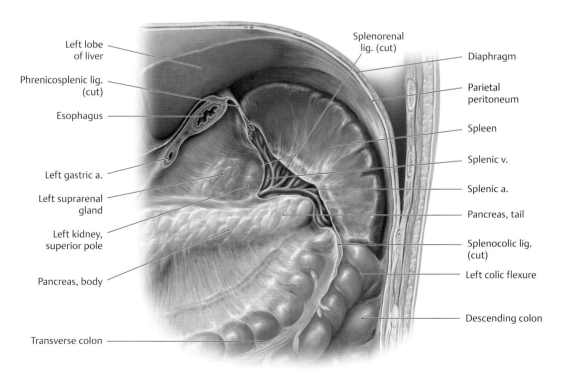

— Accessory spleens are common (20%) and are most often found within the gastrosplenic ligament, near the hilum or tail of the pancreas.

— The splenic artery, a large tortuous branch of the celiac trunk, divides within the splenorenal ligament at the splenic hilum (see **Fig. 8.11**).

— The spleen is vulnerable to infarction (interruption of the blood supply causing tissue death) because the splenic artery has no collateral arteries and is the gland's sole blood supply.

— The splenic vein courses behind the pancreas, where it joins with the superior mesenteric vein to form the portal vein (see **Fig. 8.16**).

— The splenic plexus, a derivative of the celiac plexus, innervates the spleen (see **Fig. 9.3A**).

Splenic trauma and splenectomy

Although the spleen appears to be well protected by the lower ribs on the posterior wall, it is the most frequently injured abdominal organ. It is particularly vulnerable to rupture from left-sided trauma that fractures the lower ribs. An enlarged spleen (splenomegaly) that projects below the costal margin may be vulnerable during blunt abdominal trauma that can rupture the thin splenic capsule. Splenic rupture results in severe hemorrhage and may require a total or partial splenectomy. During a total splenectomy the tail of the pancreas is vulnerable to injury where it passes through the splenorenal ligament with the splenic vessels.

Accessory spleens

Accessory spleens are small nodules of splenic tissue, usually ~1 cm in diameter, that form separate from the main spleen. They are usually located at the splenic hilum (commonly) near the tail of the pancreas, in the gastrosplenic or splenorenal ligament, in the mesentery, or near the ovary or testis.

9.4 Kidneys, Ureters, and Suprarenal Glands

9.4a The Kidneys

The **kidneys** are generally smooth-sided, reddish brown organs ~11 cm in length. They are retroperitoneal and lie anterior to the quadratus lumborum muscles on each side of the vertebral column between T12 and L3 vertebral levels (**Figs. 9.20** and **9.21**). The kidneys regulate blood pressure and the ionic balance and water content of the blood; they also eliminate metabolic waste and produce urine.

— The right kidney

  • lies anterior to the 12th rib, slightly lower than the left, because of the presence of the large right lobe of the liver.

  • lies posterior to the right suprarenal gland, liver, descending part of the duodenum, and right colic flexure of the large bowel.

— The left kidney

  • lies anterior to ribs 11 and 12.

  • lies posterior to the left suprarenal gland, spleen, tail of the pancreas, and left colic flexure.

— A **renal** (Gerota's) **fascia** surrounds each kidney and its associated suprarenal gland, renal vessels, ureter, and capsule of perirenal fat (**Fig. 9.22**). Pararenal fat lies outside this space and is thickest posteriorly.

Fig. 9.20 ▶ **Kidneys and suprarenal glands: Location**
Posterior view with the trunk wall opened.

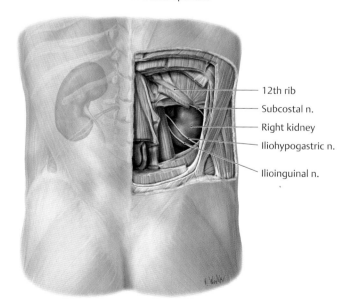

12th rib
Subcostal n.
Right kidney
Iliohypogastric n.
Ilioinguinal n.

Fig. 9.21 ► Kidneys and suprarenal glands in the retroperitoneum
Anterior view. Both the kidneys and suprarenal glands are retroperitoneal.
Removed: Intraperitoneal organs, along with portions of the ascending
and descending colon.

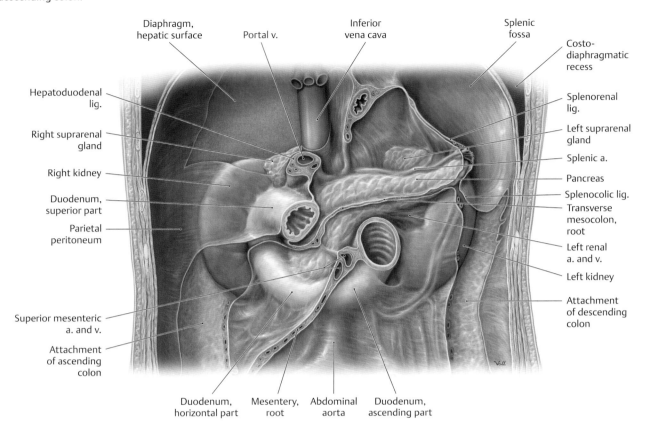

Fig. 9.22 ► Right kidney in the renal bed
Sagittal section through the right renal bed.

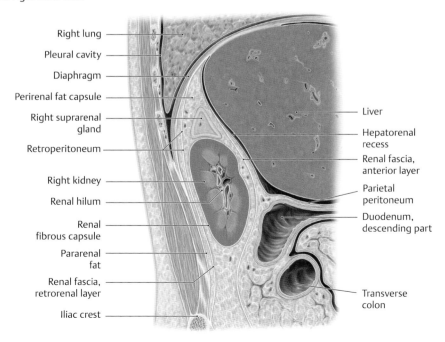

— Deep to the renal fascia, a thin, fibrous **renal capsule** completely invests each kidney.
— The lateral edge of the kidney is smooth and concave; the medial border has a vertical hilum that is pierced by the renal vein, renal artery, and renal pelvis. The hilum expands within the kidney as the **renal sinus**.
— Internally, the kidney consists of cortical and medullary regions, which contain up to 2 million nephrons, the renal functional units (**Fig. 9.23**).

  • The cortex, the outer region, lies deep to the fibrous capsule and extends into the medullary region as **renal columns**.
  • The medulla, the inner region, is arranged in **renal pyramids** with the broad base facing outward and the apex fitting into a cup-shaped **minor calyx**.

• Up to 11 minor calyces merge to form two or three **major calyces**, which combine to form the **renal pelvis**, the superior part of the ureter.

— A single renal artery, a direct branch of the abdominal aorta at L2, normally supplies each kidney (see **Figs. 8.9** and **8.12**).

  • The right renal artery is longer than the left artery and passes posterior to the inferior vena cava.
  • The artery divides near the hilum to supply anterior and posterior segments of the kidney, which are separated by an avascular longitudinal plane (Brodel's white line).

Fig. 9.23 ► **Kidney: Structure**
Right kidney. Midlongitudinal section, posterior view.

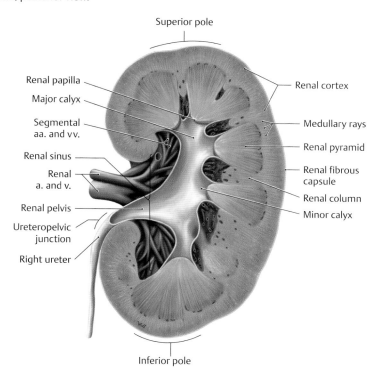

Superior pole

Renal papilla
Major calyx
Segmental aa. and vv.
Renal sinus
Renal a. and v.
Renal pelvis
Ureteropelvic junction
Right ureter

Renal cortex
Medullary rays
Renal pyramid
Renal fibrous capsule
Renal column
Minor calyx

Inferior pole

– A single renal vein from each kidney drains to the inferior vena cava (see **Fig. 8.15**).

  • Both renal veins receive a tributary from the ureter, but only the left renal vein receives the left suprarenal and left testicular or ovarian veins. On the right these veins drain directly into the inferior vena cava.

  • The left renal vein is longer than the right vein and passes anterior to the aorta immediately inferior to the origin of the superior mesenteric artery.

  • The longer length of the left renal vein makes the left kidney the preferred choice for organ donation.

Renal vein entrapment

The left renal vein crosses the midline in the narrow angle between the downwardly directed superior mesenteric artery and the abdominal aorta. Pathological conditions (atherosclerosis, aneurysms) of the arteries or downward pressure on the superior mesenteric artery can compress the renal vein. This is sometimes called the nutcracker syndrome.

– The renal plexus, an extension of the celiac plexus, forms a dense periarterial plexus along the renal arteries (**Fig. 9.24**).

  • Pain from renal disease is referred along the T12–L2 dermatomes to the lumbar and inguinal regions and the upper part of the anterior thigh.

Renal variations

Variations in renal vessels are common and usually asymptomatic. Kidneys develop in the pelvis and ascend to their location in the lumbar region between the 6th and 9th fetal weeks. As they ascend, more superior renal arteries and veins replace the inferior renal vessels. In ~30% of the population, failure of these inferior vessels to degenerate results in multiple renal arteries and veins.

During ascent, the inferior poles of the kidneys may fuse to form a single U-shaped structure, although they remain functionally separate. These "horseshoe kidneys" get trapped in their ascent under the inferior mesenteric artery and remain at the L3 or L4 level.

Fig. 9.24 ► **Autonomic innervation of the kidneys and upper ureters**

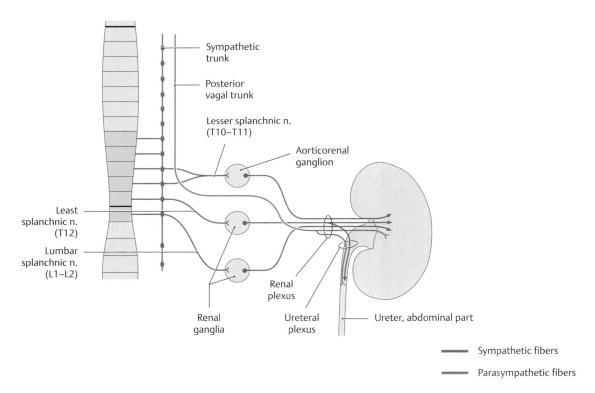

9.4b The Ureters

The **ureters** are muscular tubes, 25 to 30 cm in length, that convey urine from the kidneys to the bladder through peristaltic (wavelike) action (**Fig. 9.25**). Both the abdominal and the pelvic parts of the ureters are retroperitoneal along their entire course. The pelvic ureter is discussed further with the pelvic viscera in Chapter 11.

— Near the hilum of the kidney, the renal pelvis narrows to join with the origin of the ureter at the **ureteropelvic junction** (see **Fig. 9.23**).
— The abdominal part of the ureter descends along the anterior surface of the psoas muscle where it is crossed by the gonadal vessels.

Fig. 9.25 ▶ **Ureters in situ**
Retroperitoneum of male abdomen, anterior view. *Removed:* Nonurinary organs and rectal stump.

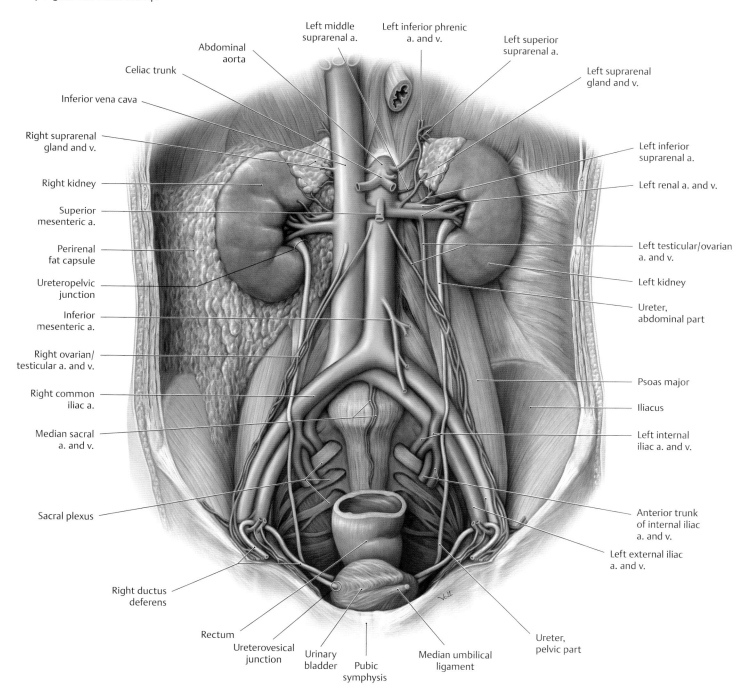

165

— The ureter crosses over the pelvic brim to enter the pelvis at the bifurcation of the common iliac artery into internal and external iliac branches.

— The pelvic part of the ureter travels anteriorly along the lateral pelvic wall before it enters the urinary bladder at the **uretero-vesical junction**.

— Constrictions of the ureter, caused by ureteral narrowing or compression by adjacent structures, can occur near its origin and along its length (**Fig. 9.26**).

— Branches from several arteries form a delicate anastomosis along the length of the ureter (see **Fig. 8.15**).

• In the abdomen, this network of vessels usually includes contributions from the abdominal aorta and the renal, gonadal (testicular or ovarian), and common iliac arteries.

• Branches of the superior vesical, inferior vesical, and uterine arteries supply the pelvic ureter.

— The veins of the ureter accompany the arteries.

— Contributions from the renal, aortic, and superior hypogastric plexuses innervate the abdominal ureter. The inferior hypogastric plexus innervates the pelvic ureter.

— Pain from the ureter is relayed along sympathetic routes to spinal cord segments T11–L2 and is referred to the corresponding dermatomes of the lower abdominal wall, inguinal region, and medial aspects of the thigh.

■ Calculi of the kidney and ureter

Calculi (stones) formed in the urine can become lodged in the renal calyces, renal pelvis, or ureter. Calculi lodged in the ureters distend the ureteric walls and cause intense intermittent pain as peristaltic contractions move the calculi inferiorly. As the calculi move toward the pelvis, pain moves from the lumbar to inguinal regions (T11–L2 dermatomes) and may extend into the scrotum and anterior thigh with branches of the genitofemoral nerve.

Fig. 9.26 ▶ **Anatomic constrictions of the ureter**
Right side, anterior view.

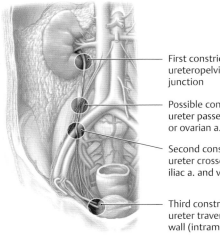

First constriction: ureteropelvic junction

Possible constriction where ureter passes behind testicular or ovarian a. and v.

Second constriction: ureter crosses over external iliac a. and v. (at the pelvic brim)

Third constriction: ureter traverses the bladder wall (intramural part)

9.4c Suprarenal Glands

The paired **suprarenal** (adrenal) **glands** are located in the retroperitoneum, where they cap the superior pole of each kidney and lie anterior to the crura of the diaphragm (see **Fig. 9.25**). The suprarenal glands are neuroendocrine glands that respond to stress.

— Perirenal fat and renal fascia surround both glands; a septum of the fascia separates them from the kidney.

— The right suprarenal gland is pyramidal, and the left is crescent shaped.

— The glands are composed of an outer cortex and an inner medulla. Both parts act as endocrine glands (i.e., secrete hormones) but differ from each other developmentally and functionally.

— The **cortex**

• is derived from mesoderm;

• is stimulated by hormones such as adrenocorticotrophic hormone (ACTH); and

• secretes hormones (corticosteroids and androgens), which influence blood pressure and blood volume by regulating sodium and water retention in the kidneys.

— The **medulla**

• is primarily composed of nervous tissue that is derived from neural crest cells (embryonic cells that migrate from the developing neural tube and give rise to a variety of structures associated with the peripheral nervous system);

• is stimulated by preganglionic sympathetic fibers from the celiac plexus; and

• contains **chromaffin cells** that function like sympathetic ganglia and secrete hormones (catecholamines) that increase heart rate, blood pressure, blood flow, and respiration.

— Veins and lymphatic vessels exit at the hilum on the anterior surface, but arteries and nerves access the glands at multiple points.

— Each suprarenal gland has multiple superior, middle, and inferior suprarenal arteries, which branch from the inferior phrenic, abdominal aorta, and renal arteries, respectively.

— A single suprarenal vein drains each gland. The right vein drains to the inferior vena cava; the left vein may join with the inferior phrenic vein before draining to the left renal vein.

— Preganglionic sympathetic fibers of the greater splanchnic nerve combine with fibers of the celiac plexus to form the suprarenal plexus, but they do not synapse on the celiac ganglia. These preganglionic fibers, which may be considered homologous with postganglionic sympathetic neurons, terminate directly on the chromaffin cells of the medulla.

Review Questions: Abdomen

1. An arteriogram performed on one of your patients revealed significant arterial disease (atherosclerosis) of the proximal 3 cm of the superior mesenteric artery, which narrowed the angle between the artery and the aorta. What structure normally crosses the aorta below the artery and is at risk of compression in this patient?
   A. Left renal vein
   B. Second part of the duodenum
   C. Jejunum
   D. Transverse colon
   E. Pancreas

2. A 12-year-old girl is seen in the emergency department for the suspicion of appendicitis. However, her pain is vague, and she doesn't complain when you gently press on her abdominal wall in the lower right quadrant. You are undeterred in your diagnosis, however, because you know that pain from an inflamed appendix refers first to another area of the abdomen based on its embryonic origins. Which of the following is true regarding referred pain from the appendix?
   A. As part of the embryonic foregut, pain is referred to the epigastric region.
   B. As part of the embryonic midgut, pain is referred to the epigastric region.
   C. As part of the embryonic midgut, pain is referred to the periumbilical region.
   D. As part of the embryonic hindgut, pain is referred to the hypogastric region.
   E. As part of the embryonic hindgut, pain is referred to the periumbilical region.

3. A renal abscess can irritate the nerves of the posterior abdominal wall. This is often referred to the dermatome that runs just above the inguinal ligament from the iliac crest to the pubis. Which nerves transmit this irritation?
   A. Lateral femoral cutaneous nerve
   B. Ilioinguinal and iliohypogastric nerves
   C. Femoral nerve
   D. Inferior phrenic nerve
   E. T10 intercostal nerve

4. Which of the following is true regarding the renal vessels?
   A. The right renal artery passes posterior to the inferior vena cava.
   B. Both renal veins receive tributaries from the suprarenal glands.
   C. The left renal vein is shorter than the right renal vein.
   D. Renal arteries are the most anterior structure in the renal hilum.
   E. Renal arteries arise from the aorta at the L4 vertebral level.

5. During a colectomy on a patient with colon cancer, you ask a medical student to describe characteristics of the descending colon. Her correct answer would include that it
   A. is supplied primarily by branches of the superior mesenteric artery
   B. receives parasympathetic innervation by the vagus nerve
   C. is marked by three teniae coli on its outer surface
   D. is primarily retroperitoneal
   E. is derived from the embryonic midgut

6. The external oblique muscle and aponeurosis contribute to the formation of all except which of the following structures?
   A. Umbilical ring
   B. Linea alba
   C. Conjoined tendon
   D. Inguinal ligament
   E. Superficial inguinal ring

7. Which of the following is true regarding the relations of the pancreas?
   A. The splenic artery runs along its inferior border.
   B. The portal vein forms anterior to the neck and body.
   C. The neck crosses the midline slightly superior to the transpyloric plane.
   D. The accessory pancreatic duct drains inferiorly to the horizontal part of the duodenum.
   E. It lies on the posterior wall of the omental bursa.

8. The artery that supplies blood directly to the pyloric region of the stomach is the
   A. left gastric artery
   B. short gastric artery
   C. right gastric artery
   D. left gastro-omental artery
   E. superior pancreaticoduodenal artery

9. Inferior to the arcuate line, the posterior layer of the rectus sheath is composed of the
   A. aponeurosis of the external oblique muscle
   B. aponeurosis of the internal oblique muscle
   C. aponeurosis of the transversus abdominis muscle
   D. transversalis fascia
   E. All of the above

10. One of your elderly patients has lost significant weight and complains of abdominal pain following meals. You know that his inferior mesenteric artery was ligated several years ago as part of an aortic aneurysm repair, and imaging reveals that his superior mesenteric artery is now severely narrowed at its origin. As a result, anastomosing vessels between the celiac trunk and the superior mesenteric artery are enlarged. What vessels are involved in this anastomosis?
    A. Marginal artery
    B. Pancreaticoduodenal arteries
    C. Gastro-omental artery
    D. Proper hepatic arteries
    E. Left gastric artery

11. A 46-year-old waitress is admitted to the emergency department with acute abdominal pain due to peritonitis from a ruptured duodenal ulcer. Imaging reveals an abscess in one of the peritoneal recesses. Which of the following is the lowest space within the peritoneal cavity where fluid accumulation and abscess formation are most likely to occur in a bedridden patient?
    A. Omental bursa
    B. Infracolic compartment
    C. Left paracolic gutter
    D. Subphrenic recess
    E. Hepatorenal recess

12. A young mother is determined to get into shape following the birth of her first child. She was humiliated in aerobics class when she could no longer do the required sit-ups. Strengthening which of the following muscles would help her accomplish this exercise?
    A. External oblique
    B. Internal oblique
    C. Rectus abdominis
    D. Psoas major
    E. All of the above

13. Which of the following vessels are involved in the venous drainage of the liver?
    A. Portal vein
    B. Hepatic vein
    C. Ductus venosus
    D. Umbilical vein
    E. All of the above

14. In patients who have conditions that affect the peritoneal cavity, such as an inflammation due to a perforated gastric ulcer, the abdominal wall muscles, in a "defense" reflex, become rigid and can be encountered as such during physical examination. Which of the following nerves contribute sensory and motor branches to this defense mechanism?
    A. Phrenic nerve
    B. Vagus nerve
    C. Intercostal nerves
    D. Lumbar splanchnic nerves.
    E. Greater splanchnic nerve

15. A pediatric surgeon is performing an appendectomy on a 10-year-old child, but upon entering the abdomen he finds a healthy appendix. With further exploration he finds an inflamed finger of bowel originating from the ileum ~2 feet from the ileocecal valve. It is connected to the umbilicus by a fibrous stalk. What embryonic structure failed to degenerate in this patient?
    A. Ductus venosus
    B. Umbilical vein
    C. Umbilical artery
    D. Omphalomesenteric duct
    E. Urachus

16. One of your patients suffers from multisystem disease as a result of his poor diet and long-term alcoholism. He exhibits many symptoms of chronic portal hypertension, but you suspect that some of his other symptoms have a different underlying cause. Which of the following symptoms are probably not associated with his portal hypertension?
    A. Esophageal varices
    B. Enlarged spleen
    C. Rectal varices
    D. Renal calculi
    E. Ascites (fluid in the peritoneal cavity)

17. A 6-month-old boy underwent surgery for an indirect inguinal hernia. The surgeon opened the superficial inguinal ring and located the hernia sac, which protruded through the abdominal wall
    A. below the inguinal ligament
    B. medial to the inferior epigastric vessels
    C. within the inguinal triangle
    D. at the deep inguinal ring
    E. above the conjoined tendon

18. Which of the following arteries supply branches to the stomach?
    A. Splenic artery
    B. Superior mesenteric artery
    C. Renal artery
    D. Marginal artery
    E. Middle colic artery

19. Your neighbor was recently diagnosed with liver cancer. His doctor explained that, because the primary tumor was in the bare area, it metastasized quickly to the posterior mediastinum and supraclavicular nodes. You recall that, although most lymph from the liver drains toward the celiac nodes and intestinal trunks, the bare area drains to bronchomediastinal trunks in the thorax. What is the bare area?
    A. An area on the diaphragmatic surface bounded by coronary and triangular ligaments
    B. The area of liver that lines the gallbladder fossa
    C. An area on the visceral surface surrounding the porta hepatis
    D. The space between the leaflets of the falciform ligament
    E. A subperitoneal fibrous capsule that covers the surface of the liver

20. A 58-year-old postal worker complained to his physician that he noticed a swelling in his scrotum that felt similar to "a bag of worms," that was present during the day but disappeared in the morning. On examination you are able to diagnose a varicocele of the pampiniform plexus that drains his left testis. What is the venous drainage of the testes?
    A. The right testis drains to the inferior vena cava; the left testis drains to the left common iliac vein.
    B. The right testis drains to the inferior vena cava; the left testis drains to the left renal vein.
    C. The right testis drains to the right renal vein; the left testis drains to the inferior vena cava.
    D. Both testes drain to ipsilateral renal veins.
    E. Both testes drain to the inferior vena cava.

21. In portal hypertension portocaval anastomoses allow portal blood to divert into the systemic system. These anastomoses might involve the
    A. pancreaticoduodenal vein
    B. periumbilical veins
    C. renal vein
    D. testicular vein
    E. None of the above

22. The bile duct is most often formed by the
    A. right and left hepatic ducts
    B. cystic duct and common hepatic duct
    C. main pancreatic duct and common hepatic duct
    D. hepatopancreatic duct and cystic duct
    E. main pancreatic duct and cystic duct

23. Within the testis, sperm are produced in the
    A. epididymis
    B. tunica albuginea
    C. ductus deferens
    D. rete testis
    E. seminiferous tubules

24. Lateral aortic lymph nodes
    A. drain to intestinal trunks
    B. include superior mesenteric nodes
    C. receive lymph from the ovaries and testes
    D. receive lymph from the pancreas
    E. bypass the cisterna chyli (chyle cistern) and drain directly into the thoracic duct

25. A man presented to his physician's office with the complaint of severe intermittent pain in the upper right quadrant of his abdomen. You recognize his condition as biliary colic due to gallstones lodged at the entrance to the gallbladder. What valve or sphincter maintains the opening of the cystic duct?
    A. Spiral valve
    B. Ileocecal valve
    C. Pyloric sphincter
    D. Sphincter of Oddi
    E. Major duodenal papilla

26. You routinely perform vasectomies at the free clinic in your area. You make a small incision at the top of the scrotum to access the spermatic cord. Ligation of which of the cord structures would be most effective in preventing the transmission of sperm?
    A. Testicular artery
    B. Pampiniform plexus
    C. Urachus
    D. Ductus deferens
    E. Epididymis

27. Sympathetic innervation of abdominal viscera is provided by
    A. pelvic splanchnic nerves
    B. vagus nerve
    C. lumbar splanchnic nerves
    D. subcostal nerve
    E. lumbar plexus

28. Which of the following structures forms as an intraperitoneal organ but becomes secondarily retroperitoneal during later development?
    A. Aorta
    B. Pancreas
    C. Spleen
    D. Transverse colon
    E. Kidney

29. Which of the following are reflections or remnants of peritoneum?
    A. Gerota's fascia
    B. Tunica albuginea
    C. Glisson's capsule
    D. Lesser omentum
    E. Medial umbilical ligament

30. Which of the following are tributaries of the inferior vena cava?
    A. Inferior mesenteric vein
    B. Lumbar vein
    C. Left gastric vein
    D. Inferior mesenteric vein
    E. Superior rectal vein

Answers and Explanations

1. **A** The left renal vein passes under the superior mesenteric artery as it crosses the aorta and can be compressed in the narrow angle (Section 9.4a).
   B The second part of the duodenum lies on the right side of the vertebral column and doesn't cross the aorta.
   C The jejunum is suspended by the mesentery that contains the superior mesenteric artery.
   D The transverse colon is suspended from the transverse mesocolon and lies anterior to the superior mesenteric artery.
   E The pancreas lies anterior to the superior mesenteric artery.

2. **C** The appendix is derived from the embryonic midgut, which refers pain to the periumbilical region (Section 9.1).
   A The appendix is derived from the embryonic midgut, not the foregut.
   B Midgut structures refer pain to the periumbilical region; foregut structures refer pain to the epigastric region.
   D The appendix is derived from the embryonic midgut, not the hindgut.
   E Pain from the appendix is referred to the periumbilical region, but it is not part of the embryonic hindgut.

3. **B** The pain is felt in the L1 dermatome innervated by the ilioinguinal and iliohypogastric nerves (Section 7.2d).
   A The lateral femoral cutaneous nerve transmits sensation from the lateral thigh.
   C The femoral nerve transmits sensation from the anterior thigh.
   D The inferior phrenic nerve transmits sensation from the inferior surface of the diaphragm.
   E The T10 intercostal nerve transmits sensation from the T10 dermatome at the level of the umbilicus.

4. **A** The right renal artery is longer than the left and passes posterior to the inferior vena cava (Section 9.4a).
   B The left suprarenal gland drains into the left renal vein, but the right suprarenal gland drains into the inferior vena cava.
   C The left renal vein crosses the aorta and is longer than the right renal vein.
   D At the renal hilum the renal veins are anterior to the renal arteries. The renal pelvis is the most posterior structure.
   E Renal arteries arise from the aorta at the L1/L2 vertebral level.

5. **C** The teniae coli, three longitudinal bands of muscle, are characteristics of the entire large intestine (Section 9.2c).
   A Branches of the inferior mesenteric artery supply the descending colon.
   B Pelvic splanchnic nerves provide parasympathetic innervation to the descending colon.
   D The descending colon forms with the gastrointestinal tract as an intraperitoneal organ and loses its mesentery during later development, becoming secondarily retroperitoneal.
   E The descending colon is part of the embryonic hindgut.

6. **C** The conjoined tendon is formed by the aponeuroses of the internal oblique and transversus abdominis muscles (Section 7.1b).
   A The umbilical ring, a remnant of the opening for the umbilical cord, interrupts the linea alba at the L4 vertebral level.
   B The linea alba is a tendinous raphe formed in the midline by the aponeuroses of the three anterior abdominal wall muscles.
   D The lower edge of the external oblique muscle is thickened and curved inward to form the inguinal ligament.
   E The superficial inguinal ring is a defect in the aponeurosis of the external oblique muscles that allows passage of the spermatic cord.

7. **E** The pancreas lies behind the stomach on the posterior wall of the omental bursa (Section 9.3c).
   A The splenic artery runs along the superior border of the pancreas.
   B The portal vein forms by the union of the splenic and superior mesenteric veins posterior to the neck of the pancreas.
   C The neck and body cross the midline slightly below the transpyloric plane at approximately the L2 vertebral level.
   D The accessory pancreatic duct drains into the descending part of the duodenum, superior to the drainage of the main pancreatic duct.

8. **C** The right gastric artery, a branch of the proper hepatic artery, supplies the pyloric region (Sections 8.2a and 9.2a).
   A The left gastric artery supplies blood to the cardiac part of the stomach and the gastroesophageal sphincter.
   B The short gastric arteries supply blood to the fundus of the stomach.
   D The left gastro-omental artery supplies blood to the greater curvature of the stomach and the greater omentum.
   E The superior pancreaticoduodenal artery supplies blood to the descending duodenum and the head of the pancreas.

9. **D** Inferior to the arcuate line, the posterior wall of the rectus sheath is composed of transversalis fascia (Section 7.1b).
   A The external oblique muscle only contributes to the anterior layer of the rectus sheath.
   B The internal oblique muscle forms part of the posterior layer of the rectus sheath above the arcuate line and part of the anterior layer of the rectus sheath below the arcuate line.
   C The transversus abdominis forms part of the anterior layer of the rectus sheath below the arcuate line.
   E Not applicable.

10. **B** The superior pancreaticoduodenal arteries arise from the gastroduodenal artery (a secondary branch of the celiac trunk). The inferior pancreaticoduodenal arteries arise from the superior mesenteric artery. These vessels anastomose within the head of the pancreas and can enlarge significantly to form an effective collateral pathway (Section 8.2a).
    A The marginal artery establishes a collateral circulation between the superior mesenteric and inferior mesenteric arteries but does not communicate directly with branches of the celiac trunk.
    C The gastro-omental arteries anastomose with the gastroduodenal and splenic arteries but do not communicate with the superior mesenteric artery.
    D The proper hepatic artery anastomoses with the left gastric artery through its right gastric branch but it does not communicate directly with the superior mesenteric artery.
    E The left gastric artery anastomoses with the hepatic and splenic arteries but does not communicate directly with the superior mesenteric artery.

11. **E** The hepatorenal recess, which is continuous with the subphrenic recess, is the lowest and most gravity-dependent space in the peritoneal cavity. Therefore, it is a common site for fluid collection and abscess formation (Section 8.1d).
    A Fluid from the omental bursa flows into the hepatorenal recess.
    B The infracolic compartment lies below the transverse mesocolon and is separated into right and left sides by the mesentery of the small intestine. Fluid in this space can drain to the paracolic gutters and the pelvis.
    C Fluid in the left paracolic gutter would likely drain to the pelvis.
    D Fluid in the subphrenic recess drains to the more gravity-dependent hepatorenal recess in the supine patient.

12. **E** The external oblique, internal oblique, and rectus abdominis muscles flex the trunk when acting bilaterally and help stabilize the pelvis. The psoas major assists in raising the trunk from the supine position (Section 7.1b).
    A The external oblique muscles flex the trunk when acting bilaterally and help stabilize the pelvis. B through D are also correct (E).
    B The internal oblique muscles flex the trunk when acting bilaterally and help stabilize the pelvis. A, C, and D are also correct (E).
    C The rectus abdominis flexes the trunk, compresses the abdomen, and stabilizes the pelvis. A, B, and D are also correct (E).
    D The psoas major flexes the hip and assists in raising the trunk from the supine position. A through C are also correct (E).

13. **B** Three hepatic veins of the liver drain into the inferior vena cava immediately below the diaphragm (Section 9.3a).
    A The portal vein carries blood from the gastrointestinal organs into the liver.
    C During fetal life, the ductus venosus shunts placental blood from the umbilical vein to the inferior vena cava, allowing it to bypass the liver circulation.
    D The umbilical vein is part of the fetal circulation that transports oxygenated blood from the placenta to the ductus venosus in the liver.
    E Only the hepatic veins are involved in venous drainage of the liver.

14. **C** The intercostal nerves are instrumental in the ability to sense, and react to, abdominal pain as they innervate the parietal peritoneum (sensory branches) and the abdominal wall muscles (motor branches). Inflammation of the parietal peritoneum can cause severe pain. The visceral peritoneum is not very sensitive (Section 8.1c).
    A The phrenic nerve innervates the diaphragm but does not contribute to the innervation of the abdominal wall muscles.
    B The vagus nerve innervates neither the peritoneum nor the abdominal wall muscles.
    D Lumbar splanchnic nerves carry sympathetic fibers that innervate abdominal viscera.
    E The greater splanchnic nerve carries only sympathetic fibers, which innervate abdominal viscera.

15. **D** The omphalomesenteric duct (yolk stalk) has failed to regress and remains as an ileal (Meckel's) diverticulum (Section 9.1).
A The ductus venosus diverts blood in the umbilical vein into the inferior vena cava in the fetus.
B The remnant of the umbilical vein, the round ligament (ligamentum teres), runs in the inferior edge of the falciform ligament, which connects the liver to the anterior abdominal wall.
C The medial umbilical ligament on the anterior abdominal wall is the remnant of the umbilical artery.
E The urachus, the remnant of the fetal allantois, extends superiorly on the anterior abdominal wall from the apex of the bladder to the umbilicus, as the median umbilical ligament.

16. **D** Renal calculi form in the kidney from concentrated urine and are associated with inflammatory bowel disease and other pathology but are not a symptom of portal hypertension (Section 9.3a).
A Esophageal veins that drain superiorly to the azygos (systemic) system and inferiorly to the portal system form an important portocaval anastomosis. Varices of these veins are a typical symptom of portal hypertension.
B In portal hypertension, flow through the splenic vein slows, causing the spleen to enlarge abnormally (splenomegaly).
C Rectal veins drain superiorly to the portal system and inferiorly to the systemic system. In portal hypertension they enlarge (forming varices) to accommodate the greater flow into the systemic system.
E Ascites is a typical symptom of portal hypertension due to liver disease.

17. **D** Indirect inguinal hernias pass through the deep inguinal ring, which is lateral to the inferior epigastric vessels and superior to the inguinal ligament (Section 7.3a).
A Inguinal hernias are located above the inguinal ligament; femoral hernias are located below the ligament.
B Indirect inguinal hernias are located lateral to the inferior epigastric vessels; direct inguinal hernias are located medial to the vessels.
C Direct inguinal hernias protrude through the inguinal triangle; indirect inguinal hernias protrude through the deep inguinal ring lateral to the triangle.
E The aponeuroses of the internal oblique and transversus abdominis muscles form the conjoined tendon where they attach to the pubic ramus. This is not a common site for hernias.

18. **A** Short gastric and left gastro-omental arteries that supply the wall of the stomach are branches of the splenic artery (Sections 8.2a and 9.2a).
B The superior mesenteric artery supplies the midgut and does not normally supply the stomach.
C The renal arteries supply no branches to gastrointestinal organs.
D The marginal artery is an anastomotic connection between branches of the superior mesenteric and inferior mesenteric arteries but has no branches that supply the stomach.
E The middle colic artery is a branch of the superior mesenteric artery that supplies the transverse colon.

19. **A** The bare area is an area devoid of peritoneum adjacent to the inferior surface of the diaphragm bounded by the coronary and triangular ligaments (Section 9.3a).
B The fossa of the gallbladder on the visceral surface of the liver is also devoid of peritoneum but is not known as the bare area.
C Peritoneum covers the surface of the liver around the porta hepatis, the entry site for the structures of the portal triad.
D The leaflets of the falciform ligament do not contain the bare area, but on the surface of the liver the leaflets separate to form the coronary ligaments, which surround the bare area.
E The subperitoneal fibrous capsule of the liver is Glisson's capsule, not the bare area.

20. **B** The right testicular vein drains into the inferior vena cava, but the left vein drains into the left renal vein. The angle at which the left testicular vein enters the left renal vein increases its susceptibility to obstruction. This is probably the reason why varicoceles are most commonly found on the left side (Section 7.3c).
A Neither testis drains to the common iliac vein.
C The right testis drains to the inferior vena cava, and the left drains to the left renal vein.
D Although the left testis drains to the ipsilateral renal vein, the right testis drains directly to the inferior vena cava.
E Although the right testis drains directly to the inferior vena cava, the left testis drains to the ipsilateral renal vein.

21. **B** Periumbilical veins anastomose with veins on the anterior abdominal wall and act as a portocaval shunt in severe portal hypertension (Section 8.2b).
A Pancreaticoduodenal veins drain to the portal vein but do not anastomose with veins of the systemic system.
C Renal veins drain into the inferior vena cava and do not connect to the portal system.
D Testicular veins drain to the systemic system and do not anastomose with the portal system.
E Not applicable.

22. **B** The common hepatic duct of the liver joins the cystic duct of the gallbladder to form the bile duct (Section 9.3b).
A The right and left hepatic ducts join to form the common hepatic duct.
C The main pancreatic duct joins the common hepatic duct to form the hepatopancreatic ampulla.
D The cystic duct does not join the hepatopancreatic duct. It joins the common hepatic duct to form the common bile duct.
E The main pancreatic duct does not join the cystic duct.

23. **E** Seminiferous tubules are highly coiled structures within the lobes of the testes where sperm are produced (Section 7.3c).
A The epididymis is a site of sperm storage and maturation.
B The tunica albuginea is the tough connective tissue capsule of the testis.
C The ductus deferens transports sperm along the spermatic cord to the deep pelvis.
D The rete testis is a network of ducts through which sperm exit the testis.

24. **C** Lateral aortic nodes drain the abdominal wall and structures of the retroperitoneum, including the gonads (Section 8.2c).
A Lateral aortic nodes drain to lumbar trunks. Preaortic nodes drain to intestinal trunks.
B Superior mesenteric, inferior mesenteric, and celiac nodes are part of the preaortic group of lymph nodes that drain the gastrointestinal tract.
D The pancreas and other organs associated with the gastrointestinal tract drain to preaortic nodes.
E Lumbar trunks, which receive lymph from the lateral aortic nodes, drain into the chyle cistern (cisterna chyli) with the intestinal trunks that drain the gastrointestinal tract. If the chyle cistern is absent, the trunks drain directly into the thoracic duct.

25. **A** The spiral valve in the neck of the gallbladder maintains the opening of the cystic duct (Section 9.3b).
B The ileocecal valve is located between the ileum and cecum.
C The pyloric sphincter is located between the pylorus of the stomach and the first part of the duodenum.
D The sphincter of Oddi surrounds the hepatopancreatic ampulla as it enters the descending part of the duodenum at the major duodenal papilla.
E The major duodenal papilla is an elevation on the medial wall of the descending part of the duodenum where the hepatopancreatic ampulla (formed by the union of the bile duct and pancreatic duct) enters.

26. **D** The ductus deferens is the structure within the spermatic cord that transmits sperm (Section 7.3d).
A The testicular artery does not transmit sperm.
B The pampiniform plexus is a venous plexus that drains the testis.
C The urachus connects the apex of the bladder to the umbilicus and transmits urine in the fetus.
E The epididymis is a site for sperm maturation and storage located within the scrotal sac on the posterior surface of the testis.

27. **C** Lumbar splanchnic nerves (T11–L2) innervate abdominal viscera (Section 8.2d).
A Pelvic splanchnic nerves carry only parasympathetic fibers.
B The vagus nerve provides parasympathetic innervation to most abdominal viscera (except hindgut structures).
D The subcostal nerve is a somatic nerve that innervates part of the abdominal wall.
E The lumbar plexus is a somatic plexus whose nerves innervate the lower abdominal wall and lower limb.

28. **B** Most of the pancreas is secondarily retroperitoneal. The tail of the pancreas lies within the splenorenal ligament and is considered intraperitoneal (Sections 8.1a and 9.3c).
A The abdominal aorta is retroperitoneal and lies on the left side of the vertebral bodies.
C The spleen is completely intraperitoneal, supported by the gastrosplenic ligament and the splenorenal ligament.
D The transverse colon is intraperitoneal, supported by its transverse mesocolon.
E The kidney is a primary retroperitoneal organ, surrounded by perirenal fat and covered by peritoneum only on its anterior surface.

29. **D** The lesser omentum is a two-layer peritoneal membrane that connects the liver to the stomach and duodenum (Section 8.1b).
A Gerota's fascia is the renal fascia that surrounds the kidney, suprarenal glands, renal vessels, and perirenal fat.
B The tunica albuginea is the tough outer fibrous membrane that surrounds the testis and invaginates to form the testicular lobes.
C Glisson's capsule is a subperitoneal fibrous capsule that surrounds the liver.
E The medial umbilical ligament is the remnant of the umbilical artery on the anterior abdominal wall.

30. **B** The four lumbar veins on each side drain the posterior abdominal wall and terminate in the inferior vena cava (Section 8.2b).
A The inferior mesenteric vein terminates either in the superior mesenteric or in the splenic veins, which are tributaries of the portal vein.
C The left gastric vein drains into the portal vein.
D The inferior mesenteric vein joins with the superior mesenteric vein to form the portal vein.
E The superior rectal vein drains superiorly to the inferior mesenteric vein, which is a tributary of the portal system.

10   Overview of the Pelvis and Perineum

The pelvic region is the area of the trunk between the abdomen and lower limb. It includes the **pelvic cavity**, the bowl-shaped space enclosed by the bony pelvis, and the **perineum**, the diamond-shaped area inferior to the pelvic floor and between the upper aspects of the thighs.

10.1 General Features

— **Table 10.1** provides an overview of the divisions of the pelvis and perineum.

  • The bony pelvis, or pelvic girdle, encloses the pelvic cavity. Its superior bony landmark is the iliac crest (**Fig. 10.1**).

  • The **pelvic brim** at the plane of the **pelvic inlet** defines the upper border of the bony **true pelvis** (birth canal) and separates it from the **false pelvis** above. A **pelvic outlet** defines the lower border of the true pelvis (**Fig. 10.2A** and **B**).

Fig. 10.1 ► **Pelvic girdle**
Anterosuperior view. The pelvic girdle consists of the two hip bones and the sacrum.

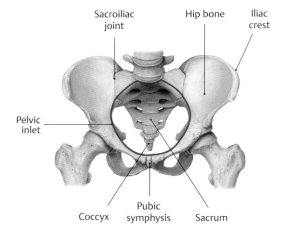

Fig. 10.2 ► **True and false pelvis**

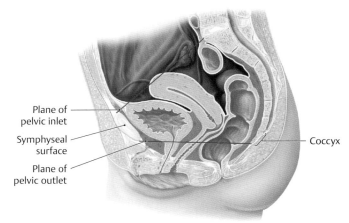

A Female.

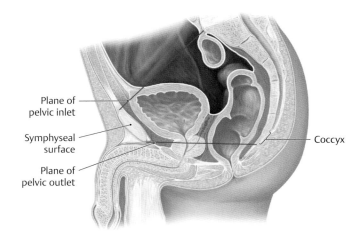

B Male.

Table 10.1 ▶ Divisions of the Pelvis and Perineum

The levels of the pelvis are determined by bony landmarks (iliac alae and pelvic inlet/brim). The contents of the perineum are separated from the true pelvis by the pelvic diaphragm and two fascial layers.

Iliac crest

Pelvis	**False pelvis**	Ileum (coils)
		Cecum and appendix
		Sigmoid colon
		Common and external iliac aa. and vv.
		Lumbar plexus (branches)
	Pelvic inlet	
	True pelvis	Distal ureters
		Urinary bladder
		Rectum
		Male: ductus deferens, seminal gland, and prostate
		Female: vagina, uterus, uterine tubes, and ovaries
		Internal iliac a. and v. and branches
		Sacral plexus
		Inferior hypogastric plexus

Pelvic diaphragm (levator ani with superior and inferior fascia of pelvic diaphragm)

Perineum	**Deep space**	External urethral sphincter and deep transverse perineal mm; Female: compressor urethrae and urethrovaginal sphincter
		Urethra (membranous)
		Vagina
		Rectum
		Bulbourethral gland
		Ischioanal fossa
		Internal pudendal a. and v., pudendal n. and branches
	Perineal membrane	
	Superficial space	Ischiocavernosus, bulbocavernosus, and superficial transverse perineal mm.
		Urethra (penile)
		Male: penis
		Female: clitoris, vestibular bulb, vestibular glands
		Internal pudendal a. and v., pudendal n. and branches
	Superficial perineal (Colles') fascia	
	Subcutaneous perineal space	Fat

Skin

• The muscular floor of the pelvic cavity, the **pelvic diaphragm**, separates the true pelvis from the perineum, which lies below it (**Fig. 10.3A** and **B**).

• The diamond-shaped perineum is subdivided into an anterior **urogenital triangle** and a posterior **anal triangle** (**Fig. 10.4A** and **B**).

• A membranous **perineal membrane** divides the urogenital triangle into two small spaces, an upper **deep space** and a lower **superficial space** (see **Fig. 11.13**). This membrane is not present in the anal triangle (see **Fig. 11.19**).

Fig. 10.3 ► **Pelvis and urogenital triangle of the perineum**
Coronal section, anterior view.

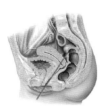

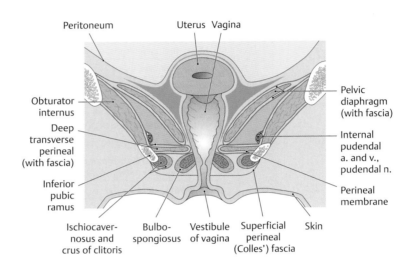

A Female.

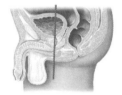

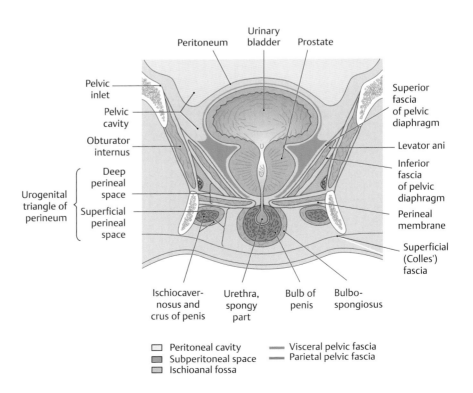

B Male.

Fig. 10.4 ► **Regions of the perineum**
Lithotomy position, caudal (inferior) view.

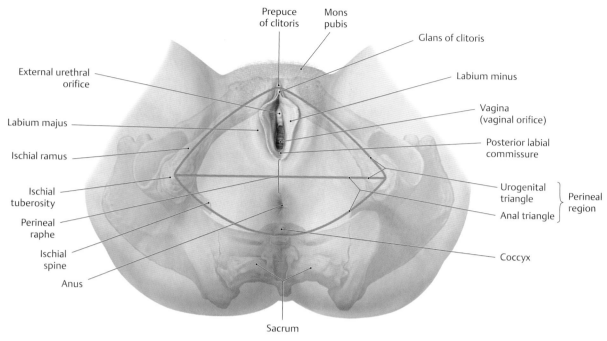

A Female.

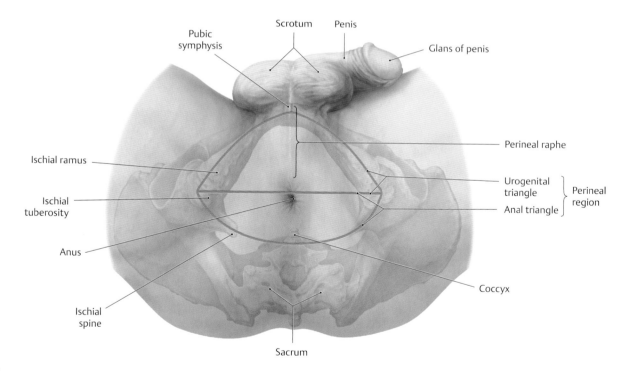

B Male.

— The pelvic inlet and pelvic outlet are apertures of the bony pelvis (**Fig. 10.5A** and **B**).

• The pelvic inlet (pelvic brim), the superior aperture, is defined by a line that extends from the promontory of the sacrum, along the arcuate line of the ilium and pectineal line of the pubic bone, to the superior border of the pubic symphysis.

• The pelvic outlet, the inferior aperture, is defined by a line that connects the coccyx, sacrotuberous ligaments, ischial tuberosities, ischiopubic rami, and inferior border of the pubic symphysis.

Fig. 10.5 ▸ **Pelvic inlet and outlet**

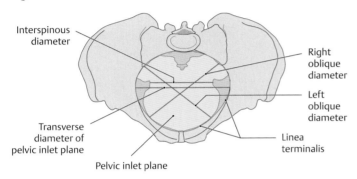

A Female pelvis, superior view. Pelvic inlet outlined in red.

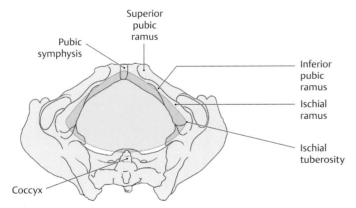

B Female pelvis, inferior view. Pelvic outlet outlined in red.

Pelvic diameters: true conjugate, diagonal conjugate

Pelvic measurements are important obstetric predictors of ease of vaginal delivery. The true conjugate, the narrowest anteroposterior diameter of the birth canal, is measured from the upper border of the pubic symphysis to the tip of the sacral promontory (~11 cm). Because this distance is difficult to measure accurately, the diagonal conjugate is used to estimate it. This is measured from the lower border of the pubic symphysis to the tip of the sacral promontory (~12.5 cm).

— The cavities of the true pelvis and the false pelvis are continuous with each other but contain different viscera.

• The **true pelvis** lies below the pelvic brim and is bounded inferiorly by the muscular pelvic floor. In the adult, this space houses the bladder, rectum, and pelvic genital structures.

• The **false pelvis** is the lower part of the abdominal cavity that lies above the pelvic brim and is bounded on each side by the iliac fossa. It contains the cecum, appendix, sigmoid colon, and loops of the small intestine.

— The peritoneum of the abdominal cavity continues into the pelvic cavity.

• The peritoneum of the anterior abdominal wall drapes over the bladder, uterus, rectum, and pelvic walls, but it does not extend as far inferiorly as the pelvic floor.

• Deep pelvic viscera that lie below the peritoneum occupy a **subperitoneal space** that is continuous with the retroperitoneum of the abdomen (see **Fig. 10.3A** and **B**).

— The perineum lies inferior to the pelvic cavity (see **Fig. 10.4A** and **B**).

• The pelvic outlet forms the perimeter of the perineum, the pelvic diaphragm forms its roof, and, inferiorly, perineal skin forms its floor.

• The urogenital triangle of the perineum contains the external genital structures and openings for the urethra and vagina (in females).

• The anal triangle of the perineum contains the anal opening and anal canal, surrounded by the external anal sphincter.

— The **ischioanal fossae**, wedge-shaped, fat-filled spaces of the anal triangle, lie on either side of the anal canal and extend anteriorly into a small recess of the urogenital triangle (see Section 12.5b).

10.2 The Bony Pelvis

The bony pelvis, or **pelvic girdle**, consists of the sacrum, the coccyx, and the two **hip (coxal) bones**. It protects the pelvic viscera, stabilizes the back, and provides an attachment site for the lower limbs. Pelvic joints create the circular configuration of the pelvic girdle, which is maintained by strong pelvic ligaments (see **Fig. 10.1**).

— The sacrum and coccyx, the lowest segments of the vertebral column, constitute the posterior wall of the pelvic girdle.

— The hip bone, the lateral part of the pelvic girdle, is formed by the fusion of three bones: the **ilium**, **ischium**, and **pubis** (**Fig. 10.6**). Features of the hip bone (**Fig. 10.7A and B**) include the following:

  • The **superior** and **inferior pubic rami**, which join anteriorly but diverge laterally around the large **obturator foramen**
  • The **ischial spine** posteriorly, which separates the **greater** and **lesser sciatic notches**
  • The **ischial ramus**, which fuses with the **inferior pubic ramus** anteriorly and ends as the **ischial tuberosity** posteriorly

  • The **iliac wing**, which is concave anteriorly, forming the **iliac fossa**. The superior edge of the iliac wing, the **iliac crest**, ends anteriorly as the **anterior superior iliac spine** and posteriorly as the **posterior superior iliac spine**.
  • An **arcuate line** on the internal surface, which bisects the ilium and continues anteriorly to join with the **pectineal line** of the pubis. Both lines form part of the pelvic inlet.
  • A deep, cup-shaped depression, the **acetabulum,** on the lateral surface, which articulates with the femur of the lower limb

— The joints of the pelvic girdle include the following (see **Fig. 10.1**):

  • The paired **sacroiliac joints,** which are synovial joints between the auricular surfaces of the sacrum and the hip bones
  • The **pubic symphysis**, an immobile cartilaginous joint in the anterior midline that joins the pubic portions of the hip bones with an intervening fibrocartilaginous disk

Fig. 10.6 ► **Triradiate cartilage of the hip bone**
Right hip bone, lateral view. The hip bone consists of the ilium, ischium, and pubis.

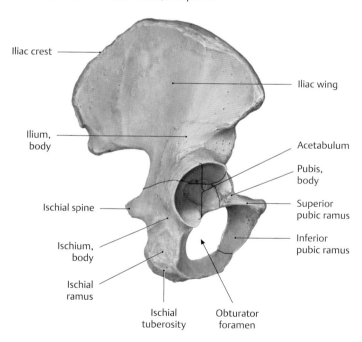

Fig. 10.7 ► **Hip bone**
Right hip bone (male).

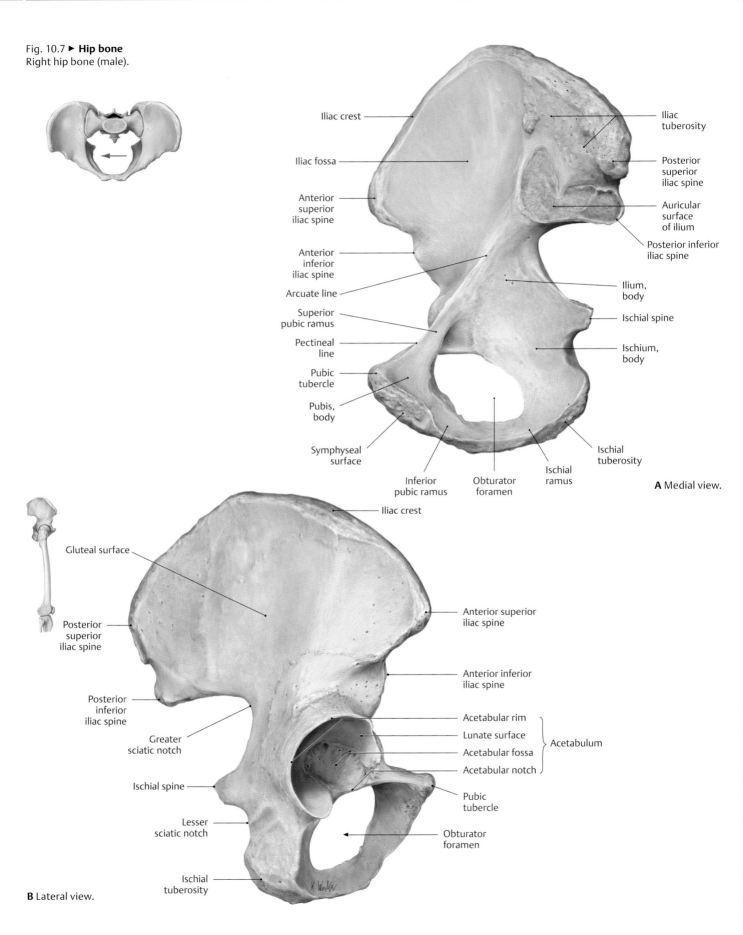

Iliac crest

Iliac tuberosity

Iliac fossa

Posterior superior iliac spine

Anterior superior iliac spine

Auricular surface of ilium

Anterior inferior iliac spine

Posterior inferior iliac spine

Arcuate line

Ilium, body

Superior pubic ramus

Ischial spine

Pectineal line

Ischium, body

Pubic tubercle

Pubis, body

Symphyseal surface

Ischial tuberosity

Inferior pubic ramus

Obturator foramen

Ischial ramus

A Medial view.

Iliac crest

Gluteal surface

Posterior superior iliac spine

Anterior superior iliac spine

Anterior inferior iliac spine

Posterior inferior iliac spine

Acetabular rim

Lunate surface

Acetabular fossa

Acetabulum

Greater sciatic notch

Acetabular notch

Ischial spine

Pubic tubercle

Lesser sciatic notch

Obturator foramen

Ischial tuberosity

B Lateral view.

— Ligaments that support pelvic joints include the following (**Fig. 10.8A** and **B**):
  • The strong **anterior**, **posterior**, and **interosseous sacroiliac ligaments** that support the sacroiliac joints
  • The **iliolumbar ligaments** that stabilize the junction between the lumbar spine and sacrum

• Two pairs of posterior ligaments that secure the sacrum and hip bone articulations and resist posterior displacement of the sacrum
  1. The **sacrotuberous ligament** originates on the sacrum and inserts on the ischial tuberosity.
  2. The **sacrospinous ligament** originates on the sacrum and inserts on the ischial spine.

Fig. 10.8 ► **Ligaments of the pelvis**
Male pelvis.

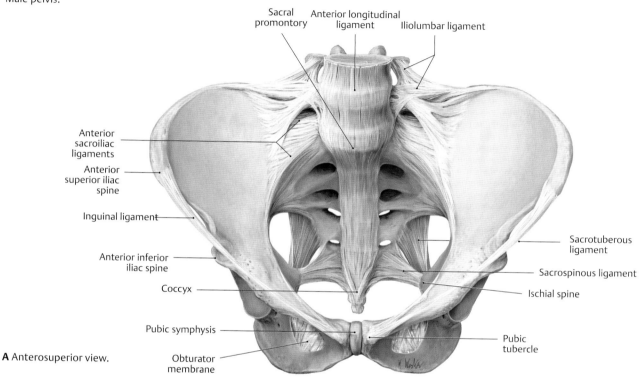

Sacral promontory
Anterior longitudinal ligament
Iliolumbar ligament
Anterior sacroiliac ligaments
Anterior superior iliac spine
Inguinal ligament
Anterior inferior iliac spine
Coccyx
Pubic symphysis
Obturator membrane
Sacrotuberous ligament
Sacrospinous ligament
Ischial spine
Pubic tubercle

A Anterosuperior view.

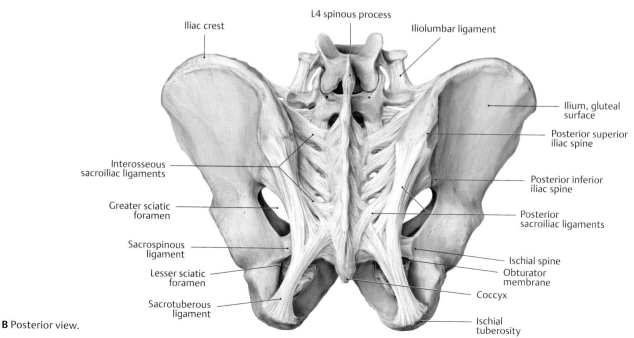

Iliac crest
L4 spinous process
Iliolumbar ligament
Ilium, gluteal surface
Posterior superior iliac spine
Posterior inferior iliac spine
Posterior sacroiliac ligaments
Interosseous sacroiliac ligaments
Greater sciatic foramen
Sacrospinous ligament
Lesser sciatic foramen
Sacrotuberous ligament
Ischial spine
Obturator membrane
Coccyx
Ischial tuberosity

B Posterior view.

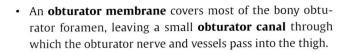

— The pelvic bones and ligaments form openings that allow pelvic vessels, nerves, and muscles to connect to adjacent regions (**Fig. 10.9**).

• The **greater sciatic foramen** is a posterior opening that connects the pelvis to the gluteal region (the buttocks).
• The **lesser sciatic foramen** is a passageway between the sacrotuberous and sacrospinous ligaments that connects the gluteal region and perineum.

Fig. 10.9 ▶ **Pelvic openings**
Right half of male pelvis, medial view.

• An **obturator membrane** covers most of the bony obturator foramen, leaving a small **obturator canal** through which the obturator nerve and vessels pass into the thigh.

10.3 Pelvic Walls and Floor (**Fig. 10.10A, B,** and **C, Table 10.2**)

— The muscles that line the pelvic walls pass into the gluteal region, where they attach to the femur (thigh bone) and act on the hip joint.

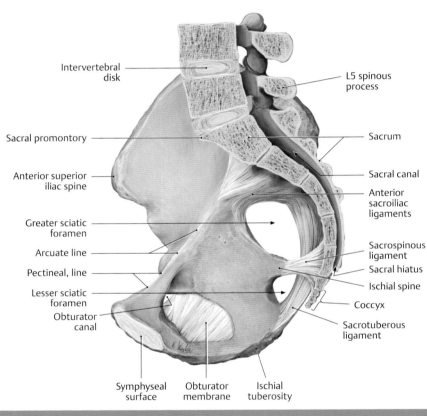

| | Intervertebral disk | L5 spinous process | Sacral promontory | Sacrum | Anterior superior iliac spine | Sacral canal | Greater sciatic foramen | Anterior sacroiliac ligaments | Arcuate line | Sacrospinous ligament | Pectineal, line | Sacral hiatus | Lesser sciatic foramen | Ischial spine | Obturator canal | Coccyx | Sacrotuberous ligament | Symphyseal surface | Obturator membrane | Ischial tuberosity |

Table 10.2 ▶ **Muscles of the Pelvic Floor**				
Muscle		**Origin**	**Insertion**	**Innervation**	**Action**

Muscle		**Origin**	**Insertion**	**Innervation**	**Action**
Muscles of the pelvic diaphragm					
Levator ani	Puborectalis	Superior pubic ramus (both sides of pubic symphysis)	Anococcygeal ligament	Direct branches of sacral plexus (S4), inferior anal n.	Pelvic diaphragm: Supports pelvic viscera
	Pubococcygeus	Pubis (lateral to origin of puborectalis)	Anococcygeal ligament, coccyx		
	Iliococcygeus	Internal obturator fascia of levator ani (tendinous arch)			
Coccygeus		Sacrum (inferior end)	Ischial spine	Direct branches from sacral plexus (S4–S5)	Supports pelvic viscera, flexes coccyx
Muscles of the pelvic wall (parietal muscles)					
Piriformis		Sacrum (pelvic surface)	Femur (apex of greater trochanter)	Direct branches from sacral plexus (S1–S2)	Hip joint: External rotation, stabilization, and abduction of flexed hip
Obturator internus		Obturator membrane and bony boundaries (inner surface)	Femur (greater trochanter, medial surface)	Direct branches from sacral plexus (L5–S1)	Hip joint: External rotation and abduction of flexed hip

- The **piriformis** lines the posterior wall of the pelvis.
  - It passes from the pelvis to the gluteal region through the greater sciatic foramen.
  - It forms the bed for the sacral plexus and internal iliac vessels on the posterior pelvic wall.
- The **obturator internus**, covered by an overlying **obturator fascia**, lines the sidewall of the pelvis and perineum.
  - Its tendon passes from the perineum to the gluteal region through the lesser sciatic foramen.
  - A thickening of the obturator fascia, the **tendinous arch of the levator ani**, runs from the body of the pubis to the ischial spine.

Fig. 10.10 ▸ **Muscles of the pelvic floor**
Female pelvis.

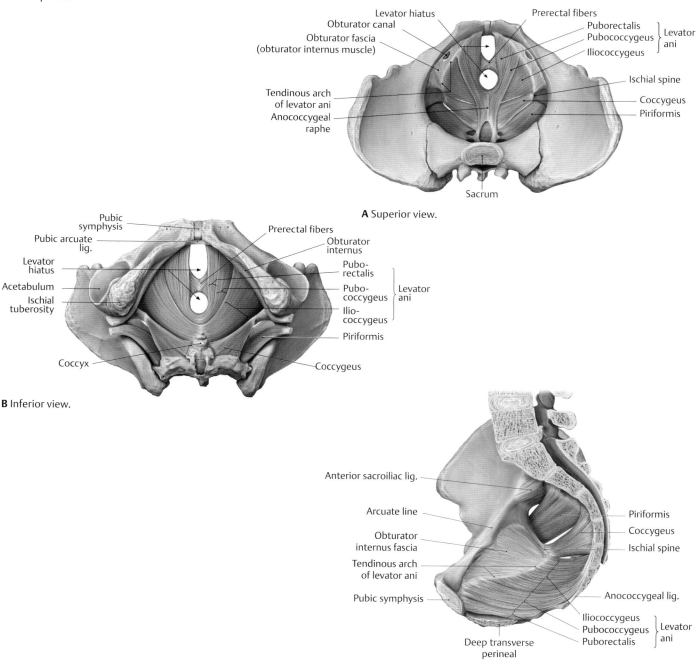

A Superior view.

B Inferior view.

C Medial view of right hemipelvis.

— The funnel-shaped pelvic floor is composed of muscles, collectively known as the **pelvic diaphragm**, that support the pelvic viscera and resist intra-abdominal pressure (i.e., pressure created during coughing, sneezing, forced expiration, defecating, and parturition). The pelvic diaphragm is composed of the **levator ani** and the **coccygeus muscles**.

- The levator ani forms the largest part of the pelvic floor. The three muscles of the levator ani arise from the superior pubic ramus and the tendinous arch. They insert in the midline on the coccyx and along a tendinous raphe, called the **anococcygeal ligament** (**levator plate**).

  ○ The **pubococcygeus** forms the anterior part of the levator ani.

  ○ The **iliococcygeus** forms the middle part of the levator ani.

  ○ The **puborectalis** forms a muscular sling that loops around the anorectum. Normal tone of the muscle maintains the anterior angle of the anorectum where it passes through the pelvic diaphragm. The muscle relaxes during defecation.

- The coccygeus muscle forms the posterior part of the pelvic diaphragm; it attaches to the sacrum and ischial spine and tightly adheres to the sacrospinous ligament along its entire length.

— The **levator** (or **genital**) **hiatus**, a gap between the puborectalis muscles on either side, allows the passage of the urethra, vagina, and rectum into the perineum.

— The inferior gluteal, superior gluteal, and lateral sacral branches of the internal iliac arteries and the median sacral branch of the abdominal aorta supply most muscles of the pelvic walls and floor (see **Fig. 10.14A**).

— Veins that accompany the arteries and drain the pelvic floor and walls ultimately drain to the internal iliac veins, although the lateral sacral veins may also drain to the internal vertebral venous plexus.

10.4 Pelvic Fascia

Pelvic fascia is a connective tissue layer located between the viscera and the muscular walls and floor of the pelvis. There are two types, **membranous fascia** and **endopelvic fascia** (**Figs. 10.11** and **10.12**; see also **Fig. 10.3A** and **B**).

— Membranous pelvic fascia, usually a thin layer that adheres to the pelvic walls and viscera, has visceral and parietal layers.

- The **visceral pelvic fascia** surrounds the individual organs, and when in contact with the peritoneum it lies between the visceral peritoneum and the organ wall.

- The **parietal pelvic fascia** lines the inner surface of the muscles of the pelvic walls and floor. It is continuous with the transversalis fascia and psoas fascia of the abdomen and is named regionally for the muscle it covers (i.e., obturator fascia).

- Where the pelvic viscera pierce the pelvic diaphragm, the parietal and visceral layers merge to form a **tendinous arch of the pelvic fascia**. This arch runs from the pubis to the sacrum on either side of the pelvic floor and attaches to, and supports, pelvic viscera.

— **Endopelvic fascia** forms a loose connective tissue matrix that fills the subperitoneal space between the visceral and parietal layers of the membranous fascia.

- Much of this fascia has a "cotton candy-like" consistency that pads the subperitoneal space but allows for distension of the pelvic viscera (e.g., vagina, rectum).

- Large supporting columns of this connective tissue extend from the pelvic wall to the rectum, the **lateral ligament of the rectum**, and from the pelvic wall to the bladder, the **lateral ligament of the bladder**.

- In some areas, the endopelvic fascia forms fibrous condensations [e.g., cardinal (transverse cervical) ligament] that support the pelvic viscera and their vascular and nerve plexuses.

Fig. 10.11 ▶ **Pelvic fascia**
Male pelvis in coronal section, anterior view.

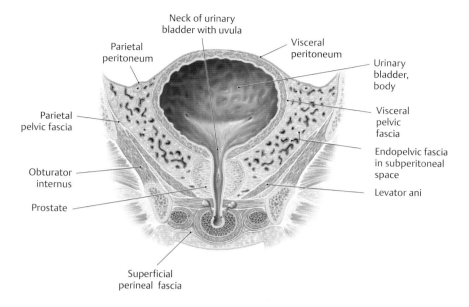

Neck of urinary
bladder with uvula

Visceral
peritoneum

Parietal
peritoneum

Urinary
bladder,
body

Parietal
pelvic fascia

Visceral
pelvic
fascia

Endopelvic fascia
in subperitoneal
space

Obturator
internus

Levator ani

Prostate

Superficial
perineal fascia

Fig. 10.12 ▶ **Fascial attachments in the female pelvis**
Transverse section through the cervix, superior view.

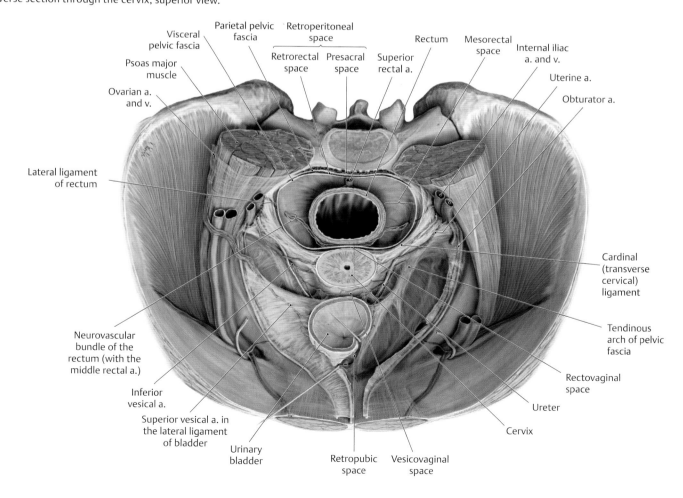

Parietal pelvic
fascia

Retroperitoneal
space

Rectum

Mesorectal
space

Visceral
pelvic fascia

Internal iliac
a. and v.

Psoas major
muscle

Retrorectal
space

Presacral
space

Superior
rectal a.

Uterine a.

Ovarian a.
and v.

Obturator a.

Lateral ligament
of rectum

Cardinal
(transverse
cervical)
ligament

Tendinous
arch of pelvic
fascia

Neurovascular
bundle of the
rectum (with the
middle rectal a.)

Rectovaginal
space

Inferior
vesical a.

Ureter

Superior vesical a. in
the lateral ligament
of bladder

Cervix

Urinary
bladder

Retropubic
space

Vesicovaginal
space

10.5 Pelvic Spaces

The peritoneum of the abdominal wall covers the superior surface of the bladder, the anterior and posterior surfaces of the uterus, and the anterolateral surfaces of the rectum. Because the peritoneum does not descend to the pelvic floor, spaces are created above the peritoneum, within the peritoneal cavity, and below the peritoneum in the subperitoneal space (**Fig. 10.13A** and **B**).

— **Peritoneal recesses**, intraperitoneal spaces that are continuous with the peritoneal cavity of the abdomen and lined by the visceral peritoneum of the pelvic organs, are normally occupied by loops of small intestine and peritoneal fluid.

  • In males, a **rectovesical pouch** between the bladder and rectum is the lowest point in the male peritoneal cavity.

  • In females, a **vesicouterine pouch** forms between the bladder and uterus, and a **rectouterine pouch** (of Douglas) forms between the uterus and rectum. The rectouterine pouch is the lowest point of the female peritoneal cavity.

Fig. 10.13 ► **Peritoneal and subperitoneal spaces in the pelvis**
Midsagittal section, viewed from the left side. Subperitoneal spaces shown in green

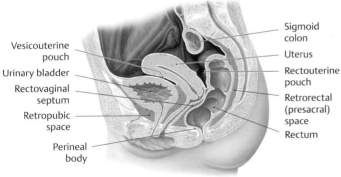

Vesicouterine pouch
Urinary bladder
Rectovaginal septum
Retropubic space
Perineal body
Sigmoid colon
Uterus
Rectouterine pouch
Retrorectal (presacral) space
Rectum

A Female.

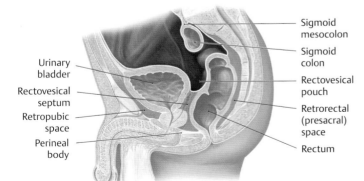

Urinary bladder
Rectovesical septum
Retropubic space
Perineal body
Sigmoid mesocolon
Sigmoid colon
Rectovesical pouch
Retrorectal (presacral) space
Rectum

B Male.

— **Subperitoneal recesses** are extraperitoneal spaces that are continuous with the retroperitoneum of the abdomen and are filled with endopelvic fascia.

  • The **retropubic space** (prevesical space, space of Retzius) lies between the pubic symphysis and the bladder.

  • The **rectorectal space** (presacral space) lies between the rectum and sacrum.

— A double-layered peritoneal septum descends from the rectovesical (or rectouterine) pouch to the perineum.

  • In males, this **rectovesical septum** separates the rectum from the seminal vesicles and prostate. Its lower part is often referred to as the **rectoprostatic fascia**.

  • In females, the **rectovaginal septum** separates the rectum from the vagina.

10.6 Neurovasculature of the Pelvis and Perineum

10.6a Arteries of the Pelvis and Perineum (Fig. 10.14)

Pelvic viscera are well vascularized, primarily by branches of the internal iliac artery, with abundant ipsilateral and contralateral communications. The superior rectal artery and paired ovarian arteries that arise in the abdomen provide an important collateral blood supply.

— The **right** and **left common iliac arteries** descend along the pelvic brim before bifurcating into the external and internal iliac arteries at the level of the L5–S1 intervertebral disk.

— Each **external iliac artery** continues along the pelvic brim, lateral to the accompanying vein, and enters the lower limb without contributing branches to pelvic viscera.

Fig. 10.14 ▶ **Blood vessels of the pelvis**
Idealized right hemipelvis, left lateral view.

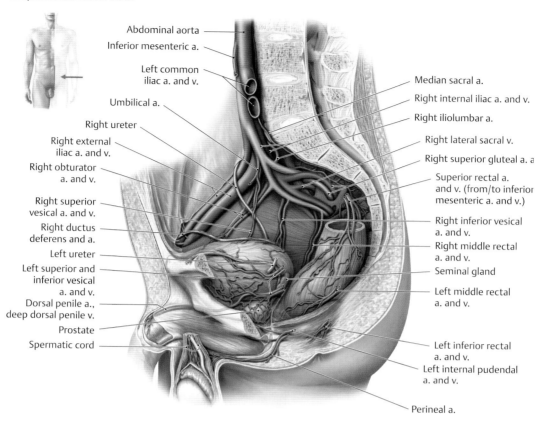

Abdominal aorta
Inferior mesenteric a.
Left common iliac a. and v.
Umbilical a.
Right ureter
Right external iliac a. and v.
Right obturator a. and v.
Right superior vesical a. and v.
Right ductus deferens and a.
Left ureter
Left superior and inferior vesical a. and v.
Dorsal penile a., deep dorsal penile v.
Prostate
Spermatic cord

Median sacral a.
Right internal iliac a. and v.
Right iliolumbar a.
Right lateral sacral v.
Right superior gluteal a. a
Superior rectal a. and v. (from/to inferior mesenteric a. and v.)
Right inferior vesical a. and v.
Right middle rectal a. and v.
Seminal gland
Left middle rectal a. and v.
Left inferior rectal a. and v.
Left internal pudendal a. and v.
Perineal a.

A Male pelvis.

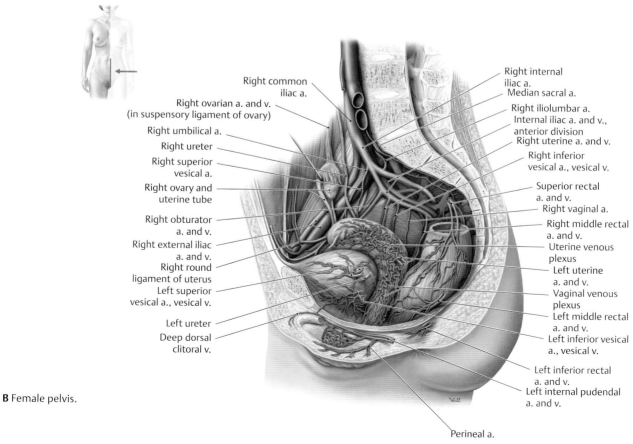

Right common iliac a.
Right ovarian a. and v. (in suspensory ligament of ovary)
Right umbilical a.
Right ureter
Right superior vesical a.
Right ovary and uterine tube
Right obturator a. and v.
Right external iliac a. and v.
Right round ligament of uterus
Left superior vesical a., vesical v.
Left ureter
Deep dorsal clitoral v.

Right internal iliac a.
Median sacral a.
Right iliolumbar a.
Internal iliac a. and v., anterior division
Right uterine a. and v.
Right inferior vesical a., vesical v.
Superior rectal a. and v.
Right vaginal a.
Right middle rectal a. and v.
Uterine venous plexus
Left uterine a. and v.
Vaginal venous plexus
Left middle rectal a. and v.
Left inferior vesical a., vesical v.
Left inferior rectal a. and v.
Left internal pudendal a. and v.
Perineal a.

B Female pelvis.

— Each **internal iliac artery** descends into the lesser pelvis along the lateral wall before branching into two divisions (**Table 10.3**)

1. The anterior division supplies most of the pelvic viscera, structures of the perineum, and some muscles in the gluteal region and thigh.
2. The posterior division contributes only parietal branches that supply muscles of the posterior abdominal wall, lower back, and gluteal region, as well as spinal branches that supply the meninges of the sacral spinal roots.

Table 10.3 ► Branches of the Internal Iliac Artery		
Anterior Division		**Posterior Division**
Visceral branches	**Parietal branches**	**Parietal branches**
*Umbilical—superior vesical	Obturator	Iliolumbar
Uterine (female)	Inferior gluteal	Lateral sacral
Vaginal (female)		Superior gluteal
Inferior vesical (male)		
Middle rectal		
Internal pudendal		

*After birth, the distal portion of the umbilical artery obliterates, but its remnant remains as the medial umbilical ligament on the anterior abdominal wall; the proximal portion remains as the superior vesical artery to the bladder.

— The **internal pudendal artery**, a branch of the internal iliac artery, supplies most structures in the perineum. It exits the pelvis through the greater sciatic foramen and then passes through the lesser sciatic foramen into the perineum where it runs along the lateral wall of the anal triangle to the perineal membrane. Its major branches (**Figs. 10.15** and **10.16**) include the following:

• The **inferior rectal artery**, which supplies the external anal sphincter and skin around the anus
• The **perineal artery**, which supplies the structures of the superficial perineal pouch through posterior scrotal or posterior labial branches
• The **dorsal penile** or **clitoral artery**, which supplies structures in the deep perineal pouch and the glans of the penis or clitoris

— The **external pudendal artery**, a branch of the femoral artery in the thigh, supplies superficial tissues of the perineum.
— The **ovarian artery** in females arises from the abdominal aorta at L2 and descends along the posterior abdominal wall. It crosses the pelvic brim and enters the pelvis within the **suspensory ligament of the ovary**. The ovarian artery supplies the ovary and uterine tube and anastomoses with the uterine artery (**Fig. 10.17**).

Fig. 10.15 ► **Neurovasculature of the female perineum**
Lithotomy position. *Removed*: Perineal membrane and left bulbospongiosus and ischiocavernosus muscles.

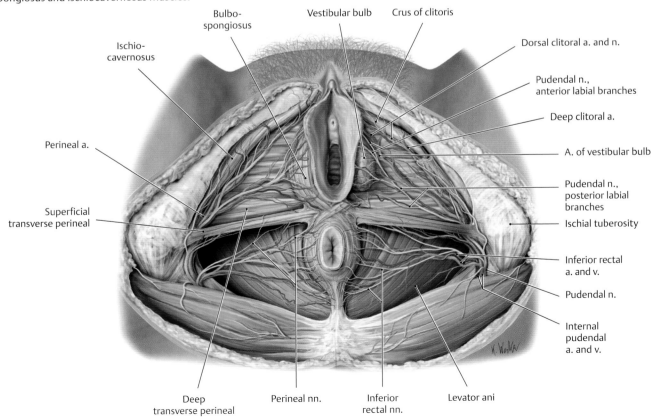

Fig. 10.16 ▶ Neurovasculature of the male perineum
Lithotomy position. *Removed from left side*: Perineal membrane,
bulbospongiosus muscle, and root of penis.

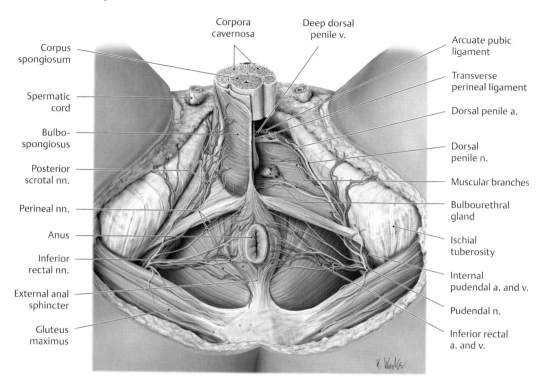

Corpora cavernosa

Deep dorsal penile v.

Corpus spongiosum

Spermatic cord

Bulbo-spongiosus

Posterior scrotal nn.

Perineal nn.

Anus

Inferior rectal nn.

External anal sphincter

Gluteus maximus

Arcuate pubic ligament

Transverse perineal ligament

Dorsal penile a.

Dorsal penile n.

Muscular branches

Bulbourethral gland

Ischial tuberosity

Internal pudendal a. and v.

Pudendal n.

Inferior rectal a. and v.

Fig. 10.17 ▶ Blood vessels of the female genitalia
Anterior view. *Removed from left side*: Peritoneum. *Displaced*: Uterus.

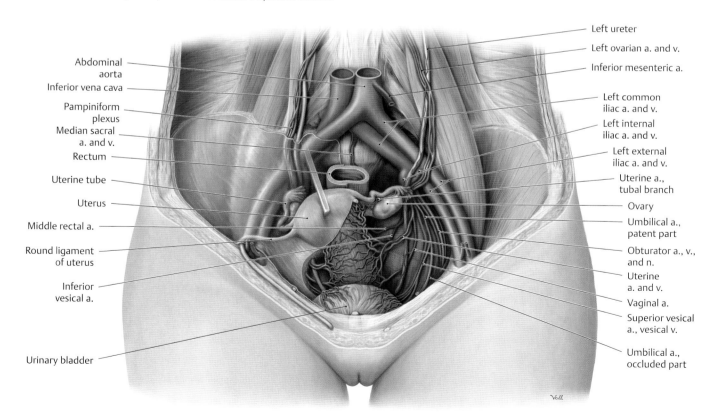

Abdominal aorta

Inferior vena cava

Pampiniform plexus

Median sacral a. and v.

Rectum

Uterine tube

Uterus

Middle rectal a.

Round ligament of uterus

Inferior vesical a.

Urinary bladder

Left ureter

Left ovarian a. and v.

Inferior mesenteric a.

Left common iliac a. and v.

Left internal iliac a. and v.

Left external iliac a. and v.

Uterine a., tubal branch

Ovary

Umbilical a., patent part

Obturator a., v., and n.

Uterine a. and v.

Vaginal a.

Superior vesical a., vesical v.

Umbilical a., occluded part

- The testicular artery passes through the inguinal canal as part of the spermatic cord to supply the testis and therefore is not a vessel of the pelvis (see Section 7.3b).

— The **superior rectal artery,** a branch of the inferior mesenteric artery, supplies the upper rectum and anal canal and anastomoses with middle and inferior rectal arteries in the pelvis and perineum (**Fig. 10.18**, see also Section 8.2a).

10.6b Veins of the Pelvis and Perineum

Blood from most pelvic viscera drains to a venous plexus contained either within the visceral fascia surrounding the organ (bladder, prostate) or within the organ wall (rectum).

— The visceral venous plexuses in the pelvis communicate freely, and most drain to the inferior vena caval system through tributaries of the internal iliac veins that accompany the arteries of similar name and vascular territory (area supplied by a vessel) (see **Fig. 10.14A** and **B**).

— The **internal pudendal vein** accompanies the internal pudendal artery and drains most structures of the perineum. However, erectile tissues in the urogenital triangle drain through **deep dorsal veins** that pass under the pubic symphysis to join with visceral venous plexuses in the pelvis.

— The **internal iliac veins** ascend from the pelvis to join with the **external iliac veins**. These join to form the **right** and **left common iliac veins**, which converge to form the inferior vena cava at the L5 vertebral level.

— There are three alternate venous drainages from pelvic viscera.

1. Ovarian veins drain directly into the inferior vena cava on the right and into the renal vein on the left, but they also communicate with other pelvic venous plexuses (uterine, vaginal), which drain to the internal iliac veins (see **Fig. 10.17**).

2. The superior rectal vein drains to the hepatic portal system through the inferior mesenteric vein. This drainage establishes an anastomosis between the portal and caval venous systems (a portosystemic anastomosis) with the middle and inferior rectal veins, which are tributaries of the internal iliac veins (see **Figs. 10.18** and **7.15**).

3. The vertebral venous plexus, which drains into the azygos system, communicates with pelvic visceral plexuses through tributaries of the internal iliac veins (see **Fig. 2.16B**).

10.6c Lymphatics of the Pelvis and Perineum

Lymph from the pelvis and perineum travels through one or more groups of lymph nodes, all of which ultimately drain into the thoracic duct (**Table 10.4**). The groups of nodes tend to be interconnected but vary in size and number.

There are several general drainage patterns.

— Within the pelvis, lymph drainage usually follows venous pathways, although structures that drain to the external iliac nodes do not follow this pattern.
— External iliac nodes receive lymph from the superior parts of the anterior pelvic viscera.
— Internal iliac nodes receive lymph from deep pelvic and deep perineal structures.
— Sacral nodes receive lymph from deep posterior pelvic viscera.
— Superficial and deep inguinal nodes drain most structures of the perineum.
— Inguinal nodes drain to external iliac nodes.
— External iliac, internal iliac, and sacral nodes drain to common iliac nodes, which in turn drain to lateral aortic nodes and lumbar trunks.

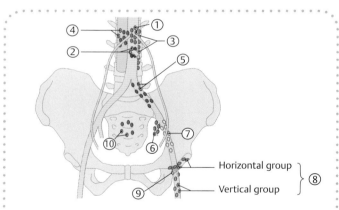

Table 10.4 ▶ **Lymph Nodes of the Pelvis**		
Preaortic l.n.	① Superior mesenteric l.n.	
	② Inferior mesenteric l.n.	
③ Left lateral aortic l.n.		
④ Right lateral aortic (caval) l.n.		
⑤ Common iliac l.n.		
⑥ Internal iliac l.n.		
⑦ External iliac l.n.		
⑧ Superficial inguinal l.n.	Horizontal group	
	Vertical group	
⑨ Deep inguinal l.n.		
⑩ Sacral l.n.		

Fig. 10.18 ► **Blood vessels of the rectum**
Posterior view. The main blood supply to the rectum is from the superior
rectal artery; the middle rectal arteries serve as an anastomosis between the
superior and inferior rectal arteries.

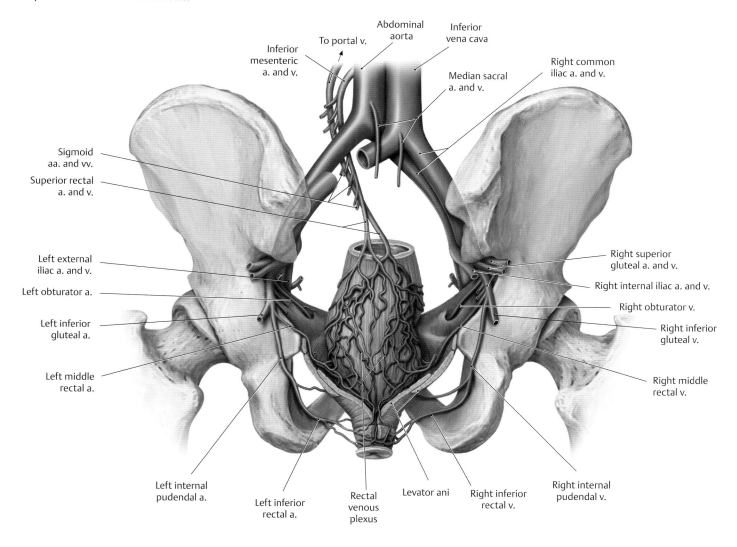

To portal v.

Abdominal
aorta

Inferior
mesenteric
a. and v.

Inferior
vena cava

Median sacral
a. and v.

Right common
iliac a. and v.

Sigmoid
aa. and vv.

Superior rectal
a. and v.

Left external
iliac a. and v.

Left obturator a.

Left inferior
gluteal a.

Left middle
rectal a.

Right superior
gluteal a. and v.

Right internal iliac a. and v.

Right obturator v.

Right inferior
gluteal v.

Right middle
rectal v.

Left internal
pudendal a.

Left inferior
rectal a.

Rectal
venous
plexus

Levator ani

Right inferior
rectal v.

Right internal
pudendal v.

10.6d Nerves of the Pelvis and Perineum (Figs. 10.19 and 10.20)

— The obturator nerve (L2–L4), a branch of the lumbar plexus, passes along the sidewall of the pelvis and exits through the obturator canal. It does not innervate structures of the pelvis but can be injured during pelvic surgery.

— The **sacral plexus** forms on the posterior wall of the pelvis from the anterior rami of L4–S4. Except for short branches to pelvic floor muscles, branches of the plexus exit the pelvis through the greater sciatic foramen, where they innervate structures in the perineum, gluteal region, and lower limb (see Section 15.4d).

Fig. 10.19 ▶ **Innervation of the female pelvis**
Right pelvis, left lateral view. *Reflected*: Uterus and rectum.

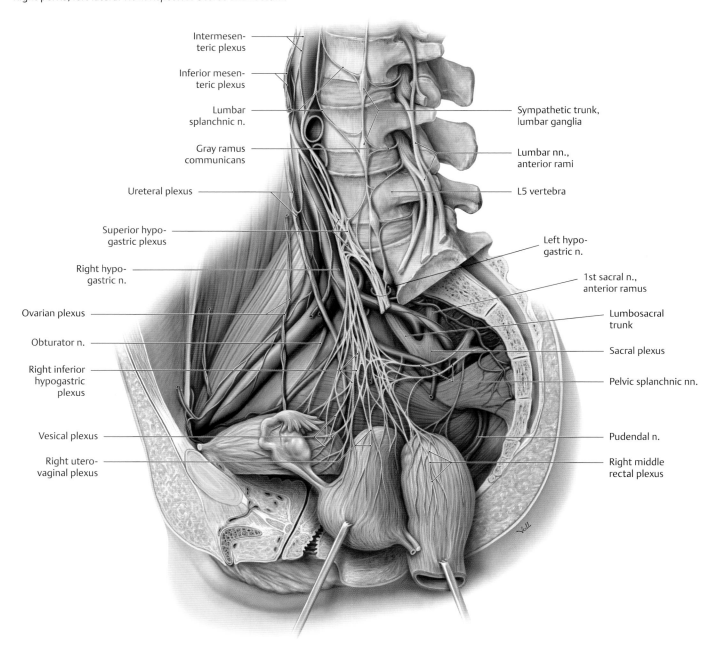

Intermesenteric plexus
Inferior mesenteric plexus
Lumbar splanchnic n.
Gray ramus communicans
Ureteral plexus
Superior hypogastric plexus
Right hypogastric n.
Ovarian plexus
Obturator n.
Right inferior hypogastric plexus
Vesical plexus
Right uterovaginal plexus

Sympathetic trunk, lumbar ganglia
Lumbar nn., anterior rami
L5 vertebra
Left hypogastric n.
1st sacral n., anterior ramus
Lumbosacral trunk
Sacral plexus
Pelvic splanchnic nn.
Pudendal n.
Right middle rectal plexus

Fig. 10.20 ▶ **Innervation of the male pelvis**
Right pelvis, left lateral view.

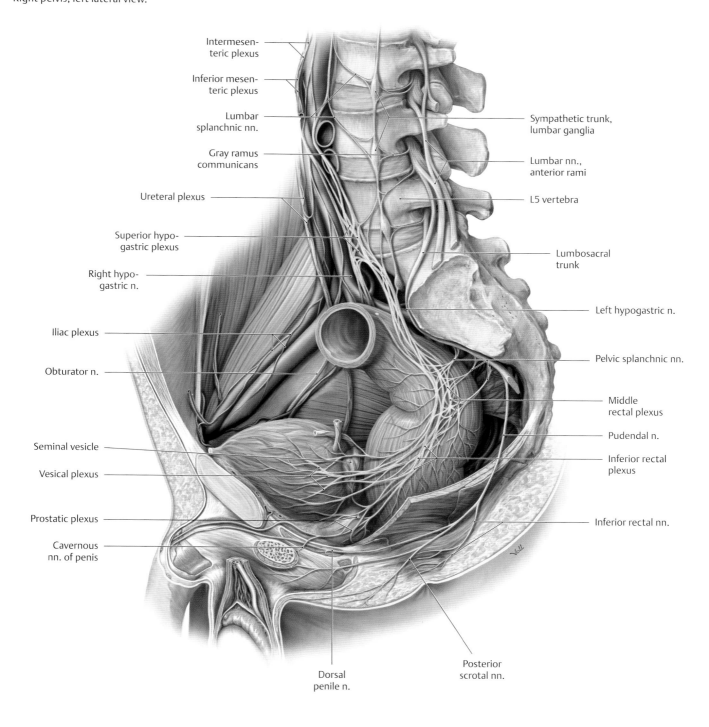

Intermesen-
teric plexus

Inferior mesen-
teric plexus

Lumbar
splanchnic nn.

Gray ramus
communicans

Ureteral plexus

Superior hypo-
gastric plexus

Right hypo-
gastric n.

Iliac plexus

Obturator n.

Seminal vesicle

Vesical plexus

Prostatic plexus

Cavernous
nn. of penis

Sympathetic trunk,
lumbar ganglia

Lumbar nn.,
anterior rami

L5 vertebra

Lumbosacral
trunk

Left hypogastric n.

Pelvic splanchnic nn.

Middle
rectal plexus

Pudendal n.

Inferior rectal
plexus

Inferior rectal nn.

Dorsal
penile n.

Posterior
scrotal nn.

— The **pudendal nerve** (S2–S4), a branch of the sacral plexus, is the primary nerve of the perineum. It passes through the greater sciatic foramen close to the ischial spine and then into the perineum through the lesser sciatic foramen, where it courses anteriorly with the internal pudendal vessels (**Figs. 10.21A** and **B** and **10.22A** and **B**; see also **Fig. 10.20**). The pudendal nerve is a mixed somatic nerve (motor and sensory) but also carries postganglionic sympathetic fibers to perineal structures. Its major branches include the following:

- The **inferior rectal nerve**, which innervates the external anal sphincter
- The **perineal nerve**, which supplies cutaneous branches to the scrotum and labia and the muscles of the deep and superficial perineal pouches
- The **dorsal penile (clitoral) nerve**, which is the primary sensory nerve to the penis and clitoris, especially to the glans

— **Sacral sympathetic trunks**, the continuations of the lumbar sympathetic trunks, provide postganglionic fibers to pelvic plexuses and to lower limb branches of the sacral plexus. The trunks descend along the anterior surface of the sacrum to the coccyx, where they merge to form a small ganglion, the ganglion impar (see **Fig. 8.21**).

◻ Ilioinguinal n. and genitofemoral n., genital branch and labial branch

◻ Pudendal n.

◻ Posterior femoral cutaneous n.

◻ Middle clunial nn.

◻ Superior clunial nn.

◻ Inferior clunial nn.

◻ Anococcygeal nn.

Pudendal nerve block

During labor, anesthesia of the pudendal nerve can ease perineal pain of delivery. A pudendal block can be administered through the posterior wall of the vagina, with the surgeon aiming the needle toward the ischial spine. The block can also be administered externally, inserting the needle through the skin medial to the ischial tuberosity. Since the pudendal nerve innervates only the perineum, the superior vagina and cervix are not affected by the block, and the mother continues to feel the uterine contractions.

Fig. 10.21 ▶ **Nerves of the female perineum and genitalia**

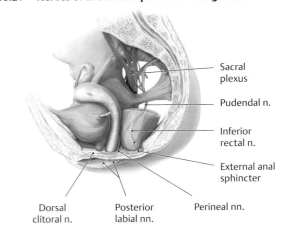

A Course of the pudendal nerve, left lateral view.

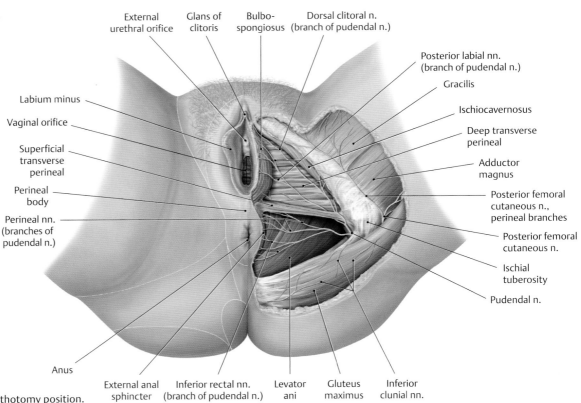

B Sensory innervation, lithotomy position.

- The **superior hypogastric plexus**, a continuation of the intermesenteric plexus in the abdomen, receives additional contributions from the two lower lumbar splanchnic nerves (sympathetic). It drapes over the bifurcation of the aorta and branches into right and left **hypogastric nerves**, which pass into the pelvis.
- The pelvic splanchnic nerves, the pelvic component of the parasympathetic nervous system, originate from the sacral spinal cord and enter the pelvis with the S2–S4 anterior rami.
- The hypogastric nerves, joined by sacral splanchnic nerves (sympathetic) nerves and pelvic splanchnic nerves (parasympathetic), form right and left **inferior hypogastric** (pelvic) **plexuses**.
- **Vesical**, **prostatic** (in males), **uterovaginal** (in females), and **rectal plexuses** are derived from the inferior hypogastric plexus and surround individual pelvic organs.
- **Cavernous nerves** from the inferior hypogastric plexus pass through the genital hiatus carrying parasympathetic nerves to perineal structures. They are responsible for erection of the penis and clitoris.
- Visceral afferent fibers from most structures in the pelvis travel with sympathetic or parasympathetic nerves depending on the relationship of the viscera to the peritoneum.

- In pelvic viscera covered by peritoneum, afferent fibers travel with sympathetic nerves to the superior hypogastric plexus and thoracic spinal cord.
- In pelvic viscera below the peritoneum, afferent fibers travel with pelvic splanchnic nerves to the sacral spinal cord.
- Although the rectum is in contact with the peritoneum on most of its surfaces, its visceral afferent fibers also travel with pelvic splanchnic nerves.

Fig. 10.22 ▶ **Nerves of the male perineum and genitalia**

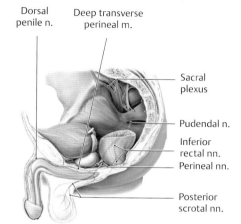

A Course of the pudendal nerve, left lateral view.

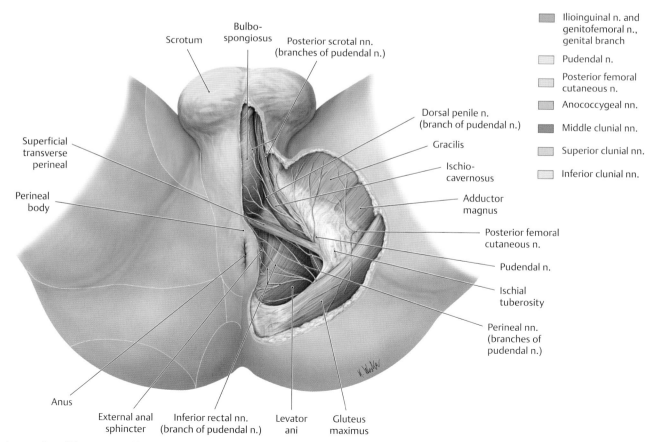

B Sensory innervation, lithotomy position.

11 Pelvic Viscera

The pelvic cavity contains the male or female genital organs, the pelvic urinary organs, and the rectum. These organs normally reside in the true pelvis, although when enlarged the bladder and uterus can extend into the abdominal cavity.

11.1 Male Genital Structures

The male gonad, the testis, is located in the inguinal region and is discussed in Chapter 7. The seminal glands (vesicles) and prostate gland are male accessory reproductive structures found in the pelvis (**Fig. 11.1**).

Fig. 11.1 ► **Male pelvis**
Parasagittal section, viewed from the right side.

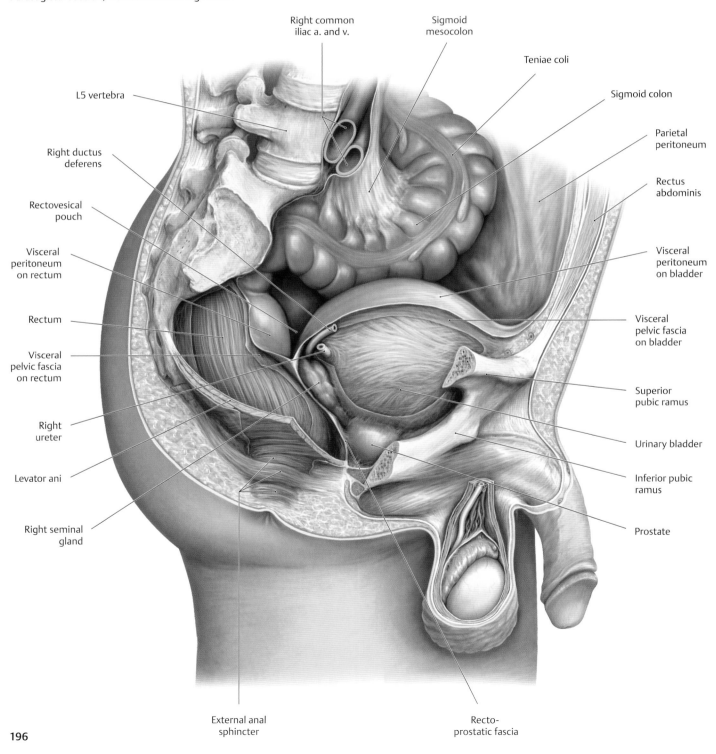

Right common iliac a. and v.

Sigmoid mesocolon

Teniae coli

Sigmoid colon

L5 vertebra

Parietal peritoneum

Right ductus deferens

Rectus abdominis

Rectovesical pouch

Visceral peritoneum on rectum

Visceral peritoneum on bladder

Rectum

Visceral pelvic fascia on bladder

Visceral pelvic fascia on rectum

Superior pubic ramus

Right ureter

Urinary bladder

Levator ani

Inferior pubic ramus

Right seminal gland

Prostate

External anal sphincter

Recto-prostatic fascia

Fig. 11.2 ▶ **Accessory sex glands**
The bladder, prostate, seminal glands, and bulbourethral glands, posterior view.

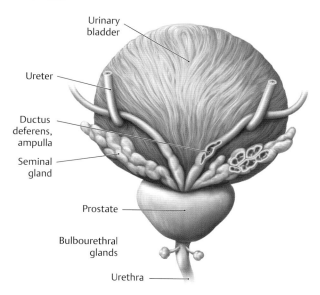

11.1a Seminal Glands (Vesicles)

The **seminal glands** are paired convoluted tubules that produce 70% of the seminal fluid (**Figs. 11.2** and **11.3**).

— They lie superior to the prostate, between the urinary bladder and the rectum.
— The seminal glands are subperitoneal, located immediately below the peritoneum of the rectovesical pouch.
— The duct of each seminal gland joins with the ampulla of the ductus deferens to form the **ejaculatory ducts**, which pierce the prostate and drain into the **prostatic urethra**.
— The middle rectal and inferior vesical arteries supply the seminal glands.

Veins of similar names accompany the arteries.

— Branches from the pelvic plexus innervate the seminal glands.

Fig. 11.3 ▶ **Prostate in situ**
Sagittal section through the male pelvis, left lateral view.

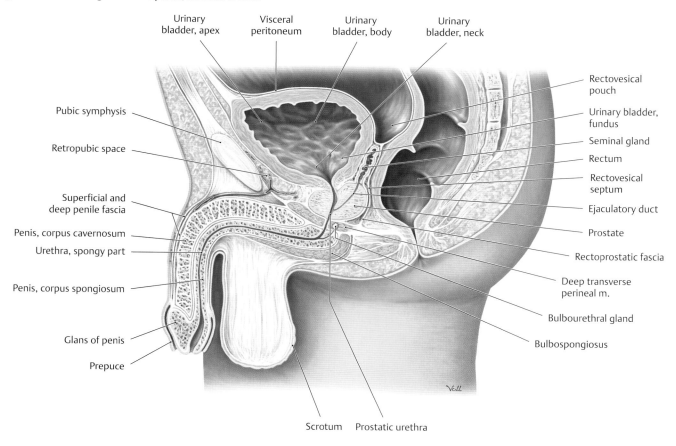

11.1b The Prostate

The **prostate** is an accessory reproductive gland that produces ~25% of the seminal fluid (**Fig. 11.4 A, B,** and **C**; see also **Figs. 11.2** and **11.3**).

— The base, or superior surface, sits directly below the bladder. The apex points inferiorly and is in contact with the external urethral sphincter.

— It is posterior to the lower part of the pubic symphysis and anterior to the **rectovesical septum**, which separates it from the rectum.

— The prostate surrounds the proximal (prostatic) part of the urethra. Secretions from prostatic glands drain into the urethra through numerous prostatic ductules.

— A fibromuscular capsule surrounds the prostate. The prostatic capsule is separated from the outer prostatic sheath (derived from endopelvic fascia) by the prostatic venous plexus.

— **Puboprostatic ligaments**, anterior extensions of the tendinous arch of the pelvic fascia, attach the apex of the prostate (and neck of the bladder) to the pubis (see **Fig. 11.14**). Posterior extensions of the tendinous arch secure it to the sacrum.

— The anatomic lobes of the prostate include the following:

  • A fibromuscular isthmus anterior to the urethra
  • Right and left lateral lobes that are subdivided into lobules. The lower posterior lobule (sometimes referred to as the posterior lobe), which lies posterior to the urethra and inferior to the ejaculatory ducts, is palpable by digital exam
  • A poorly defined middle lobe that sits above the lateral lobes between the urethra and ejaculatory ducts and is in close contact with the neck of the bladder

— For clinical purposes, the prostate is divided into three zones determined by their proximity to the urethra: **periurethral**, **central** (comparable to the anatomic middle lobe), and **peripheral**.

— Prostatic arteries are usually branches of the inferior vesical arteries. Middle rectal arteries also contribute to the prostatic blood supply (see **Fig. 10.14A**).

Benign prostatic hypertrophy (hyperplasia)

Benign prostatic hypertrophy (more accurately called hyperplasia) is the benign enlargement of the prostate gland that results from the proliferation of the epithelial and stomal tissues, particularly in the periurethral area. Although it is common in men of middle age, the incidence increases in later years and is thought to be due to the greater conversion of testosterone to the more active form, dihydrotestosterone (DHT), in the aging prostate gland. The hyperplasia constricts the internal urethral orifice, causing dysuria (difficult or painful urination), nocturia (excessive urination at night), and urgency (sudden desire to urinate). It is treated with a 5a-reductase inhibitor that blocks the conversion of testosterone to DHT by inhibiting the enzyme 5a-reductase. This may be used in combination with α-blockers that relax the muscles in the prostate and in the neck of the bladder, making urination easier. In severe cases, transurethral resection of the prostate may be necessary.

Fig. 11.4 ▶ **Prostate**
The prostate may be divided anatomically (top row) or clinically (bottom row).

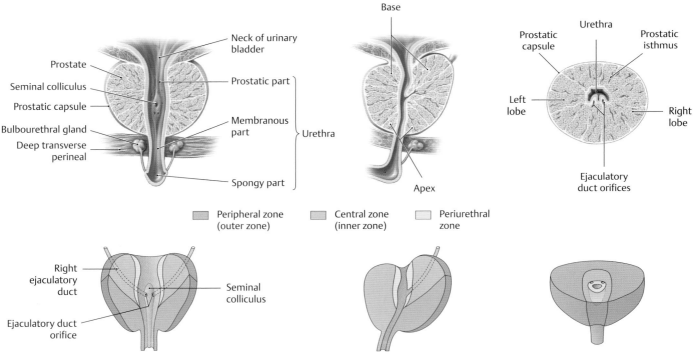

A Coronal section, anterior view. **B** Sagittal section, left lateral view. **C** Transverse section, superior view.

— The prostatic venous plexus, continuous with the vesical venous plexus of the bladder, drains to internal iliac veins. The prostatic plexus also communicates with the vertebral venous plexus (see **Fig. 2.16**).

— The lymph vessels of the prostate follow venous pathways to the internal iliac nodes.

— The prostatic nerve plexus is a derivative of the inferior hypogastric plexus. The role of parasympathetic innervation is unclear, but sympathetic nerves cause the smooth muscle of the gland to contract, expelling prostatic secretion into the prostatic urethra during ejaculation.

Carcinoma of the prostate

Carcinoma of the prostate is a slow-growing cancer affecting elderly men that commonly arises in the posterior lobe of the prostate. It metastasizes to the bony pelvis, vertebral column, skull, and brain via the vertebral venous plexus but also to the heart and lungs via drainage through the internal iliac veins and inferior vena cava. Symptoms include hesitancy (difficulty in beginning the flow of urination), frequency, and dribbling on urination (collectively known as prostatism). It can be diagnosed by digital examination of the rectum, ultrasonography, or prostate-specific antigen (PSA) levels. A PSA value greater than 4.0 ng/mL indicates disease activity.

Prostatectomy

Prostatectomy is the surgical removal of the prostate gland. Open radical prostatectomy involves removal of the prostate along with the seminal vesicles, ductus deferens, and pelvic lymph nodes via a retropubic or perineal incision. Transurethral resection of the prostate (TURP) is performed using a cystoscope that is advanced through the urethra to resect the prostate. Cavernous nerves carrying parasympathetic fibers that are responsible for penile erection run alongside the prostate and are particularly at risk during these procedures.

11.2 Female Genital Structures

Female genital structures, which include the ovaries, uterine tubes, uterus, and vagina, are located in the middle of the pelvis between the bladder anteriorly and the rectum posteriorly (**Fig. 11.5**).

Fig. 11.5 ▶ **Female pelvis**
Sagittal section viewed from the left side.

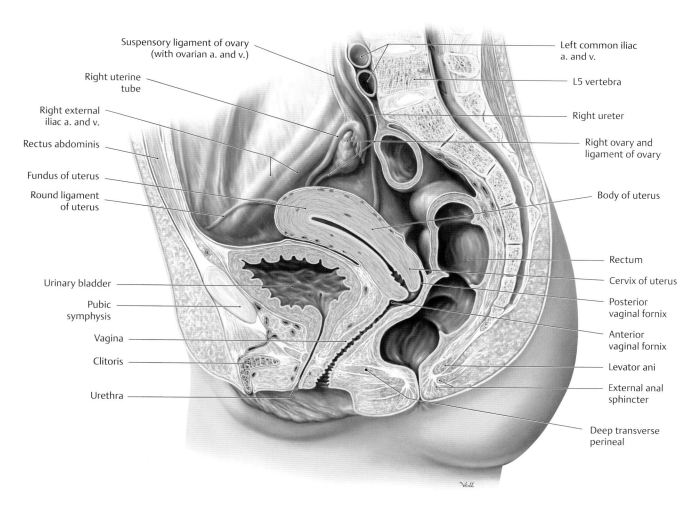

Suspensory ligament of ovary (with ovarian a. and v.)

Right uterine tube

Right external iliac a. and v.

Rectus abdominis

Fundus of uterus

Round ligament of uterus

Urinary bladder

Pubic symphysis

Vagina

Clitoris

Urethra

Left common iliac a. and v.

L5 vertebra

Right ureter

Right ovary and ligament of ovary

Body of uterus

Rectum

Cervix of uterus

Posterior vaginal fornix

Anterior vaginal fornix

Levator ani

External anal sphincter

Deep transverse perineal

11.2a The Ovary

The **ovary** is the female gonad, an ovoid structure that produces eggs and reproductive hormones and resides in the lateral wall of the pelvis (**Fig. 11.6A** and **B**).

— The **ligament of the ovary** attaches the ovary to the supralateral aspect of the uterus.
— The **suspensory ligament of the ovary** is a fold of peritoneum that encloses the ovarian vessels and nerves as they pass over the pelvic brim to the ovary.
— The **mesovarium** suspends the ovary from the posterior part of the broad ligament.
— The ovarian artery, a branch of the abdominal aorta at L2, supplies the ovary (see **Fig. 10.17**).
— A pampiniform plexus, which may converge to form a single ovarian vein, drains the ovary. The right ovarian vein is a direct tributary of the inferior vena cava; the left ovarian vein is a tributary of the left renal vein.
— Lymphatic vessels follow the ovarian vessels superiorly to the lateral aortic nodes.
— Both the ovarian nerve plexus, which follows the ovarian vessels, and the pelvic nerve plexus, which follows the uterine vessels, innervate the ovary.

11.2b The Uterine Tubes

The **uterine tubes** (fallopian tubes, oviducts), paired muscular tubes that extend laterally from the horns (supralateral corners) of the uterus, transmit ova from the ovary and sperm from the uterine cavity (see **Fig. 11.6A** and **B**).

— The uterine tubes are the normal sites of fertilization and are also the most common sites of ectopic pregnancies (implantation of a fertilized ovum outside the uterus).
— The uterine tube has four parts:
  1. The uterine (intramural) part, the segment that passes through the wall of the uterus
  2. The isthmus, the narrowest part
  3. The ampulla, the longest and widest part and normally the site of fertilization
  4. The infundibulum, the trumpet-shaped terminal part that is open to the peritoneal cavity, with fingerlike fimbriae that surround the ovary
— The uterine tube is ensheathed in the upper edge of the broad ligament, where it is supported by its mesosalpinx (see Section 11.2c).
— The uterine tube is supplied by the anastomosing ovarian and uterine arteries and drained by accompanying veins.
— Lymph vessels follow the ovarian veins to the lateral aortic nodes.
— The ovarian and uterine plexuses innervate the uterine tubes.

Ectopic pregnancy

Implantation of a fertilized ovum outside the uterus can occur anywhere, but the ampulla of the uterine tube is the most common site. Often the tube has been partially blocked by inflammation (salpingitis), preventing the blastocyst from completing its journey to the uterus. If not diagnosed early in the pregnancy, rupture of the uterine tube with consequent hemorrhage into the peritoneal cavity can result in a life-threatening situation for the mother. A ruptured ectopic pregnancy on the right side may be misdiagnosed as a ruptured appendix because both conditions irritate the parietal peritoneum and have similar presentations.

11.2c The Uterus

The **uterus** is a pear-shaped muscular organ located in the center of the pelvis, posterior to the bladder and anterior to the rectum (see **Fig. 11.5**). It is the site of implantation of the fertilized egg, subsequent development of the embryo, and parturition of the fetus.

— The uterus has two parts (see **Fig. 11.6A** and **B**).
  1. The **body** is the superior two thirds of the uterus and includes
     ○ the **fundus**, the uppermost part above the openings of the uterine tubes, and
     ○ the uterine **isthmus**, a narrow inferior segment that extends into the cervix.
  2. The **cervix** is the narrow inferior third of the uterus and its least mobile part.
     ○ A supravaginal part sits above the vagina.
     ○ A vaginal part protrudes into the upper vagina and is surrounded by the vaginal fornices (upper recesses).
— The **uterine cavity**, a narrow space within the uterine body,
  • communicates with the lumen of the uterine tubes where they enter at the uterine horns, and
  • extends inferiorly through the **internal os** (orifice) to the cervical canal and terminates where the **external os** opens into the vagina.

Fig. 11.6 ▶ **Uterus and uterine tube**

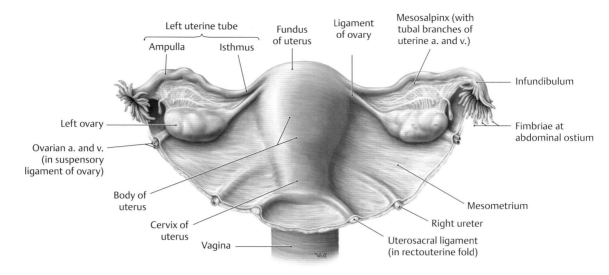

A Posterosuperior view.

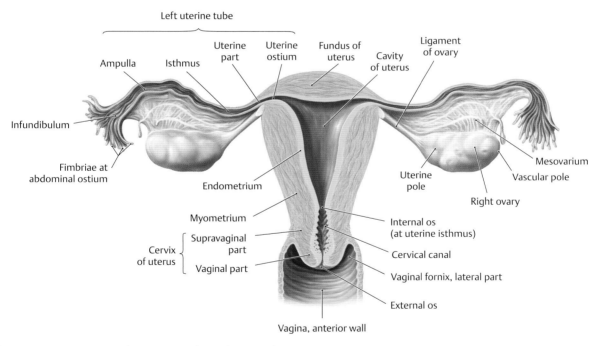

B Coronal section, posterior view with uterus straightened. *Removed:* Mesometrium.

Bicornuate uterus

The embryonic uterus is formed from the fusion of two paramesonephric ducts. When these ducts fail to fuse properly, a bicornuate uterus results in which the upper part of the uterus is bifurcated. The caudal part of the uterus is usually normal. Although a normal pregnancy is possible with this malformation, there is a higher chance of recurrent pregnancy loss, preterm birth, and malpresentation of the baby (e.g., the baby may be in a breech or transverse position).

— Although the body of the uterus is mobile, its position changes with the fullness of the bladder and rectum. Its normal position is anteflexed and anteverted (**Fig. 11.7**).

  • **Flexion** describes the angle between the uterine body and isthmus. In an anteflexed uterus, the long axis of the uterine body is tipped anteriorly; a **retroflexed** uterus is tipped posteriorly.

  • **Version** describes the angle between the cervix and vagina. In an anteverted uterus, the axis of the cervix is bent anteriorly; in a **retroverted** uterus, the cervix is bent posteriorly.

— Peritoneum covers the body of the uterus, extending as far inferiorly as the cervix on its posterior surface. The uterus is flanked anteriorly by the vesicouterine space and posteriorly by the rectouterine space (pouch) (**Fig. 11.8**).

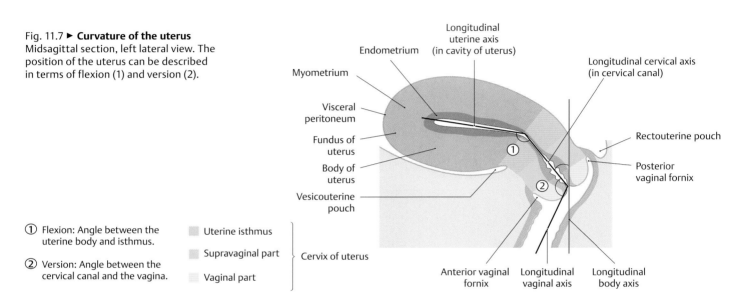

Fig. 11.7 ► **Curvature of the uterus**
Midsagittal section, left lateral view. The position of the uterus can be described in terms of flexion (1) and version (2).

① Flexion: Angle between the uterine body and isthmus.

② Version: Angle between the cervical canal and the vagina.

Uterine isthmus

Supravaginal part

Vaginal part

Cervix of uterus

Fig. 11.8 ► **Peritoneum in the female pelvis**

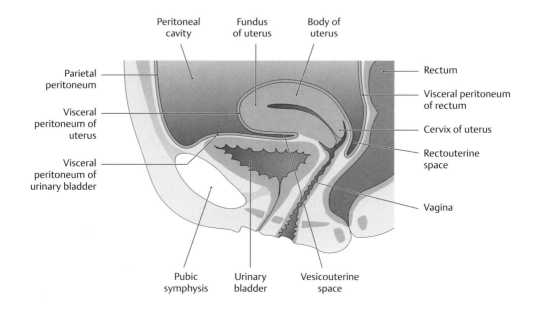

— Uterine ligaments that arise from the uterine body include the broad ligament and the round ligaments of the uterus (**Fig. 11.9**; see also **Fig. 11.6A**).

- The **broad ligament** is a double fold of peritoneum that extends laterally from each side of the uterus to the sidewalls of the pelvis. The parts of the broad ligament (**Fig. 11.10**) are

  ○ the **mesosalpinx,** which ensheaths the uterine tube;

  ○ the **mesovarium**, a posterior extension, which suspends the ovary; and

  ○ the **mesometrium,** which extends from the uterine body below the mesovarium to the sidewall of the pelvis.

- The paired **round ligaments of the uterus**, which originate near the fundus from each side of the uterus, pass through the deep inguinal rings, traverse the inguinal canal, and insert in the labia majora of the perineum.

Fig. 11.9 ▶ **Peritoneal relationships in the female pelvis**
Lesser pelvis, anterosuperior view. *Retracted:* Small intestine loops and colon (portions).

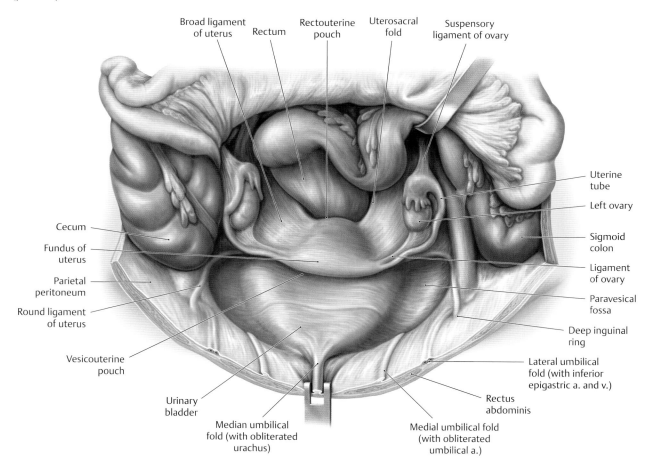

Fig. 11.10 ▶ **Mesenteries of the broad ligament**
Sagittal section. The broad ligament of the uterus is a combination of the mesosalpinx, mesovarium, and mesometrium.

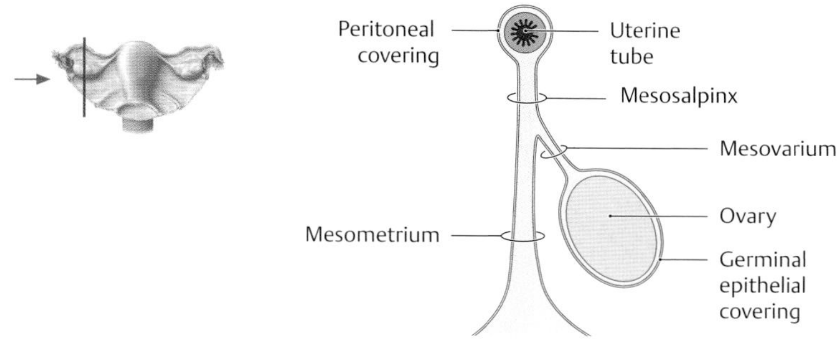

— Uterine ligaments that arise from the cervix include the transverse cervical ligaments and the uterosacral ligaments (**Fig. 11.11**).

- The paired **cardinal** (transverse cervical) **ligaments** are thickenings of endopelvic fascia that connect the uterine cervix to the pelvic sidewall. They are located at the base of the broad ligament and transmit the uterine vessels.
- The paired **uterosacral ligaments** are thickenings of endopelvic fascia that connect the uterine cervix to the sacrum and help to maintain the anteverted position of the uterus.

— The uterine artery, the primary blood supply to the uterus (see **Fig. 10.17**), traverses the cardinal ligament and anastomoses superiorly with the ovarian artery and inferiorly with the vaginal artery.

— A uterine venous plexus receives the uterine veins and drains to the internal iliac vein.

— Lymphatic drainage of the uterus is complex but generally follows the uterine veins or the uterine ligaments (see **Table 10.4**).

- The uterine fundus drains to para-aortic nodes via the ovarian veins.
- The supralateral part of the uterus drains to superficial inguinal nodes via the round ligament.
- The uterine body drains to external iliac nodes via the broad ligament.
- The cervix drains to internal iliac and sacral nodes via the cardinal and uterosacral ligaments.

— The uterovaginal nerve plexus, derived from the inferior hypogastric plexus, innervates the uterus (see **Fig. 10.19**).

11.2d The Vagina

The **vagina** is a fibromuscular tube that extends from the cervix of the uterus to the vaginal orifice in the perineum (**Figs. 11.12 and 11.13**). It serves as the inferior part of the birth canal and the conduit for menstrual fluid, and it accommodates the penis during sexual intercourse.

Fig. 11.11 ▶ **Ligaments of the female pelvis**
Superior view. *Removed:* Peritoneum, neurovasculature, and superior portion of bladder to demonstrate only the fascial condensations. Deep pelvic ligaments support the uterus within the pelvic cavity and prevent uterine prolapse, the downward displacement of the uterus into the vagina.

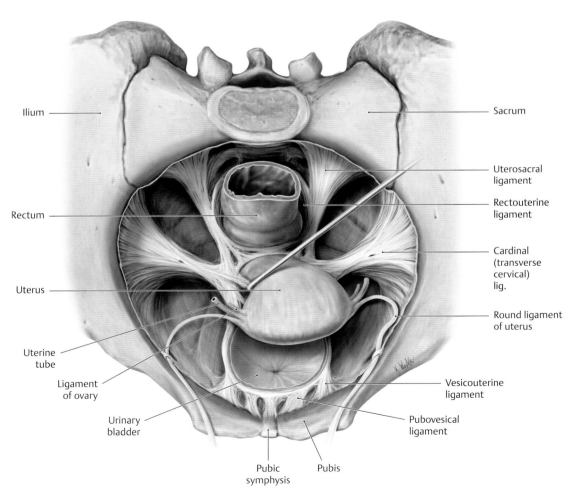

Ilium

Sacrum

Uterosacral ligament

Rectouterine ligament

Rectum

Cardinal (transverse cervical) lig.

Uterus

Round ligament of uterus

Uterine tube

Ligament of ovary

Vesicouterine ligament

Urinary bladder

Pubovesical ligament

Pubic symphysis

Pubis

Fig. 11.12 ▶ **Vagina**
Midsagittal section, left lateral view.

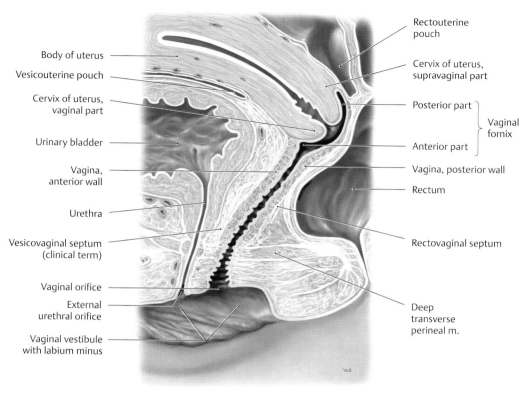

Body of uterus
Vesicouterine pouch
Cervix of uterus, vaginal part
Urinary bladder
Vagina, anterior wall
Urethra
Vesicovaginal septum (clinical term)
Vaginal orifice
External urethral orifice
Vaginal vestibule with labium minus

Rectouterine pouch
Cervix of uterus, supravaginal part
Posterior part
Anterior part
Vaginal fornix
Vagina, posterior wall
Rectum
Rectovaginal septum
Deep transverse perineal m.

Fig. 11.13 ▶ **Female pelvis**
Coronal section, anterior view.

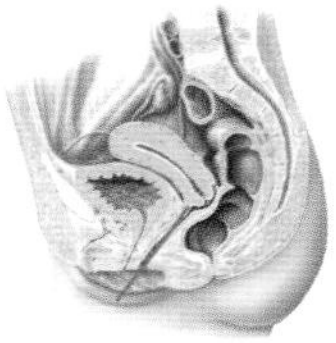

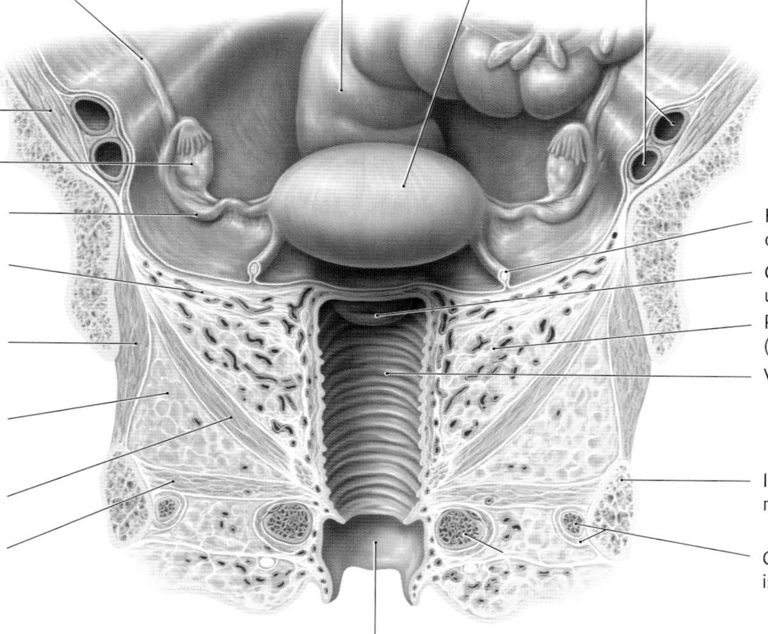

Suspensory ligament of ovary
Rectum
Fundus of uterus
External iliac a. and v.
Iliacus
Ovary
Uterine tube
Cardinal (transverse cervical) ligament
Obturator internus
Ischioanal fossa
Levator ani
Deep transverse perineal
Round ligament of uterus
Cervix of uterus
Paravaginal tissue (endopelvic fascia)
Vagina
Inferior pubic ramus
Crus of clitoris (with ischiocavernosus)
Vestibule of vagina

- The vagina is posterior to the bladder and urethra and anterior to the rectum.
- It is normally flattened with its anterior and posterior walls in contact.
- Connections to the sacrum and side wall of the pelvis via the tendinous arch of the pelvic fascia stabilize the vagina, especially during childbirth.
- The **vaginal fornix**, which has anterior, lateral, and posterior parts, is a recess that surrounds the lower cervix as it protrudes into the upper vagina (see **Figs. 11.5** and **11.6B**).
- The posterior fornix is in contact with the rectouterine pouch, thereby providing access to the peritoneal cavity. The anterior fornix is shorter and lies against the posterior wall of the bladder.
- The internal iliac artery supplies the vagina through its uterine, vaginal, and internal pudendal branches (see **Figs. 10.14B** and **10.17**).
- Veins of the vagina contribute to the uterovaginal venous plexus, which drains to the internal iliac vein.
- Lymphatic vessels of the vagina drain to several groups of nodes.
  - The superior part of the vagina drains to external or internal iliac nodes.
  - The inferior part of the vagina drains to sacral and common iliac nodes.
  - The vaginal orifice drains to superficial inguinal nodes.
- The uterovaginal nerve plexus, an extension of the inferior hypogastric plexus, innervates the superior three fourths of the vagina (see **Fig. 10.19**).
- A deep perineal branch of the pudendal nerve, a branch of the sacral plexus, innervates the lowest vaginal segment (see **Fig. 10.15**). This somatically innervated segment is the only part of the vagina that is sensitive to touch.

Culdocentesis

Culdocentesis is a procedure in which peritoneal fluid is extracted from the rectouterine pouch by needle aspiration. The needle is advanced through the posterior fornix of the vagina. No fluid or a small amount of clear fluid is normal, but purulent fluid is suggestive of pelvic inflammatory disease (PID). The presence of blood is an indication for emergency surgery.

11.3 Pelvic Urinary Organs

The pelvic urinary organs include the distal ureters, the urinary bladder, and the urethra.

11.3a The Ureters

Each ureter crosses over the brim of the pelvis at the bifurcation of the common iliac artery and descends along the lateral wall near the ischial spine. It runs anteriorly and enters the posterolateral wall of the bladder.

- In males, the ureter passes under the pelvic portion of the ductus deferens and enters the bladder lateral and superior to the free ends of the seminal vesicles (**Fig. 11.14**; see also **Fig. 11.2**).
- In females, the ureter passes inferior to the uterine arteries within the cardinal ligament, ~2 cm lateral to the vaginal part of the cervix (**Fig. 11.15**).
- The most reliable blood supply to the pelvic part of the ureter is the uterine artery in females and the inferior vesical artery in males. Veins of similar names accompany the arteries.
- The pelvic part of the ureter derives its innervation from the inferior hypogastric plexuses.
- Visceral afferent fibers follow sympathetic nerves to spinal cord levels T11–L2; therefore, ureteric pain is usually felt in the ipsilateral inguinal region.

Fig. 11.14 ▶ **Ureter and bladder in the male pelvis**
Superior view.

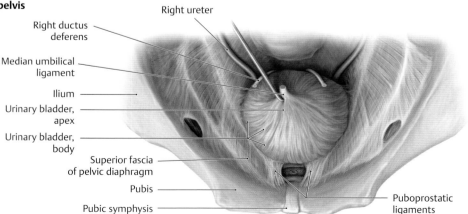

Right ureter
Right ductus deferens
Median umbilical ligament
Ilium
Urinary bladder, apex
Urinary bladder, body
Superior fascia of pelvic diaphragm
Pubis
Pubic symphysis
Puboprostatic ligaments

Fig. 11.15 ▶ **Ureter in the female pelvis**
Superior view. *Removed from right side:* Peritoneum and broad ligament of uterus.

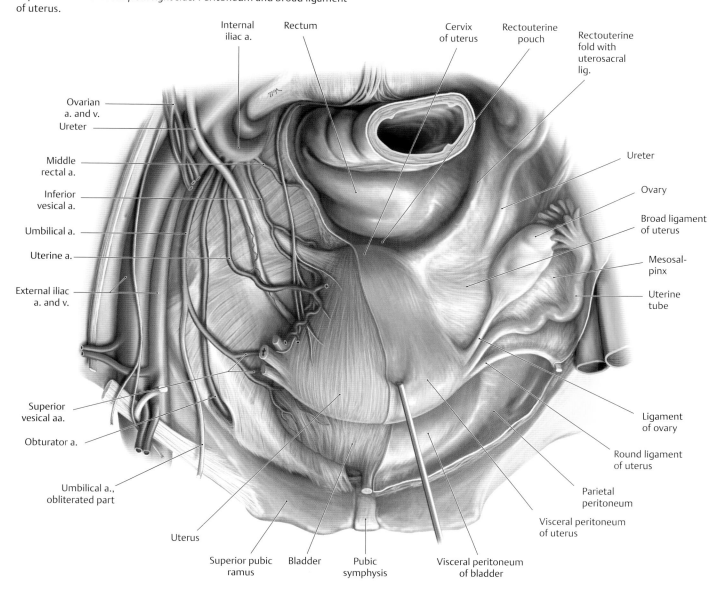

Internal iliac a.

Rectum

Cervix of uterus

Rectouterine pouch

Rectouterine fold with uterosacral lig.

Ovarian a. and v.

Ureter

Middle rectal a.

Inferior vesical a.

Umbilical a.

Uterine a.

External iliac a. and v.

Superior vesical aa.

Obturator a.

Umbilical a., obliterated part

Uterus

Superior pubic ramus

Bladder

Pubic symphysis

Visceral peritoneum of bladder

Ureter

Ovary

Broad ligament of uterus

Mesosalpinx

Uterine tube

Ligament of ovary

Round ligament of uterus

Parietal peritoneum

Visceral peritoneum of uterus

11.3b The Urinary Bladder

The bladder is a muscular reservoir for the temporary storage of urine. Although normally located in the true pelvis, when full it may extend superiorly into the abdomen.

— It lies directly posterior to the pubic symphysis, separated from it by the retropubic space. Posteriorly, it is related to the rectum in the male (see **Fig. 11.1**) and the upper vagina in the female (see **Fig. 11.5**).

— It is covered by peritoneum only on its superior surface.

— The bladder is tetrahedral with superior, posterior, and two inferolateral surfaces. It has four parts:

1. The **apex** points toward the pubic symphysis. The median umbilical ligament extends from the apex to the umbilicus.
2. The **fundus** forms the bladder base, or posterior wall.
3. The **body** makes up most of the bladder.
4. The **neck** is the lowest and least mobile region.

— The neck of the bladder is firmly attached to

• the pubis by anterior extensions of the tendinous arch of the pelvic fascia, the **pubovesical ligaments** in females and puboprostatic ligaments in males (see **Figs. 11.11** and **11.14**); and

• the lateral pelvic walls by condensations of endopelvic fascia, the **lateral vesicular ligaments** (see **Fig. 10.12**).

— The walls are made up of bundles of smooth muscle fibers. In the male, the muscle fibers near the bladder neck, which form the internal urethral sphincter, contract during ejaculation.

— The internal surface of the base of the bladder is marked by the **trigone**, a smooth triangular region (**Fig. 11.16**). The corners of the triangle are formed posterolaterally by the slitlike openings of the right and left ureters and anteriorly by the urethral orifice.

— The bladder is highly distensible and in most individuals may hold up to 600–800 mL (painfully), although micturition (urination) usually occurs at a much smaller volume. Normally, no urine remains in the bladder after voiding.

— The superior vesical arteries, with contributions from the inferior vesical arteries (in males) and vaginal arteries (in females), supply the bladder (see **Fig. 10.14A** and **B**).

— The vesical venous plexus surrounds the inferolateral surfaces of the bladder and drains to the internal iliac veins. The plexus communicates with the prostatic plexus in males, with the uterovaginal plexus in females, and with the vertebral venous plexus in both sexes.

— Lymph from the bladder drains to internal and external iliac nodes.

Fig. 11.16 ▶ **Trigone of the bladder**
Coronal section, anterior view.

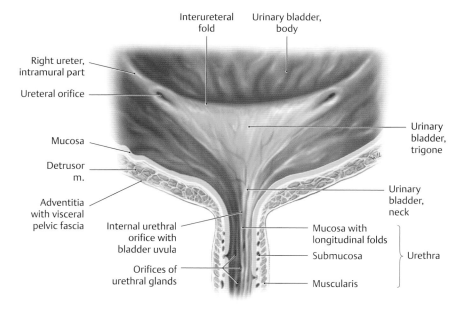

Interureteral fold

Urinary bladder, body

Right ureter, intramural part

Ureteral orifice

Mucosa

Detrusor m.

Adventitia with visceral pelvic fascia

Internal urethral orifice with bladder uvula

Orifices of urethral glands

Urinary bladder, trigone

Urinary bladder, neck

Mucosa with longitudinal folds

Submucosa

Muscularis

Urethra

— The vesical nerve plexus of the bladder is a derivative of the inferior hypogastric plexus (see **Fig. 10.19**).

- Sympathetic stimulation relaxes the detrusor muscle and contracts the internal sphincter, thus inhibiting micturition.
- Parasympathetic nerves stimulate the detrusor muscle to contract while inhibiting the internal sphincter, thereby facilitating micturition.
- Afferent fibers carrying pain from the inferior bladder follow parasympathetic routes. Pain fibers from the superior bladder follow sympathetic routes.

11.3c The Urethra

The urethra is the muscular conduit for urine in the female and for urine and semen in the male. It extends from the internal urethral orifice at the bladder neck to the external urethral orifice in the perineum.

— The male urethra extends 18 to 22 cm from the urinary bladder to the tip of the glans penis (**Fig. 11.17**). The male urethra has four parts. Although all are mentioned here, the membranous and spongy parts are located in the perineum and are discussed further in Chapter 12.

1. The **preprostatic** part at the neck of the bladder contains the internal urethral orifice. Sympathetic nerves of the superior hypogastric plexus control closure of the **internal urethral sphincter** during ejaculation.
2. The **prostatic** part is surrounded by the prostate gland and characterized by
   - the **urethral crest**, a vertical ridge on the posterior wall that contains a central eminence, the **seminal colliculus**; and
   - ejaculatory ducts that open onto the urethral crest, and prostatic ductules from the prostate that open into recesses on either side of the crest.
3. The **membranous** part passes through the perineal membrane in the urogenital triangle and is surrounded by the external urethral sphincter.
4. The **spongy** part passes through the corpus spongiosum, one of the vascular erectile bodies of the penis.

Urethral rupture in males

Fractures of the pelvic girdle may be accompanied by a rupture of the membranous part of the urethra. This allows the extravasation (escape) of urine and blood into the deep perineal space and superiorly through the genital hiatus to the subperitoneal spaces around the prostate and bladder. Rupture of the bulbous part of the spongy urethra may occur from a straddle injury in which there is a forceful blow to the perineum, or from the false passage of a transurethral catheter. In this case urine can leak into the superficial peritoneal space, which is continuous with the scrotal sac, the space around the penis, and the space on the inferior anterior abdominal wall between the abdominal muscles and the membranous layer of the superficial fascia. The attachment of the superficial perineal fascia to the fascia lata (fascia enclosing the thigh muscles) prevents urine from spreading laterally into the thighs. Similarly, it is prevented from spreading into the anal triangle by the attachment of the fascia to the deep perineal fascia and perineal membrane.

Fig. 11.17 ▶ **Male urethra**
Longitudinal section, anterior view.

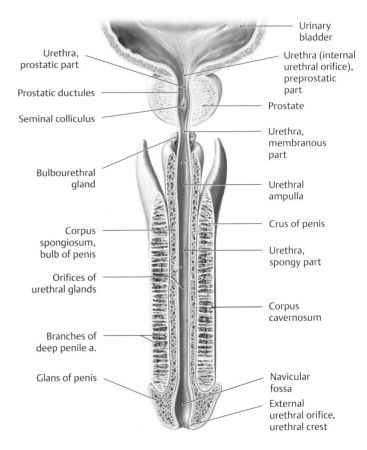

— The female urethra extends 4 cm from the internal urethral orifice at the bladder neck to the external urethral orifice in the perineum (**Fig. 11.18**).

    • Within the pelvis it lies anterior to the vagina, forming an elevation within the anterior vaginal wall.

    • It passes through the genital hiatus of the pelvic diaphragm, the external urethral sphincter (there is no organized internal urethral sphincter), and the perineal membrane.

    • In the perineum, the urethra opens within the vestibule of the vagina directly anterior to the vaginal orifice (see **Fig. 12.8**).

— Branches of the pudendal artery, as well as the inferior vesical artery in the male and vaginal artery in the female, supply the urethra. In both sexes, a venous plexus that accompanies the arteries drains the urethra.

— The female urethra and proximal parts of the male urethra (preprostatic, prostatic, and membranous) drain to the internal iliac nodes. The spongy urethra of the male (the perineal part) drains to deep inguinal nodes.

— Nerves to the urethra arise from the prostatic nerve plexus in the male and comparable vesical nerve plexus in the female. Sympathetic nerves control the closure of the external urethral sphincter in males.

— Visceral afferent fibers from the pelvic urethra travel with pelvic splanchnic nerves; somatic afferent fibers from the perineal urethra travel with the pudendal nerve.

Fig. 11.18 ▶ **Female urethra**
Coronal section tilted slightly posterior, anterior view.

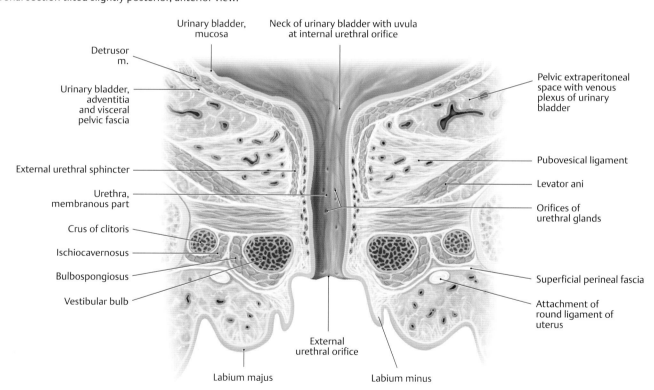

Urinary bladder, mucosa

Neck of urinary bladder with uvula at internal urethral orifice

Detrusor m.

Urinary bladder, adventitia and visceral pelvic fascia

Pelvic extraperitoneal space with venous plexus of urinary bladder

External urethral sphincter

Pubovesical ligament

Urethra, membranous part

Levator ani

Crus of clitoris

Orifices of urethral glands

Ischiocavernosus

Bulbospongiosus

Superficial perineal fascia

Vestibular bulb

Attachment of round ligament of uterus

External urethral orifice

Labium majus

Labium minus

11.4 The Rectum

The rectum is the continuation of the gastrointestinal tract in the pelvis and functions as a temporary storage site for fecal matter. It is continuous with the sigmoid colon superiorly and the anal canal inferiorly (see Section 12.5a; **Figs. 11.19** and **11.20**).

— It lies anterior to the lower sacrum and coccyx and rests on the anococcygeal ligament of the pelvic floor.
— Anteriorly, the rectum is related to the bladder, seminal glands, and prostate in males and to the vagina in females. A rectovesical or rectovaginal septum separates the rectum from these anterior structures.

— The rectum has no mesentery. Its superior two thirds are retroperitoneal and form the posterior surface of the rectovesical and rectouterine pouches. The distal third is subperitoneal.
— Unlike the colon, the rectum lacks taeniae coli, haustra, and epiploic appendices.
— The rectum begins at the **rectosigmoid junction**, the point at which the teniae coli disappear. At this junction, muscle fibers of the bands spread out evenly over the surface of the rectum. This junction usually occurs anterior to the S3 vertebra.

Rectal examination

A rectal examination is performed by inserting a gloved, lubricated finger into the rectum, while the other hand is used to press on the lower abdomen or pelvic region. Palpable structures include the prostate, seminal vesicles, ampulla of the ductus deferens, bladder, uterus, cervix, and ovaries. Pathological anomalies such as hemorrhoids, tumors, enlargements, and changes in consistency of the tissues can be felt. The tonicity of the anal sphincter, mediated by the pudendal nerve (S2–S4), can also be assessed.

Fig. 11.19 ▶ **Rectum in situ**
Female pelvis, coronal section, anterior view.

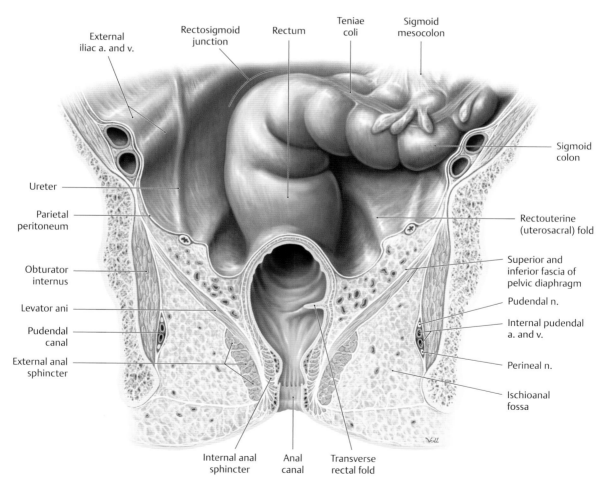

— The rectum terminates at the **anorectal junction** (its junction with the anal canal), where it passes through the pelvic diaphragm adjacent to the tip of the coccyx.

— The internal wall of the rectum has three transverse **rectal folds**, one on the right and two on the left, which create lateral flexures that are visible externally.

— The **ampulla**, the most distal segment of the rectum, stores accumulating fecal material until defecation and has an important role in fecal continence. It narrows abruptly as it joins with the anal canal and passes through the pelvic diaphragm.

Fig. 11.20 ▶ **Rectum**
Coronal section, anterior view.

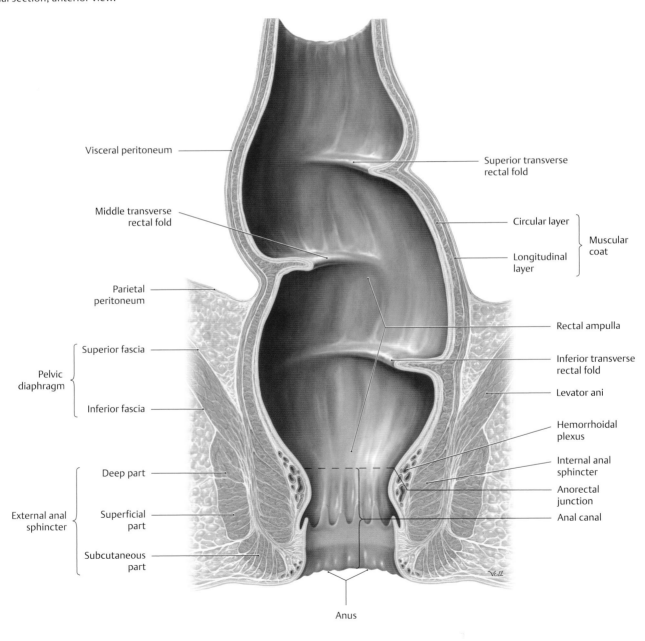

— The rectum has a dual blood supply:

- The superior rectal artery, the unpaired terminal branch of the inferior mesenteric artery, supplies the upper rectum (see **Fig. 10.18**).
- Right and left middle rectal arteries, branches of the internal iliac arteries, supply the lower rectum.

— The rectal veins drain a submucosal rectal venous plexus, which has internal and external (subcutaneous) components.

- The external plexus communicates with other visceral venous plexuses in the pelvis.
- The internal plexus communicates with branches from the rectal arteries (an arteriovenous anastomosis), forming a thickened vascular tissue (**hemorrhoidal plexus**) that surrounds the anorectal junction. This tissue forms prominent anal cushions in the left lateral, right anterolateral, and right posterolateral positions.

Hemorrhoids

External hemorrhoids are thrombosed veins of the external venous plexus, commonly associated with pregnancy or chronic constipation. They lie below the dentate line and are covered by skin. Because they are somatically innervated, they are more painful than internal hemorrhoids.

Internal hemorrhoids contain dilated veins of the internal rectal plexus. With a breakdown of the muscularis layer, these vascular cushions prolapse into the anal canal and may become ulcerated. Because they lie above the dentate line and are viscerally innervated, these hemorrhoids are painless. They are generally not associated with portal hypertension, but bleeding is characteristically bright red due to the anastomoses between the venous plexus and branches of the rectal arteries.

— Venous blood from the rectum drains into the portal and caval (systemic) venous systems (see **Fig. 10.18**).

- A superior rectal vein, which drains the upper rectum, is a tributary of the portal system via the inferior mesenteric vein.
- The paired middle and inferior rectal veins that drain the lower rectum (and anal canal) are tributaries of the inferior vena cava via the internal iliac veins.
- Communications between the superior, middle, and inferior rectal veins form clinically important portocaval anastomoses that enlarge in portal hypertension.

— Lymphatic drainage follows venous pathways.

- The upper rectum drains to inferior mesenteric nodes along the course of the superior rectal artery. It eventually drains to lumbar nodes, although some lymph may drain first to sacral nodes.
- The lower rectum drains primarily to sacral nodes or directly to internal iliac nodes.

— Sympathetic innervation to the rectum is carried by lumbar splanchnic nerves to the hypogastric plexuses, as well as by nerves of the inferior mesenteric nerve plexus traveling along the superior rectal artery (see **Figs. 10.19** and **10.20**).

— Parasympathetic innervation originates in pelvic splanchnic nerves, which also carry visceral afferent fibers.

12 The Perineum

The perineum is the space inferior to the pelvic floor, which is divided into a urogenital triangle and an anal triangle. The urogenital triangle contains the male and female external genital structures, and the anal triangle contains the anal canal and anus.

12.1 Perineal Spaces (**Figs. 12.1** and **12.2**; see also **Figs. 10.3** and **10.4**)

— The boundaries of the diamond-shaped perineum are
  - the pelvic outlet (pubic symphysis, ischiopubic rami, sacrotuberous ligaments, and coccyx), which forms the perimeter;
  - the lower parts of the obturator internus muscles and their obturator fasciae, which line the lateral walls;
  - the inferior surface of the pelvic diaphragm, which forms the roof; and
  - the skin of the perineum, which forms the floor.

— A line connecting the ischial tuberosities separates the perineum into an anterior urogenital triangle and a posterior anal triangle (see **Fig. 10.4A** and **B**).

— The **perineal membrane**, a tough, fibrous sheet, stretches between the ischiopubic rami, extending anteriorly almost to the pubic symphysis and posteriorly to the ischial tuberosities.
  - It separates the urogenital triangle into the **deep perineal** and **superficial perineal spaces**.
  - It forms a platform for the attachment of the cavernous bodies (which become engorged during arousal) of the external genitalia.

— The superficial perineal space is a potential space bounded above by the perineal membrane and below by the **superficial perineal fascia** (Colles' fascia), the extension of the membranous layer of superficial fascia (Scarpa's fascia) on the abdominal wall.
  - In both sexes it contains
    - the **bulbocavernosus, ischiocavernosus,** and **superficial transverse perineal muscles** and
    - the **deep perineal branches** of the internal pudendal vessels and pudendal nerve.
  - In males it also contains
    - the **root** of the penis and
    - the proximal portion of the spongy urethra.
  - In females it also contains (see **Fig. 12.8**)
    - the **clitoris** and associated muscles,
    - the **vestibular bulb,** and
    - the **greater vestibular glands**.

— The deep perineal space is bounded inferiorly by the perineal membrane and superiorly by the pelvic diaphragm.
  - In both sexes it contains
    - part of the urethra and inferior part of the **external urethral sphincter**.
    - the anterior recesses of the **ischioanal fat pads,** and
    - neurovascular structures to the penis or clitoris.
  - In males it also contains
    - the membranous part of the urethra,
    - the **bulbourethral glands,** and
    - the **deep transverse perineal muscles**.
  - In females it also contains
    - compressor urethrae and urethrovaginal sphincter,
    - the proximal part of the urethra, and
    - smooth muscle associated with the **perineal body**.

Fig. 12.1 ► **Muscles and fascia of the female perineum**
Lithotomy position, caudal (inferior) view. The green arrow is pointing forward to the anterior recess of the ischioanal fossa.

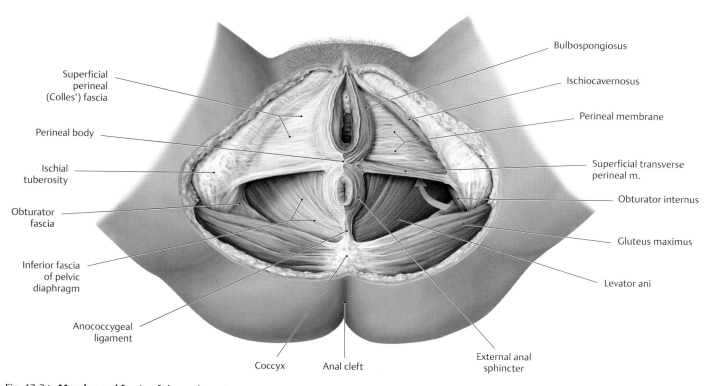

Superficial perineal (Colles') fascia
Perineal body
Ischial tuberosity
Obturator fascia
Inferior fascia of pelvic diaphragm
Anococcygeal ligament
Coccyx
Anal cleft
Bulbospongiosus
Ischiocavernosus
Perineal membrane
Superficial transverse perineal m.
Obturator internus
Gluteus maximus
Levator ani
External anal sphincter

Fig. 12.2 ► **Muscles and fascia of the male perineum**
Lithotomy position, caudal (inferior) view. The green arrow is pointing forward to the anterior recess of the ischioanal fossa.

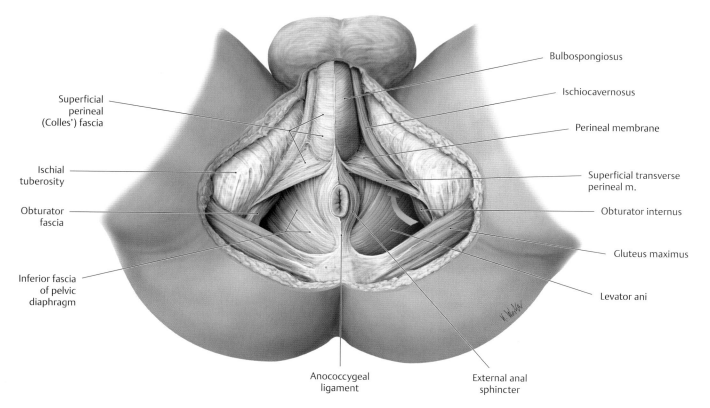

Superficial perineal (Colles') fascia
Ischial tuberosity
Obturator fascia
Inferior fascia of pelvic diaphragm
Anococcygeal ligament
External anal sphincter
Bulbospongiosus
Ischiocavernosus
Perineal membrane
Superficial transverse perineal m.
Obturator internus
Gluteus maximus
Levator ani

12.2 Muscles of the Perineum

- Muscles of the perineum support the pelvic floor, surround the orifices of the urethra and anus, and assist in the erection of genital structures (**Table 12.1**, **Fig. 12.3A** and **B**; see also **Figs. 12.1** and **12.2**).
- The **perineal body** is an irregular subcutaneous mass of fibromuscular tissue formed by converging fibers of the levator ani, the deep transverse perineal and bulbospongiosus muscles, and the external anal sphincter.
  - It lies between the rectum and bulb of the penis in males and between the rectum and vagina in females.
  - It supports the pelvic diaphragm and pelvic viscera.
- **Perineal branches** of the internal pudendal artery supply muscles of the perineum. Venous blood drains to the internal pudendal vein and the internal iliac vein.
- The pudendal nerve (S2–S4) innervates the muscles of the perineum.

Fig. 12.3 ► **Muscles of the perineum**
Inferior view.

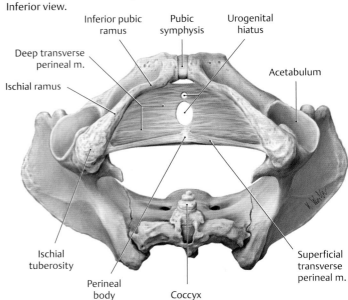

A Superficial and deep transverse perineal muscles.

Table 12.1 ► **Muscles of the Perineum**				
Muscle	**Origin**	**Insertion**	**Innervation**	**Action**
Deep perineal space				
External urethral sphincter		Encircles urethra	Pudendal n. (S2–S4)	Compresses urethra
Compressor urethrae (females)	Ischiopubic ramus	Part of external urethral sphincter		Compresses urethra
Urethrovaginal sphincter (females)	Anterior urethra	Interdigitates with opposite side posterior to vagina		Compresses urethra and vagina
Deep transverse perineal	Inferior pubic ramus, ischial ramus	Wall of vagina or prostate, perineal body		Supports the prostate
Superficial perineal space				
Bulbospongiosus	Runs anteriorly from perineal body to clitoris (female) or penile raphe (male)		Pudendal n. (S2–S4)	Females: compresses greater vestibular gland Males: assists in erection
Ischiocavernosus	Ischial ramus	Crus of clitoris or penis	Pudendal n. (S2–S4)	Maintains erection by squeezing blood into the corpus cavernosum of the clitoris or penis
Superficial transverse perineal	Ischial ramus	Perineal body	Pudendal n. (S2–S4)	Stabilizes the perineal body
Anal triangle				
External anal sphincter	Encircles anus (runs posteriorly from perineal body to anococcygeal ligament)		Pudendal n. (S2–S4)	Closes the anus

■ Episiotomy

During vaginal delivery, pressure on the perineum risks tearing the perineal muscles. A clean incision through the posterior vaginal orifice into the perineal body, known as an episiotomy, is often performed to enlarge the opening and prevent damage to perineal muscles. A median episiotomy extends only into the perineal body, but if further traumatic tearing occurs to extend the cut, it can damage the external anal sphincter (resulting in fecal incontinence) or create an anovaginal fistula. Mediolateral episiotomies often replace the midline incisions. These extend laterally from the vaginal orifice to the superficial perineal muscles, thus avoiding the perineal body and the possible sequelae from extensive tearing.

■ Prolapse of pelvic organs

The pelvic diaphragm, pelvic ligaments, and perineal body provide important structural support for the pelvic viscera. Stretching or disruption of these tissues often occurs during childbirth and results in prolapse of the uterus into the vagina. A widening of the genital hiatus from an atrophic pelvic floor or a weakened perineal body can allow the bladder (cystocele), rectum (rectocele), or rectovesical pouch (enterocele) to bulge into the vaginal wall.

Fig. 12.3 ▶ **Muscles of the perineum** (*continued*)

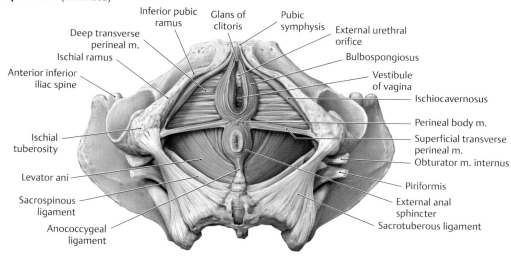

B Sphincter and erector muscles, female.

12.3 Male Urogenital Triangle

The male urogenital triangle contains the scrotum, penis, bulbourethral glands, perineal muscles, and associated neurovasculature (see **Figs. 10.3** and **11.3**).

12.3a The Scrotum

— The **scrotum** is a saccular extension of the anterior abdominal wall that encloses the testes and spermatic cord (see Section 7.3).

— The subcutaneous layer of the skin over the scrotum is devoid of fat, but the **dartos fascia** that underlies the skin is continuous with the deep membranous layer of the superficial fascia (Scarpa's fascia) of the abdomen and with the superficial perineal fascia (Colles' fascia) of the perineum.

— An extension of dartos fascia divides the scrotum into right and left compartments and is visible externally as the **scrotal raphe**.

— Scrotal branches of the internal pudendal and external pudendal arteries, and cremasteric branches of the inferior epigastric artery supply the scrotum. Veins of similar names accompany the arteries (**Figs. 12.4A** and **B** and **12.5**).

Fig. 12.4 ▶ **Blood vessels of the male genitalia**
Left lateral view.

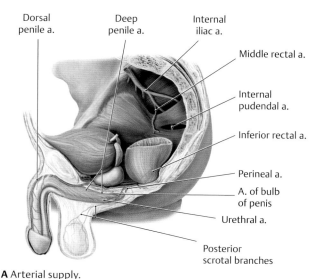

A Arterial supply.

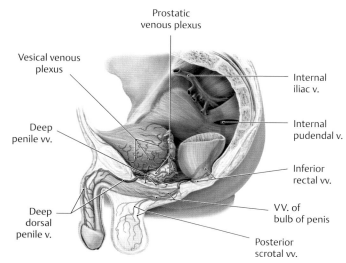

B Venous drainage.

Fig. 12.5 ▶ **Neurovasculature of the penis and scrotum**
Anterior view. *Partially removed:* Skin and fascia.

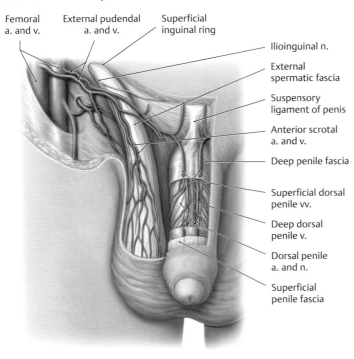

Femoral a. and v.
External pudendal a. and v.
Superficial inguinal ring
Ilioinguinal n.
External spermatic fascia
Suspensory ligament of penis
Anterior scrotal a. and v.
Deep penile fascia
Superficial dorsal penile vv.
Deep dorsal penile v.
Dorsal penile a. and n.
Superficial penile fascia

— Lymph from the scrotum drains to superficial inguinal nodes. Recall that lymph from the contents within the scrotum (i.e., the testis and epididymis) drains directly to the para-aortic nodes.

— Innervation of the scrotum (see **Fig. 10.22B**) is supplied by

  • the ilioinguinal and genitofemoral (genital branch) nerves, which innervate the anterior scrotum, and

  • the pudendal and posterior femoral cutaneous nerves of the thigh, which innervate the posterior scrotum.

12.3b   The Penis

The **penis** is the male copulatory organ, transmitting semen during sexual intercourse. It contains the spongy part of the urethra and therefore also transmits urine from the bladder (**Fig. 12.6A** and **B**).

— It has three parts:

  1. The **root**, attached to the perineal membrane and covered by muscles, is composed of

    ○ paired **crura** that are attached to the ischiopubic rami and covered by the ischiocavernosus muscles, and

    ○ the **bulb of the penis**, which is attached to the perineal membrane and covered by the bulbospongiosus muscle. The spongy urethra enters on its dorsal surface.

2. The **body**, pendulous and not covered by muscle, is made up of three cylindrical bodies of erectile tissue. A **tunica albuginea**, a dense fibrous coat, surrounds each erectile body, and distally a **deep penile fascia** (Buck's fascia) binds the three bodies together. The three erectile bodies include

  ○ two **corpora cavernosa**, continuations of the crura, which lie side by side on the dorsum of the penis, and

  ○ one **corpus spongiosum**, a continuation of the bulb of the penis, which lies ventral to the two corpora cavernosa and is traversed by the penile urethra.

3. The **glans penis** (also known as the **glans**), an expansion of the distal end of the corpus spongiosum, is characterized by

  ○ the **corona**, which overhangs the distal ends of the corpora cavernosa, and

  ○ the **external urethral orifice** at its tip.

— The external pudendal artery supplies the skin and subcutaneous tissue of the penis. Venous drainage of this tissue passes through the **superficial dorsal veins**, which drain to the external pudendal veins (see **Fig. 12.5**).

— The internal pudendal artery supplies the deep penile structures. Its branches (**Fig. 12.7**; see also **Fig. 12.6B**) include

  • the **artery of the bulb of the penis**, which supplies the bulb of the penis, the urethra within the bulb, and the bulbourethral glands;

  • the **dorsal penile artery**, which runs between the deep penile fascia and tunica albuginea to supply the penile fascia and skin and the glans; and

  • the **deep penile artery**, which runs within the corpus cavernosum and gives off **helicine arteries** that supply the erectile tissue and are responsible for engorgement of the corpora during erection.

— The erectile bodies are drained by a venous plexus that empties into the single **deep dorsal vein**, which passes under the pubic symphysis to join the prostatic venous plexus in the pelvis.

— Lymphatic drainage areas of the penis include

  • the erectile bodies of the penis, which drain to internal iliac nodes;

  • the glans penis, which drains to deep inguinal nodes; and

  • the urethra, which drains to internal iliac and deep inguinal nodes.

— The glans of the penis is richly innervated by sensory fibers via the **dorsal penile nerve**, a branch of the pudendal nerve. Sympathetic fibers from the hypogastric nerve plexus are also carried along this route.

Fig. 12.6 ▶ **Penis**

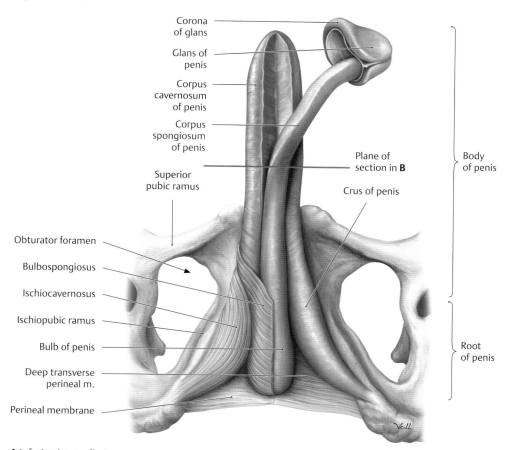

A Inferior (ventral) view.

Fig. 12.7 ▶ **Neurovasculature on the dorsum of the penis**
Superior (dorsal) view. *Removed:* Skin.

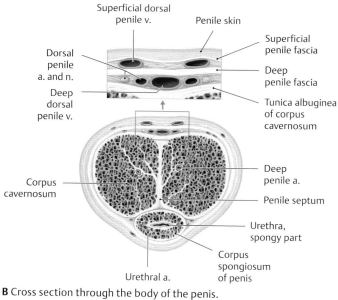

B Cross section through the body of the penis.

— Parasympathetic fibers carried by the cavernous nerves derived from the prostatic plexus innervate the helicine arteries within the erectile tissue and are responsible for penile erection.

12.3c Bulbourethral Glands

The bulbourethral glands are paired mucus-secreting glands (see **Figs. 11.2** and **11.3**).

— They lie on either side of the urethra below the prostate surrounded by the urethral sphincter.
— Their ducts open into the proximal part of the spongy urethra.
— They are active during sexual arousal.

12.3d Erection, Emission, and Ejaculation

The sexual responses of **erection**, **emission**, and **ejaculation** involve sympathetic, parasympathetic, and somatic (via the pudendal nerve) pathways.

— During erection
  • constriction of the helicine arteries, normally maintained by sympathetic innervation, is inhibited by parasympathetic stimulation. As the arteries relax, the cavernous spaces dilate and become engorged, and
  • contractions of the bulbocavernosus and ischiocavernosus muscles, innervated by the pudendal nerve, impede venous outflow and maintain the erection.

— During emission
  • parasympathetic stimulation mediates the secretion of seminal fluid from the seminal glands, bulbourethral glands, and prostate gland, and
  • sympathetic stimulation mediates emission, the movement of seminal fluid through the ducts, by initiating peristalsis of the ductus deferens and seminal glands. This propels the seminal fluid into the prostatic urethra, where additional fluid is added as the prostate contracts.

— During ejaculation
  • sympathetic stimulation constricts the internal urethral sphincter, which prevents the seminal fluid from entering the bladder (retrograde ejaculation);
  • parasympathetic stimulation contracts the urethral muscles; and
  • the pudendal nerve contracts the bulbospongiosus muscle.

▌ Retrograde ejaculation

Relaxation of the detrusor muscle and contraction of the internal urethral sphincter in males are controlled by sympathetic fibers from the superior hypogastric plexus. Closure of the sphincter occurs during ejaculation, preventing the retrograde flow of semen into the bladder. Disruption of the sympathetic nerves can result in retrograde ejaculation. This can occur during the repair of an abdominal aortic aneurysm, for example, if the aneurysm involves the bifurcation of the aorta.

12.4 Female Urogenital Triangle

As in the male perineum, the female perineum contains erectile bodies, secretory glands, and their associated neurovasculature. In addition, it contains paired folds of skin that surround the urethral and vaginal orifices. These external genitalia are known collectively as the **vulva** (**Figs. 12.8, 12.9,** and **12.10**).

— The **mons pubis**, a superficial mound of fatty subcutaneous tissue that is continuous with the superficial fatty layer of the abdominal wall, lies anterior to the pubic symphysis and is continuous with the **labia majora**.
— **Labia majora**, bilateral folds of fatty subcutaneous tissue, flank the **pudendal cleft**, the opening between the labia. The labia join anteriorly at the **anterior commissure** and posteriorly at the **posterior commissure**. Pigmented skin and coarse pubic hair cover the labia's outer surface; the inner surface is smooth and hairless.

Fig. 12.8 ► **Female external genitalia**
Lithotomy position with labia minora separated.

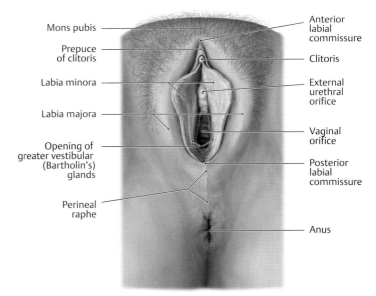

— **Labia minora**, bilateral folds of hairless skin within the pudendal cleft, flank the vestibule of the vagina.
— The **clitoris**, a highly sensitive erectile organ, is located at the anterior junction of the paired labia minora.
- Paired erectile bodies, the **corpora cavernosa**, make up the crura, which join to form the **body** of the clitoris. The **prepuce** (hood) covers the body.
- The **glans** at the tip of the clitoris is its most sensitive part.

— The **vestibule** of the vagina is a space surrounded by the two labia minora. It contains the urethral and vaginal orifices and the openings of the ducts of the greater vestibular and lesser vestibular glands.
— **Vestibular bulbs** are paired masses of erectile tissue that lie deep to the labia minora and are covered by the bulbospongiosus muscles.

Fig. 12.9 ▶ **Vestibule and vestibular glands**
Lithotomy position with labia separated.

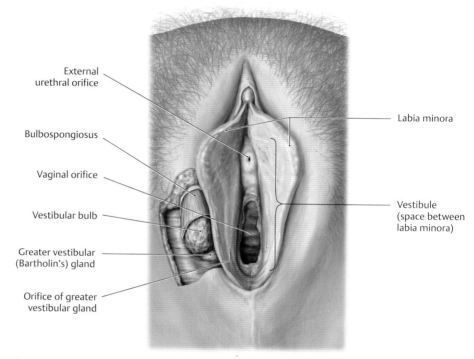

Fig. 12.10 ▶ **Erectile muscles and tissue of the female genitalia**
Lithotomy position. *Removed:* Labia, skin, and perineal membrane; *Removed from left side:* Ischiocavernosus and bulbospongiosus muscles; greater vestibular (Bartholin's) gland.

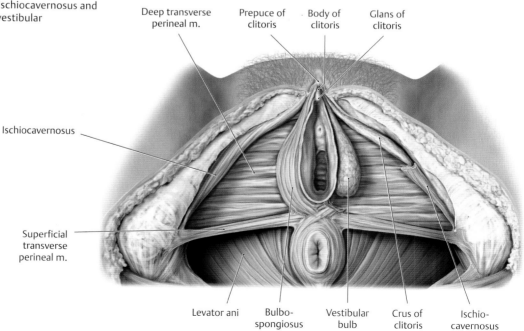

— **Greater vestibular** (Bartholin's) **glands**, small glands that lie under the posterior end of the vestibular bulbs, help to lubricate the vestibule during sexual arousal.

— Small **lesser vestibular glands** lie on each side of the vestibule and secrete mucus to moisten the labia and vestibule.

— The external pudendal artery supplies the skin over the mons pubis and labia majora. Similar to those in the male, these superficial structures drain to the external pudendal vein.

— The internal pudendal artery supplies most of the external genitalia through branches that are similar to those in the male perineum (**Fig. 12.11A**).

• The **perineal artery** supplies perineal muscles and labia minora.

• The **artery of the vestibular bulb** supplies the bulb of the vestibule and greater vestibular gland.

• The **dorsal clitoral artery** supplies the glans of the clitoris.

• The **deep clitoral artery** supplies the corpus cavernosum and is responsible for their engorgement during arousal.

— Tributaries of the pudendal vein drain most perineal structures and accompany the arteries. A single **deep dorsal clitoral vein** drains the venous plexuses of the erectile tissue and passes under the pubic symphysis to join the venous plexus in the pelvis (**Fig. 12.11B**).

— Most lymph from the female perineum drains to superficial inguinal lymph nodes. Exceptions include

• the clitoris, bulbs of the vestibule, and anterior labia, which drain to deep inguinal or internal iliac nodes; and

• the urethra, which drains to sacral or internal iliac nodes.

— The pudendal nerve is the primary nerve of the perineum (see **Fig. 10.21B**). It supplies

• the **perineal nerve** to the vaginal orifice and superficial perineal muscles;

• the **dorsal clitoral nerve** to deep perineal muscles and sensation from the clitoris, especially the glans; and

• the **posterior labial nerves** to the posterior vulva.

— As in the innervation of the male scrotum, the anterior vulva receives sensory innervation (see **Fig. 10.21B**) from

• the ilioinguinal nerve and genital branch of the genitofemoral nerve, which supply branches to the mons pubis and anterior labia; and

• the posterior femoral cutaneous nerve, which supplies the posterolateral vulva.

— Sympathetic fibers to the perineum travel with the hypogastric nerve plexus; parasympathetic fibers travel with cavernous nerves of the uterovaginal plexus. Both innervate the erectile tissue of the clitoris and bulbs of the vestibule.

Fig. 12.11 ▶ **Blood vessels of the female external genitalia** Inferior view.

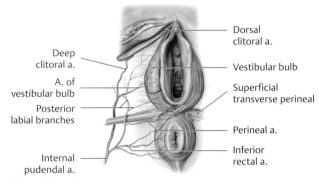

A Arterial supply.

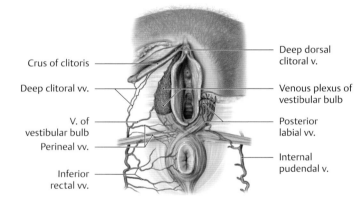

B Venous drainage.

12.5 Anal Triangle

The anal triangle contains the anal canal and ischioanal fossae.

12.5a The Anal Canal

The **anal canal**, the terminal part of the gastrointestinal tract, controls fecal continence and the defecation response. It extends from the anorectal junction at the pelvic diaphragm to the **anus** (**Fig. 12.12**).

— The puborectalis muscle forms a sling around the anorectal junction, pulling it anteriorly and creating the **perineal flexure** (**Fig. 12.13**). From this angle the anal canal descends inferiorly and posteriorly between the anococcygeal ligament (levator plate) and the perineal body (see **Fig. 12.1A** and **B**).

Fig. 12.12 ▶ **Anal canal**
Coronal section, anterior view.

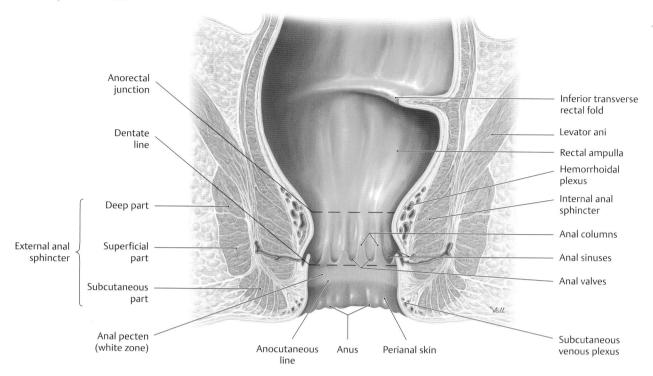

Fig. 12.13 ▶ **Closure of the rectum**
Left lateral view. The puborectalis acts as a muscular sling that kinks the anorectal junction. It functions in the maintenance of fecal continence.

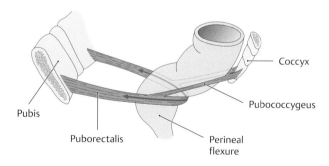

— Two sphincters surround the anal canal:

1. The **internal anal sphincter** is a thickening of the circular muscular layer that surrounds the upper part of the anal canal.

   ○ It is an involuntary sphincter.
   ○ It remains contracted via sympathetic innervation except in response to distension of the rectal ampulla. Parasympathetic innervation relaxes the sphincter.

2. The **external anal sphincter** is a broad band of muscle that extends anteriorly to merge with the perineal body, posteriorly to attach to the coccyx (through the anococcygeal ligament), and superiorly to merge with the puborectalis muscle of the pelvic floor (see also **Figs. 11.1, 12.1,** and **12.2**).

   ○ It is a voluntary sphincter.
   ○ Although the anal sphincter is described as having deep, superficial, and subcutaneous parts, they are functionally, and often anatomically, indistinct.
   ○ The inferior rectal nerve, a branch of the pudendal nerve, innervates this sphincter.

— The inner surface of the anal canal is characterized by

- **anal columns**, vertical ridges formed by underlying branches of the superior mesenteric vessels;
- **anal valves** that connect the inferior edges of the anal columns; and
- **anal sinuses**, recesses at the base of the anal columns that secrete mucus to facilitate defecation.

— The **dentate** (**pectinate) line** is an irregular ridge at the base of the anal columns.

  • It divides the anal canal into a superior part derived from the embryonic hindgut and an inferior part derived from the ectoderm.

  • It divides the anal canal in its blood supply, lymphatic drainage, and innervation.

— Below the dentate line, a smooth lining devoid of glands and hair, the **anal pecten**, extends down to the **anocutaneous line**, or intersphincteric groove.

— Below the anocutaneous line, the anal canal is lined by hair-bearing skin that is continuous with **perianal skin** that surrounds the anus.

> **■ Anal fissures**
>
> Anal fissures are tears in the mucosa around the anus (usually in the posterior midline) that are caused by the passing of hard or large stools. Because they are below the pectinate line and innervated by the inferior rectal nerves, these lesions are painful. Most anal fissures heal spontaneously within a few weeks if care is taken to prevent constipation. Perianal abscesses that develop from the fissures can spread into the adjacent ischioanal fossae.

— Above the dentate line the neurovasculature of the anal canal is similar to that of the distal gastrointestinal tract (see **Figs. 10.18** and **10.20**).

  • It receives its blood supply from the superior rectal artery, a branch of the inferior mesenteric artery.

  • The rectal venous plexus drains through the superior rectal vein into the portal venous system.

  • Lymph drains to the internal iliac nodes.

  • Visceral innervation is transmitted via rectal plexuses to the inferior hypogastric plexus.

    ○ Sympathetic stimulation maintains the tone of the sphincter.

    ○ Parasympathetic innervation relaxes the sphincter and stimulates peristalsis of the rectum.

    ○ Visceral afferent fibers travel with pelvic splanchnic (parasympathetic) nerves and convey only sensation of stretching (no sensitivity to pain).

— Below the dentate line the neurovasculature of the anal canal is similar to that of the perineum (see **Fig. 10.15**).

  • It receives its blood supply from the right and left **inferior rectal arteries**, branches of the internal iliac arteries.

  • The rectal venous plexus drains into **inferior rectal veins**, which in turn drain to internal iliac veins of the venae caval system.

  • Lymph drains to superficial inguinal nodes.

  • Somatic innervation is transmitted via the **inferior rectal nerve**, a branch of the pudendal nerve.

    ○ Somatic efferent fibers stimulate contraction of the external anal sphincter.

    ○ Somatic afferent fibers transmit pain, touch, and temperature.

12.5b Ischioanal Fossae and Pudendal Canal

— The ischioanal fossae are paired wedge-shaped spaces on either side of the anal canal bounded by the pelvic diaphragm superiorly and the skin of the anal region inferiorly (see **Fig. 11.19**).

  • Fat and loose connective tissue, strengthened by strong, fibrous bands, fill the fossae. These tissues support the anal canal but can be displaced readily when the anal canal distends with feces.

  • The inferior rectal vessels and nerve, branches of the internal pudendal vessels and pudendal nerve, traverse the fossae.

  • The ischioanal fossae extend anteriorly into the urogenital triangle superior to the perineal membrane.

— The pudendal canal is a passageway formed by the splitting of the fascia of the obturator internus muscle on the lateral wall of the ischioanal fossa.

  • The internal pudendal artery and vein and the pudendal nerve enter the canal after exiting the lesser sciatic foramen and giving off inferior rectal branches.

Review Questions: Pelvis and Perineum

1. During a practice match, a heavyweight prizefighter endured an illegal hit to the left flank. Following the match, a focused assessment with sonography for trauma (FAST) exam revealed that blood from a renal laceration had tracked inferiorly and accumulated in the groove between the psoas major and iliacus muscles. What nerve would you expect to be irritated by blood in this location?
   A. Sciatic
   B. Femoral
   C. Obturator
   D. Superior gluteal
   E. Lateral femoral cutaneous

2. Which one of the following statements best describes the muscles of the pelvis?
   A. The obturator internus muscle leaves the pelvis through the greater sciatic foramen.
   B. The levator ani muscle is composed of the pubococcygeus, puborectalis, and iliococcygeus.
   C. The pelvic diaphragm is a sling of muscle that separates the true pelvis from the false pelvis.
   D. The piriformis muscle forms the lateral wall of the pelvis.
   E. The coccygeus muscle attaches to the sacrotuberous ligament.

3. Typically, the posterior division of the internal iliac artery supplies
   A. structures of the perineum
   B. muscles of the medial thigh
   C. meninges of the sacral spinal roots
   D. uterus and uterine tubes
   E. prostate

4. The components of the pelvic splanchnic nerves are most similar to the components of the
   A. lumbar splanchnic nerves
   B. sacral splanchnic nerves
   C. pudendal nerve
   D. vagus nerve
   E. hypogastric nerves

5. Carcinoma of the prostate can metastasize to bone and the brain through its connections with the vertebral venous plexus. Which other structures communicate with this venous plexus?
   A. Breast
   B. Spinal cord
   C. Intercostal muscles
   D. Esophagus
   E. All of the above

6. Although branches of the uterine artery anastomose extensively throughout the pelvis, the main stem of the vessel travels within the
   A. proper ovarian ligament
   B. cardinal ligament
   C. uterosacral ligament
   D. ovarian suspensory ligament
   E. round ligament

7. Which of the following statements accurately describes the relations of the ureter?
   A. It is crossed anteriorly by the gonadal vessels on the posterior abdominal wall.
   B. It crosses the brim of the pelvis at the bifurcation of the common iliac artery.
   C. In females it passes under the uterine artery ~2 cm lateral to the cervix.
   D. It enters the bladder at the posterolateral aspect of the trigone.
   E. All of the above

8. During a routine physical exam on a male patient, you test the integrity of the external anal sphincter. What spinal cord segments are involved in this?
   A. T12–L1
   B. L2–L4
   C. L4–L5
   D. S1–S2
   E. S2–S4

9. The superficial perineal fascia is continuous with the
   A. perineal membrane
   B. dartos fascia
   C. deep penile fascia
   D. tunica albuginea of the penis
   E. endopelvic fascia

10. The boundary of the pelvic inlet
   A. provides the attachment site for the pelvic diaphragm
   B. includes the iliac crests
   C. includes the ramus of the ischium
   D. is crossed by the ovarian and testicular arteries
   E. separates the cavity of the true pelvis from the abdominal cavity

11. Several years after delivering her twin boys, Laura experienced mild uterine prolapse and urinary incontinence. Her gynecologist was able to confirm that the angle of her anococcygeal ligament had changed, suggesting a laxity in her pelvic floor muscles. Which muscles insert on the anococcygeal ligament?
    A. Coccygeus
    B. Iliococcygeus
    C. Piriformis
    D. Deep transverse perineal
    E. Obturator internus

12. Tumors that metastasize via the bloodstream often form metastases in the first capillary bed that the cells reach after they enter the bloodstream. Based on their venous drainage, tumors in which of the following locations are likely to reach the lung before they reach the liver?
    A. Ascending colon
    B. Sigmoid colon
    C. Pancreas
    D. Superior (proximal) rectum
    E. Inferior (distal) rectum

13. Which one of the following structures passes through the genital hiatus?
    A. Ductus deferens
    B. Cavernous nerves
    C. Round ligament
    D. Obturator nerve
    E. External iliac artery

14. A 44-year-old woman undergoes a total hysterectomy for painful fibroids. The ovaries will not be removed during the procedure. Which of the following ligaments must be preserved?
    A. Suspensory ligament
    B. Ovarian ligament
    C. Uterosacral ligament
    D. Transverse cervical ligament
    E. Round ligament

15. Which of the following statements best describes the uterine cervix?
    A. In a normally anteflexed uterus, the cervix is tilted posteriorly.
    B. Vaginal fornices surround its supravaginal part.
    C. It is the attachment site for the round ligament.
    D. It makes up the inferior third of the uterus.
    E. It communicates with the uterine cavity through the external os.

16. A 53-year-old man had an aortic aneurysm that extended through his aortic bifurcation into his common iliac arteries. During the open repair, the surgeon opened the vessels longitudinally and fixed a synthetic graft to the walls of the vessels above and below the aneurysm. Following surgery, the man experienced retrograde ejaculation because of damage to nerves that innervated his internal urethral sphincter. Which nerves were damaged?
    A. Sympathetic nerves of the superior hypogastric plexus
    B. Parasympathetic nerves of the superior hypogastric plexus
    C. Somatic nerves of the sacral plexus
    D. Pelvic splanchnic nerves
    E. Sympathetic trunk

17. You are treating a 34-year-old woman for hemorrhoids. Although she does not complain of pain, the hemorrhoids protrude into her anal canal and are becoming ulcerated. There is no evidence of portal hypertension, but blood from the ulcers is bright red. Based on her brief history, what can you surmise about her condition?
    A. The prolapsed tissue contains the dilated veins of the external rectal plexus.
    B. The hemorrhoids originate from below the dentate line.
    C. The dilated veins in the hemorrhoids drain to the inferior rectal veins.
    D. The dilated veins communicate with the rectal arteries to form an arteriovenous hemorrhoidal plexus.
    E. All of the above

18. During a robotic prostatectomy on a 41-year-old man, the cavernous nerves were inadvertently damaged. What symptoms would you expect in this patient?
    A. Loss of tone in his external anal sphincter
    B. Urinary incontinence
    C. Inability to ejaculate
    D. Inability to form an erection
    E. Loss of sensation at the tip of the penis

19. Structures that pass through the greater sciatic foramen include the
    A. obturator internus
    B. coccygeus
    C. iliopsoas
    D. piriformis
    E. obturator nerve

20. The tendinous arch of the pelvic fascia
    A. is a condensation of endopelvic fascia
    B. includes the lateral rectal ligament
    C. supports the pelvic viscera
    D. provides an attachment site for the pelvic diaphragm
    E. All of the above

21. Structures that drain (directly or indirectly) into the deep inguinal lymph nodes include the
    A. glans of the penis
    B. perianal skin
    C. supralateral part of the uterus via the round ligament
    D. scrotum
    E. all of the above

22. During the national championships an Olympic gymnast fell backward off the balance beam, fracturing the tip of her coccyx and subluxing (dislocating) her sacroiliac joint. The team physician was concerned about damage to her sacral plexus and its branches that exit the pelvis. Nerves of the sacral plexus pass through the
    A. posterior sacral foramina
    B. obturator canal
    C. lesser sciatic foramen
    D. superficial inguinal ring
    E. deep inguinal ring

23. A young, pregnant woman in her third trimester was alarmed when she experienced a sharp pain in the anterior part of her labia majora when she stood up. Her obstetrician assured her that this was a common problem in late pregnancy and was most likely caused by
    A. stretching of the round ligament
    B. tightening of the inguinal ligament
    C. pressure on the obturator nerve
    D. irritation of the perineal branch of the pudendal nerve
    E. stretching of the iliohypogastric nerve

24. A vascular surgeon is repairing an aneurysm of the aortic bifurcation that extends along the right common iliac artery to its division into internal iliac and external iliac branches. What structure does the surgeon encounter that is at risk as it crosses over the pelvic brim at this distal end of the aneurysm?
    A. Ureter
    B. Testicular artery
    C. Lumbosacral trunk
    D. Sciatic nerve
    E. Ductus deferens

25. Similar to other sections of the large intestine, the rectum is characterized by
    A. teniae coli
    B. haustra
    C. a mesentery
    D. epiploic appendices
    E. None of the above

26. Which of the following are found within the superficial perineal space?
    A. Bulbourethral glands
    B. External urethral sphincter
    C. Bulbospongiosus muscle
    D. Anterior extension of ischioanal fat pad
    E. Inferior rectal nerve

Answers and Explanations

1. **B** The femoral nerve runs in the groove between the psoas and iliacus muscles (Sections 10.1 and 15.4d).
   A The blood accumulated above the pelvic brim in a muscular pocket of the false pelvis. The sciatic nerve does not pass through the false pelvis.
   C The obturator nerve passes medial to the psoas muscle and not in the groove between the psoas and iliacus muscles.
   D The superior gluteal nerve is a branch of the sacral plexus and does not pass through the false pelvis where the blood accumulated.
   E The lateral femoral cutaneous nerve crosses the iliacus muscle in the iliac fossa and passes under the inguinal ligament close to the anterior superior iliac spine to innervate the skin of the lateral thigh.

2. **B** The levator ani muscle is composed of the pubococcygeus, puborectalis, and iliococcygeus muscles (Section 10.3).
   A The obturator internus muscle covers the sidewall of the pelvis and perineum. Its tendon passes from the perineum to the gluteal region through the lesser sciatic foramen.
   C The pelvic diaphragm separates the true pelvis from the perineum, which lies below it.
   D The piriformis muscle forms the posterior muscular wall of the pelvis.
   E The coccygeus muscle attaches to the sacrospinous ligament along its entire length.

3. **C** The posterior division supplies parietal branches to the posterior abdominal wall, some gluteal muscles, and the meninges of the sacral spinal roots (Section 10.6a).
   A The internal pudendal artery, a branch of the anterior division of the internal iliac artery, supplies most structures of the perineum.
   B The obturator artery, a branch of the anterior division of the internal iliac artery, supplies muscles of the medial thigh.
   D The uterine artery, a branch of the anterior division of the internal iliac artery, supplies the uterus and uterine tubes.
   E The prostatic arteries, usually branches of the inferior vesical arteries, are derived from the anterior division of the internal iliac artery.

4. **D** The pelvic splanchnic nerves represent the sacral component of the parasympathetic system; the vagus nerve represents the cranial component of the parasympathetic system (Section 10.6d).
   A Lumbar splanchnic nerves arise from the lumbar sympathetic trunk and carry postganglionic sympathetic fibers.
   B Sacral splanchnic nerves arise from the sacral sympathetic trunk and carry postganglionic sympathetic fibers.
   C The pudendal nerve arises from the sacral plexus and carries somatic sensory and motor fibers.
   E Hypogastric nerves derive from the superior hypogastric plexus carrying postganglionic sympathetic fibers to the pelvic plexus.

5. **E** The vertebral venous system is a tributary of the azygos system. The breast, intercostal muscles, and esophagus drain via intercostal veins to the azygos system, and the spinal cord drains directly into the vertebral venous plexus (Section 11.1b and Thorax unit).
   A Blood from the breast drains to intercostal veins and the azygos system, which communicates with the vertebral venous plexus. B through D are also correct (E).
   B The veins of the spinal cord drain to the vertebral venous plexus. A, C, and D are also correct (E).
   C The intercostal veins that drain intercostal muscles terminate in the azygos system, which also receives the vertebral venous plexus. A, B, and D are also correct (E).
   D Veins of the lower esophagus drain to the portal system, but in the thorax esophageal veins drain to the azygos system, which also receives the vertebral venous plexus. A through C are also correct (E).

6. **B** The uterine artery and vein travel within the cardinal ligament at the base of the broad ligament (Section 11.2c).
   A The proper ovarian ligament connects the ovary to the uterus and does not contain any major vessels.
   C The uterosacral ligament is a thickening of endopelvic fascia that connects the cervix of the uterus to the sacrum. It does not contain any major vessels.
   D The ovarian suspensory ligament is a fold of peritoneum that contains the ovarian vessels as they cross over the pelvic brim.
   E The round ligament extends from the uterus through the inguinal canal to the labia majora. Although it is accompanied by small vessels, it does not contain any major arteries.

7. **E** All are correct (Section 11.3a).
   A The gonadal vessels cross anterior to the ureter as it descends along the posterior abdominal wall. B through D are also correct (E).
   B The bifurcation of the common iliac artery is a useful landmark for locating the ureter as it crosses the pelvic brim. A, C, and D are also correct (E).
   C The ureter passes under the uterine artery lateral to the uterine cervix and therefore is at risk of injury during a hysterectomy. A, B, and D are also correct (E).
   D The ureteral openings posterolaterally and the urethral opening in the anterior midline define the apexes of the trigone. A through C are also correct (E).

8. **E** The pudendal nerve (S2–S4) provides motor innervation to the external sphincter (Sections 11.4 and 10.6d).
A T12–L1 nerve roots contribute to the subcostal, iliohypogastric, and ilioinguinal nerves, which innervate muscles of the anterior abdominal wall.
B The L2–L4 nerve roots form the femoral and obturator nerves, which innervate muscles of the anterior and medial thigh.
C Nerves from L4–L5 spinal cord segments form the lumbosacral trunk, which joins the sacral plexus to innervate muscles of the lower limb.
D S1–S2 nerve roots contribute to the sacral plexus, which innervates muscles of the lower limb.

9. **B** The superficial perineal fascia is continuous with the dartos fascia that lines the scrotum and with the membranous layer (Scarpa's fascia) of the superficial fascia of the abdominal wall (Section 12.1).
A The perineal membrane is a fibrous sheet that forms the roof of the superficial perineal space.
C Deep penile fascia is a fibrous layer that binds the three erectile bodies of the penis.
D Each of the three erectile bodies of the penis is surrounded by the dense, fibrous tunica albuginea.
E Endopelvic fascia is the loose connective tissue matrix that fills the subperitoneal spaces of the pelvis.

10. **E** The pelvic inlet separates the true pelvis from the false pelvis. The cavity of the false pelvis is the lower part of the abdominal cavity and contains abdominal viscera (Section 10.1).
A The pelvic diaphragm attaches to the superior pubic ramus, tendinous arch of the levator ani, and sacrospinous ligament.
B The iliac crests form the upper boundary of the false pelvis. The pelvic inlet forms its lower boundary.
C The ramus of the ischium forms part of the pelvic outlet but not the pelvic inlet.
D The ovarian arteries cross the pelvic inlet, but the testicular arteries pass along the brim of the pelvis (pelvic inlet) to the deep inguinal ring, where they enter the inguinal canal as part of the spermatic cord.

11. **B** The anococcygeal ligament (also known as the levator plate) is a midline raphe between the anus and coccyx that serves as the insertion for the pubococcygeus and iliococcygeus muscles (Section 10.3).
A The coccygeus inserts on the ischial spine.
C The piriformis inserts on the greater trochanter of the femur.
D Deep transverse perineal muscles insert on the vagina (or prostate) and perineal body.
E The obturator internus inserts on the greater trochanter of the femur.

12. **E** The inferior rectal veins drain through the caval system (via the internal iliac vein and inferior vena cava) back to the heart and pulmonary circulation. All other choices are tributaries of the portal system, which drains through the liver before returning to the heart (Sections 8.2b and 11.4).
A Veins of the ascending colon are tributaries of the portal system. Therefore, blood passes through the liver before returning to the heart and pulmonary circulation.
B Veins of the sigmoid colon, and all parts of the gastrointestinal tract, are tributaries of the portal system. Therefore, blood passes through the liver before returning to the heart and pulmonary circulation.
C Veins of the pancreas are tributaries of the portal system. Therefore, blood from the pancreas drains through the liver before returning to the heart and pulmonary circulation.
D The superior rectal vein that drains the superior rectum is a tributary of the portal system. Therefore, this blood passes through the liver before returning to the heart and pulmonary circulation.

13. **B** The cavernous nerves carry parasympathetic innervation from the pelvic plexus to the perineum by passing through the genital hiatus (Section 10.6d).
A The ductus deferens passes through the deep inguinal ring and inguinal canal of the male.
C The round ligament traverses the female inguinal canal and terminates in the labia majora.
D The obturator nerve passes through the obturator canal into the medial thigh.
E The external iliac artery passes below the inguinal ligament into the anterior thigh.

14. **A** The suspensory ligament contains the ovarian vessels and is removed only during the removal of the ovary (Section 11.2a).
B The ovarian ligament attaches the ovary to the uterus and must be ligated to extract the uterus.
C The uterosacral ligament connects the cervix to the sacrum.
D The transverse cervical ligament contains the uterine arteries, which are ligated during a hysterectomy.
E The round ligament passes through the inguinal canal and connects the uterus to the labia majora.

15. **D** The uterus comprises a body that forms the superior two thirds and a cervix that forms the inferior one third (Section 11.2c).
A In an anteflexed uterus, the cervix is tilted anteriorly.
B The vaginal part of the cervix is surrounded by the vaginal fornices.
C The round ligaments arise from the upper part of the uterus.
E The cervix communicates with the body of the uterus through the internal os.

16. **A** The superior hypogastric plexus, a sympathetic nerve plexus, drapes over the aortic bifurcation as it enters the pelvis. It is frequently cut during surgery for the repair of an aneurysm at the location. The sympathetic nerves stimulate closure of the internal urethral sphincter during ejaculation, preventing the retrograde flow of seminal fluid into the bladder. Damage to these nerves can result in retrograde ejaculation (Sections 10.6d and 12.3d).
B The superior hypogastric plexus is a sympathetic nerve plexus derived from the intermesenteric plexus and lumbar splanchnic nerves.
C Somatic nerves do not stimulate visceral responses such as closure of the sphincter.
D Pelvic splanchnic nerves do not innervate the internal urethral sphincter.
E The paired sympathetic trunks run along the vertebral bodies on either side and would not be damaged in this procedure.

17. **D** The submucosal venous plexus of the anorectal region communicates with branches of the rectal arteries in an arteriovenous anastomosis, creating a thickened vascular tissue known as the hemorrhoidal plexus. As a result of these anastomoses, bleeding from the internal rectal plexus appears bright red (Section 11.4).
A Prolapsed internal hemorrhoids contain the dilated veins of the internal rectal plexus and are painless. External hemorrhoids, containing the external rectal plexus, are covered by skin and sensitive to pain.
B External hemorrhoids that occur below the dentate line are somatically innervated and therefore very painful, but internal hemorrhoids are viscerally innervated and painless.
C Veins of painless internal hemorrhoids lie above the dentate line and therefore drain to the superior rectal vein, a tributary of the portal system.
E A, B, and C are incorrect.

18. **D** The cavernous nerves carry parasympathetic nerves that are responsible for engorgement of the erectile tissue of the penis (Sections 10.6d and 12.3b).
A The external anal sphincter is innervated by the pudendal nerve, a branch of the sacral plexus.
B The external urethral sphincter that regulates urinary continence is innervated by the pudendal nerve, a branch of the sacral plexus.
C Ejaculation is a sympathetically mediated response. The cavernous nerves carry parasympathetic nerves from the inferior hypogastric plexus.
E The pudendal nerve carries sensation from perineal structures such as the tip of the penis.

19. **D** The piriformis passes through the greater sciatic foramen to insert on the trochanter of the femur (Section 10.3).
A The tendon of the obturator internus muscle passes through the lesser sciatic foramen from the perineum to the gluteal region.
B The coccygeus muscle lies along the sacrospinous ligament and forms the lower border of the greater sciatic foramen.
C The iliopsoas muscle passes under the inguinal ligament into the thigh.
E The obturator nerve passes along the sidewall of the pelvis and through the obturator canal into the thigh.

20. **C** The tendinous arch of the pelvic fascia is a thickening of the membranous fascia on the floor of the pelvis where visceral and parietal fascial layers meet. It provides support for pelvic viscera (Section 10.4).
A The tendinous arch of the pelvic fascia is a thickening of the membranous fascia, which lines the pelvic walls and viscera. Endopelvic fascia is a loose connective tissue layer that fills the subperitoneal spaces.
B The lateral rectal ligaments, like the lateral vesicular ligaments, are supporting columns of endopelvic fascia that connect the viscera to the pelvic walls.
D The tendinous arch of the levator ani, a condensation of the fascia over the obturator internus muscle, is the attachment site for the levator ani part of the pelvic diaphragm.
E A, B, and D are incorrect.

21. **E** The superficial and deep inguinal nodes drain most structures of the perineum, including the glans of the penis, perianal skin, and scrotum. The supralateral parts of the uterus drain along the round ligaments (which terminate in the labia majora) to superficial inguinal nodes. These nodes drain to the deep inguinal nodes (Section 10.6c).
A Lymph from the glans of the penis drains to deep inguinal nodes. B through D are also correct (E).
B Lymph from perianal skin, like all skin of the perineum, drains to superficial inguinal nodes, which drain to deep inguinal nodes. A, C, and D are also correct (E).
C Lymph from the supralateral parts of the uterus drain along the round ligaments (which terminate in the labia majora) to superficial inguinal nodes. These nodes drain to the deep inguinal nodes. A, B, and D are also correct (E).
D Lymph from the scrotum drains to superficial inguinal nodes, which drain to deep inguinal nodes. A through C are also correct (E).

22. **C** The pudendal nerve is a branch of the sacral plexus that passes through the lesser sciatic foramen (Section 10.6d).
A Only posterior rami of sacral spinal nerves pass through the posterior sacral foramina. The sacral plexus is formed by anterior rami of sacral spinal nerves.
B The obturator nerve, which passes through the obturator canal, is a branch of the lumbar plexus.
D The ilioinguinal and genitofemoral nerves, which pass through the superficial inguinal ring, are branches of the lumbar plexus.
E The genitofemoral nerve, a branch of the lumbar plexus, passes through the deep inguinal ring.

23. **A** The round ligament originates on the superior aspect of the anterolateral uterus and inserts in the labia majora. As the uterus enlarges and stretches the ligament, pain is felt in the labia (Section 11.2c).
B During late pregnancy pelvic ligaments are more relaxed in preparation for the passage of the child through the birth canal.
C Pressure on the obturator nerve would be felt on the medial thigh.
D The anterior part of the labia majora is innervated by the labial branches of the genitofemoral nerve, not the pudendal nerve.
E The iliohypogastric nerve innervates the skin above the pubic crest and does not extend inferiorly to the labia.

24. **A** The ureter crosses the pelvic brim at the bifurcation of the common iliac artery into its internal iliac and external iliac branches (Section 11.3a).
B The testicular artery does not cross the pelvic brim but enters the deep inguinal ring.
C The lumbosacral trunk crosses the pelvic brim posterior to the common iliac vessels and anterior to the sacroiliac joint. It enters the pelvis to join the sacral plexus.
D The sciatic nerve passes through the greater sciatic foramen and does not cross the pelvic brim.
E The ductus deferens courses around the inferior epigastric vessels and over the distal end of the external iliac vessels to descend into the pelvis.

25. **E** The rectum is devoid of ta eniae coli, haustra, a mesentery, and epiploic appendices (Section 11.4).
A The taeniae coli of the large intestine converge to form a uniform layer surrounding the rectum.
B The haustra of the large intestine disappear at the rectosigmoid junction.
C The rectum has no mesentery. The upper rectum is covered anteriorly by peritoneum, but the lower rectum lies in the subperitoneal space.
D Epiploic appendices are not present in the rectum.

26. **C** The bulbospongiosus muscle is found within the superficial perineal space (Section 12.1).
A The bulbourethral glands are found in the deep perineal space.
B The external urethral sphincter is located in the deep perineal space.
D The anterior extensions of the ischioanal fat pads are found in the deep perineal space.
E The inferior rectal nerve is found in the anal triangle, not the deep perineal or the superficial perineal spaces of the urogenital triangle.

13 Overview of the Upper Limb

The upper limb is designed for mobility and dexterity. Actions at the shoulder and elbow joints that allow positioning of the limb complement fine movements of the hands and fingers. Some stability is sacrificed for this extensive mobility, particularly in the shoulder, which makes the upper limb vulnerable to injury.

13.1 General Features

— In the anatomic position, the upper limbs hang vertically with the elbow joint pointing posteriorly and the palm of the hand facing anteriorly.

— The major regions of the upper limb (**Fig. 13.1A, B,** and **C**) are

- the **shoulder region**, which includes the **pectoral**, **scapular**, **deltoid**, and **lateral cervical regions** and overlies the **pectoral** (**shoulder**) **girdle**;
- the **axilla** (**axillary region**), the armpit;
- the **arm** (**brachial region**), between the shoulder and elbow;
- the **cubital region**, at the elbow;
- the **forearm** (**antebrachial region**), between the elbow and wrist;
- the **carpal region**, at the wrist; and
- the **hand**, which has palmar and dorsal surfaces.

— Movements at joints of the upper limb include

- **flexion**, bending the joint;
- **extension**, straightening the joint;
- **abduction**, movement away from a central axis;
- **adduction**, movement toward a central axis;
- **external** (**lateral**) **rotation**, outward rotation around a longitudinal axis;
- **internal** (**medial**) **rotation**, inward rotation around a longitudinal axis;
- **circumduction**, circular motion around the point of articulation;
- **supination**, turning the palm up;
- **pronation**, turning the palm down;

Fig. 13.1 ▶ **Regions of the upper limb**

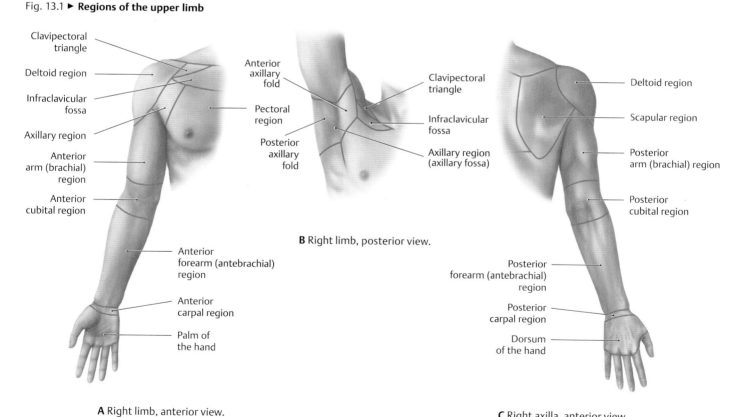

A Right limb, anterior view.

B Right limb, posterior view.

C Right axilla, anterior view.

- **radial** or **ulnar deviation**, angling the wrist toward the radius or ulnar side (also abduction or adduction of the wrist); and
- **opposition**, movement of the thumb or 5th digit to oppose the other fingers.
— Muscles of the upper limb are categorized as
  - **intrinsic muscles**, whose origin and insertion are near the joint (e.g., intrinsic muscles of the hand originate and insert on bones of the wrist and hand), and

- **extrinsic muscles**, whose origin is distant from the area of movement but insert near the joint via a long tendon (e.g., forearm muscles that flex the fingers are extrinsic muscles of the hand).
  - ○ The tendons of extrinsic muscles are often referred to as **long flexor** (or **extensor**) **tendons**.
  - ○ **Synovial tendon sheaths**, which surround tendons of extrinsic muscles at the wrist and fingers, provide a lubricated surface that facilitates movement of these tendons across the joint.

Fig. 13.2 ▶ **Skeleton of the upper limb**
Right limb. The upper limb is subdivided into three regions: arm, forearm, and hand. The pectoral (shoulder) girdle (clavicle and scapula) joins the upper limb to the thorax at the sternoclavicular joint.

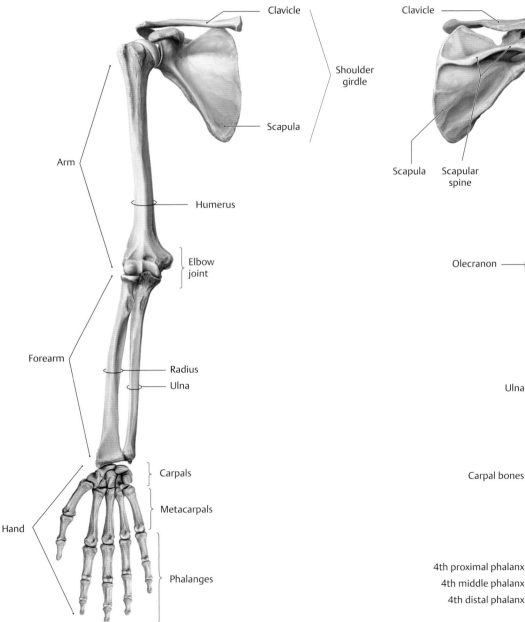

A Anterior view.

B Posterior view.

13.2 Bones of the Upper Limb
(Fig. 13.2A and B)

— The **clavicle** is an S-shaped bone that forms the anterior part of the pectoral girdle (**Fig. 13.3**).

- It articulates with the manubrium medially and the scapula laterally.
- It is palpable along its entire length.

Clavicular fractures

Fractures of the clavicle are common, particularly in children. A midclavicular fracture may be displaced by the upward pull of the proximal segment by the sternocleidomastoid muscle and the downward pull of the distal fragment by the weight of the upper limb. Distal clavicular fractures may disrupt the acromioclavicular joint or the coracoclavicular ligaments.

Fig. 13.3 ► **Clavicle**
Right clavicle, superior view.

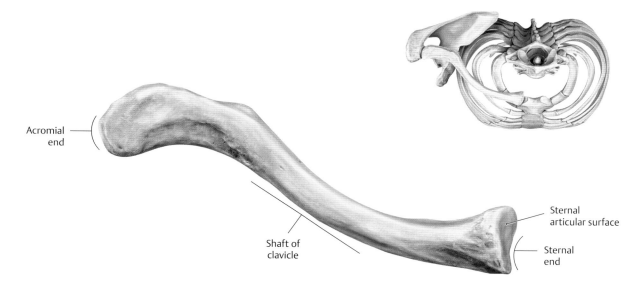

Acromial end

Shaft of clavicle

Sternal articular surface

Sternal end

— The **scapula** is a flat triangular bone that forms the posterior part of the pectoral girdle (**Fig. 13.4A**, **B**, and **C**).

- It overlies the 2nd to 7th ribs on the posterior thoracic wall.
- It has medial, lateral, and superior borders and a superior and inferior angle.
- Laterally, a shallow depression, the **glenoid cavity**, articulates with the humerus.
- A narrow **neck** separates the glenoid cavity from the large body of the scapula.
- A **subscapular fossa** lies on the anterior surface against the rib cage.
- The **spine** of the scapula on the posterior surface separates the **supraspinous** and **infraspinous fossae**. Laterally, the spine expands to form the **acromion**.
- A **coracoid process** extends anteriorly and superiorly over the glenoid cavity.

Fig. 13.4 ▶ **Scapula**
Right scapula.

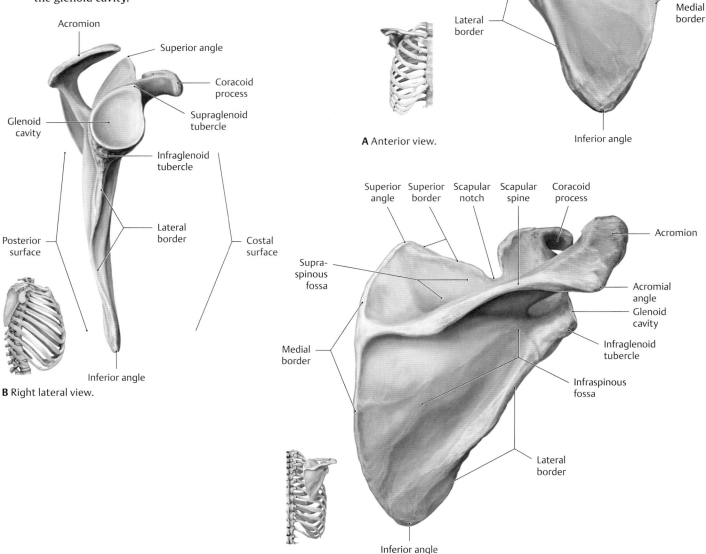

A Anterior view.

B Right lateral view.

C Posterior view.

— The **humerus** is the long bone of the arm (**Fig. 13.5A and B**).

- Proximally, the **head** articulates with the glenoid cavity of the scapula.
- Anteriorly, an **intertubercular groove** separates the **greater** and **lesser tubercles**.
- An **anatomic neck** separates the head from the greater and lesser tubercles. The **surgical neck** is the narrow part of the shaft immediately distal to the head and tubercles.

- A **deltoid tuberosity** on the midshaft is a site for attachment of the deltoid muscle.
- A **radial groove** runs obliquely around the posterior and lateral surfaces.
- Distally, the humerus articulates with the radius at the **capitullum** and with the ulna at the **trochlea**.
- A large **medial epicondyle** and smaller **lateral epicondyle** are attachment sites for muscles.
- An **ulnar groove** separates the medial epicondyle and trochlea.

Fig. 13.5 ▶ Humerus
Right humerus. The head of the humerus articulates with the scapula at the glenohumeral joint. The capitellum and trochlea of the humerus articulate with the radius and ulna, respectively, at the elbow (cubital) joint.

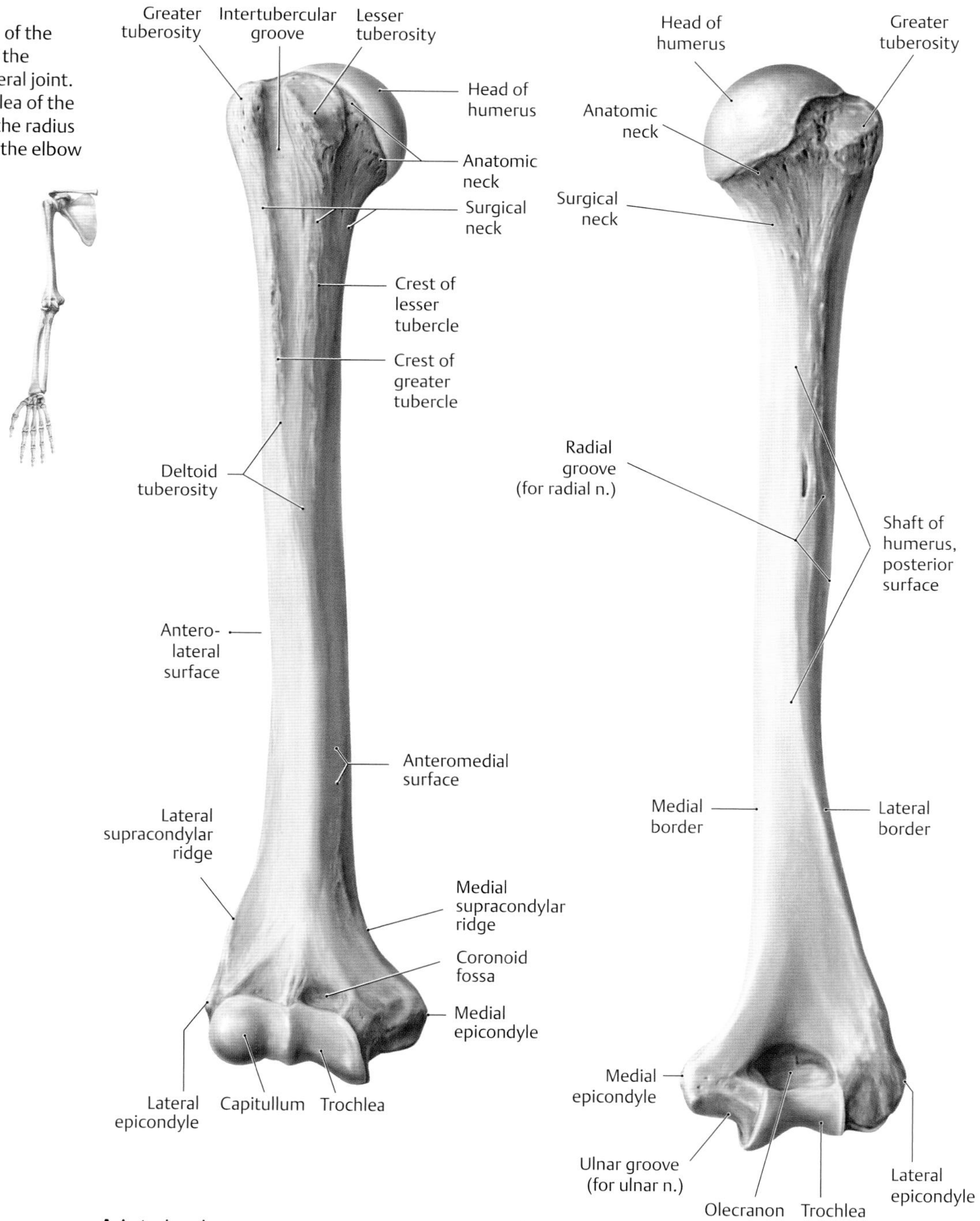

A Anterior view.

B Posterior view.

237

Fig. 13.6 ▶ **Radius and ulna**
Right forearm, anterosuperior view.

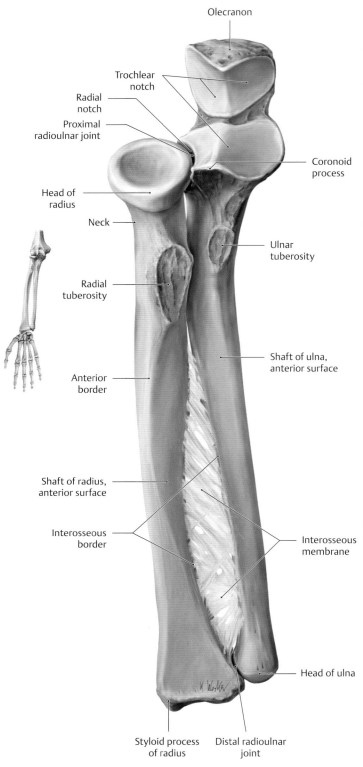

Olecranon

Trochlear
notch

Radial
notch

Proximal
radioulnar joint

Head of
radius

Neck

Coronoid
process

Ulnar
tuberosity

Radial
tuberosity

Anterior
border

Shaft of ulna,
anterior surface

Shaft of radius,
anterior surface

Interosseous
border

Interosseous
membrane

Head of ulna

Styloid process   Distal radioulnar
of radius   joint

Humeral fractures

Fractures of the humerus are very common and are often associated with injury to blood vessels and nerves. A proximal fracture at the anatomic neck can damage the posterior circumflex artery and axillary nerve, at the midshaft the radial nerve may be injured in the radial groove, and distally the median and ulnar nerves are vulnerable in supracondylar fractures.

— The **ulna** is the medial bone of the forearm (**Fig. 13.6**).
  • A C-shaped **trochlear notch**, formed by the **olecranon** posteriorly and the **coronoid process** anteriorly, articulates with the trochlea of the humerus.
  • The ulna articulates with the radius at the **radial notch**.
  • An **interosseous membrane** joins the shafts of the radius and ulna.
  • An **ulnar styloid process** projects from its distal end.
— The **radius** is the lateral bone of the forearm (see **Fig. 13.6**).
  • A round **radial head** articulates with the humerus and ulna and sits on top of a narrow **neck**.
  • A **radial tuberosity** on the anterior surface provides attachments for the biceps brachii muscle.
  • Distally, the radius is triangular in cross section with a flattened anterior surface.
  • The radius articulates with the ulna proximally at the elbow and distally at the wrist. The interosseous membrane attaches the radius to the shaft of the ulna.
  • A **radial styloid process** projects from the distal end and extends farther than the styloid process of the ulna.
  • The radius articulates with carpal bones at the wrist.

Colles' fractures

A Colles' fracture, a transverse fracture through the distal 2 cm of the radius, is the most common forearm fracture and results from a fall on an outstretched hand. The distal segment of bone is displaced dorsally and proximally, and with shortening of the radius, the styloid process appears proximal to the styloid of the ulna. The resulting appearance is referred to as the "dinner fork" deformity.

— The **carpal bones** consist of eight short bones that are arranged in two curved rows at the wrist (**Figs. 13.7** and **13.8**). From lateral to medial, they are
  • in the proximal row, the **scaphoid**, **lunate**, **triquetrum**, and **pisiform**; and,
  • in the distal row, the **trapezium**, **trapezoid**, **capitate**, and **hamate**.

Lunate dislocation

The lunate is the most commonly displaced of the carpal bones. Normally located in the floor of the carpal tunnel, a displaced bone moves toward the palmar surface and can compress structures of the carpal tunnel.

— The **metacarpal bones** consist of five long bones that form the hand.
  • Proximally, their **bases** articulate with the carpal bones.
  • Distally, their **heads**, the knuckles of the hand, articulate with the proximal phalanges.

— The **phalanges** are small long bones that form the fingers.
  • They are designated as proximal, middle, and distal in each finger except in the thumb, which has only a proximal and a distal phalanx.

— Fingers and their corresponding metacarpals and phalanges are designated as 1st through 5th, with the thumb as the 1st digit and the little finger as the 5th digit.

Fig. 13.7 ► **Bones of the hand**
Right hand, palmar view.

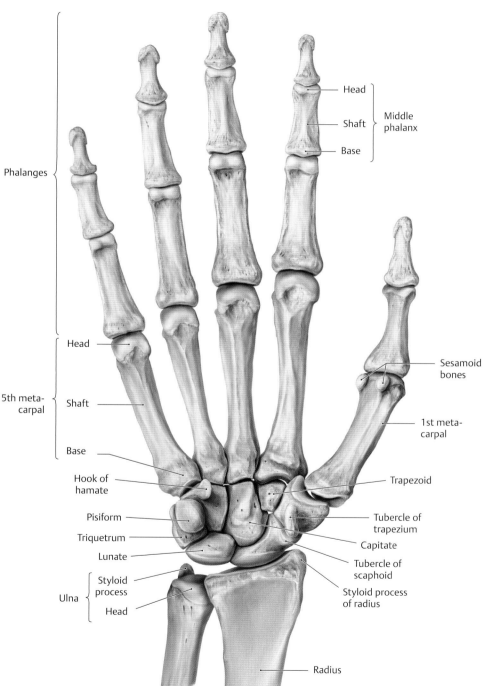

Scaphoid fractures

Scaphoid fractures are the most common carpal bone fractures, generally occurring at the narrow waist between the proximal and distal poles. Because the blood supply to the bone is transmitted via the distal segment, fractures at the waist can compromise the supply to the proximal segment, often resulting in nonunion and avascular necrosis.

Fig. 13.8 ► **Bones of the hand**
Right hand, dorsal view.

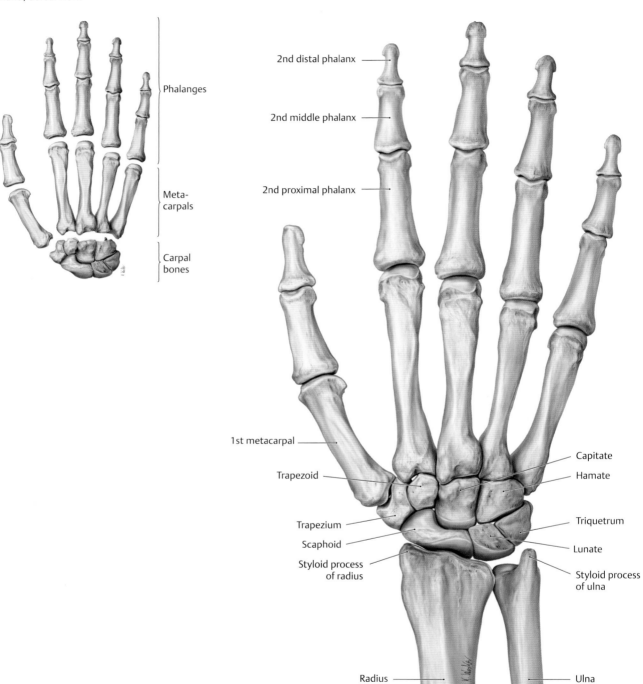

Phalanges

Meta-carpals

Carpal bones

2nd distal phalanx

2nd middle phalanx

2nd proximal phalanx

1st metacarpal

Trapezoid

Capitate

Hamate

Trapezium

Triquetrum

Scaphoid

Lunate

Styloid process of radius

Styloid process of ulna

Radius

Ulna

13.3 Fascia and Compartments of the Upper Limb

— Deep fascia snugly encloses muscles of the upper limb. It is continuous over the pectoral girdle, the axilla, and the upper limb but has regional designations.

- **Pectoral fascia** invests the pectoralis major muscle.
- **Clavipectoral fascia** invests the subclavius and pectoralis minor muscles.
- **Axillary fascia** forms the floor of the **axilla**.
- **Brachial fascia** invests muscles of the arm.
- **Antebrachial fascia** invests muscles of the forearm and extends onto the wrist as transverse thickened bands, the **flexor** and **extensor retinacula**.
- Fascia of the hand is continuous over the dorsum and palm, but in the center of the palm it forms a thickened fibrous sheet, the **palmar aponeurosis**.
- **Digital fibrous sheaths**, extensions of the palmar aponeurosis onto the fingers, surround the flexor tendons.

— Intermuscular septa arising from the deep fascia attach to the bones of the arm, forearm, and hand, separating the limb musculature into discrete compartments. The muscles within each compartment usually share a similar function, innervation, and blood supply. The compartments of the upper limb (see **Figs. 14.34A** and **B** and **14.35A** and **B**) are

- the **anterior** and **posterior compartments** of the arm;
- the **anterior** and **posterior compartment**s of the forearm; and
- the **thenar**, **hypothenar**, **central**, **adductor**, and **interosseous compartments** of the palm of the hand.

13.4 Neurovasculature of the Upper Limb

13.4a Arteries of the Upper Limb

— The **subclavian artery** and its branches supply structures in the neck, part of the thoracic wall, and the entire upper limb (**Fig. 13.9**).

- The right subclavian artery is a branch of the brachiocephalic trunk, which arises from the aortic arch. The left subclavian artery arises directly from the aortic arch.
- The subclavian arteries enter the neck through the superior thoracic aperture, pass laterally toward the shoulder, and terminate as they pass over the 1st rib.
- The subclavian artery branches that supply the neck and thoracic wall (discussed further in Section 17.3) include
  - the **vertebral artery**;
  - the internal thoracic artery; and
  - the **thyrocervical trunk**, whose branches are the **suprascapular**, **ascending cervical**, **inferior thyroid**, and **transverse cervical arteries**.
- The branches of the thyrocervical trunk that supply muscles and skin of the scapular region include
  - the transverse cervical artery and its **dorsal scapular branch** and
  - the suprascapular artery.

Fig. 13.9 ▶ **Branches of the subclavian artery**
Right side, anterior view.

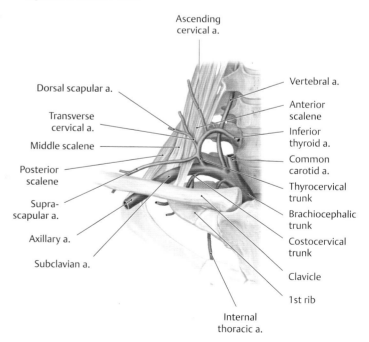

Fig. 13.10 ▶ **Axillary artery**
Right limb, anterior view.

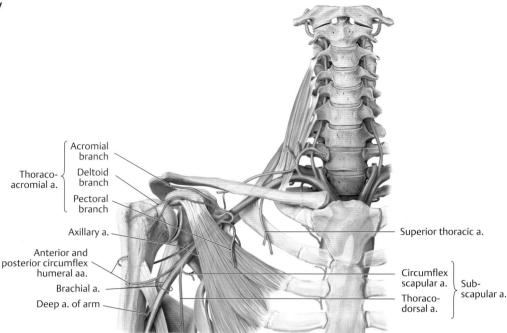

- The **axillary artery**, the continuation of the subclavian artery, begins at the lateral edge of the 1st rib and terminates at the lateral border of the axilla (the lower border of the teres major muscle).

  Within the axilla, the **pectoralis minor** muscle lies anterior to the middle third of the axillary artery. Branches of the axillary artery, therefore, are described as arising from its proximal, middle, or distal thirds (**Fig. 13.10**).

  - The proximal third has one branch:
    - The **superior thoracic** branch supplies the muscles of the first intercostal space.
  - The middle third has two branches:
    - The **thoracoacromial artery** divides into deltoid, pectoral, clavicular, and acromial branches.
    - The **lateral thoracic artery** supplies the lateral thoracic wall, including the serratus anterior muscle and the breast.
  - The distal third has three branches:
    - The **subscapular artery** further divides into a **thoracodorsal artery**, supplying the latissimus dorsi muscle, and a **circumflex scapular artery**, supplying muscles of the scapula.
    - The **anterior circumflex humeral** and the **posterior circumflex humeral arteries** encircle the humeral neck to supply the deltoid region.

- A **scapular arcade**, formed by the anastomoses of the dorsal scapular and suprascapular branches of the subclavian artery, and the circumflex scapular and thoracodorsal branches of the axillary artery provides an important collateral circulation to the scapular region when the axillary artery is injured or ligated (**Fig. 13.11**).

Fig. 13.11 ▶ **Scapular arcade**
Right side, posterior view.

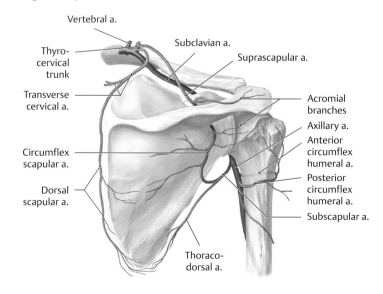

Fig. 13.12 ▶ **Arteries of the upper limb**
Right limb, anterior view.

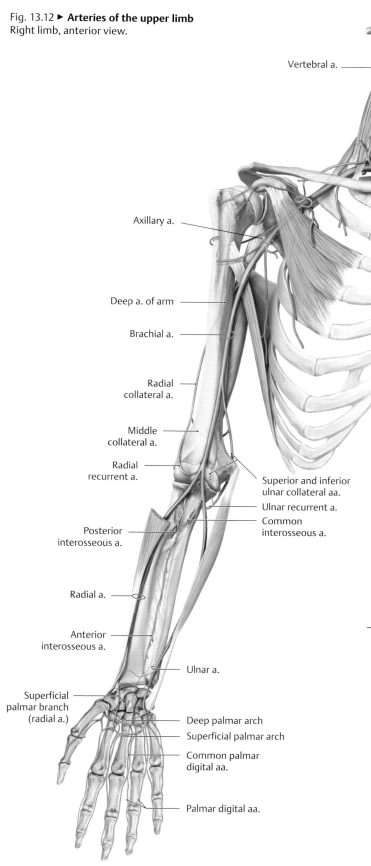

Vertebral a.

Axillary a.

Deep a. of arm

Brachial a.

Radial
collateral a.

Middle
collateral a.

Radial
recurrent a.

Posterior
interosseous a.

Radial a.

Anterior
interosseous a.

Superficial
palmar branch
(radial a.)

Superior and inferior
ulnar collateral aa.

Ulnar recurrent a.

Common
interosseous a.

Ulnar a.

Deep palmar arch

Superficial palmar arch

Common palmar
digital aa.

Palmar digital aa.

— The **brachial artery**, the continuation of the axillary artery, begins after the lateral border of the axilla (the lower margin of the tendon of the teres major), runs superficially along the medial border of the **biceps brachii muscle**, and terminates at its bifurcation in the cubital fossa (anterior elbow region). Its branches include (**Fig. 13.12**)

• the **deep artery of the arm** (deep brachial artery, profunda brachii), which arises proximally, descends on the posterior surface of the humerus, and supplies muscles of the posterior arm;

• the **superior** and **inferior ulnar collateral arteries**, distal branches, which anastomose with the deep artery of the arm and arteries of the forearm to supply the elbow joint; and

• the **radial** and **ulnar arteries**, the terminal branches of the brachial artery, which supply the forearm and hand.

— The ulnar artery originates in the cubital fossa, descends along the medial side of the forearm, and crosses through a narrow space at the wrist, the **ulnar canal**. It terminates as the **superficial palmar arch** of the hand. The major branches of the ulnar artery in the forearm (see **Fig. 13.12**) are

• the **ulnar recurrent artery**, which anastomoses with ulnar collateral arteries to supply the elbow joint, and

• the **common interosseous artery**, which arises in the proximal forearm and branches into **anterior** and **posterior interosseous arteries**. These interosseous branches descend on either side of the interosseous membrane and supply the anterior and posterior muscle compartments of the forearm.

— The radial artery, the smaller lateral branch of the brachial artery, descends from the cubital fossa along the lateral side of the forearm to the wrist. It crosses the wrist through the **anatomic snuffbox** on the dorsal side, pierces the muscles between the 1st and 2nd digits, and enters the palm of the hand, where it ends as the **deep palmar arch**. Its branches (see **Fig. 13.12**) include

• the **radial recurrent artery**, which anastomoses with collateral branches of the deep artery of the arm to supply the elbow joint, and

• the **palmar** and **dorsal carpal arteries**, which anastomose with branches of the ulnar artery in the wrist and hand.

— Arteries of the wrist and hand (**Fig. 13.13A and B**) include
- the **palmar** and **dorsal carpal networks**, which form by contributions from radial, ulnar, and anterior interosseous arteries;
- the superficial and deep palmar arches, which arise from the ulnar and radial arteries, respectively. A **deep palmar branch** of the ulnar artery connects the two palmer arches;
- the **princeps pollicis artery**, a branch of the radial artery, which follows the ulnar surface of the 1st metatarsal to the base of the thumb, where it divides into two digital branches;
- the **radialis indicis,** which arises from the princeps pollicis or radial artery and courses along the radial side of the index finger;
- the **palmar metacarpal** and **digital arteries**, which arise from the superficial and deep palmar arches in the palm of the hand; and
- the **dorsal metacarpal** and **digital arteries**, which arise from the dorsal carpal arch on the dorsum of the hand.

13.4b Veins of the Upper Limb

Veins of the limbs, similar to veins of the trunk, are more variable than the arteries, and they often form anastomoses that surround the arteries they accompany. Veins of the limbs have unidirectional valves that prevent pooling of blood in the extremities and facilitate the movement of blood back to the heart. The limbs have both deep and superficial veins.

— Deep veins accompany the major arteries and their branches and have similar names (**Fig. 13.14**).
- In the distal limb, the deep veins, referred to as **accompanying veins** (venae comitantes), are paired and surround the artery. Proximally, the pairs merge to form a single vessel.
- The **axillary vein** drains the shoulder, arm, forearm, and hand and receives additional contributions from
  ○ the lateral chest wall, including the breast, and
  ○ the thoracoepigastric vein of the anterolateral abdominal wall.
- The **subclavian vein**, the continuation of the axillary vein, also receives the venous drainage from the scapular region.

Fig. 13.13 ► **Arteries of the forearm and hand**
Right limb. The ulnar and radial arteries are interconnected by the superficial and deep palmar arches, the perforating branches, and the dorsal carpal network.

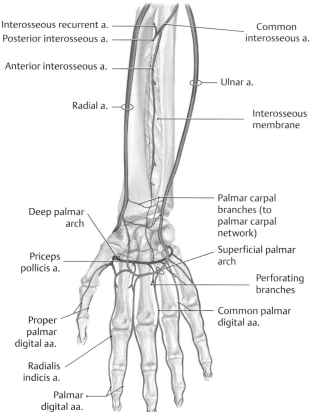

Interosseous recurrent a.
Posterior interosseous a.
Anterior interosseous a.
Common interosseous a.
Radial a.
Ulnar a.
Interosseous membrane
Deep palmar arch
Palmar carpal branches (to palmar carpal network)
Priceps pollicis a.
Superficial palmar arch
Perforating branches
Proper palmar digital aa.
Common palmar digital aa.
Radialis indicis a.
Palmar digital aa.

A Anterior (palmar) view.

Common interosseous a.
Posterior interosseous a.
Anterior interosseous a.
Interosseous membrane
Anterior interosseous a. (posterior branch)
Ulnar a. (dorsal carpal branch)
Dorsal carpal network
Perforating branches
Radial a.
Dorsal carpal a.
Dorsal metacarpal aa.
Dorsal digital aa.

B Posterior (dorsal) view.

— The superficial veins are found in the subcutaneous tissue and drain into the deep venous system via **perforating** (connecting) **veins** (**Fig. 13.15A** and **B**).

- The **dorsal venous network** on the dorsum of the hand drains into two large superficial veins, the **cephalic** and **basilic veins**.
- The **cephalic vein** originates on the lateral side of the dorsum of the hand and ascends on the lateral side of the forearm and arm. In the shoulder, it passes through the **deltopectoral groove** (formed by the borders of the deltoid and pectoralis major muscles) before emptying into the axillary vein.
- The **basilic vein** arises on the medial side of the dorsum of the hand and runs posteromedially to pass anterior to the medial epicondyle of the humerus. In the arm, it pierces the brachial fascia (at the **basilic hiatus**) and joins the paired **deep brachial veins** to form the axillary vein.

- The **median cubital vein** connects the cephalic and basilic veins anterior to the cubital fossa.
- The **median antebrachial vein** arises from the venous network of the palm, ascends on the anterior forearm, and terminates in the basilic or median cubital vein.

Fig. 13.15 ▶ **Superficial veins of the upper limb**
Right limb.

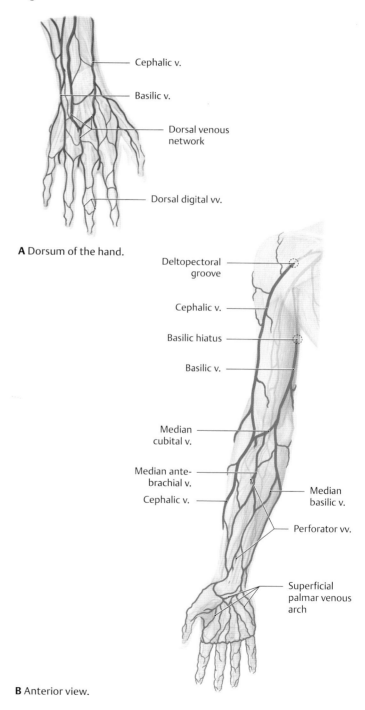

Cephalic v.

Basilic v.

Dorsal venous network

Dorsal digital vv.

A Dorsum of the hand.

Deltopectoral groove

Cephalic v.

Basilic hiatus

Basilic v.

Median cubital v.

Median antebrachial v.

Cephalic v.

Median basilic v.

Perforator vv.

Superficial palmar venous arch

B Anterior view.

Fig. 13.14 ▶ **Deep veins of the upper limb**
Right limb, anterior view.

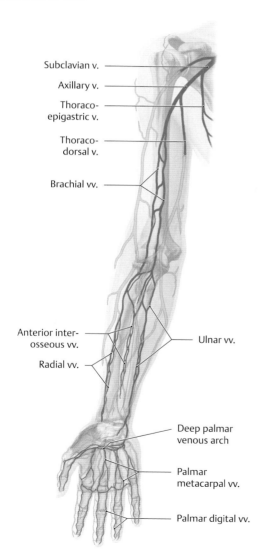

Subclavian v.

Axillary v.

Thoraco-epigastric v.

Thoraco-dorsal v.

Brachial vv.

Anterior inter-osseous vv.

Radial vv.

Ulnar vv.

Deep palmar venous arch

Palmar metacarpal vv.

Palmar digital vv.

13.4c Lymphatic Drainage of the Upper Limb

Lymphatic vessels of the upper limb drain toward the axilla. They usually accompany the veins of the superficial system (cephalic and basilic veins), although there are numerous connections between the deep and superficial drainages.

— Axillary lymph node groups, each containing four to seven large nodes, are described in relation to the pectoralis minor muscle (**Fig. 13.16**).

- The lower axillary group lies lateral and deep to the pectoralis minor.

  o **Pectoral** (anterior) **nodes** on the anterior wall of the axilla drain the anterior thoracic wall, including the breast (75% of lymph from the breast drains to axillary nodes).

  o **Subscapular nodes** along the posterior axillary fold drain the posterior thoracic wall and scapular region.

  o **Humeral** (posterior) **nodes** lie medial and posterior to the axillary vein and receive lymphatic vessels that accompany the basilic vein and the deep veins of the arm.

  o **Central nodes** lie deep to the pectoralis minor muscle and receive lymph from the pectoral, subscapular, and humeral nodes.

- The middle axillary group lies on the surface of the pectoralis minor muscle.

  o **Interpectoral nodes** lie between the pectoralis major and pectoralis minor muscles and drain to the apical nodes.

- The upper axillary group lies medial to the pectoralis minor muscle.

  o **Apical nodes** lie along the axillary vein adjacent to the first part of the axillary artery in the apex of the axilla. They receive lymph from the central nodes as well as from lymphatic vessels traveling along the cephalic vein.

— Apical lymph vessels unite to form the subclavian lymph trunks, which usually drain to the right lymphatic trunk and the thoracic duct (left lymphatic duct).

13.4d Nerves of the Upper Limb: The Brachial Plexus

The upper limb is innervated almost entirely by the nerves of the **brachial plexus**, which originates from the lower cervical and upper thoracic spinal cord (**Table 13.1**; **Figs. 13.17**, **13.18**, **13.19**, **13.20**, and **13.21**). (One exception, the intercostobrachial nerve, formed by the anterior rami of T1 and T2, is sensory to the medial arm but is not part of the plexus.)

Fig. 13.16 ► **Axillary lymph nodes**
Anterior view.

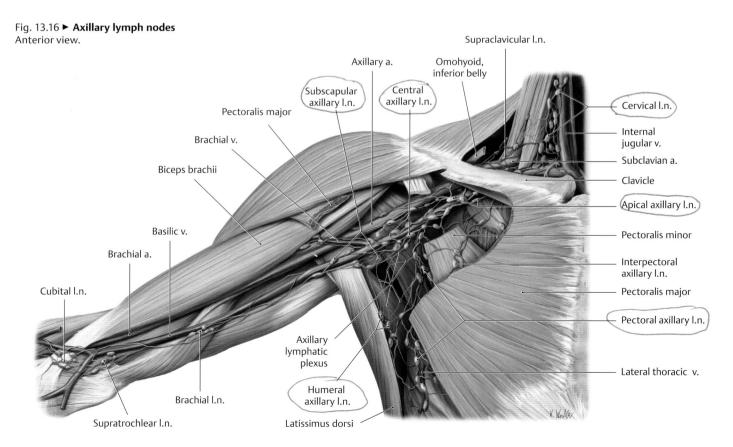

— Roots of the brachial plexus emerge from the vertebral column between the anterior and middle scalene muscles (interscalene groove) in the neck.

— Formation of the plexus begins in the neck (**supraclavicular part**), where it accompanies the subclavian artery, and continues into the axilla (**infraclavicular part**), where it accompanies the axillary artery.

— The roots, trunks, and divisions of the plexus are **supraclavicular** (above the clavicle); the cords form at the level of the clavicle, and their branches are **infraclavicular** (below the clavicle).

— **Fig. 13.17** shows the architecture of the brachial plexus.

  • Anterior rami of spinal nerves C5–T1 form five **roots**.

    ○ Within the plexus, upper roots form nerves that innervate muscles of the proximal limb; lower roots form nerves that innervate muscles of the distal limb.

    ○ The terms **pre-fixed** or **post-fixed plexus** indicate that the plexus includes anterior rami from one spinal level above (C4) or below (T2) the normal levels, respectively.

• Roots C5 to T1 combine to form three **trunks**:

  1. C5 and C6 form the **upper trunk**.
  2. C7 forms the **middle trunk**.
  3. C8 and T1 form the **lower trunk**.

• Anterior and posterior divisions (components of the anterior rami of all spinal nerves), which are bundled together in the roots and trunks of the plexus, separate to form three **cords**:

  1. Anterior divisions of the upper and middle trunk (C5–C7) form the **lateral cord**.
  2. Anterior divisions of the lower trunk (C8–T1) form the **medial cord**.
  3. Posterior divisions of all trunks (C5–T1) form the **posterior cord**.

• The three cords divide to form the five **terminal nerves** of the plexus.

  ○ Medial and lateral cords form the **musculocutaneous, median**, and **ulnar nerves**, which innervate the anterior muscles of the arm and forearm, and all muscles of the palm.

  ○ The posterior cord forms the **axillary** and **radial nerves**, which innervate muscles of the scapular and deltoid regions and posterior muscles of the arm and forearm.

Fig. 13.17 ▶ **Structure of the brachial plexus**
Right side, anterior view.

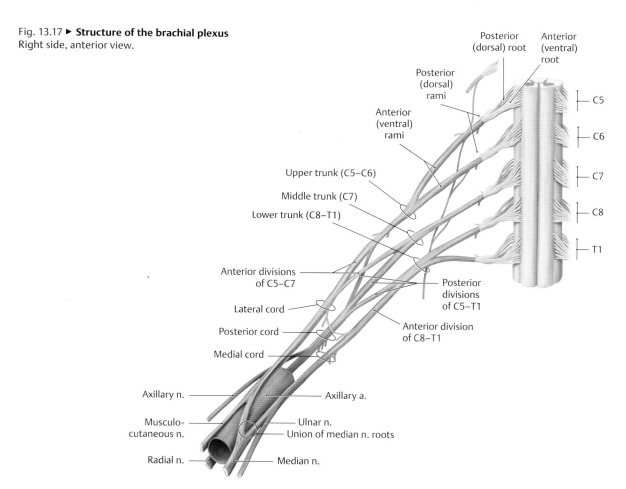

Fig. 13.18 ► **Brachial plexus**
Right side, anterior view.

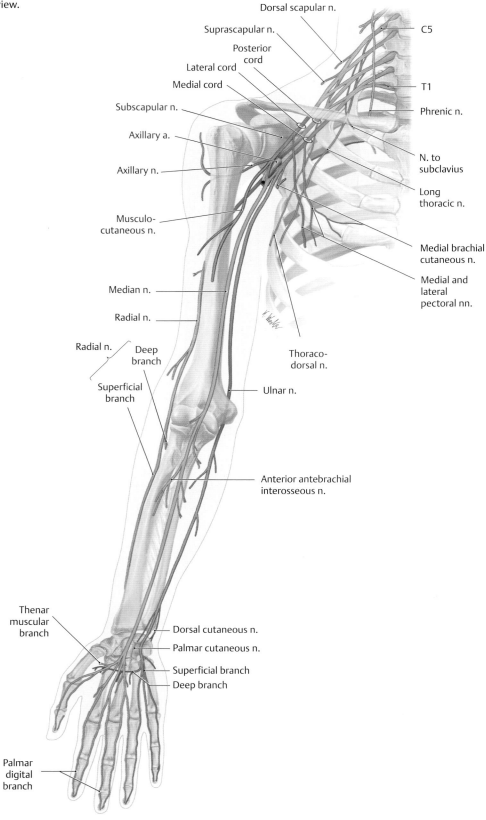

Dorsal scapular n.

Suprascapular n.

C5

Posterior cord

Lateral cord

Medial cord

T1

Subscapular n.

Phrenic n.

Axillary a.

N. to subclavius

Axillary n.

Long thoracic n.

Musculo-cutaneous n.

Medial brachial cutaneous n.

Median n.

Medial and lateral pectoral nn.

Radial n.

Radial n.

Deep branch

Thoraco-dorsal n.

Superficial branch

Ulnar n.

Anterior antebrachial interosseous n.

Thenar muscular branch

Dorsal cutaneous n.

Palmar cutaneous n.

Superficial branch

Deep branch

Palmar digital branch

Table 13.1 ▶ Nerves of the Brachial Plexus

Nerve			Level	Area of Innervation
Supraclavicular part				
Direct branches from the anterior rami or plexus trunks				
	Dorsal scapular n.		C4–C5	Levator scapulae, rhomboid major and minor
	Suprascapular n.		C4–C6	Supraspinatus, infraspinatus
	N. to the subclavius		C5–C6	Subclavius m.
	Long thoracic n.		C5–C7	Serratus anterior
Infraclavicular part				
Short and long branches from the plexus cords				
Lateral cord	Lateral pectoral n.		C5–C7	Pectoralis major
	Musculocutaneous n.			Coracobrachialis, biceps brachii, brachialis; skin of lateral forearm
	Median n.	Lateral root	C6–C7	Pronator teres, flexor carpi radialis, palmaris longus, flexor digitorum superficialis, pronator quadratus, flexor pollicis longus, flexor digitorum profundus (radial half), abductor pollicis brevis, flexor pollicis brevis (superficial head), opponens pollicis, 1st and 2nd lumbricals; skin of radial half of palm and palmar surface and distal dorsal segment of 2nd and 3rd digits and half of 4th digit
Medial cord		Medial root	C8–T1	
	Medial pectoral n.			Pectoralis major and minor
	Medial antebrachial cutaneous n.			Skin of medial forearm
	Medial brachial cutaneous n.		T1	Skin of medial arm
	Ulnar n.		C7–T1	Flexor carpi ulnaris, flexor digitorum profundus (ulnar half), palmaris brevis, abductor digiti minimi, flexor digiti minimi, opponens digiti minimi, 3rd and 4th lumbricals, interossei, adductor pollicis, flexor pollicis brevis (deep head); skin of ulnar half of the dorsum and palm of the hand, dorsum and palmar surface of the 4th and 5th digits and half of the 3rd digit
Posterior cord	Upper subscapular n.		C5–C6	Subscapularis (upper part)
	Thoracodorsal n.		C6–C8	Latissimus dorsi
	Lower subscapular n.		C5–C6	Subscapularis (lower part), teres major
	Axillary n.			Deltoid, teres minor; skin of lower deltoid region
	Radial n.		C5–T1	Muscles of posterior arm and forearm; skin of posterior and inferolateral arm, posterior forearm, radial half of dorsum of hand, dorsum of 1st, 2nd, 3rd digits and half of 4th digit

Fig. 13.19 ▶ Sensory innervation of the hand
Right hand. Extensive overlap exists between adjacent areas. Exclusive nerve territories indicated with darker shading.

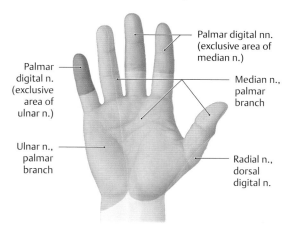

Palmar digital nn. (exclusive area of median n.)

Palmar digital n. (exclusive area of ulnar n.)

Median n., palmar branch

Ulnar n., palmar branch

Radial n., dorsal digital n.

A Anterior (palmar) view.

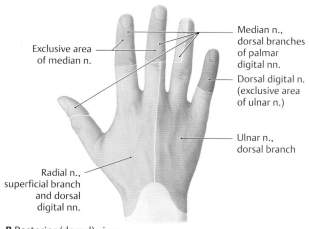

Exclusive area of median n.

Median n., dorsal branches of palmar digital nn.

Dorsal digital n. (exclusive area of ulnar n.)

Ulnar n., dorsal branch

Radial n., superficial branch and dorsal digital nn.

B Posterior (dorsal) view.

Fig. 13.20 ▶ **Cutaneous innervation of the upper limb**

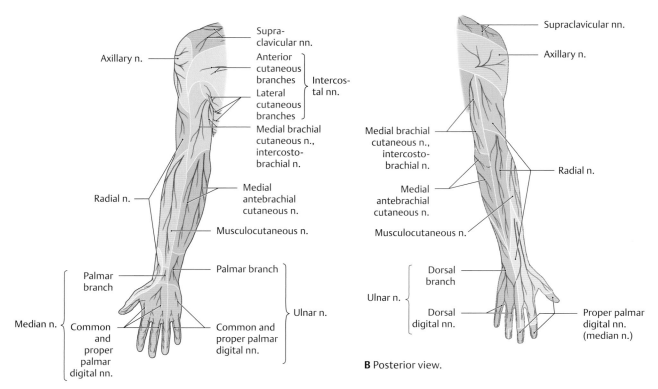

A Anterior view.

B Posterior view.

Fig. 13.21 ▶ **Dermatomes of the upper limb**

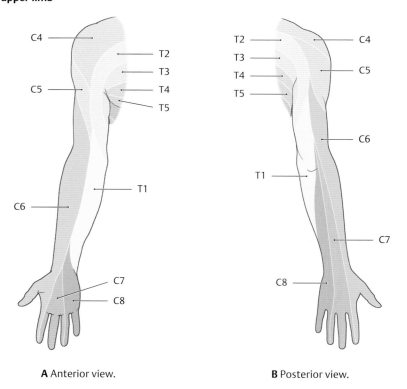

A Anterior view.

B Posterior view.

— The musculocutaneous nerve (C5–C7) pierces and innervates the coracobrachialis muscle of the arm as it leaves the axilla and then descends within the anterior compartment of the arm between the biceps brachii and brachialis muscles.

• In the arm, its **muscular branches** innervate the muscles of the anterior compartment, the biceps brachii and the brachialis muscles.

• It enters the forearm at the lateral edge of the cubital fossa as the **lateral antebrachial cutaneous nerve** to supply the skin of the lateral forearm.

▮▮▮▮ Musculocutaneous nerve injury

The musculocutaneous nerve is protected on the medial side of the arm, and isolated injuries are uncommon, but they would affect the coracobrachialis, biceps brachii, and brachialis muscles. Flexion and supination at the elbow would be weakened but not absent because the brachioradialis and supinator muscles, which are innervated by the radial nerve, also provide those movements.

— The median nerve (C6–T1) is formed by contributions from the medial and lateral cords.

• In the arm, the median nerve descends with the brachial vessels, medial to the biceps brachii, but it does not innervate any arm muscles.

• In the forearm, it travels deep within the anterior compartment but becomes superficial at the wrist before passing through the caspal tunnel into the hand. It innervates most muscles in the anterior forearm (except the flexor carpi ulnaris and the medial half of the flexor digitorum profundus).

◦ Its largest branch in the forearm is the **anterior antebrachial interosseous nerve**.

◦ A **palmar branch** arises distally and crosses the wrist superficial to the carpal tunnel to supply the skin of the palm.

• In the hand, the median nerve has motor and sensory functions.

◦ A thenar muscular branch, the **recurrent nerve**, innervates most muscles of the thenar compartment (intrinsic muscles of the thumb).

▮▮▮▮ Median nerve injury

Injury at the distal humerus is often caused by a supracondylar fracture and results in

• loss of sensation in the palm and palmar surface of the lateral three and a half digits,
• loss of flexion of 1st to 3rd digits,
• weakened flexion of 4th and 5th digits,
• loss of thenar opposition,
• loss of pronation,
• an "ape hand" produced by flattening of the thenar eminence, and
• the "hand of benediction" produced by flexing the hand in a fist (2nd and 3rd digits remain partly extended).

◦ **Palmar digital branches** innervate the lateral two lumbricals (intrinsic muscles of the central compartment) and the skin of the 1st through 3rd fingers and lateral half of the 4th finger.

— The ulnar nerve [C7(C8–T1)] is a branch of the medial cord.

• In the arm, it descends on the medial side with the brachial artery. At the midarm, it pierces the intermuscular septum to enter the posterior compartment. It crosses the elbow joint behind the medial epicondyle, where it is subcutaneous and vulnerable to injury. It does not innervate any muscles in the arm.

• In the forearm, it runs deep to the flexor muscles but becomes superficial just proximal to the wrist.

◦ In the arm, its **muscular branches** innervate the flexors on the medial side (flexor carpi ulnaris and medial half of the flexor digitorum profundus).

◦ **Palmar** and **dorsal cutaneous nerves** arise in the wrist but are distributed to the skin of the medial half of the hand, proximal parts of the 5th digit, and medial half of the 4th digit.

• It crosses the wrist with the ulnar artery within a narrow space, the **ulnar canal**, where it splits into deep and superficial branches.

◦ Its **deep branch** supplies most of the intrinsic muscles of the palm (except two of the thenar muscles and the 1st and 2nd lumbricals).

◦ Its **superficial branch** innervates a small superficial muscle of the palm (palmaris brevis) and contributes to sensory innervation of the 4th and 5th digits.

▮▮▮▮ Ulnar nerve injury

The ulnar nerve may be injured at the elbow by a fracture of the medial epicondyle, compressed in the cubital fossa between the two heads of the flexor carpi ulnaris, or compressed in the ulnar canal at the wrist. These result in the following:

• Paresthesia of the palmar and dorsal side of the medial hand and the medial one and a half digits
• Loss of thumb adduction
• Hyperextension of the metacarpophalangeal (MCP) joints
• Loss of extension of interphalangeal (IP) joints
• Weakened adduction and flexion of the wrist (for lesions at the elbow)
• Inability to form a fist due to "claw hand" deformity

— The axillary nerve (C5–C6), a branch of the posterior cord, passes to the posterior shoulder region with the posterior circumflex humeral vessels.

• In the shoulder region, it innervates scapular and deltoid muscles and skin of the deltoid region.

■■■■■■ Axillary nerve injury

The axillary nerve is most vulnerable as it courses around the neck of the humerus and can be injured by fractures at the surgical neck or dislocation of the glenohumeral joint. These result in the following:

- Weakened lateral rotation at the shoulder
- Inability to abduct the shoulder even to the horizontal position
- Loss of sensation over the deltoid region
- A flattened shoulder contour

— The radial nerve (C5–T1) forms from the posterior cord.
  - In the arm, it runs posteriorly around the humerus in the radial groove with the deep brachial artery and descends within the posterior compartment.
    - Its **muscular branches** innervate all of the muscles of the posterior arm, the triceps brachii and anconeus muscles.
    - Its sensory branches of the arm include the **posterior brachial cutaneous** and **inferior lateral brachial cutaneous nerves**.
    - A **posterior antebrachial cutaneous nerve** arises in the arm but innervates skin over the posterior forearm.
  - In the cubital region, it passes through the lateral intermuscular septum into the anterior compartment, where it runs anterior to the medial epicondyle. As it enters the proximal forearm, it splits into deep and superficial branches.
    - The deep branch becomes the **posterior interosseous nerve** as it circles around the radius into the posterior forearm compartment. It innervates all muscles of this compartment.
    - The **superficial branch** descends along the lateral forearm to the wrist.

- In the hand, the radial nerve has no motor branches.
  - At the wrist, the superficial branch runs posteriorly to innervate the skin on the dorsum of the hand and proximal segments of the1st through 3rd digits and half of the 4th digit.

■■■■■■ Radial nerve injury

The radial nerve is most vulnerable to injury from a midhumeral fracture where the nerve courses along the radial groove. Because radial branches to the triceps brachii are usually proximal to the injury, elbow flexion is unaffected. Other effects include the following:

- Loss of wrist extension
- Loss of extension at the metacarpophalangeal (MCP) joints
- Weakened pronation
- Flexed wrist and fingers producing the "wrist drop" position

■■■■■■ Brachial plexus injuries

Injuries to the proximal segments of the brachial plexus, involving the avulsion of the roots or stretching or compression of the trunks, have classic presentations that represent the distribution of the affected nerves.

Upper plexus injuries (Erb-Duchenne palsy) involve the C5 and C6 roots or the upper trunk and are usually caused by trauma that forcefully separates the head and shoulder. The resulting deformity includes an adducted shoulder and medially rotated limb that is extended at the elbow.

Injuries of the lower plexus (Klumpke's palsy) are far less common than those of the upper plexus, but a violent upward pull of the limb can avulse the C8 and T1 roots or damage the lower trunk. This affects the intrinsic muscles of the hand and creates a "claw hand" deformity. Because C8 and T1 are the superiormost contributions to the sympathetic trunk, avulsion of these nerve roots also affects the sympathetic innervation in the head. The manifestation of this is known as Horner's syndrome (see Section 20.1e).

14 Functional Anatomy of the Upper Limb

The upper limb is characterized by its wide range of movement and fine motor ability. Coordinated movements at the pectoral girdle, as well as the shoulder, elbow, radioulnar, and wrist joints, position the hand for performing work as vital as eating and as complicated as playing a violin.

Schematics of upper limb muscles accompany the muscle tables (origin, attachment, innervation, and action) in the appropriate chapter sections. To see the muscles in situ, view the gallery of topographic images in Section 14.7 at the end of the chapter.

14.1 The Pectoral Girdle

The **pectoral girdle**, formed by the clavicle and scapula, attaches the upper limb to the trunk (see **Fig. 13.2A and B**). The clavicle, acting as a strut, holds the scapula and humerus away from the trunk, allowing the free range of motion necessary for upper limb function.

14.1a Joints of the Pectoral Girdle

The joints of the pectoral girdle include articulations of the clavicle with the sternum and scapula, and a nonosseous joint that permits gliding movement between muscles of the trunk and scapula.

— The **sternoclavicular joint** is a strong but highly mobile synovial joint between the sternal end of the clavicle and the manubrium and 1st costal cartilage (**Fig. 14.1**).

- It is the only bony articulation between the upper limb and the trunk.
- An articular disk separates the articulating surfaces.
- **Anterior** and **posterior sternoclavicular**, **costoclavicular**, and **interclavicular ligaments** strengthen the joint.
- The joint allows the clavicle to elevate and rotate in conjunction with limb movements.

Fig. 14.1 ▶ **Sternoclavicular joint**
Anterior view with sternum coronally sectioned (left). *Note:* A fibrocartilaginous articular disk compensates for the mismatch of surfaces between the two saddle-shaped articular facets of the clavicle and the manubrium.

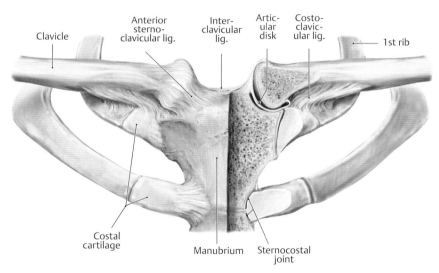

— The **acromioclavicular joint** is a plane type of synovial joint between the acromion of the scapula and acromial end of the clavicle (**Fig. 14.2**).

- An articular disk separates the articulating surfaces.
- An **acromioclavicular ligament** supports the joint superiorly.
- The **coracoclavicular ligament**, an extrinsic ligament (distant from the joint), strengthens the joint by anchoring the clavicle to the coracoid process. Its two parts are the **conoid** and **trapezoid ligaments**.

— The **scapulothoracic joint** is not a bony articulation but a functional relationship between the serratus anterior and subscapularis muscles that allows the scapula to glide and pivot on the chest wall (**Fig. 14.3**).

Injury to the long thoracic nerve

The superficial course of the long thoracic nerve (C5–C7) along the medial wall of the axilla puts it at risk of injury during regional surgeries such as axillary node dissection. Nerve damage results in the inability of the serratus anterior to laterally rotate the scapula, which is necessary to abduct the arm above the horizontal plane. The serratus anterior is also unable to support the scapula against the thoracic wall, which creates a "winged" scapula, especially noticeable when the subject presses the outstretched arm against a hard surface.

14.1b Muscles of the Pectoral Girdle

Muscles of the pectoral girdle attach the upper limb to the trunk and move and stabilize the pectoral girdle in response to movements of the glenohumeral joint at the shoulder (**Table 14.1**).

Fig. 14.2 ▶ **Acromioclavicular joint**
Anterior view. The acromioclavicular joint is a plane joint. Because the articulating surfaces are flat, they must be held in place by strong ligaments, greatly limiting the mobility of the joint.

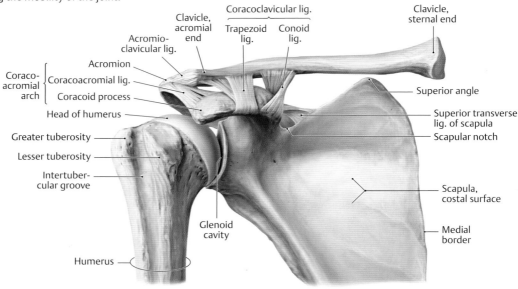

Fig. 14.3 ▶ **Scapulothoracic joint**
Right side, superior view. In all movements of the shoulder girdle, the scapula glides on a curved surface of loose connective tissue between the serratus anterior and the subscapularis muscles. This surface can be considered a scapulothoracic joint.

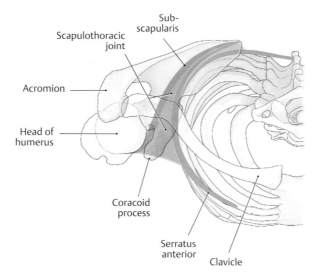

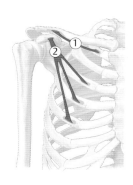

A Subclavius and pectoralis minor, right, anterior view.

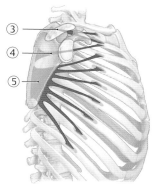

B Serratus anterior, right lateral view.

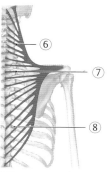

C Trapezius, right posterior view.

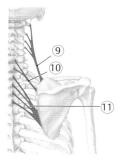

D Levator scapulae with rhomboids major and minor, right posterior view.

Table 14.1 ► Pectoral Girdle Muscles

Muscle		Origin	Insertion	Innervation	Action
① Subclavius		1st rib	Clavicle (inferior surface)	N. to subclavius (C5–C6)	Steadies the clavicle in the sternoclavicular joint
② Pectoralis minor		3rd to 5th ribs	Coracoid process	Medial and lateral pectoral nn. (C6–T1)	Draws scapula downward, causing inferior angle to move posteromedially; rotates glenoid inferiorly; assists in respiration
Serratus anterior	③ Superior part	1st to 9th ribs	Scapula (medial border)	Long thoracic n. (C5–C7)	Superior part: lowers the raised arm
	④ Intermediate part				Entire muscle: draws scapula laterally forward; elevates ribs when shoulder is fixed
	⑤ Inferior part				Inferior part: rotates scapula laterally
Trapezius	⑥ Descending part	Occipital bone; spinous process of C1–C7	Clavicle (lateral one third)	Accessory n. (CN X); C3–C4 of the cervical plexus	Draws scapula obliquely upward; rotates glenoid cavity superiorly; tilts head to same side and rotates it to opposite
	⑦ Transverse part	Aponeurosis at T1–T4 spinous processes	Acromion		Draws scapula medially
	⑧ Ascending part	Spinous process of T5–T12	Scapular spine		Draws scapula medially downward
					Entire muscle: steadies scapula on thorax
⑨ Levator scapulae		Transverse process of C1–C4	Scapula (superior angle)	Dorsal scapular n. (C4–C5)	Draws scapula medially upward while moving inferior angle medially; inclines neck to same side
⑩ Rhomboid minor		Spinous process of C6, C7	Medial border of scapula above (minor) and below (major) scapular spine		Steadies scapula; draws scapula medially upward
⑪ Rhomboid major		Spinous process of T1–T4 vertebrae			

Abbreviation: CN, cranial nerve.

— Anterior muscles of the pectoral girdle, which lie on the anterior and lateral thoracic wall,
  - include the **subclavius**, **pectoralis minor**, and **serratus anterior** and
  - are anchored to the ribs, as well as to the bones of the pectoral girdle.
— Posterior muscles of the pectoral girdle, which are part of the superficial muscular layer of the back,
  - include the **trapezius**, **levator scapulae**, **rhomboid major**, and **rhomboid minor** and
  - arise from cervical and thoracic vertebrae and insert on the scapula.
— Movements of the pectoral girdle and the muscles that provide them are listed in **Table 14.2**.

Table 14.2 ► Movements of the Pectoral Girdle

Action	Muscle
Elevation	Trapezius (descending part) Levator scapulae
Depression	Pectoralis minor Trapezius (ascending part)
Protraction	Pectoralis minor Serratus anterior
Retraction	Trapezius (transverse part) Rhomboid minor Rhomboid major
Lateral rotation	Serratus anterior (inferior part) Trapezius (descending part)
Medial rotation	Levator scapulae Rhomboid minor Rhomboid major

Fig. 14.4 ▶ **Walls of the axilla**
Right side, inferior view.

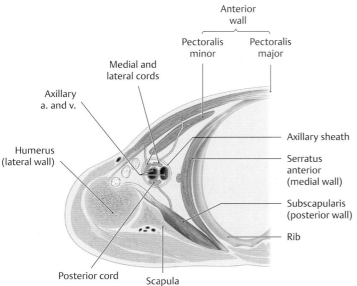

14.2 The Shoulder Region

The shoulder region includes the axilla, a passageway for neuro-vascular structures between the trunk and upper limb, and the glenohumeral joint, the largest joint of the upper limb. Muscles of the pectoral, scapular, and deltoid regions support the joint.

14.2a The Axilla

The **axilla** is a four-sided pyramidally shaped region between the upper parts of the arm and lateral thoracic wall (**Fig. 14.4**; see also **Fig. 13.1A** and **C**).

— Its boundaries are

- the **cervicoaxillary canal**, the narrow space between the clavicle and 1st rib, which forms the apex;
- the axillary fascia and axillary skin between the upper arm and the lateral thoracic wall, which form the base, or floor;

Fig. 14.5 ▶ **Dissection of the axilla**
Right shoulder, anterior view. *Removed:* Pectoralis major and clavipectoral fascia.

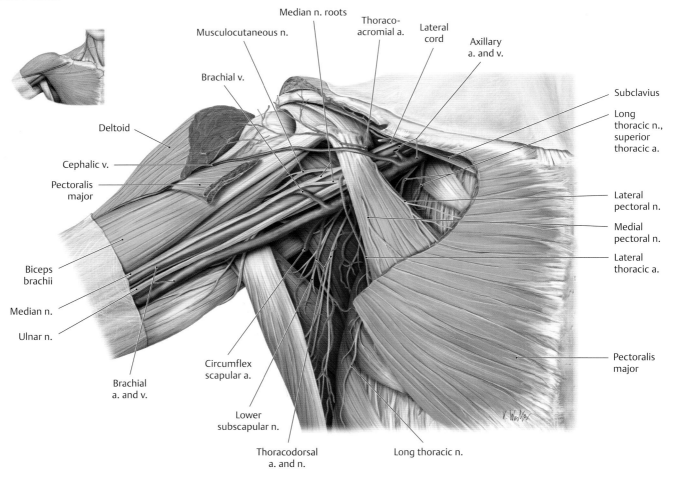

- the pectoralis major and pectoralis minor muscles, which form the anterior axillary wall (the lower edge of the pectoralis major forms a prominent ridge called the **anterior axillary fold**);
- the subscapularis, latissimus dorsi, and teres major muscles, which form the posterior axillary wall (the lower edge of the latissimus dorsi and teres major form a prominent ridge called the **posterior axillary fold**); and
- the lateral thoracic wall and the humerus of the arm, which form the medial and lateral walls, respectively.

— The contents of the axilla (**Fig. 14.5**), which are embedded in axillary fat, include
- the axillary artery and its branches,
- the axillary vein and its tributaries,
- axillary lymph nodes and vessels, and
- the cords and terminal nerves of the brachial plexus.

— An extension of the fascia of the neck forms a sleevelike **axillary sheath** that encloses the axillary vessels and the brachial plexus.

14.2b The Glenohumeral (Shoulder) Joint (Fig. 14.6A and B)

The **glenohumeral joint** is a ball-and-socket type of synovial joint between the shallow glenoid cavity of the scapula and the large head of the humerus.

— The **glenoid labrum**, a rim of fibrocartilage attached to the glenoid cavity, deepens the articular surface.

Glenohumeral dislocation

The glenohumeral joint is the most mobile but least stable joint of the body, and dislocations are frequent. Rotator cuff muscles provide the greatest stability, supporting the joint anteriorly, posteriorly, and superiorly, but inferior support is lacking. The coracoacromial arch, coracohumeral ligament, and capsular glenohumeral ligaments add further support. The majority of dislocations (90%) occur inferiorly, although most are labeled "anterior" dislocations based on the position of the displaced humeral head relative to the glenoid. These injuries can damage the axillary nerve and lead to a flattened shoulder profile. Posterior dislocations are rare and most often associated with seizures or electrocutions.

Fig. 14.6 ► **Glenohumeral joint: Bony elements**
Right shoulder, anterior view.

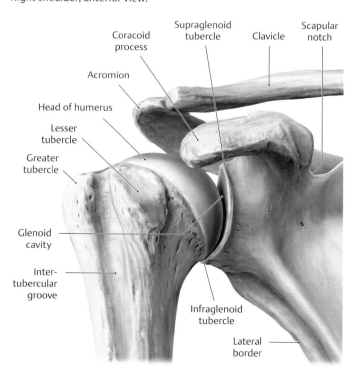

A Anterior view.

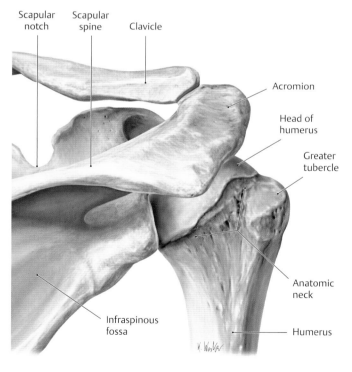

B Posterior view.

Fig. 14.7 ▶ **Glenohumeral joint: Capsule and ligaments**
Right shoulder, anterior view.

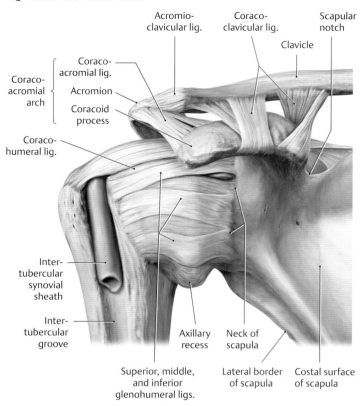

— A fibrous capsule, lined by a synovial membrane, surrounds the joint (**Fig. 14.7**). Ligaments that support the joint capsule include

- anteriorly, three thickenings of the capsule, the **superior, middle,** and **inferior glenohumeral ligaments,** and
- superiorly, a **coracohumeral ligament,** that extends between the coracoid process of the scapula and lesser tuberosity of the humerus.

— A synovial membrane lines the joint space (synovial cavity) (**Fig. 14.8**).

- It forms a tubular sheath around the tendon of the biceps brachii as the tendon passes through the joint space.
- The synovial cavity communicates with a bursa under the subscapularis tendon (subtendinous bursa of the subscapularis).

— The **coracoacromial ligament** between the coracoid process and acromion prevents superior dislocation of the humerus.

Fig. 14.8 ▶ **Glenohumeral joint cavity**
Right shoulder, anterior view.

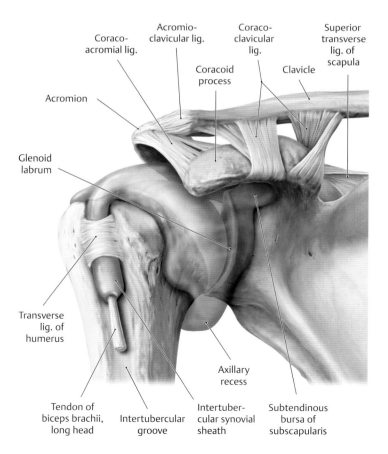

— Three large bursae are associated with the glenohumeral joint (**Fig. 14.9**).

1. Anteriorly, the **subtendinous bursa of the subscapularis**, which lies between the tendon of the subscapularis and the neck of the scapula, communicates with the synovial cavity of the joint.
2. Superiorly, the **subacromial bursa** lies under the coracoacromial ligament and above the supraspinatus tendon and glenohumeral joint capsule.
3. Laterally, the **subdeltoid bursa** lies deep to the deltoid muscle and above the subscapularis tendon. It communicates with the subacromial bursa.

Fig. 14.9 ▶ **Bursae of the shoulder region**
Right shoulder, anterior view.

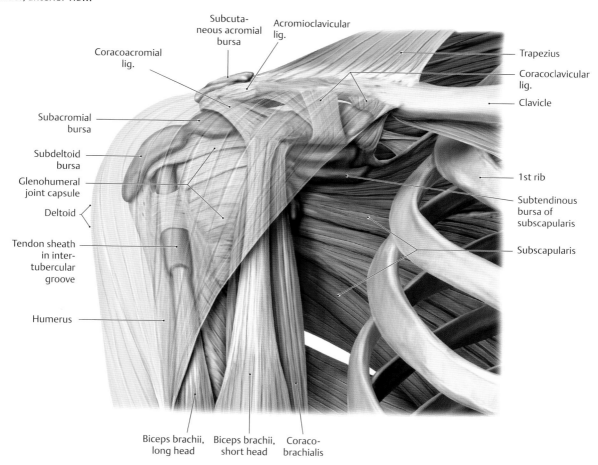

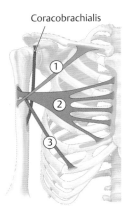

Coracobrachialis

A Pectoralis major and coracobrachialis, right side, anterior view.

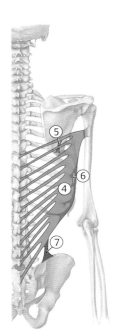

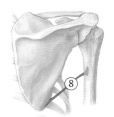

B Latissimus dorsi, right side, posterior view.

C Teres major, right side, posterior view.

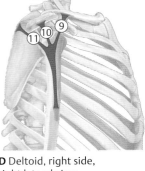

D Deltoid, right side, right lateral view.

E Rotator cuff (supraspinatus, infraspinatus, and teres minor), right shoulder, posterior view.

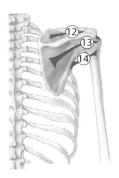

F Rotator cuff (subscapularis), right shoulder, anterior view.

Table 14.3 ► Shoulder Muscles

Muscle		Origin	Insertion	Innervation	Action
Pectoralis major	① Clavicular part	Clavicle (medial half)	Humerus (crest of greater tubercle)	Medial and lateral pectoral nn. (C5–T1)	Entire muscle: adduction, internal rotation Clavicular and sternocostal parts: flexion; assist in respiration when shoulder is fixed
	② Sternocostal part	Sternum and costal cartilages 1–6			
	③ Abdominal part	Rectus sheath (anterior layer)			
Latissimus dorsi	④ Vertebral part	Spinous process of T7–T12 vertebrae; thoracolumbar fascia	Crest of lesser tubercle of the humerus (anterior angle)	Thoracodorsal n. (C6–C8)	Internal rotation, adduction, extension, respiration ("cough muscle")
	⑤ Scapular part	Scapula (inferior angle)			
	⑥ Costal part	9th to 12th ribs			
	⑦ Iliac part	Iliac crest (posterior one third)			
⑧ Teres major		Scapula (inferior angle)		Lower subscapular n. (C5–C7)	Internal rotation, adduction, extension
Deltoid	⑨ Clavicular part	Lateral one third of clavicle	Humerus (deltoid tuberosity)	Axillary n. (C5–C6)	Flexion, internal rotation, adduction
	⑩ Acromial part	Acromion			Abduction
	⑪ Spinal part	Scapular spine			Extension, external rotation, adduction
⑫ Supraspinatus		Supraspinous fossa of scapula	Humerus (greater tubercle)	Suprascapular n. (C4–C6)	Abduction
⑬ Infraspinatus		Infraspinous fossa of scapula			External rotation
⑭ Teres minor		Lateral border of scapula		Axillary n. (C5–C6)	External rotation, weak adduction
⑮ Subscapularis		Subscapular fossa of scapula	Humerus (lesser tubercle)	Subscapular n. (C5–C6)	Internal rotation

14.2c Muscles of the Shoulder Region

Muscles that cross the glenohumeral joint stabilize the head of the humerus in the glenoid cavity and assist in movements of the arm (**Table 14.3**)

— Two muscles of the trunk, the **pectoralis major** and **latissimus dorsi**, extend from the axial skeleton to the humerus and together provide strong adduction and medial rotation of the arm.

  • The pectoralis major is a strong flexor of the arm.
  • The latissimus dorsi is a strong extensor of the arm.

— Scapulohumeral muscles attach the humerus to the scapula and provide stability for the glenohumeral joint.

  • The **deltoid**, which forms the rounded contour of the shoulder, abducts, flexes, and extends the arm.
  • The **teres major** adducts and medially rotates the arm.
  • The **supraspinatus** initiates abduction of the arm and assists the deltoid in the first 15 degrees of movement.
  • The **infraspinatus** externally rotates the arm.
  • The **teres minor** externally rotates the arm.
  • The **subscapularis** on the anterior surface of the scapula internally rotates the arm.

— A musculotendinous **rotator cuff** around the glenohumeral joint includes four of the scapulohumeral muscles, which are the important dynamic stabilizers of the joint.

  • The rotator cuff muscles include the **supraspinatus, infraspinatus, teres minor**, and **subscapularis**.

• Their tendons insert on, and reinforce, the fibrous capsule of the joint, forming a supportive cuff around the anterior, posterior, and superior aspects of the joint.

▌ Rotator cuff tears

Rotator cuff tears can occur at any age but are most common in the older patient and usually involve the supraspinatus tendon. Degenerative changes and chronic inflammation from repetitive use (baseball pitchers are a good example) can cause the tendon to fray and rupture. When the subacromial and subdeltoid bursae tear in conjunction with the ruptured tendon, they become continuous with the cavity of the glenohumeral joint.

— A few muscles of the arm cross the glenohumeral joint and support its movements (see **Table 14.5**).

  • The tendon of the long head of the **biceps brachii** passes through the intertubercular groove of the humerus and enters the joint cavity, where it is ensheathed by the synovial layer of the capsule. It prevents dislocation of the humerus during abduction and flexion.
  • The short head of the biceps brachii and the **coracobrachialis** muscles cross the joint anteriorly and assist in flexion of the arm.
  • The long head of the **triceps brachii** crosses the joint posteriorly and assists in adduction and extension.

— Movements at the glenohumeral joint and the muscles that provide them are listed in **Table 14.4**.

Table 14.4 ▶ Movements at the Glenohumeral Joint	
Action	**Muscles**
Flexion	Deltoid (clavicular part) Pectoralis major (clavicular and sternocostal parts) Coracobrachialis Biceps brachii (short head)
Extension	Deltoid (spinal part) Latissimus dorsi Teres major Triceps brachii (long head)
Abduction	Deltoid (acromial part) Supraspinatus
Adduction	Deltoid (clavicular and spinal parts) Pectoralis major Latissimus dorsi Teres major Triceps brachii (long head)
Internal rotation	Deltoid (clavicular part) Pectoralis major (clavicular part) Latissimus dorsi Teres major Subscapularis
External rotation	Deltoid (spinal part) Infraspinatus Teres minor

14.2d Spaces of the Posterior Shoulder Region

Spaces formed between muscles of the shoulder and the scapula allow nerves and vessels to pass between the axilla and the posterior scapular and humeral regions (**Fig. 14.10**).

— The **scapular notch**, limited superiorly by the superior transverse scapular ligament, lies deep to the supraspinatus muscle. The suprascapular nerve passes below the ligament, and the suprascapular artery passes above it.

— The **quadrangular space**, bounded by the long head of the triceps, the humerus, and the teres major and teres minor muscles, transmits the posterior circumflex humeral artery and axillary nerve.

— The **triangular space**, bounded by the long head of the triceps and the teres major and teres minor muscles, transmits the circumflex scapular artery.

— The **triceps hiatus**, between the long and lateral heads of the triceps and below the teres major muscle, transmits the radial nerve and deep brachial artery.

Fig. 14.10 ▶ **Spaces of the posterior shoulder region**
Right shoulder, posterior view. The course of arteries and nerves through the spaces are shown by red and yellow arrows in the schematic.

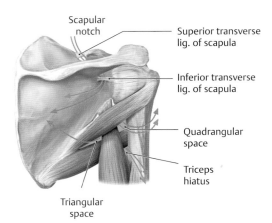

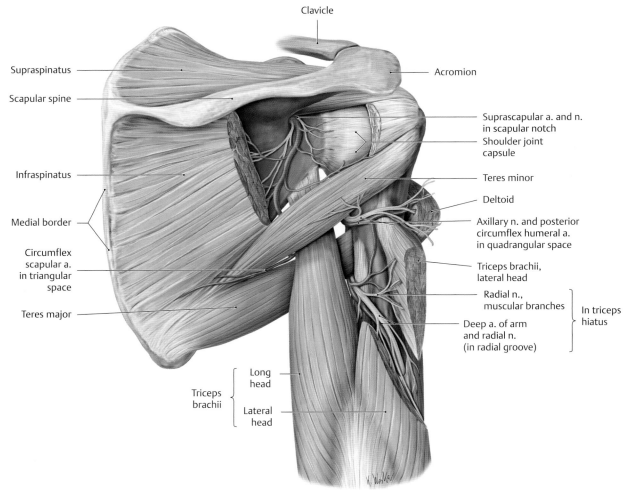

14.3 The Arm and Cubital Region

The arm (brachial region) extends from the shoulder to the elbow and contains the humerus and muscles of the arm. The cubital region contains the cubital fossa and the elbow joint.

14.3a Muscles of the Arm

Muscles of the arm move the shoulder and elbow joints. Brachial fascia that surrounds the arm divides these muscles into anterior and posterior compartments (**Table 14.5**).

— The anterior compartment contains
  - muscles that flex the glenohumeral and elbow joints and supinate the radioulnar joint,
  - the musculocutaneous nerve, and
  - the brachial artery and vein.
— The posterior compartment contains
  - muscles that extend the glenohumeral and elbow joints,
  - the radial nerve, and
  - the deep brachial artery and vein.
— The median and ulnar nerves descend along the medial side of the arm between the anterior and posterior compartments but do not innervate muscles of the arm.

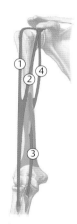

A Biceps brachii, brachialis, and corachobrachialis, right arm, anterior view.

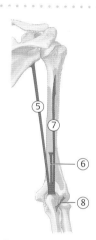

B Triceps brachii and anconeus, right arm, posterior view.

Table 14.5 ▶ **Arm Muscles, Anterior and Posterior Compartments**

Muscle		Origin	Insertion	Innervation	Action
Anterior compartment					
Biceps brachii	① Long head	Supraglenoid tubercle of scapula	Radial tuberosity	Musculocutaneous n. (C5–C6)	Elbow joint: flexion; supination*
	② Short head	Coracoid process of scapula			Shoulder joint: flexion; stabilization of humeral head during deltoid contraction; abduction and internal rotation of the humerus
③ Brachialis		Humerus (distal half of anterior surface)	Ulnar tuberosity	Musculocutaneous n. (C5–C6) and radial n. (C7, minor)	Flexion at the elbow joint
④ Coracobrachialis		Scapula (coracoid process)	Humerus (in line with crest of lesser tuberosity)	Musculocutaneous n. (C6, C7)	Flexion, adduction, internal rotation
Posterior compartment					
Triceps brachii	⑤ Long head	Scapula (infraglenoid tubercle)	Olecranon of ulna	Radial n. (C6–C8)	Elbow joint: extension
	⑥ Medial head	Posterior humerus, distal to radial groove; medial intermuscular septum			Shoulder joint, long head: extension and adduction
	⑦ Lateral head	Posterior humerus, proximal to radial groove; lateral intermuscular septum			
⑧ Anconeus		Lateral epicondyle of humerus (variance: posterior joint capsule)	Olecranon of ulna (radial surface)		Extends the elbow and tightens its joint

*Note: When the elbow is flexed, the biceps brachii acts as a powerful supinator because the lever arm is almost perpendicular to the axis of pronation/supination.

14.3b The Cubital Fossa

The **cubital fossa** is a shallow depression anterior to the elbow joint (**Fig. 14.11A** and **B**).

— Its boundaries are,

- medially, the pronator teres;
- laterally, the brachioradialis; and
- superiorly, a line that connects the medial and lateral epicondyles of the humerus.

Fig. 14.11 ▶ **Cubital region**
Right elbow, anterior view.

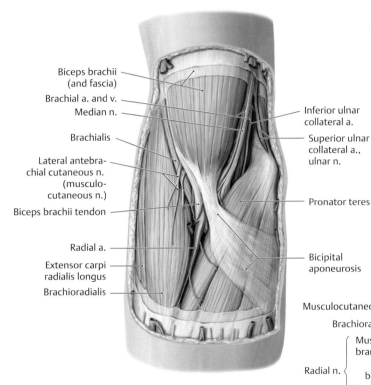

A Superficial cubital fossa. *Removed:* Fasciae and epifascial neurovascular structures.

— The cubital fossa contains
- the tendon of the biceps brachii,
- the brachial artery and vein,
- the proximal part of radial and ulnar arteries and veins, and
- the median and radial nerves and the cutaneous branch of the musculocutaneous nerve (lateral antebrachial cutaneous nerve).

— The **bicipital aponeurosis**, a fascial extension of the biceps brachii, forms the root of the fossa, and the medial cubital vein crosses the fossa superficially.

14.3c The Elbow Joint

The elbow joint is made up of three separate synovial joints contained within a single joint capsule (**Figs. 14.12A** and **B** and **14.13**).

— The hinge-type **humeroulnar joint** is an articulation between the trochlea of the humerus and the trochlear notch of the ulna.

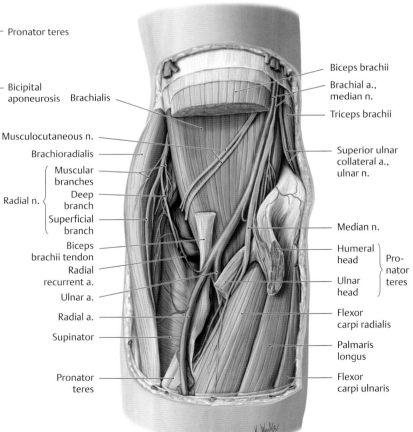

B Deep cubital fossa. *Removed:* Biceps brachii (distal muscle belly). *Retracted:* Brachioradialis.

Fig. 14.12 ▶ Elbow (cubital) joint

Right elbow in extension. The elbow consists of three articulations: the humeroulnar, humeroradial, and proximal radioulnar.

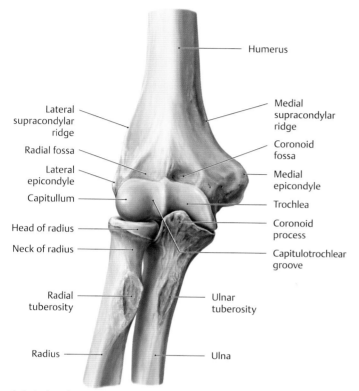

A Anterior view.

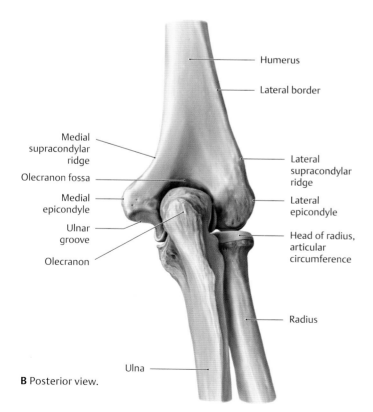

B Posterior view.

- The **ulnar** (medial) **collateral ligament**, which supports the joint medially, connects the coronoid process and olecranon with the medial epicondyle of the humerus.

— The hinge-type **humeroradial joint** is an articulation between the capitullum of the humerus and the head of the radius.

- The **radial** (lateral) **collateral ligament**, which supports the joint laterally, extends from the lateral epicondyle of the humerus to the **annular ligament** of the radius that encircles the radial neck.

— The proximal radioulnar joint, the articulation between the head of the radius and the radial notch of the ulna, is discussed further with the radioulnar joints of the forearm.

— Movements at the humeroulnar and humeroradial joints and the muscles that provide them are listed in **Table 14.6**.

Table 14.6 ▶ **Movements at the Humeroulnar and Humeroradial Joints**	
Action	**Muscle**
Flexion	Biceps brachii Brachialis Brachioradialis
Extension	Triceps brachii

Fig. 14.13 ▶ Joint capsule of the elbow

Right elbow in extension, anterior view.

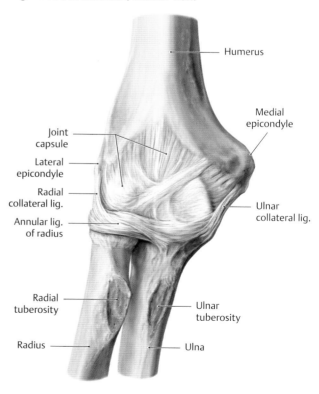

14.4 The Forearm

The forearm (antebrachial region) extends from the elbow to the wrist and contains the radius and ulna and the muscles of the forearm.

14.4a Radioulnar Joints

The radioulnar joints connect the bones of the forearm proximally at the elbow and distally at the wrist. Movement at these joints allows rotation of the distal radius around the ulna, causing supination (palm up) and pronation (palm down) of the hand (**Figs. 14.14** and **14.15**). These movements and the muscles of the arm and forearm that provide them are listed in **Table 14.7**.

Table 14.7 ▶ Movements at the Radioulnar Joints	
Action	**Muscle**
Supination	Supinator Biceps brachii
Pronation	Pronator teres Pronator quadratus

— The **proximal radioulnar joint** is a synovial joint that allows rotation of the radial head within the cuff formed by the annular ligament and the radial notch of the ulna. This articulation is contained within the elbow joint capsule.

> **Subluxation of the radial head (nursemaid's elbow)**
>
> In young children the immature radial head can be subluxated when the child's arm is jerked upward. The movement tears the lax distal attachment of the annular ligament around the neck of the radius and allows the distal displacement of the radial head. The injured arm is held in a flexed and pronated position. Supination of the flexed elbow returns the joint to the correct orientation.

— The **distal radioulnar joint** has an L-shaped joint cavity with a triangular articular disk that separates the radioulnar joint from the cavity of the wrist joint.
— An **interosseous membrane** connects the shafts of the radius and ulna and transfers energy absorbed by the distal radius to the proximal ulna.

Fig. 14.14 ▶ **Forearm in supination**
Right forearm, anterior view.

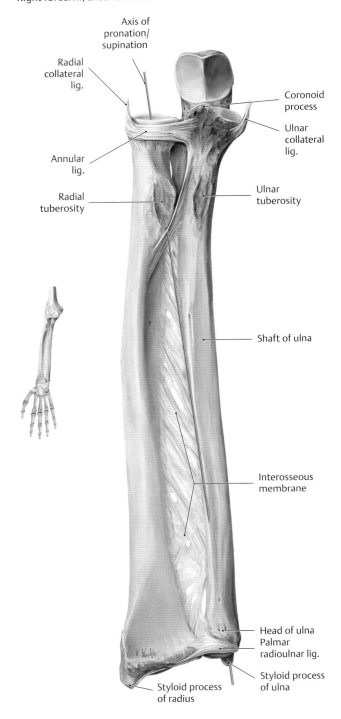

Axis of pronation/supination

Radial collateral lig.

Coronoid process

Ulnar collateral lig.

Annular lig.

Radial tuberosity

Ulnar tuberosity

Shaft of ulna

Interosseous membrane

Head of ulna
Palmar radioulnar lig.

Styloid process of ulna

Styloid process of radius

Fig. 14.15 ▶ **Forearm in pronation**
Right forearm, anterior view.

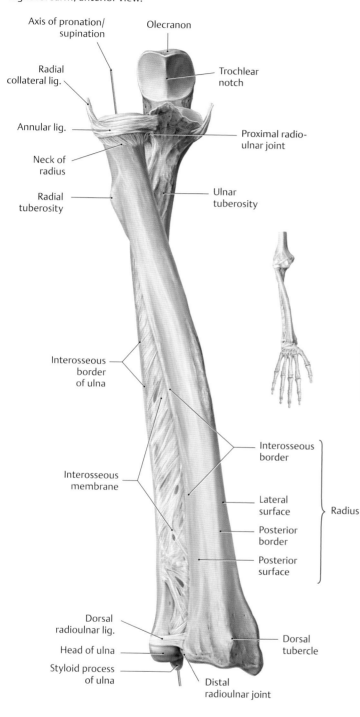

Axis of pronation/supination

Olecranon

Radial collateral lig.

Trochlear notch

Annular lig.

Proximal radio-ulnar joint

Neck of radius

Radial tuberosity

Ulnar tuberosity

Interosseous border of ulna

Interosseous membrane

Interosseous border

Lateral surface

Posterior border

Posterior surface

⎱ Radius

Dorsal radioulnar lig.

Head of ulna

Styloid process of ulna

Dorsal tubercle

Distal radioulnar joint

14.4b Muscles of the Forearm

Muscles of the forearm move joints of the elbow, wrist, and hand. Most forearm flexors and extensors have long tendons that cross the wrist and extend into the fingers. Intermuscular septa and the interosseous membrane create anterior and posterior muscular compartments.

— The anterior forearm compartment (**Table 14.8**) contains

 • muscles that flex and pronate joints of the elbow, wrist, and hand;
 • the median and ulnar nerves; and
 • the ulnar and anterior interosseous arteries and veins.

— The posterior forearm compartment (**Table 14.9**) contains

 • muscles that extend joints of the elbow, wrist, and hand and supinate the radioulnar joint (one muscle, the brachioradialis, passes anterior to the elbow and therefore acts as a flexor, instead of an extensor of this joint);
 • the radial nerve; and
 • the radial and posterior interosseous arteries and veins.

Lateral epicondylitis

Repetitive use of the forearm extensors can inflame the attachment of the common extensor tendon at the lateral epicondyle (lateral epicondylitis). Pain is focused over the tendon insertion but radiates along the extensor forearm and is exacerbated by stretching of the extensor tendons by pronation and wrist flexion.

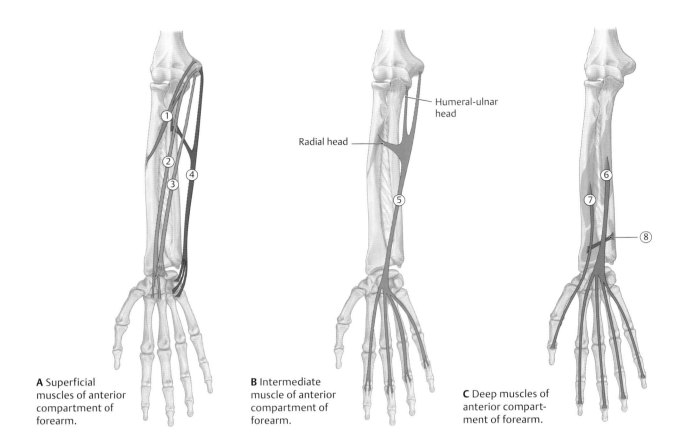

A Superficial muscles of anterior compartment of forearm.

B Intermediate muscle of anterior compartment of forearm.

C Deep muscles of anterior compartment of forearm.

Table 14.8 ► **Forearm Muscles, Anterior Compartment**

Muscle	Origin	Insertion	Innervation	Action
Superficial group				
① Pronator teres	Humeral head: medial epicondyle of humerus Ulnar head: coronoid process	Lateral radius (distal to supinator insertion)	Median n. (C6–C7)	Elbow: weak flexor Forearm: pronation
② Flexor carpi radialis	Medial epicondyle of humerus	Base of 2nd metacarpal (variance: base of 3rd metacarpal)		Wrist: flexion and abduction (radial deviation) of hand
③ Palmaris longus		Palmar aponeurosis	Median n. (C7–C8)	Elbow: weak flexion Wrist: flexion tightens palmar aponeurosis
④ Flexor carpi ulnaris	Humeral head: medial epicondyle Ulnar head: olecranon	Pisiform; hook of hamate; base of 5th metacarpal	Ulnar n. (C7–T1)	Wrist: flexion and adduction (ulnar deviation) of hand
Intermediate group				
⑤ Flexor digitorum superficialis	Humeral-ulnar head: medial epicondyle of humerus Radial head: upper half of anterior border of radius	Sides of middle phalanges of 2nd to 5th digits	Median n. (C8–T1)	Elbow: weak flexor Wrist, MCP, and PIP joints of 2nd to 5th digits: flexion
Deep group				
⑥ Flexor digitorum profundus	Ulna (two thirds of flexor surface) and interosseous membrane	Distal phalanges of 2nd to 5th digits (palmar surface)	Median n. (C8–T1) Ulnar n. (C8–T1)	Wrist, MCP, PIP, and DIP of 2nd to 5th digits: flexion
⑦ Flexor pollicis longus	Radius (midanterior surface) and adjacent interosseous membrane	Distal phalanx of thumb (palmar surface)	Median n. (C7–C8)	Wrist: flexion and abduction (radial deviation) of hand Carpometacarpal of thumb: flexion MCP and IP of thumb: flexion
⑧ Pronator quadratus	Distal quarter of ulna (anterior surface)	Distal quarter of radius (anterior surface)		Hand: pronation Distal radioulnar joint: stabilization

Abbreviations: DIP, distal interphalangeal; IP, interphalangeal; MCP, metacarpophalangeal; PIP, proximal interphalangeal.

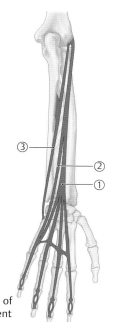

A Superficial muscles of posterior compartment of forearm.

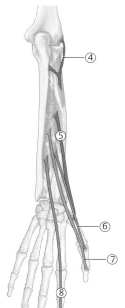

B Deep muscles of posterior compartment of forearm.

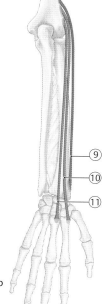

C Radialis muscle group of posterior compartment of forearm.

Table 14.9 ▶ Forearm Muscles, Posterior Compartment: Superficial, Deep, and Radialis Groups

Muscle	Origin	Insertion	Innervation	Action
Superficial group				
① Extensor digitorum	Common head (lateral epicondyle of humerus)	Dorsal digital expansion of 2nd to 5th digits	Radial n. (C7–C8)	Wrist: extension MCP, PIP, and DIP of 2nd to 5th digits: extension/abduction of fingers
② Extensor digiti minimi		Dorsal digital expansion of 5th digit		Wrist: extension, ulnar abduction of hand MCP, PIP, and DIP of 5th digit: extension and abduction of 5th digit
③ Extensor carpi ulnaris	Common head (lateral epicondyle of humerus) Ulnar head (dorsal surface)	Base of 5th metacarpal		Wrist: extension, adduction (ulnar deviation) of hand
Deep group				
④ Supinator	Olecranon, lateral epicondyle of humerus, radial collateral ligament, annular ligament of radius	Radius (between radial tuberosity and insertion of pronator teres)	Radial n. (C6–C7)	Radioulnar joints: supination
⑤ Abductor pollicis longus	Radius and ulna (dorsal surfaces, interosseous membrane)	Base of 1st metacarpal	Radial n. (C7–C8)	Radiocarpal joint: abduction of the hand Carpometacarpal joint of thumb: abduction
⑥ Extensor pollicis brevis	Radius (posterior surface) and interosseous membrane	Base of proximal phalanx of thumb		Radiocarpal joint: abduction (radial deviation) of hand Carpometacarpal and MCP of thumb: extension
⑦ Extensor pollicis longus	Ulna (posterior surface) and interosseous membrane	Base of distal phalanx of thumb		Wrist: extension and abduction (radial deviation) of hand Carpometacarpal of thumb: adduction MCP and IP of thumb: extension
⑧ Extensor indicis	Ulna (posterior surface) and interosseous membrane	Posterior digital extension of 2nd digit		Wrist: extension MCP, PIP, and DIP of 2nd digit: extension
Radialis group				
⑨ Brachioradialis	Distal humerus (distal surface), lateral intermuscular septum	Styloid process of the radius	Radial n. (C5–C6)	Elbow: flexion Forearm: semipronation
⑩ Extensor carpi radialis longus	Lateral supracondylar ridge of distal humerus, lateral intermuscular septum	2nd metacarpal (base)	Radial n. (C6–C7)	Elbow: weak flexion Wrist: extension and abduction
⑪ Extensor carpi radialis brevis	Lateral epicondyle of humerus	3rd metacarpal (base)	Radial n. (C7–C8)	

Abbreviations: DIP, distal interphalangeal; IP, interphalangeal; MCP, metacarpophalangeal; PIP, proximal interphalangeal.

14.5 The Wrist

The wrist, the narrow space between the forearm and hand, contains the carpal bones and the tendons of forearm muscles that move the wrist and fingers.

14.5a Joints of the Wrist

Joints of the wrist include the articulations between the distal radius and bones of the proximal row of carpals, articulations between adjacent carpal bones, and articulations between the distal carpal bones and the metacarpals of the hand (**Fig. 14.16**). Movements at the wrist joints and the muscles that provide them are listed in **Table 14.10**.

Table 14.10 ▸ Movements at the Wrist Joints	
Action	**Muscle**
Flexion	Flexor carpi radialis Flexor carpi ulnaris
Extension	Extensor carpi radialis longus Extensor carpi radialis brevis Extensor carpi ulnaris
Abduction (radial deviation)	Flexor carpi radialis Extensor carpi radialis longus Extensor carpi radialis brevis
Adduction (ulnar deviation)	Flexor carpi ulnaris Extensor carpi ulnaris

Fig. 14.16 ▸ **Joints of the wrist and hand**
Right hand, posterior (dorsal) view.

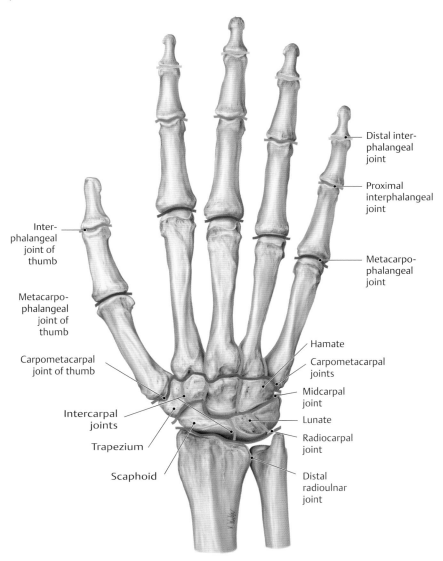

Distal inter-
phalangeal
joint

Proximal
interphalangeal
joint

Metacarpo-
phalangeal
joint

Inter-
phalangeal
joint of
thumb

Metacarpo-
phalangeal
joint of
thumb

Carpometacarpal
joint of thumb

Hamate

Carpometacarpal
joints

Midcarpal
joint

Intercarpal
joints

Lunate

Trapezium

Radiocarpal
joint

Scaphoid

Distal
radioulnar
joint

— The **radiocarpal joint** is an articulation of the distal radius and articular disk of the distal radioulnar joint with the scaphoid and lunate.

- • Palmar and dorsal radiocarpal ligaments and radial and ulnar collateral ligaments strengthen the joint.

— **Intercarpal joints** are the articulations between the carpal bones within each row; the **midcarpal joint** is the articulation between the bones of the proximal and distal carpal rows.

- • Movements at these joints augment movements at the wrist joint.

— **Carpometacarpal joints** are the synovial articulations between the distal row of carpal bones and the metacarpals.

- • Little or no movement occurs at the plane-type joints of the 2nd, 3rd, and 4th digits.
- • The joint of the 5th digit between the metacarpus and the hamate is moderately mobile.
- • The saddle-type joint between the metacarpus of the thumb and the trapezium in the distal carpal row allows movement in all directions, which is essential for thumb opposition (**Fig. 14.17**).

Fig. 14.17 ▶ Carpometacarpal joint of the thumb
Radial view. The 1st metacarpal bone has been moved slightly distally to expose the articular surface of the trapezium. Two cardinal axes of motion are shown here: (a) abduction/adduction and (b) flexion/extension.

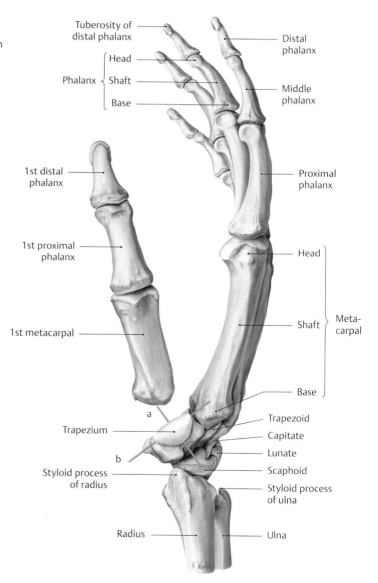

14.5b Spaces of the Wrist

Neurovascular structures and the long tendons of the forearm muscles pass between the forearm and hand through narrow spaces that are usually defined by fascial thickenings.

— The **carpal tunnel** is a fascio-osseous space on the anterior wrist (**Figs. 14.18A** and **B** and **14.19**).

- Carpal bones form the floor and sides; the flexor retinaculum forms the roof.
- The tendons of the flexor pollicis longus, flexor digitorum superficialis, and flexor digitorum profundus, and the median nerve pass through the tunnel.

Fig. 14.18 ► **Carpal tunnel**
Right hand, proximal view. The tight fit of sensitive neurovascular structures with closely apposed, frequently moving tendons in the carpal tunnel often causes problems (carpal tunnel syndrome) when any of the structures swell or degenerate.

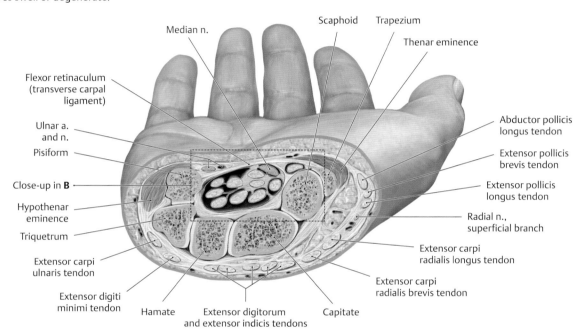

A Cross section through the right wrist.

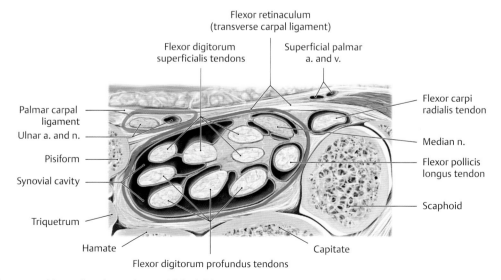

B Structures in the ulnar tunnel (green) and carpal tunnel (blue). Blow-up of area enclosed by dash lines in **A**.

- A **common flexor synovial tendon sheath** encloses the flexor tendons as they pass through the carpal tunnel (see **Fig. 14.32A**).
- The palmar carpal ligament and flexor retinaculum prevent bowing of the flexor tendons as they cross the wrist.

Carpal tunnel syndrome

The carpal tunnel, defined by inflexible fibrous and osseous boundaries, can be compromised by the swelling of its contents, infiltration of fluid from inflammation or infection, protrusion of a dislocated carpal bone, or pressure from an external source. The median nerve is most sensitive to the increased pressure, and signs of carpal tunnel syndrome reflect the nerve's distribution. These include tingling or numbness on the palmar surface of the lateral three and a half digits and weakness and eventual atrophy of the thenar muscles. The palmar cutaneous branch of the median nerve arises proximal to the canal and passes over the flexor retinaculum, so sensation of the palm remains intact.

— The **ulnar tunnel** (Guyon's canal) is a narrow passageway on the medial side of the anterior wrist (see **Figs. 14.18** and **14.19**).

- The flexor retinaculum forms the floor, and the **palmar carpal ligament** forms the roof. The pisiform and hamate form the medial and lateral borders.
- The ulnar artery and nerve pass through the tunnel into the palm of the hand.

Ulnar nerve compression

Compression of the ulnar nerve at the wrist affects the innervation of most intrinsic hand muscles. When the patient attempts to form a fist, it results in a deformity known as a "claw hand"—the metacarpophalangeal joints are hyperextended due to the loss of the interossei muscles, and the interphalangeal joints are flexed.

Fig. 14.19 ▶ **Anterior carpal region**
Right hand, anterior (palmar) view. Ulnar tunnel and deep palm. Carpal tunnel with flexor retinaculum transparent. *Removed*: Palmaris brevis, palmaris longus, palmar aponeurosis, and palmar carpal ligament.

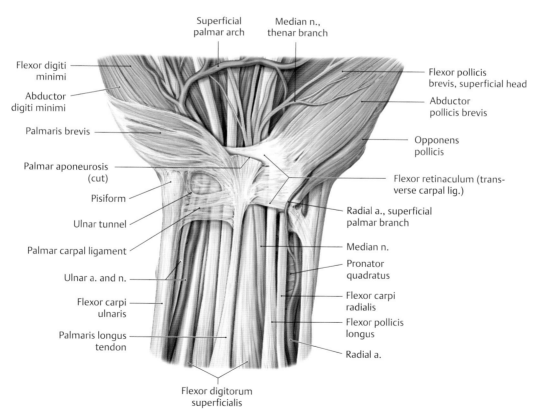

Fig. 14.20 ▶ **Anatomic snuffbox**
Right hand, radial view. The three-sided "anatomic snuffbox" (shaded light yellow) is bounded by the tendons of insertion of the abductor pollicis longus and the extensor pollicis brevis and extensor pollicis longus.

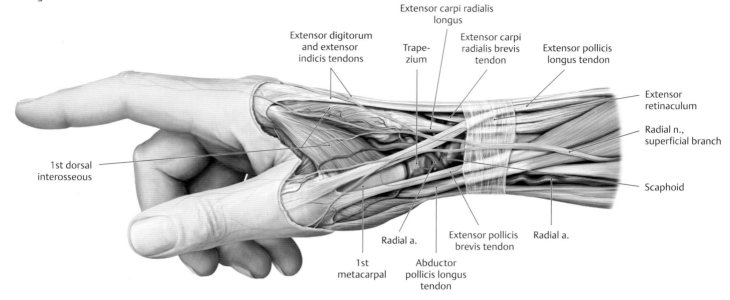

Extensor carpi radialis longus
Extensor digitorum and extensor indicis tendons
Trape-zium
Extensor carpi radialis brevis tendon
Extensor pollicis longus tendon
Extensor retinaculum
Radial n., superficial branch
Scaphoid
1st dorsal interosseous
Radial a.
Extensor pollicis brevis tendon
Radial a.
1st metacarpal
Abductor pollicis longus tendon

Fig. 14.21 ▶ **Extensor retinaculum and dorsal compartments**
Right hand.

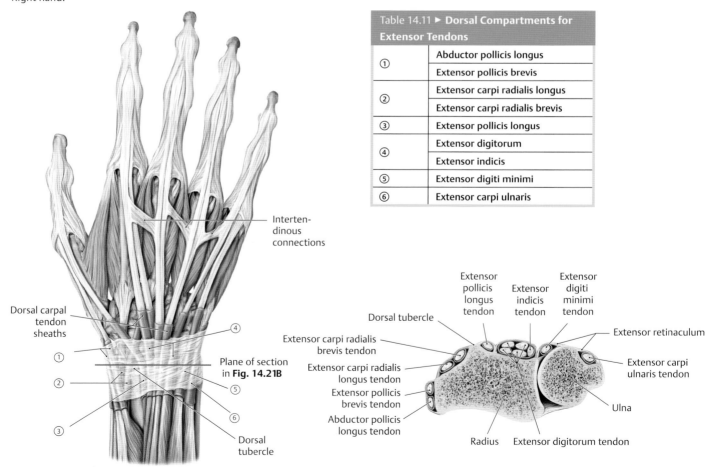

Table 14.11 ▶ Dorsal Compartments for Extensor Tendons	
①	Abductor pollicis longus
	Extensor pollicis brevis
②	Extensor carpi radialis longus
	Extensor carpi radialis brevis
③	Extensor pollicis longus
④	Extensor digitorum
	Extensor indicis
⑤	Extensor digiti minimi
⑥	Extensor carpi ulnaris

Interten-dinous connections

Dorsal carpal tendon sheaths
①
②
③
Plane of section in **Fig. 14.21B**
④
⑤
⑥
Dorsal tubercle

Extensor pollicis longus tendon
Extensor indicis tendon
Extensor digiti minimi tendon
Dorsal tubercle
Extensor carpi radialis brevis tendon
Extensor retinaculum
Extensor carpi radialis longus tendon
Extensor carpi ulnaris tendon
Extensor pollicis brevis tendon
Abductor pollicis longus tendon
Ulna
Radius
Extensor digitorum tendon

A Posterior (dorsal) view.

B Proximal view of section indicated in **A**.

— The **anatomic snuffbox** is a small triangular depression on the radial side of the dorsum of the wrist (**Fig. 14.20**).

- Tendons of the extensor pollicis longus, extensor pollicis brevis, and abductor pollicis longus form the borders. The scaphoid and trapezium form its floor.
- The radial artery passes through the snuffbox.
- The cephalic vein and superficial branch of the radial nerve cross the snuffbox superficially.

— Six small **dorsal compartments** (designated as 1st through 6th) form on the posterior surface of the wrist (**Table 14.11**; **Fig. 14.21A** and **B**).

- The extensor retinaculum forms their roof, and the dorsal surfaces of the distal radius and ulna form their floor.
- Extensor tendons of forearm muscles pass through the compartments onto the dorsum of the hand.
- **Dorsal carpal synovial tendon sheaths** enclose the extensor tendons as they pass through the dorsal compartments.

14.6 The Hand

The muscles and joints of the hand create a flexible tool that is adept at fine motor movements. The ability to grasp objects by positioning the thumb in opposition to the other fingers is a feature that is unique to humans and apes.

14.6a Joints of the Hand and Fingers

Joints of the hand and fingers are the articulations between the metacarpal bones of the palm and the proximal phalanges and between the proximal, middle, and distal phalanges of each digit (see **Fig. 14.16**). Movements at these joints and the muscles of the forearm and hand that provide them are listed in **Tables 14.12** and **14.13**.

Table 14.12 ▸ Movements at the Joints of the Fingers (Digits 2 through 5)	
Action	**Muscle**
Flexion at MCP	Lumbricals Interossei Flexor digiti minimi (only 5th digit)
Flexion at DIP	Flexor digitorum superficialis Lumbricals
Flexion at PIP	Flexor digitorum profundus
Extension at MCP	Extensor digitorum Extensor indicis (only 3rd digit) Extensor digiti minimi (only 5th digit)
Extension at DIP and PIP	Lumbricals Interossei
Abduction at MCP	Dorsal interossei Abductor digiti minimi (only 5th digit)
Adduction	Palmer interossei (digits 2, 4, and 5 only)
Opposition	Opponens digiti minimi (only 5th digit)

Abbreviations: DIP, distal interphalangeal; MCP, metacarpophalangeal; PIP, proximal interphalangeal.

Table 14.13 ▸ Movements at Joints of the Thumb	
Action	**Muscle**
Flexion	Flexor pollicis longus Flexor pollicis brevis
Extension	Extensor pollicis longus Extensor pollicis brevis
Abduction	Abductor pollicis longus Abductor pollicis brevis
Adduction	Adductor pollicis
Opposition	Opponens pollicis

— **Metacarpophalangeal (MCP) joints** are condyloid synovial joints between the heads of the metacarpals and bases of the proximal phalanges.

- Movement in two planes, flexion-extension and abduction-adduction, occurs in digits 2 through 5.
- Only flexion and extension occur at the MCP joint of the thumb.

— **Interphalangeal (IP) joints** are hinge-type synovial joints between phalanges.

- Digits 2 through 4 have proximal interphalangeal (PIP) and distal interphalangeal (DIP) joints.
- The thumb has only a single IP joint.
- IP joints permit only flexion and extension.

— MCP and IP joints are surrounded by a fibrous capsule and supported by medial and lateral collateral ligaments.

Fig. 14.22 ▶ **Surface anatomy of the dorsum of the hand**
Right hand.

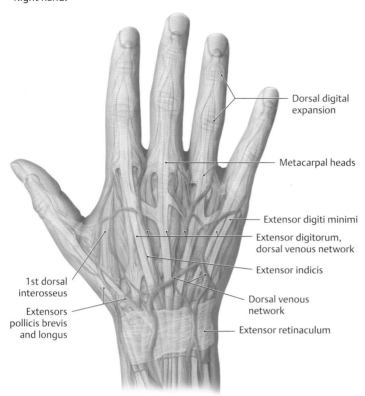

1st dorsal interosseus

Extensors pollicis brevis and longus

Dorsal digital expansion

Metacarpal heads

Extensor digiti minimi

Extensor digitorum, dorsal venous network

Extensor indicis

Dorsal venous network

Extensor retinaculum

Fig. 14.23 ▶ **Dorsal digital expansion**
Right hand, middle finger, posterior view. The dorsal digital expansion permits the long digital flexors and the short muscles of the hand to act on all three finger joints.

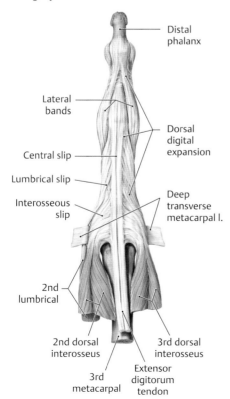

Lateral bands

Central slip

Lumbrical slip

Interosseous slip

2nd lumbrical

2nd dorsal interosseus

3rd metacarpal

Extensor digitorum tendon

3rd dorsal interosseus

Deep transverse metacarpal l.

Dorsal digital expansion

Distal phalanx

14.6b The Dorsum of the Hand and Fingers

— The dorsum of the hand has the following surface anatomy (**Fig. 14.22**):
  - The skin is thin and loose.
  - A prominent superficial dorsal venous network gives rise to the cephalic and basilic veins.
  - The heads of the metacarpals of the 2nd through 5th digits form distinct "knuckles" when the hand is flexed into a fist.
  - The extensor tendons fan out from the wrist to the fingers.

— On the dorsum of the fingers, the long extensor tendons (of the posterior forearm compartment) flatten to form a **dorsal digital expansion** (extensor expansion, extensor hood), a triangular tendinous aponeurosis (**Fig. 14.23**). The dorsal digital expansion
  - forms a hood that wraps around the sides of the distal metacarpus and proximal phalanx and holds the extensor tendon in place;
  - inserts onto the middle and distal phalanges via a **central slip** and paired **lateral bands**; and
  - is reinforced by the lumbricals and interossei muscles of the palm, which connect to the lateral bands and assist in extension of the interphalangeal joints of the fingers.

■ Extensor tendon rupture

Traumatic finger injuries can cause tendon ruptures that result in a variety of deformities. Rupture of the extensor tendon at the distal phalanx prohibits extension of the distal interphalangeal (DIP) joint. The unopposed action of the flexor digitorum profundus produces the characteristic "mallet finger" deformity in which the distal phalanx remains flexed.

14.6c The Palm of the Hand and Fingers

— The palm of the hand has the following surface anatomy (**Fig. 14.24**):
  - The skin is thickened, firmly attached to the underlying fascia, and supplied with numerous sweat glands.
  - A central concavity separates a **thenar eminence** at the base of the thumb from a **hypothenar eminence** at the base of the 5th digit.
  - Longitudinal and transverse **flexion creases** form where the skin is tightly bound to the palmar fascia.

— Deep fascia over the central palm forms a tough, thickened palmar aponeurosis (**Fig. 14.25**), which
  - firmly adheres to the skin of the palm,
  - is continuous proximally with the flexor retinaculum and palmaris longus muscle, and
  - is continuous distally with a **transverse metacarpal ligament** and the four digital fibrous sheaths of the fingers that surround the long flexor tendons and their synovial digital tendon sheaths.

Fig. 14.24 ► **Surface anatomy of the palm of the hand**
Left hand. DIP, distal interphalangeal; IP, interphalangeal; MCP, meta-carpophalangeal; PIP, proximal interphalangeal.

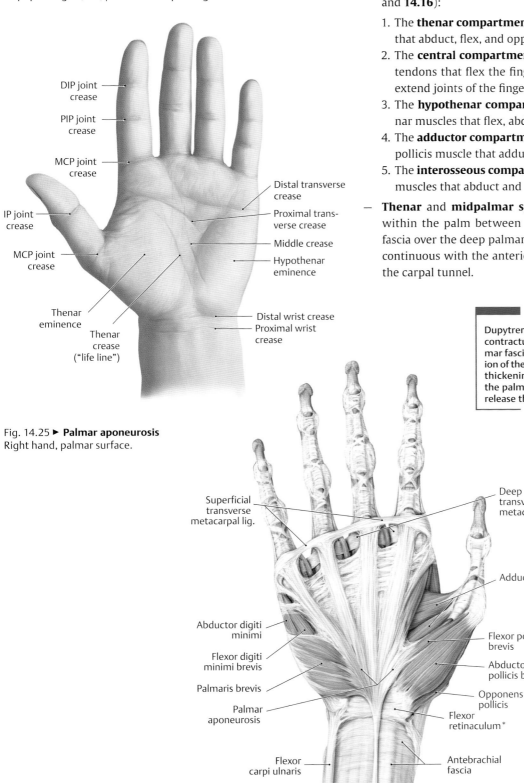

DIP joint crease
PIP joint crease
MCP joint crease
IP joint crease
MCP joint crease
Thenar eminence
Thenar crease ("life line")

Distal transverse crease
Proximal transverse crease
Middle crease
Hypothenar eminence
Distal wrist crease
Proximal wrist crease

— The palmar aponeurosis and deep palmar fascia divide the palm into five muscular compartments (**Tables 14.14, 14.15, and 14.16**):

1. The **thenar compartment**, which contains thenar muscles that abduct, flex, and oppose the thumb.
2. The **central compartment**, which contains forearm flexor tendons that flex the fingers and lumbricals that flex and extend joints of the fingers.
3. The **hypothenar compartment**, which contains hypothenar muscles that flex, abduct, and oppose the 5th digit.
4. The **adductor compartment**, which contains the adductor pollicis muscle that adducts the thumb.
5. The **interosseous compartment**, which contains interossei muscles that abduct and adduct the fingers.

— **Thenar** and **midpalmar spaces** are potential spaces deep within the palm between the long flexor tendons and the fascia over the deep palmar muscles. The midpalmar space is continuous with the anterior forearm compartment through the carpal tunnel.

Dupytren's disease

Dupytren's disease is the progressive fibrosis and contracture of the longitudinal bands of the palmar fascia to the 4th and 5th digits, causing flexion of these fingers. It presents as painless nodular thickenings that progress to raised ridges on the palm. Surgical excision is usually required to release the bands.

Fig. 14.25 ► **Palmar aponeurosis**
Right hand, palmar surface.

Superficial transverse metacarpal lig.
Deep transverse metacarpal lig.
Adductor pollicis
Abductor digiti minimi
Flexor digiti minimi brevis
Palmaris brevis
Palmar aponeurosis
Flexor pollicis brevis
Abductor pollicis brevis
Opponens pollicis
Flexor retinaculum*
Flexor carpi ulnaris
Antebrachial fascia
Palmaris longus tendon

* Also known as tranverse carpal ligament

— On the palmar surface of the fingers (see **Fig. 14.33A**),

- tendons of the flexor digitorum superficialis (FDS) split into two bands that insert on the middle phalanx,
- tendons of the flexor digitorum profundus pass between the bands of the FDS to insert on the distal phalanx, and
- **synovial tendon sheaths** surround the flexor tendons as they enter the **fibrous tendon sheaths** of the fingers (see **Fig. 14.32A**).
    - The digital synovial sheath of the 5th digit normally communicates with the common flexor sheath at the wrist.
    - The synovial sheath of the thumb extends into the wrist and may communicate with the sheath of the 5th digit and with the common synovial sheath.
    - The synovial sheaths of the 2nd, 3rd, and 4th digits usually remain independent from the common synovial sheath and other digital synovial sheaths.

— Muscles of the forearm and intrinsic muscles of the hand move the joints of the hand and fingers (see **Tables 14.12** and **14.13**).

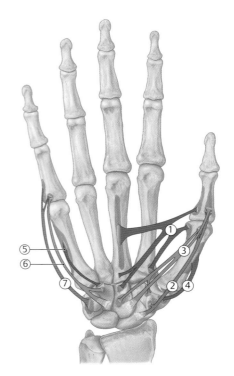

Thenar and hypothenar muscles, right hand, anterior (palmar) view.

Table 14.14 ▶ Thenar Muscles

Muscle	Origin	Insertion	Innervation	Action
① Adductor pollicis	Transverse head: 3rd metacarpal (palmar surface)	Thumb (base of proximal phalanx) via the ulnar sesamoid	Ulnar n. (C8–T1)	CMC joint of thumb: adduction MCP joint of thumb: flexion
	Oblique head: capitate bone, 2nd and 3rd metacarpals (bases)			
② Abductor pollicis brevis	Scaphoid bone and trapezium, flexor retinaculum	Thumb (base of proximal phalanx) via the radial sesamoid	Median n. (C8–T1)	CMC joint of thumb: abduction
③ Flexor pollicis brevis	Superficial head: flexor retinaculum		Superficial head: median n. (C8–T1)	CMC joint of thumb: flexion
	Deep head: capitate bone, trapezium		Deep head: ulnar n. (C8–T1)	
④ Opponens pollicis	Trapezium	1st metacarpal (radial border)	Median n. (C8–T1)	CMC joint of thumb: opposition

Abbreviations: CMC, carpometacarpal; MCP, metacarpophalangeal.

Table 14.15 ▶ Hypothenar Muscles

Muscle	Origin	Insertion	Innervation	Action
⑤ Opponens digiti minimi	Hook of hamate, flexor retinaculum	5th metacarpal (ulnar border)	Ulnar n. (C8–T1)	Draws metacarpal in palmar direction (opposition)
⑥ Flexor digiti minimi brevis		5th proximal phalanx (base)		MCP joint of little finger: flexion
⑦ Abductor digiti minimi	Pisiform bone	5th proximal phalanx (ulnar base) and dorsal digital expansion of 5th digit		MCP joint of little finger: flexion and abduction of little finger PIP and DIP joints of little finger: extension
Palmaris brevis	Palmar aponeurosis (ulnar border)	Skin of hypothenar eminence		Tightens the palmar aponeurosis (protective function)

Abbreviations: DIP, distal interphalangeal; MCP, metacarpophalangeal; PIP, proximal interphalangeal.

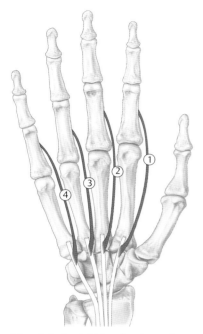

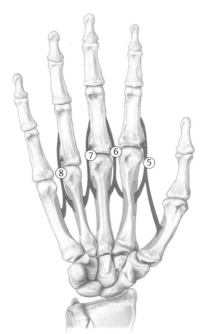

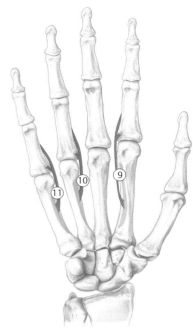

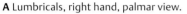

A Lumbricals, right hand, palmar view.

B Dorsal interossei, right hand, palmar view.

C Palmar interossei, right hand, palmar view.

Table 14.16 ▶ Metacarpal Muscles

Muscle Group	Muscle	Origin	Insertion	Innervation	Action
Lumbricals	① 1st	Tendons of flexor digitorum profundus (radial sides)	2nd digit (dde)	Median n. (C8–T1)	2nd to 5th digits: • MCP joints: flexion • Proximal and distal IP joints: extension
	② 2nd		3rd digit (dde)		
	③ 3rd	Tendons of flexor digitorum profundus (bipennate from medial and lateral sides)	4th digit (dde)		
	④ 4th		5th digit (dde)		
Dorsal interossei	⑤ 1st	1st and 2nd metacarpals (adjacent sides, two heads)	2nd digit (dde) 2nd proximal phalanx (radial side)	Ulnar n. (C8–T1)	2nd to 4th digits: • MCP joints: flexion • Proximal and distal IP joints: extension and abduction from 3rd digit
	⑥ 2nd	2nd and 3rd metacarpals (adjacent sides, two heads)	3rd digit (dde) 3rd proximal phalanx (radial side)		
	⑦ 3rd	3rd and 4th metacarpals (adjacent sides, two heads)	3rd digit (dde) 3rd proximal phalanx (ulnar side)		
	⑧ 4th	4th and 5th metacarpals (adjacent sides, two heads)	4th digit (dde) 4th proximal phalanx (ulnar side)		
Palmar interossei	⑨ 1st	2nd metacarpal (ulnar side)	2nd digit (dde) 2nd proximal phalanx (base)		2nd, 4th, and 5th digits: • MCP joints: flexion • Proximal and distal IP joints: extension and adduction toward 3rd digit
	⑩ 2nd	4th metacarpal (radial side)	4th digit (dde) 4th proximal phalanx (base)		
	⑪ 3rd	5th metacarpal (radial side)	5th digit (dde) 5th proximal phalanx (base)		

Abbreviations: dde, dorsal digital expansion; IP, interphalangeal; MCP, metacarpophalangeal.

Tenosynovitis

A puncture wound of the finger can initiate an infection in the digital synovial sheaths (tenosynovitis). Swelling of the tissue is painful and inhibits movement. Although synovial sheath connections vary, sheaths of the 2nd, 3rd, and 4th digits are usually independent and can confine the infection to that digit (unless the sheath ruptures).

The sheath of the 5th digit, however, normally communicates with the common synovial sheath in the palm and wrist. Infection can track via this route through the carpal tunnel and into the anterior compartment. Likewise, infection in the thumb can track into the wrist and palm.

14.7 Topographic Views of Upper Limb Musculature

14.7a Shoulder and Arm

Fig. 14.26 ▶ **Anterior shoulder muscles**
Right side, anterior view. Muscle origins are shown in red, insertions in gray.

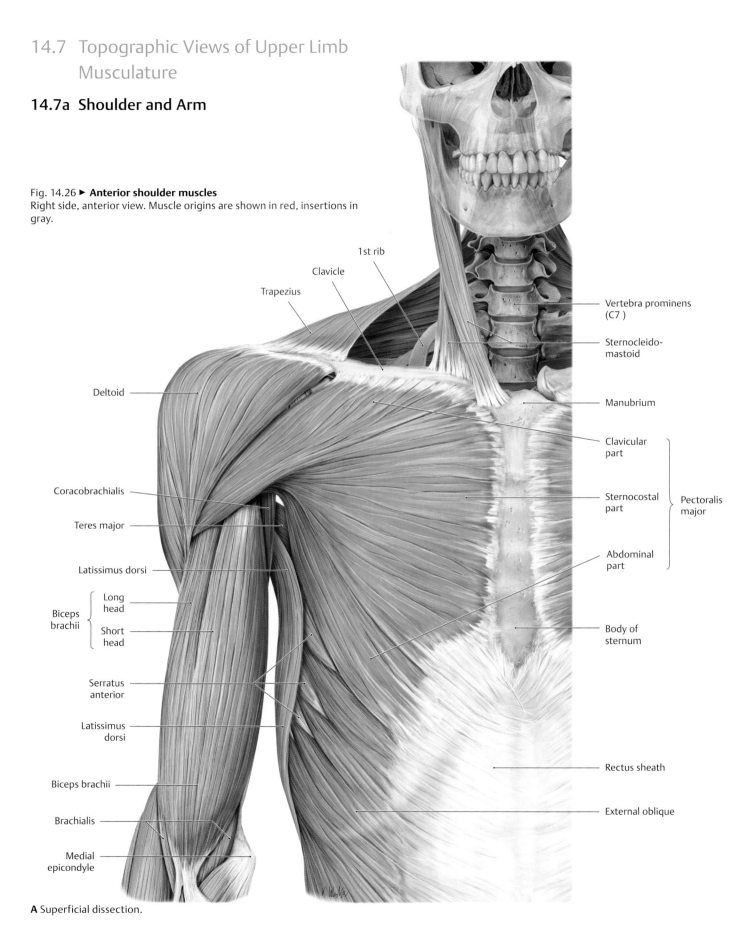

1st rib

Clavicle

Trapezius

Deltoid

Coracobrachialis

Teres major

Latissimus dorsi

Biceps brachii { Long head Short head }

Serratus anterior

Latissimus dorsi

Biceps brachii

Brachialis

Medial epicondyle

Vertebra prominens (C7)

Sternocleido-mastoid

Manubrium

Clavicular part

Sternocostal part } Pectoralis major

Abdominal part

Body of sternum

Rectus sheath

External oblique

A Superficial dissection.

Fig. 14.26 ▶ **Anterior shoulder muscles** (*continued*)

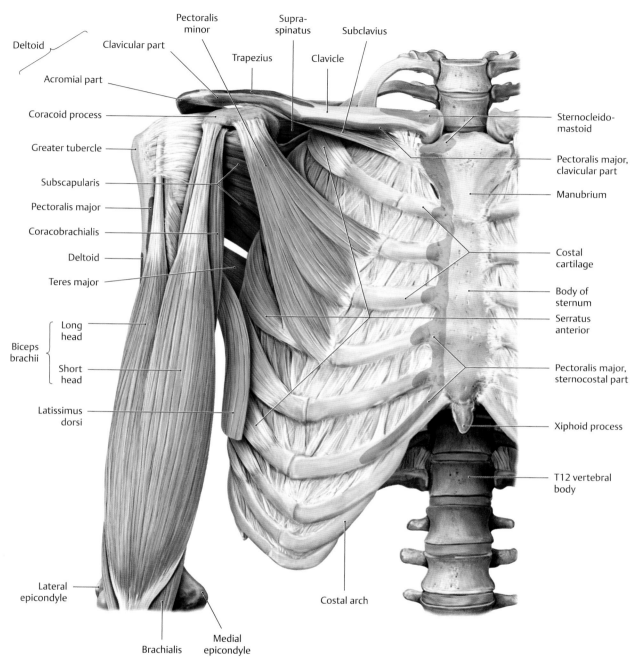

B Deep dissection. *Removed:* Sternocleidomastoid, trapezius, pectoralis major, deltoid, and external oblique muscles.

Fig. 14.27 ▶ **Anterior dissection of arm**
Right arm, anterior view. Muscle origins are shown in red, insertions in gray.

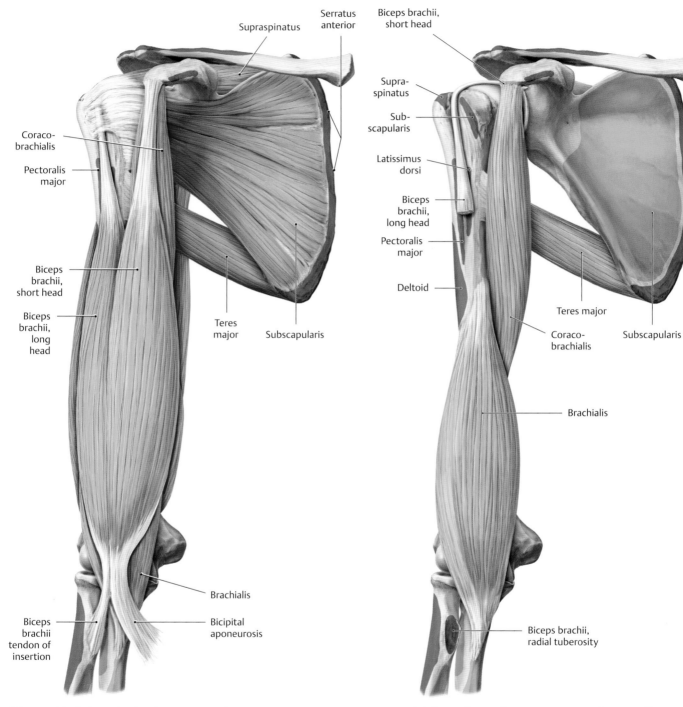

A *Removed:* Latissimus dorsi and serratus anterior.

B *Removed:* Subscapularis and supraspinatus muscles. *Partially removed:* Biceps brachii.

Fig. 14.28 ▶ **Posterior shoulder muscles**
Right side, posterior view.

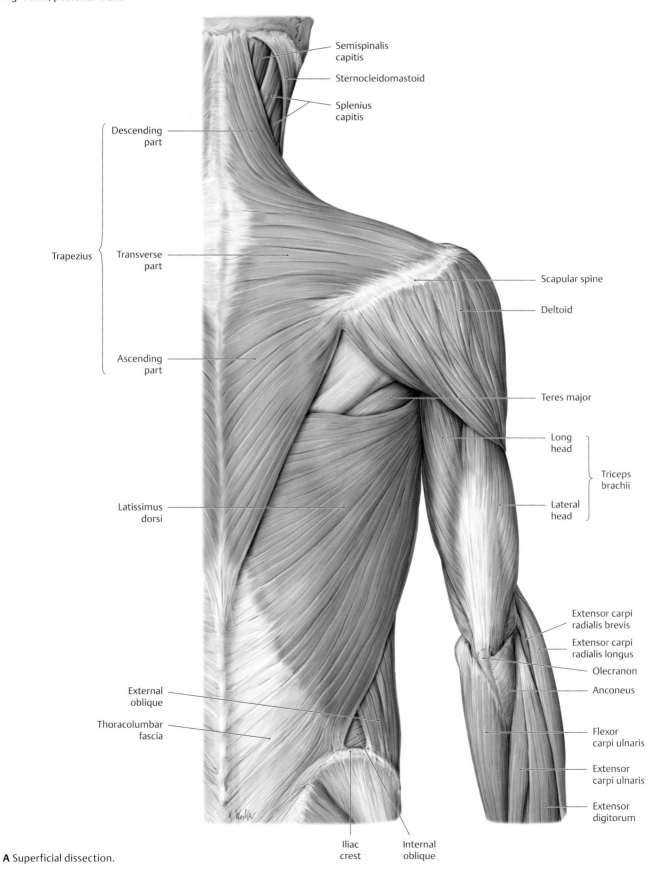

Semispinalis
capitis

Sternocleidomastoid

Splenius
capitis

Descending
part

Trapezius

Transverse
part

Scapular spine

Deltoid

Ascending
part

Teres major

Long
head

Triceps
brachii

Lateral
head

Latissimus
dorsi

Extensor carpi
radialis brevis

Extensor carpi
radialis longus

Olecranon

Anconeus

External
oblique

Thoracolumbar
fascia

Flexor
carpi ulnaris

Extensor
carpi ulnaris

Extensor
digitorum

Iliac
crest

Internal
oblique

A Superficial dissection.

Fig. 14.28 ▶ **Posterior shoulder muscles** (*continued*)
Right side, posterior view.

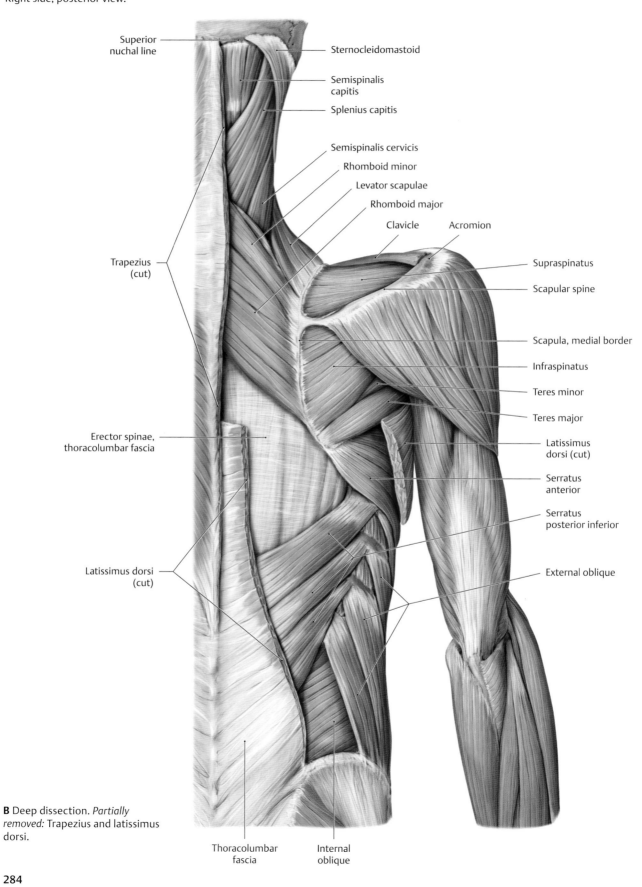

Superior
nuchal line

Sternocleidomastoid

Semispinalis
capitis

Splenius capitis

Semispinalis cervicis

Rhomboid minor

Levator scapulae

Rhomboid major

Clavicle   Acromion

Supraspinatus

Trapezius
(cut)

Scapular spine

Scapula, medial border

Infraspinatus

Teres minor

Teres major

Erector spinae,
thoracolumbar fascia

Latissimus
dorsi (cut)

Serratus
anterior

Serratus
posterior inferior

Latissimus dorsi
(cut)

External oblique

B Deep dissection. *Partially
removed:* Trapezius and latissimus
dorsi.

Thoracolumbar
fascia

Internal
oblique

284

Fig. 14.29 ▶ **Posterior dissection of arm**
Right arm, posterior view. Muscle origins are shown in red, insertions in gray. *Removed:* Deltoid and forearm muscles.

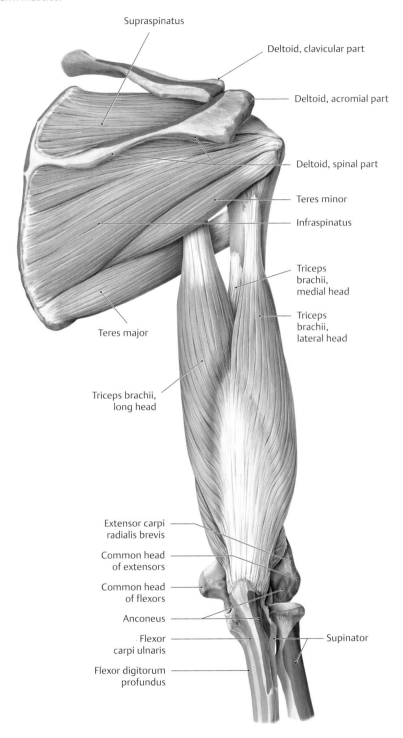

Supraspinatus

Deltoid, clavicular part

Deltoid, acromial part

Deltoid, spinal part

Teres minor

Infraspinatus

Triceps brachii, medial head

Triceps brachii, lateral head

Teres major

Triceps brachii, long head

Extensor carpi radialis brevis

Common head of extensors

Common head of flexors

Anconeus

Flexor carpi ulnaris

Supinator

Flexor digitorum profundus

14.7b Forearm and Wrist

Fig. 14.30 ▸ Anterior forearm muscles
Right forearm, anterior view. Muscle origins are shown in red, insertions in gray.

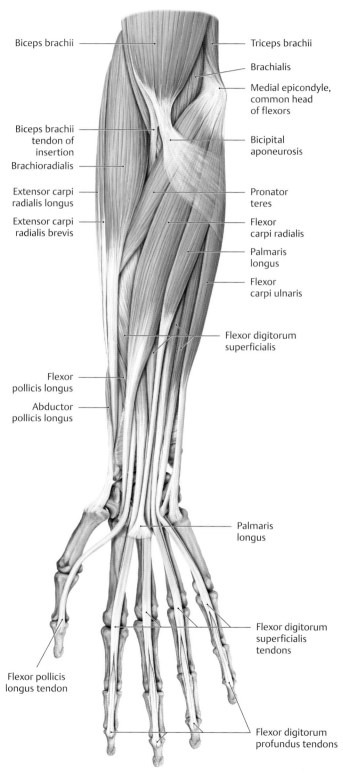

Biceps brachii

Biceps brachii tendon of insertion

Brachioradialis

Extensor carpi radialis longus

Extensor carpi radialis brevis

Flexor pollicis longus

Abductor pollicis longus

Flexor pollicis longus tendon

Triceps brachii

Brachialis

Medial epicondyle, common head of flexors

Bicipital aponeurosis

Pronator teres

Flexor carpi radialis

Palmaris longus

Flexor carpi ulnaris

Flexor digitorum superficialis

Palmaris longus

Flexor digitorum superficialis tendons

Flexor digitorum profundus tendons

A Superficial flexors and radialis group.

Fig. 14.30 ▶ Anterior forearm muscles (*continued*)
Right forearm, anterior view. Muscle origins are shown in red, insertions in gray.

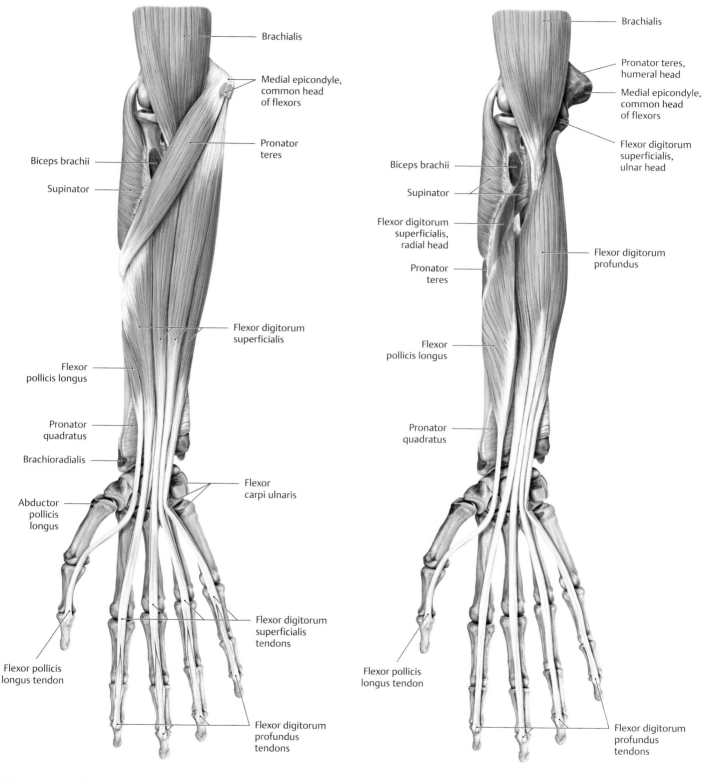

Brachialis

Medial epicondyle, common head of flexors

Pronator teres

Biceps brachii

Supinator

Flexor digitorum superficialis

Flexor pollicis longus

Pronator quadratus

Brachioradialis

Flexor carpi ulnaris

Abductor pollicis longus

Flexor digitorum superficialis tendons

Flexor pollicis longus tendon

Flexor digitorum profundus tendons

Brachialis

Pronator teres, humeral head

Medial epicondyle, common head of flexors

Flexor digitorum superficialis, ulnar head

Biceps brachii

Supinator

Flexor digitorum superficialis, radial head

Flexor digitorum profundus

Pronator teres

Flexor pollicis longus

Pronator quadratus

Flexor pollicis longus tendon

Flexor digitorum profundus tendons

B *Removed:* Radialis group (brachioradialis, extensor carpi radialis longus, and extensor carpi radialis brevis), flexor carpi radialis, flexor carpi ulnaris, abductor pollicis longus, palmaris longus, and biceps brachii.

C *Removed:* Pronator teres and flexor digitorum superficialis.

Fig. 14.31 ▶ **Posterior forearm muscles**
Right forearm, posterior view. Muscle origins are shown in red, insertions in gray.

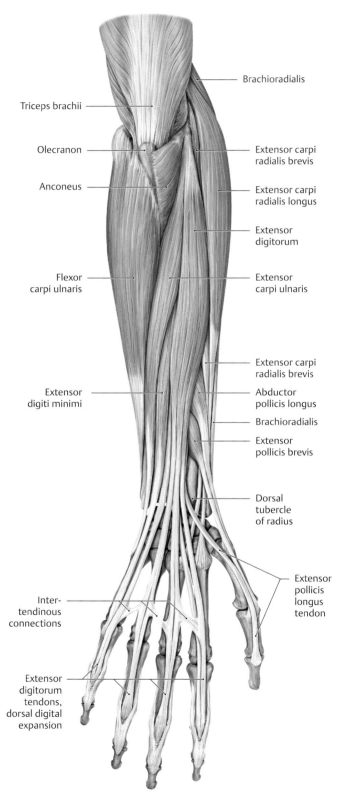

Brachioradialis

Triceps brachii

Olecranon

Anconeus

Extensor carpi radialis brevis

Extensor carpi radialis longus

Extensor digitorum

Flexor carpi ulnaris

Extensor carpi ulnaris

Extensor digiti minimi

Extensor carpi radialis brevis

Abductor pollicis longus

Brachioradialis

Extensor pollicis brevis

Dorsal tubercle of radius

Inter-tendinous connections

Extensor pollicis longus tendon

Extensor digitorum tendons, dorsal digital expansion

A Superficial extensors and radialis group.

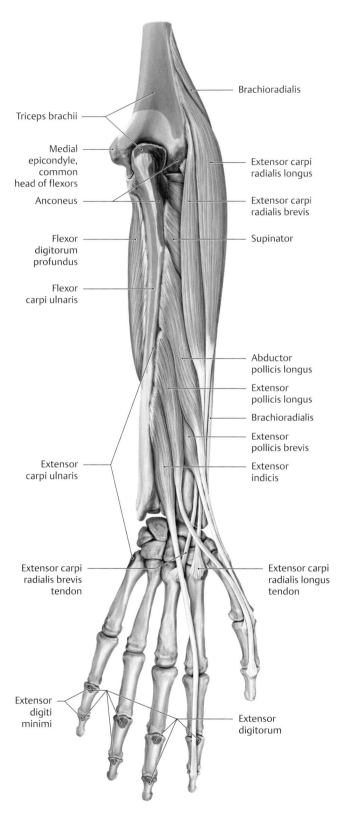

Brachioradialis

Triceps brachii

Medial epicondyle, common head of flexors

Anconeus

Extensor carpi radialis longus

Extensor carpi radialis brevis

Supinator

Flexor digitorum profundus

Flexor carpi ulnaris

Abductor pollicis longus

Extensor pollicis longus

Brachioradialis

Extensor pollicis brevis

Extensor indicis

Extensor carpi ulnaris

Extensor carpi radialis brevis tendon

Extensor carpi radialis longus tendon

Extensor digiti minimi

Extensor digitorum

B *Removed:* Triceps brachii, anconeus, flexor carpi ulnaris, extensor carpi ulnaris, and extensor digitorum.

14.7c Hand

Fig. 14.32 ▶ **Intrinsic muscles of the hand: Superficial and middle layers**
Right hand, palmar surface.

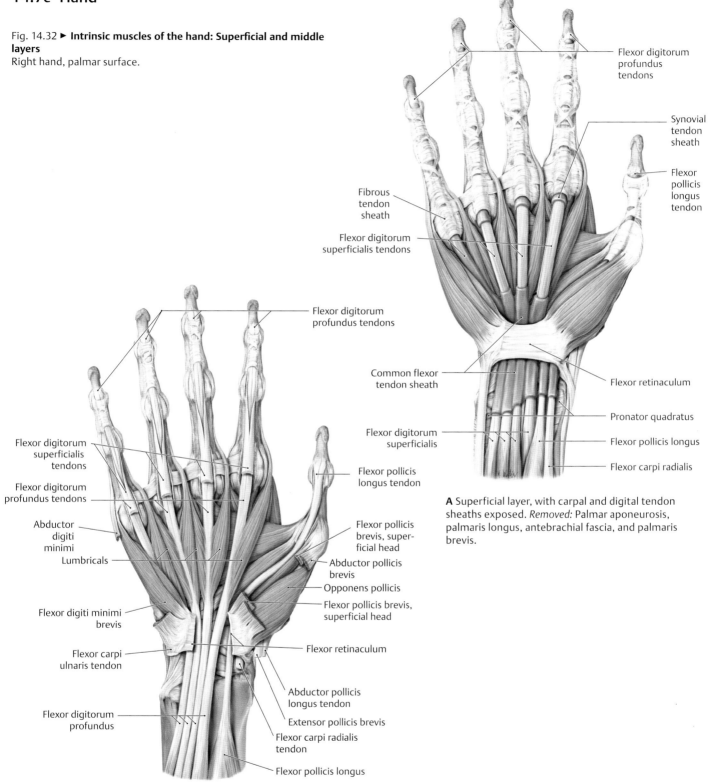

Flexor digitorum profundus tendons

Synovial tendon sheath

Flexor pollicis longus tendon

Fibrous tendon sheath

Flexor digitorum superficialis tendons

Common flexor tendon sheath

Flexor retinaculum

Pronator quadratus

Flexor digitorum superficialis

Flexor pollicis longus

Flexor carpi radialis

A Superficial layer, with carpal and digital tendon sheaths exposed. *Removed:* Palmar aponeurosis, palmaris longus, antebrachial fascia, and palmaris brevis.

Flexor digitorum profundus tendons

Flexor digitorum superficialis tendons

Flexor digitorum profundus tendons

Abductor digiti minimi

Lumbricals

Flexor digiti minimi brevis

Flexor carpi ulnaris tendon

Flexor digitorum profundus

Flexor pollicis longus tendon

Flexor pollicis brevis, superficial head

Abductor pollicis brevis

Opponens pollicis

Flexor pollicis brevis, superficial head

Flexor retinaculum

Abductor pollicis longus tendon

Extensor pollicis brevis

Flexor carpi radialis tendon

Flexor pollicis longus

B Middle layer. *Removed:* Flexor digitorum superficialis, flexors carpi radialis and ulnaris, and pronator quadratus.

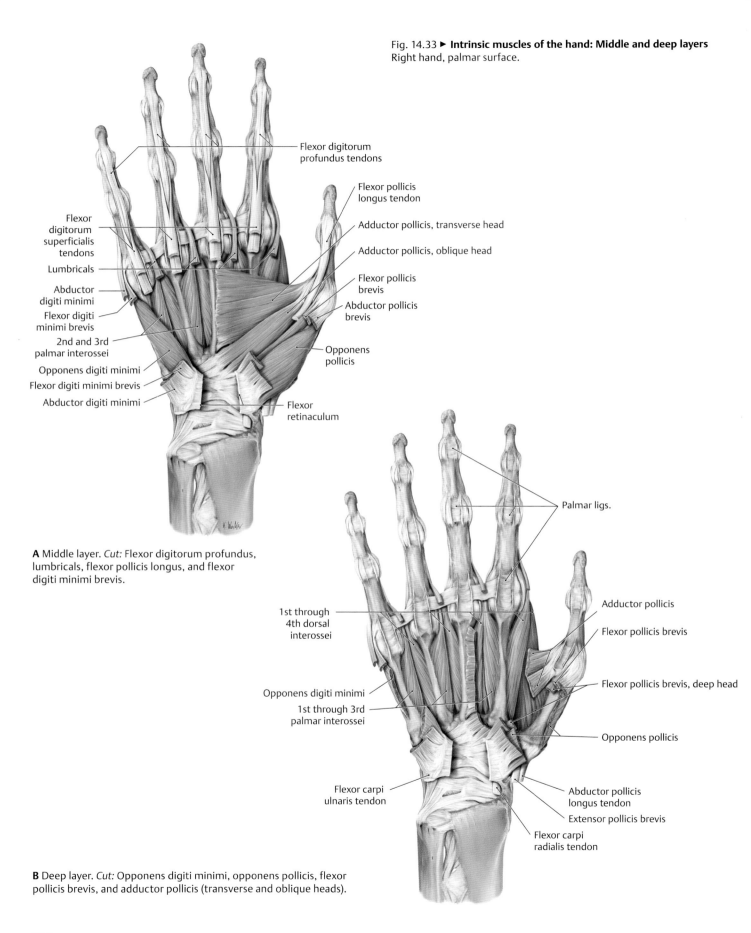

Fig. 14.33 ▶ Intrinsic muscles of the hand: Middle and deep layers
Right hand, palmar surface.

Flexor digitorum profundus tendons

Flexor pollicis longus tendon

Adductor pollicis, transverse head

Adductor pollicis, oblique head

Flexor pollicis brevis

Abductor pollicis brevis

Opponens pollicis

Flexor digitorum superficialis tendons

Lumbricals

Abductor digiti minimi

Flexor digiti minimi brevis

2nd and 3rd palmar interossei

Opponens digiti minimi

Flexor digiti minimi brevis

Abductor digiti minimi

Flexor retinaculum

A Middle layer. *Cut:* Flexor digitorum profundus, lumbricals, flexor pollicis longus, and flexor digiti minimi brevis.

Palmar ligs.

Adductor pollicis

Flexor pollicis brevis

Flexor pollicis brevis, deep head

Opponens pollicis

Abductor pollicis longus tendon

Extensor pollicis brevis

1st through 4th dorsal interossei

Opponens digiti minimi

1st through 3rd palmar interossei

Flexor carpi ulnaris tendon

Flexor carpi radialis tendon

B Deep layer. *Cut:* Opponens digiti minimi, opponens pollicis, flexor pollicis brevis, and adductor pollicis (transverse and oblique heads).

14.7d Compartments in Arm and Forearm

Fig. 14.34 ▶ **Windowed dissection**
Right limb, anterior view.

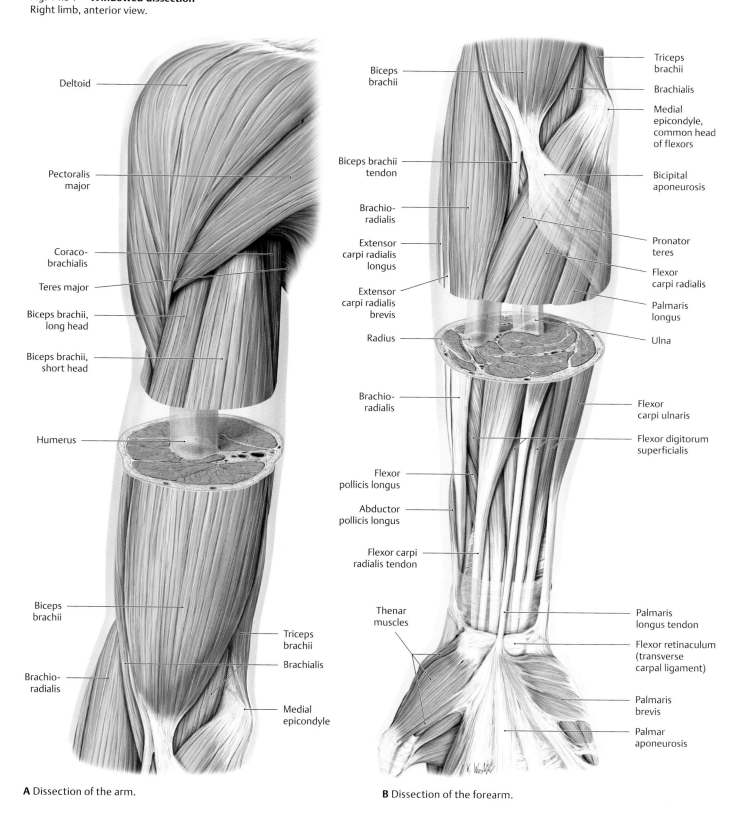

A Dissection of the arm.

B Dissection of the forearm.

Fig. 14.35 ▶ **Transverse sections**
Right limb, proximal (superior) view.
The anterior compartment is outlined in pink and the posterior compartment in green.

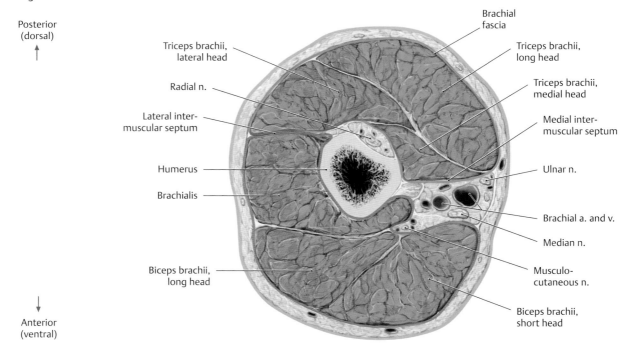

A Arm (plane of section in **Fig. 14.34A**).

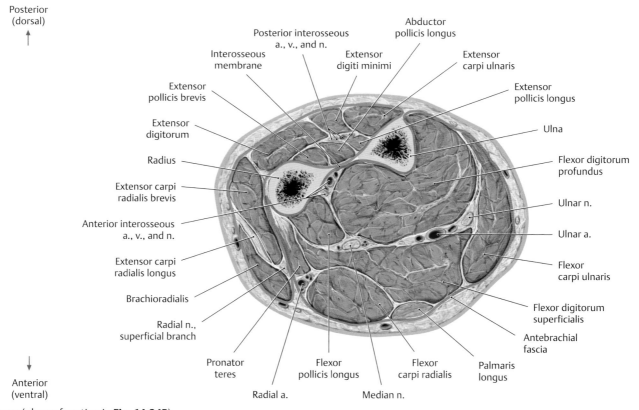

B Forearm (plane of section in **Fig. 14.34B**).

Review Questions: Upper Limb

1. A patient complains of tingling and pain in the upper arm. Upon further examination and additional tests, you determine that the axillary artery has been occluded by atherosclerosis. The patient, however, still has a radial pulse at the wrist. Which of the following arteries could provide a collateral circulation around the occlusion?
   A. Suprascapular and circumflex scapular arteries
   B. Suprascapular and lateral thoracic arteries
   C. Posterior circumflex humeral and anterior circumflex humeral arteries
   D. Superior thoracic and lateral thoracic arteries
   E. Posterior intercostals and lateral thoracic arteries

2. The deep palmar arch of the hand is formed mainly by the
   A. ulnar artery
   B. radial artery
   C. brachial artery
   D. palmar digital arteries
   E. palmar metacarpal arteries

3. Each cord of the brachial plexus
   A. contains nerve fibers from C5 to T1 levels of the spinal cord
   B. is formed from the junction of one anterior and one posterior division
   C. gives a branch to the median nerve
   D. lies within the axilla
   E. gives rise to a subscapular nerve (upper, middle, and lower)

4. Nerves often pair with arteries to travel as neurovascular bundles. Which of the following is *not* an accurate pairing?
   A. Axillary nerve and posterior circumflex humeral artery
   B. Median nerve and brachial artery
   C. Musculocutaneous nerve and circumflex scapular artery
   D. Radial nerve and deep brachial artery
   E. Long thoracic nerve and lateral thoracic artery

5. During a radical mastectomy on a 50-year-old woman, the surgeon does a careful but thorough axillary node dissection. What nerve lies along the medial wall of the axilla and is particularly vulnerable during this procedure?
   A. Lateral branch of posterior intercostal
   B. Musculocutaneous
   C. Lateral pectoral
   D. Long thoracic
   E. Dorsal scapular

6. One of your patients ruptured the tendon of the long head of the biceps brachii. Although he is bothered by the unattractive bulge that formed in his anterior arm, he is surprised to find that he has lost little flexor strength. You confirm that the brachialis muscle has greater leverage at the joint and therefore is the more powerful flexor of the elbow. Where does the brachialis insert?
   A. Radial tuberosity
   B. Ulnar tuberosity
   C. Coronoid process
   D. Bicipital aponeurosis
   E. Olecranon

7. Which part(s) of the triceps brachii crosses/cross the glenohumeral joint?
   A. Medial head
   B. Lateral head
   C. Long head
   D. Lateral and medial heads
   E. Lateral and long heads

8. Structures that pass through the quadrangular space of the upper limb include the
   A. radial nerve
   B. suprascapular nerve
   C. posterior humeral circumflex artery
   D. anterior humeral circumflex artery
   E. deep brachial artery

9. Which of the following bones articulates with the radius at the wrist?
   A. Pisiform
   B. Hamate
   C. Capitate
   D. Trapezium
   E. Scaphoid

10. The flexor retinaculum
    A. forms the floor of the ulnar tunnel
    B. forms the roof of the carpal tunnel
    C. is continuous with the palmar aponeurosis
    D. is continuous with the palmaris longus
    E. All the above

11. As a second-year resident doing a pediatric surgery rotation, you set up an arterial line on your 6-year-old patient prior to surgery. You choose the radial artery of her left (nondominant) hand. Because you know that the procedure can result in occlusion of the artery, you verify that the collateral circulation to the hand is patent. The radial artery
    A. forms the superficial arch of the hand
    B. passes superficial to the anatomic snuffbox
    C. supplies the muscles of the posterior compartment through its posterior interosseous branch
    D. supplies the princeps pollicis artery of the thumb
    E. lies medial to the tendon of the flexor carpi radialis in the wrist

12. During your first training session as a phlebotomist, you are relieved to find that your "patient" is a 24-year-old weight lifter whose superficial veins stand out dramatically against his overdeveloped muscles. Superficial veins of the upper limb
    A. include a basilic vein that runs in the deltopectoral groove
    B. include a cephalic vein that joins the brachial veins in the arm
    C. drain into the veins of the deep venous system via perforating veins
    D. course with the arteries as paired accompanying veins
    E. have bidirectional valves that allow flow in either direction.

13. An injury to the lower brachial plexus (Klumpke's palsy) would affect
    A. sensation in the nail bed of the 5th digit
    B. abduction of the 2nd through 5th digits
    C. adduction of the thumb
    D. adduction of the wrist
    E. All of the above

14. While moonlighting in the emergency department one night, you treat a 14-year-old gang member who was stabbed in the supraclavicular region of the neck 2 cm above the middle third of the clavicle. A chest X-ray confirms that he has a pneumothorax. What other structure could be injured in this area?
    A. Axillary nerve
    B. Pectoralis minor
    C. Subscapular artery
    D. Posterior cord of the brachial plexus
    E. Cephalic vein

15. The serratus anterior muscle
    A. forms a scapulothoracic joint with the external intercostal muscles
    B. is innervated by a branch of the posterior cord
    C. elevates the scapula off the thoracic wall
    D. rotates the scapula laterally during abduction of the arm above the horizontal plane
    E. originates from the subscapular fossa

16. A professional rodeo cowboy fell off his horse and fractured his humerus at the anatomic neck and the lesser tubercle. Which of the following muscles inserts on this tubercle?
    A. Supraspinatus
    B. Infraspinatus
    C. Subscapularis
    D. Coracobrachialis
    E. Teres major

17. Damage to which nerve would most affect elbow flexion?
    A. Radial nerve
    B. Ulnar nerve
    C. Median nerve
    D. Musculocutaneous nerve
    E. Axillary nerve

18. At a neighborhood block party several children engage in a tug-of-war. Suddenly, Jason, a 5-year-old boy, hugs his right elbow and cries out in pain. The inconsolable child is eventually taken to the local clinic, where the pediatrician recognizes that Jason has subluxed (partially dislocated) his radial head. By gently supinating the flexed arm, the doctor restores it to its normal position. Which of the following is true regarding the proximal radioulnar joint?
    A. The radial head rotates within the annular ligament.
    B. It includes a hinge-type joint between the head of the radius and capitellum of the humerus.
    C. The biceps brachii pronates the joint.
    D. An articular disk separates the radius and ulna.
    E. The subluxation of the radial head results from a tear of the radial collateral ligament.

19. On your first day of shadowing in your preceptor's office, you are asked to get some baseline information on each patient. You start by taking their pulse. The radial artery is easiest to palpate in the wrist where it lies immediately lateral to the tendon of the
    A. flexor carpi radialis
    B. flexor digitorum
    C. flexor pollicis longus
    D. palmaris longus
    E. extensor carpi radialis

20. You examine a 14-year-old girl in the emergency department. She has a puncture wound from a dog bite in the flesh over the middle phalange of her 5th digit. The incident occurred 2 days ago, and the finger is inflamed and likely infected. What are your thoughts regarding possible spread of the infection via the synovial sheath?
    A. It will spread into the superficial space on the dorsum of the hand.
    B. It will spread to the common flexor sheath in the wrist.
    C. It will spread to the adjacent finger.
    D. It will remain confined to the sheath of the infected finger.
    E. A and B are correct.

21. The axillary artery
    A. begins at the lateral border of the 1st rib
    B. lies anterior to the axillary vein
    C. ends by dividing into brachial and deep brachial arteries
    D. passes through the axilla between the pectoralis major and pectoralis minor muscles
    E. branches include the thyrocervical trunk

22. Axillary lymph nodes that lie medial to the pectoralis minor include
    A. pectoral nodes
    B. humeral nodes
    C. apical nodes
    D. central nodes
    E. subscapular nodes

23. The C4 anterior ramus is a component of
    A. the pre-fixed plexus
    B. the upper trunk
    C. the posterior cord
    D. the axillary nerve
    E. All the above

24. A young man suffered a crushing injury to his right arm, fracturing his humerus at midshaft and damaging the nerve that runs in the posterior compartment. What functional loss would you expect from this injury?
    A. Inability to extend the elbow
    B. Inability to supinate the hand
    C. Inability to abduct the thumb
    D. Inability to extend the wrist
    E. All of the above

25. One of your orthopedic colleagues introduces you, an anatomist, to his patient, a famous baseball pitcher, who suffers from chronic rotator cuff pain. He asks you to demonstrate the rotator cuff on a cadaver specimen and explain the anatomy of this type of injury. You tell him the following:
    A. Tendons of the rotator cuff muscles insert onto the capsule of the glenohumeral joint.
    B. The supraspinatus tendon passes through the subacromial space between the shoulder joint and the coracoacromial arch.
    C. An abnormal communication between the subacromial bursa and glenohumeral joint cavity can result from rupture of the supraspinatus tendon.
    D. Rupture of the supraspinatus tendon will impair the patient's ability to initiate abduction of the arm.
    E. All the above

26. Which of the following muscles has no attachment on the humerus?
    A. Deltoid
    B. Coracobrachialis
    C. Flexor digitorum superficialis
    D. Pronator teres
    E. Biceps brachii

27. Which muscle provides strong adduction of the glenohumeral joint?
    A. Teres minor
    B. Pectoralis major
    C. Pectoralis minor
    D. Short head of the biceps brachii
    E. Subscapularis

28. A young woman riding a 10-speed bicycle accidentally engaged the front brake, was thrown over the handlebars, and landed on her outstretched hands. In the emergency department, imaging of the elbow revealed a subtle fracture of the radial neck that allowed proximal movement of the radius relative to the ulna, which also suggested a tear in the interosseous membrane. Which movements were most impaired by this injury?
    A. Flexion of the wrist
    B. Extension of the elbow
    C. Extension of the digits
    D. Abduction of the thumb
    E. Adduction of the thumb

29. An elderly man had injured his wrist in a fall and is now experiencing tingling in his fingers and a weakened grip. A lateral X-ray of the wrist shows that his lunate has dislocated and is pressing on the structures within the carpal tunnel. Which of the following structures pass through the carpal tunnel?
    A. Ulnar artery
    B. Radial artery
    C. Flexor carpi radialis
    D. Flexor pollicis longus
    E. Palmaris longus

30. In the anatomy lab you are fascinated by the deep dissection of the hand because as a professional violinist you appreciate that the intrinsic muscles of the palm are important for the fine movements of the hand. Which of the following is true for both the lumbricals and the interossei muscles?
    A. All are innervated by the median nerve.
    B. All are innervated by the ulnar nerve.
    C. They flex the metacarpophalangeal joints.
    D. They arise from the tendons of the flexor digitorum profundus.
    E. They abduct or adduct the fingers.

Answers and Explanations

1. **A** The suprascapular and transverse cervical branches of the subclavian artery and the thoracodorsal and circumflex scapular branches of the distal segment of the axillary artery participate in a scapular arcade that provides a collateral circulation that would circumvent the occlusion (Section 13.4a).
B The lateral thoracic artery does not supply the scapula, nor does it anastomose with the suprascapular artery.
C The anterior and posterior humeral circumflex arteries anastomose around the neck of the humerus but do not anastomose with arteries proximal to the occlusion.
D Neither the superior thoracic artery nor the lateral thoracic artery supplies the scapular region.
E Posterior intercostal arteries supply the medial scapular region, but they do not anastomose with the lateral thoracic artery.

2. **B** The deep palmar arch is formed mainly by the radial artery (Section 13.4a).
A The ulnar artery forms the superficial palmar arch.
C The brachial artery begins at the lateral border of the axilla and terminates in the cubital fossa.
D The palmar digital arteries are branches of the superficial and deep palmar arches in the palm of the hand.
E The palmar metacarpal arteries arise from the superficial and deep palmar arches in the palm of the hand.

3. **D** Each cord of the brachial plexus lies within the axilla (Section 13.4d).
A The posterior cord contains fibers from C5 to T1; the medial cord contains fibers from C8 and T1; the lateral cord contains fibers from C5 to C7.
B The posterior divisions form the posterior cord; only anterior divisions form the medial and the lateral cords.
C The median nerve is formed from the medial and lateral cords.
E The subscapular nerves arise from the posterior cord.

4. **C** The musculocutaneous nerve passes from the axilla to pierce the coracobrachialis of the anterior arm. The circumflex scapular artery passes through the triangular space into the scapular region (Section 14.2d).
A The axillary artery and posterior circumflex humeral artery pass through the quadrangular space to the deltoid region.
B The median nerve and brachial artery descend on the medial side of the biceps brachii and enter the cubital fossa.
D The radial nerve and deep brachial artery wind around the posterior humerus through the triceps hiatus.
E The long thoracic nerve and lateral thoracic artery descend on the medial wall of the axilla to supply the serratus anterior muscle.

5. **D** The long thoracic nerve runs superficial to, and innervates, the serratus anterior, which forms the medial wall of the axilla. Injury to this nerve can result in a "winged" scapula (Section 14.1a).
A In the axilla the intercostal nerves run deep to the serratus anterior and external intercostal muscles and are not vulnerable to injury.
B The musculocutaneous nerve leaves the axilla just inferior to the glenohumeral joint where it enters the coracobrachialis muscle.
C The lateral pectoral nerve passes anteriorly to penetrate the pectoralis major muscle.
E The dorsal scapular nerve descends posteriorly from the upper roots of the plexus to innervate the levator scapulae and rhomboid muscles.

6. **B** The brachialis muscle inserts on the ulnar tuberosity of the ulna (Section 14.3a).
A The biceps brachii inserts on the radial tuberosity.
C The coronoid process forms the anterior lip of the trochlear notch of the ulna and is the origin of the ulnar head of the pronator teres.
D The bicipital aponeurosis is a fascial extension of the biceps brachii.
E The olecranon of the ulna forms the posterior prominence of the elbow and is the insertion for the triceps brachii and anconeus muscles.

7. **C** The long head of the triceps brachii crosses the glenohumeral joint to attach to the infraglenoid tubercle, where it contributes to extension of the joint (Section 14.2c).
A The medial head arises from the medial aspect of the humeral shaft. It joins with the lateral and long heads to insert on the olecranon of the ulna.
B The lateral head arises from the lateral aspect of the humeral shaft. It joins with the medial and long heads to insert on the olecranon of the ulna.
D The medial and lateral heads arise from the humeral shaft and cross only the elbow joint.
E The lateral head arises from the shaft of the humerus and crosses the elbow joint. The long head originates on the infraglenoid tubercle of the scapula and crosses the glenohumeral and elbow joints.

8. **C** The posterior humeral circumflex artery and the axillary nerve pass through the quadrangular space (Section 14.2d).
A The radial nerve passes through the triceps hiatus.
B The suprascapular nerve passes through the scapular notch.
D The anterior humeral circumflex artery runs horizontally beneath the coracobrachialis and the short head of the biceps brachii to encircle the neck of the humerus.
E The deep brachial artery passes through the triceps hiatus with the radial nerve.

9. **E** The radius articulates distally with the scaphoid and lunate bones of the wrist (Section 14.5a).
A The pisiform on the medial side of the wrist articulates with the triquetrum.
B The hamate articulates with the capitate, lunate, triquetrum, and 4th and 5th metacarpal bones.
C The capitate articulates with the hamate, trapezoid, scaphoid, lunate, and 3rd metacarpal.
D The trapezium articulates with the trapezoid, scaphoid, and 1st metacarpal.

10. **E** The flexor retinaculum forms the roof of the carpal tunnel and floor of the ulnar tunnel. As a thickening of the deep fascia of the palm, it is continuous with the palmar aponeurosis, palmaris longus, transverse metacarpal ligament, and fibrous digital sheaths (Sections 14.5b and 14.6c).
A The flexor retinaculum forms the floor of the ulnar tunnel; the palmar carpal ligament form its roof. B through D are also correct (E).
B The carpal tunnel is a fascio-osseous tunnel. Carpal bones form the floor and sides; the flexor retinaculum forms the roof. A, C, and D are also correct (E).
C The flexor retinaculum is continuous with the tough palmar aponeurosis of the hand. A, B, and D are also correct (E).
D The palmaris longus passes over the carpal tunnel and inserts on the flexor retinaculum and palmar aponeurosis. A through C are also correct (E).

11. **D** The princeps pollicis arises from the radial artery at the base of the 1st metacarpal and divides into two digital arteries of the thumb (Section 13.4a).
A The ulnar artery forms the superficial palmar arch. The radial artery forms the deep palmar arch.
B The radial artery courses along the floor of the anatomic snuffbox.
C The posterior interosseous artery, which supplies muscles of the posterior forearm compartment, arises from the common interosseous artery, a branch of the ulnar artery in the cubital fossa.
E The radial artery lies lateral to the tendon of the flexor carpi radialis at the wrist.

12. **C** The veins of the superficial venous system drain into the deep veins via perforating veins (Section 13.4b).
A The cephalic vein courses along the deltopectoral groove before terminating in the axillary vein.
B The basilic vein joins with the paired brachial veins to form the axillary vein.
D Veins of the deep venous system travel with the arteries as paired accompanying veins. There is no superficial arterial system that accompanies the superficial veins.
E Veins of the limbs have unidirectional valves that prevent pooling of blood and facilitate flow back toward the heart.

13. **E** The ulnar nerve arises from the lower part of the plexus. Its dorsal cutaneous branch in the hand supplies the palmar and dorsal surfaces of the 4th (half) and 5th digits, and its deep branch supplies the dorsal interossei muscles that abduct the fingers and the adductor pollicis that adducts the thumb. It also innervates the flexor carpi ulnaris that assists in adduction of the wrist (Section 13.4d).
A The ulnar nerve's (C8–T1) dorsal cutaneous branch in the hand supplies the palmar and dorsal surfaces of the 4th (half) and 5th digits. B through D are also correct (E).
B The ulnar nerve's (C8–T1) deep branch in the hand supplies the dorsal interossei muscles that abduct the fingers. A, C, and D are also correct (E).
C The ulnar nerve's (C8–T1) deep branch in the hand supplies the adductor pollicis muscle that adducts the thumb. A, B, and D are also correct (E).
D The ulnar nerve (C8–T1) innervates the flexor carpi ulnaris that assists the extensor carpi ulnaris (radial nerve) in adduction of the wrist. A through C are also correct (E).

14. **D** The posterior cord is part of the supraclavicular brachial plexus and could be injured in the area (Section 13.4d).
A The terminal nerves of the brachial plexus form below the clavicle. Although damage to the supraclavicular plexus could affect the axillary nerve, the stab wound would not directly damage the nerve itself.
B The pectoralis minor attaches to the coracoid process, which lies below the middle part of the clavicle.
C The subscapular artery is a branch of the distal part of the axillary artery, which is infraclavicular.
E The cephalic vein drains into the axillary vein below the clavicle and most likely would not be affected by this injury.

15. **D** The serratus anterior pulls the inferior angle of the scapula laterally when the glenohumeral joint is abducted above the horizontal plane (Sections 14.1a and 14.1b).
A The scapulothoracic joint is a functional relationship between the serratus anterior and subscapularis muscles.
B The long thoracic nerve, which innervates the serratus anterior muscle, arises directly from the C5–C7 roots of the brachial plexus.
C The serratus anterior supports the scapula against the thoracic wall. Denervation of the muscle allows the scapula to lift away from the thoracic wall, a condition known as a "winged" scapula.
E The serratus anterior originates from the entire medial border of the scapula.

16. **C** The subscapularis inserts on the lesser tubercle of the humerus and fibrous capsule of the glenohumeral joint (Section 14.2c).
A The supraspinatus inserts on the greater tubercle of the humerus.
B The infraspinatus inserts on the greater tubercle of the humerus.
D The coracobrachialis inserts on the shaft of the middle part of the humerus.
E The teres major inserts on the crest that extends inferiorly from the lesser tuberosity.

17. **D** The musculocutaneous nerve innervates the biceps brachii and brachialis muscles, the primary flexors of the elbow. There would also be loss of sensation to the skin of the lateral forearm (Sections 14.2c and 14.3a).
A Damage to the radial nerve results in wrist drop and loss of sensation to the dorsum of the hand and the proximal segments of the 1st through 3rd digits and half of the 4th digit.
B Damage to the ulnar nerve may cause paresthesia (numbness and tingling) in the forearm, 4th and 5th fingers, or paralysis of the intrinsic muscles of the hand (so-called claw hand deformity).
C Damage to the median nerve above the cubital fossa will cause the inability to flex the proximal interphalangeal joint of the 1st to 3rd digits and the inability to flex the distal interphalangeal joints of the 2nd and 3rd digits. This results in "benediction hand" (2nd and 3rd finger are partially extended) when trying to form a fist. It also causes the inability to flex the terminal phalanx of the thumb (due to damage of flexor pollicis longus) and loss of sensation over the lateral aspect of the hand.
E Damage to the axillary nerve causes paralysis of the deltoid muscle resulting in weakened flexion and extension of the shoulder and the inability to abduct the arm above the horizontal.

18. **A** The annular ligament forms a circular cuff around the radial head that allows the bone to rotate in the joint (Section 14.4a).
B The hinge-type joint between the radius and capitullum of the humerus is the humeroradial joint.
C The biceps brachii inserts on the tuberosity of the radius and therefore supinates the joint when contracted.
D In the proximal radioulnar joint the radius articulates at the radial notch of the ulna. An articular disk separates the radius and ulna in the distal radioulnar joint.
E Subluxation of the radial head results from a laxity of the annular ligament.

19. **A** The radial artery descends on the lateral side of the forearm and at the wrist lies immediately lateral to the tendon of the flexor carpi radialis (Section 14.5b).
B The tendons of the flexor digitorum lie in the middle of the wrist, medial to the radial artery.
C The tendon of the flexor pollicis longus lies lateral to the median nerve and medial to the tendon of the flexor carpi radialis and to the radial artery.
D The palmaris longus runs superficial to the flexor retinaculum and medial to the flexor pollicis longus.
E The radial artery lies medial (palmar) to the extensor carpi radialis tendon.

20. **B** The synovial sheath of the 5th digit normally communicates with the common synovial sheath (Section 14.6c).
A The synovial sheath of the 5th digit communicates with the common synovial sheath and with that of the thumb, but it does not normally communicate with the superficial space on the dorsum of the hand.
C The synovial sheaths of the 2nd, 3rd, and 4th digits do not normally communicate with any other tendon sheaths. It is unlikely the infection will spread to these fingers.
D Although the infection may remain confined to the infected finger, the synovial sheath of the 5th digit communicates with that of the thumb and with the common tendon sheath. Therefore, the concern is that it will spread via this route to the thumb, wrist, and forearm.
E The synovial sheath of the 5th digit normally communicates with the common flexor sheath at the wrist but not with the superficial space on the dorsum of the hand.

21. **A** The subclavian artery continues as the axillary artery at the lateral border of the 1st rib (Section 13.4a).
B The axillary artery lies posterior to the axillary vein.
C The brachial artery is a continuation of the axillary artery in the axilla. The deep brachial artery is one of the branches of the brachial artery.
D The axillary artery passes through the axilla posterior to the pectoralis minor muscle.
E The thyrocervical trunk is a branch of the subclavian artery.

22. **C** The apical nodes are the nodes of the upper infraclavicular group. These lie medial to the pectoralis minor muscle along the axillary vein and adjacent to the proximal part of the axillary artery (Section 13.4c).
A Pectoral nodes are part of the lower axillary group that lies lateral to the pectoralis minor.
B Interpectoral nodes are part of the middle axillary group that lies between the pectoralis major and pectoralis minor muscles.
D Central nodes are part of the lower axillary group that lies lateral to the pectoralis minor.
E The subscapular nodes are part of the lower axillary group that lies lateral to the pectoralis minor.

23. **A** The brachial plexus contains the anterior rami of C5 to T1. A prefixed plexus also contains the C4 anterior ramus (Section 13.4d).
B The upper trunk contains C5 and C6 anterior rami.
C The posterior cord contains the anterior rami of C5 to T1.
D The axillary nerve contains the anterior rami of C5 and C6.
E B, C, and D are incorrect.

24. **D** Damage to the radial nerve from a midhumeral fracture results in loss of innervation to the extensor carpi radialis and extensor carpi ulnaris (Sections 13.4d and 14.4b).
A The branches of the radial nerve to the triceps brachii arise high in the arm, so a midhumeral lesion of the nerve would not affect the function of this muscle.
B The radial nerve innervates only one of the muscles that supinate the hand, the supinator. The biceps brachii, also a supinator, is innervated by the musculocutaneous nerve.
C Abduction of the thumb is weakened by damage to the radial nerve.
E A, B, and C are incorrect.

25. **E** All of the rotator cuff muscles insert on the fibrous capsule of the glenohumeral joint. The supraspinatus muscle, the most frequently involved in rotator cuff tears, passes through the narrow subacromial space and, with repetitive use, becomes frayed. Rupture of the tendon allows the overlying bursa to communicate with the joint cavity and impairs the initial phase of abduction. Later phases of abduction remain intact through the action of the deltoid muscle (Sections 14.2b and 14.2c).
A The tendons of the rotator cuff muscles insert on, and reinforce, the fibrous capsule of the joint. B through D are also correct (E).
B The supraspinatus tendon and subacromial bursa pass through the narrow subacromial space between the capsule of the shoulder joint and the coracoacromial arch. A, C, and D are also correct (E).
C The supraspinatus tendon separates the subacromial and subdeltoid bursae from the joint cavity. With rupture of the tendon, a communication between the bursae and joint cavity may result. A, B, and D are also correct (E).
D The deltoid is the primary abductor of the glenohumeral joint, but the supraspinatus assists in the first 15 degrees of abduction. A through C are also correct (E).

26. **E** The two heads of the biceps brachii originate on the supraglenoid tubercle and coracoid process of the scapula and insert on the radial tuberosity of the radius (Sections 14.2c and 14.3a).
A The deltoid originates along the scapular spine and clavicle and inserts on the deltoid tuberosity of the humerus.
B The coracobrachialis originates on the coracoid process of the scapula and inserts on the shaft of the humerus.
C The flexor digitorum superficialis originates on the medial epicondyle of the humerus and upper part of the radius and inserts on the middle phalanx of the 2nd through 4th digits.
D The pronator teres originates on the medial epicondyle of the humerus and coronoid process of the ulna and inserts on the lateral radius.

27. **B** The broad origin of the pectoralis major on the anterior trunk wall allows it to strongly adduct the arm (Section 14.2c).
A As part of the rotator cuff, the teres minor supports the head of the humerus in the glenohumeral joint. It also weakly adducts and laterally rotates the arm.
C The pectoralis minor draws the scapula forward and down, causing the scapula to rotate medially.
D The short head of the biceps brachii provides some flexion, abduction, and internal rotation of the glenohumeral joint.
E The subscapularis supports the head of the humerus in the glenohumeral joint and medially rotates the arm.

28. **D** The function of the abductor pollicis muscle, the primary abductor of the thumb, would be greatly impaired because it originates on the interosseous membrane (Section 14.4b).
A The flexor carpi radialis and flexor carpi ulnaris originate from the medial epicondyle of the humerus and olecranon of the ulna and would be unaffected by this injury.
B The triceps brachii, which extends the elbow, inserts on the olecranon. It would not be impaired by this injury.
C The extensor digitorum originates from the humerus and ulna and would be unaffected by this injury.
E The adductor of the thumb, adductor pollicis, attaches to the 2nd and 3rd metacarpals and the capitate. It would not be affected by this injury.

29. **D** The flexor pollicis longus passes through the carpal tunnel with the flexor digitorum superficialis, flexor digitorum profundus, and median nerve (Section 14.5b).
A The ulnar artery and ulnar nerve pass through the ulnar canal at the wrist.
B At the wrist the radial artery turns dorsally to run through the floor of the anatomic snuffbox.
C The flexor carpi radialis crosses the wrist lateral to the carpal tunnel and inserts on the base of the 1st metacarpal.
E The palmaris longus passes superficial to the flexor retinaculum to insert into the palmar aponeurosis.

30. **C** The interossei and lumbricals flex the metacarpophalangeal joints and extend the interphalangeal joints (Section 14.6c).

A Only the lateral two lumbricals are innervated by the median nerve. The medial lumbricals and all of the interossei are innervated by the ulnar nerve.

B The ulnar nerve innervates all of the interossei and the medial two lumbricals. The lateral two lumbricals are innervated by the median nerve.

D Only the lumbricals arise from the flexor tendons. The interossei arise from the shafts of the metacarpal bones.

E The palmar interossei adduct the fingers, the dorsal interossei abduct the fingers. The lumbricals have no effect on these movements.

15 Overview of the Lower Limb

The lower limb supports the weight of the entire body and therefore is designed for strength and stability. Bones, muscles, and tendons tend to be more robust and joints more stable than those found in the upper limb.

15.1 General Features

— In the anatomic position, the body is upright and supported by the lower limb. The feet are together and pointed forward.
— The regions of the lower limb (**Fig. 15.1A** and **B**) include

- the **gluteal region**, which includes the buttocks and lateral hip region and overlies the **pelvic girdle**;
- the **thigh**, between the hip and the knee;
- the **popliteal** and **genual regions**, at the knee;
- the **leg**, between the knee and ankle; and
- the **foot**, which has dorsal and plantar surfaces. The plantar surface is also called the **sole** of the foot.

— Movements of the joints of the lower limb are similar to movements of the upper limb, with some variations. They include

- flexion—**plantar flexion** indicates flexing the foot or toes downward;
- extension—**dorsiflexion** indicates extension of the foot, as when lifting the foot or toes upward;
- abduction and adduction—the axis for abduction and adduction of the toes is the 2nd digit;
- external rotation and internal rotation—movement around a longitudinal axis;
- **inversion**, or supination of the foot—lifting the medial edge of the sole; and
- **eversion**, or pronation of the foot lifting the lateral edge of the sole.

— As in the upper limb, muscles of the lower limb can be described as intrinsic or extrinsic.

- Intrinsic muscles of the foot originate and insert on bones of the foot and ankle.
- Extrinsic flexor and extensor muscles of the foot originate in the leg.

  ○ Synovial tendon sheaths surround the long flexor and extensor tendons as they cross the ankle joint.

Fig. 15.1 ▶ **Regions of the lower limb** Right limb.

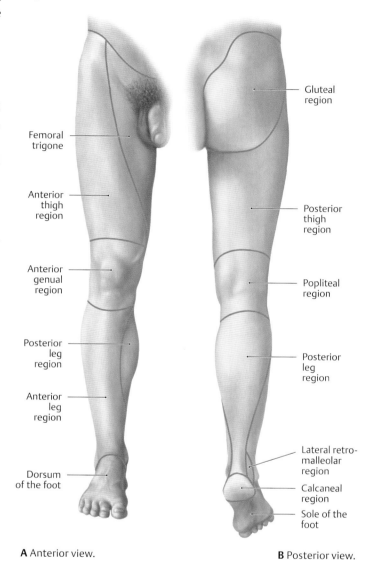

Gluteal region

Femoral trigone

Posterior thigh region

Anterior thigh region

Anterior genual region

Popliteal region

Posterior leg region

Posterior leg region

Anterior leg region

Lateral retro-malleolar region

Dorsum of the foot

Calcaneal region

Sole of the foot

A Anterior view.

B Posterior view.

Fig. 15.2 ▶ Bones of the lower limb
Right limb. The skeleton of the lower limb consists of a limb girdle and an attached free limb. The free limb is divided into the thigh (femur), leg (tibia and fibula), and foot. It is connected to the pelvic girdle by the hip joint.

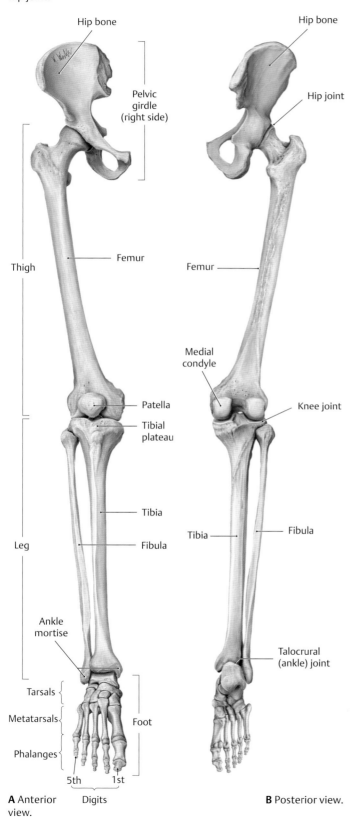

A Anterior view.

B Posterior view.

15.2 Bones of the Lower Limb (**Fig. 15.2A** and **B**)

— The **hip** (**coxal**) **bone** forms the lateral part of the pelvic girdle. The features of the hip bone are discussed in Section 10.2 with the bony pelvis.

— The **femur** is the long bone of the thigh (**Fig. 15.3A** and **B**).

   • Proximally, its large ball-shaped **head** articulates with the acetabulum of the hip bone.

   • The **neck**, angled inferolaterally, connects the head with the shaft.

   • **Greater** and **lesser trochanters**, sites for muscle attachments, are separated by an **intertrochanteric crest** posteriorly and an **intertrochanteric line** anteriorly.

   • The **shaft** is slightly bowed anteriorly and, in the anatomic position, is angled medially.

   • **Linea aspera**, paired ridges on the posterior surface of the shaft, diverge distally as the **medial** and **lateral supracondylar lines**.

   • Distally, the **medial** and **lateral epicondyles** are attachment sites for ligaments of the knee, and the **adductor tubercle** is an attachment site for muscle.

   • The femur articulates with the tibia at the **medial** and **lateral condyles**, which are separated by th e **intercondylar notch**.

   • The femur articulates with the patella anteriorly at the **patellar surface**.

Fig. 15.3 ▶ **Right femur**

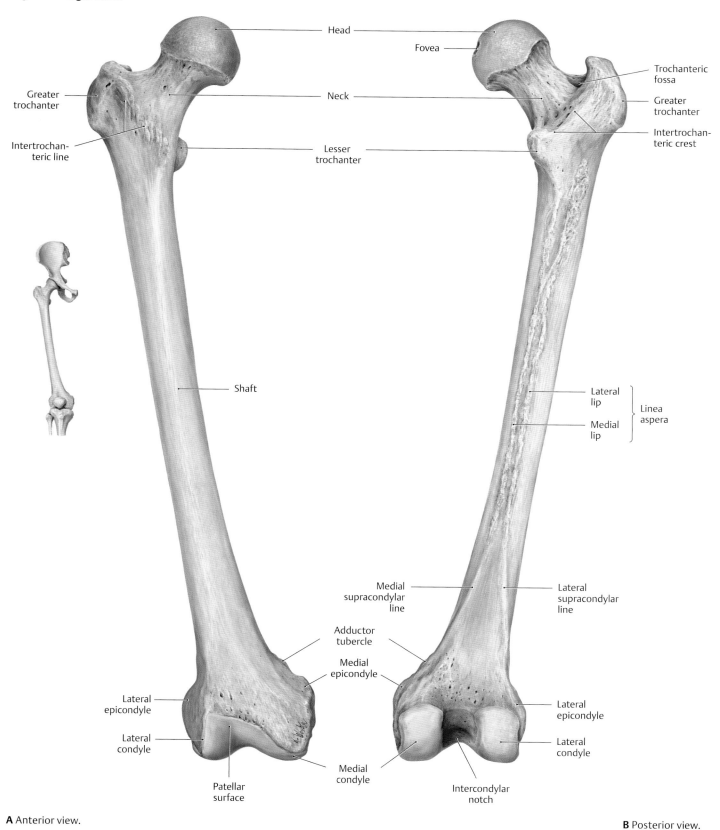

Head

Fovea

Trochanteric fossa

Greater trochanter

Neck

Intertrochanteric crest

Greater trochanter

Intertrochanteric line

Lesser trochanter

Shaft

Lateral lip

Medial lip

Linea aspera

Medial supracondylar line

Lateral supracondylar line

Adductor tubercle

Medial epicondyle

Lateral epicondyle

Lateral epicondyle

Lateral condyle

Lateral condyle

Patellar surface

Medial condyle

Intercondylar notch

A Anterior view.

B Posterior view.

— The **patella,** a large sesamoid bone, forms the kneecap (**Fig. 15.4A** and **B**; see also **Fig. 16.8**).

- It articulates with the distal femur at the knee joint.
- Superiorly, its **base** is attached to the **quadriceps tendon**.
- Inferiorly, its **apex** is attached to the **patellar ligament**.

— The **tibia** is the large medial long bone of the leg (**Fig. 15.5A** and **B**).

- Proximally, it articulates with the femur at the **tibial plateau**, which has flat **medial** and **lateral condyles** separated by an **intercondylar eminence**.
- It articulates with the fibula proximally at the **tibiofibular joint** and distally at the **tibiofibular syndesmosis**.
- A **tibial tuberosity** on the anterior surface below the tibial plateau is an attachment site for thigh muscles.
- Distally, the **medial malleolus** forms part of the mortise of the ankle joint.
- The sharp anterior border of the **shaft** is palpable between the knee and ankle.
- An **interosseous membrane** connects the shaft of the tibia and fibula.

— The **fibula** is the lateral bone of the leg (see **Fig. 15.5A** and **B**).

- Proximally, the **head** articulates with the lateral condyle of the tibia at the proximal tibiofibular joint.
- A narrow **neck** connects the head to the shaft.
- A distal tibiofibular syndesmosis binds the fibula to the distal tibia.
- Distally, the **lateral malleolus** forms the lateral wall of the mortise of the ankle joint.

Fig. 15.4 ▶ **Patella**
Right limb.

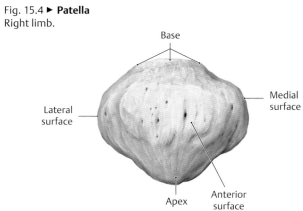

A Anterior view.

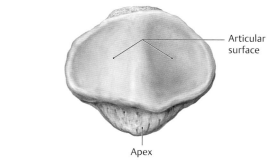

B Posterior view.

Fig. 15.5 ▶ **Tibia and fibula**
Right leg.

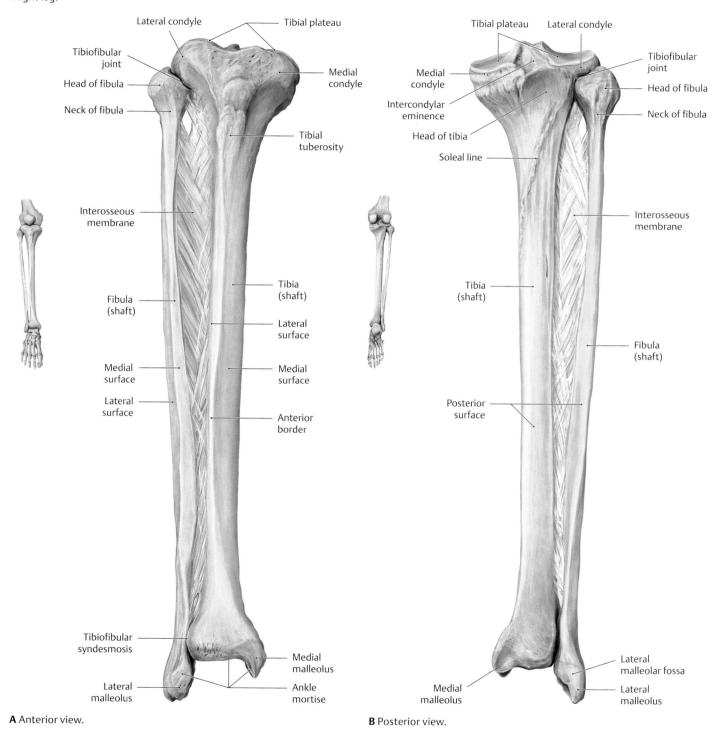

Lateral condyle
Tibial plateau
Tibiofibular joint
Medial condyle
Head of fibula
Neck of fibula
Tibial tuberosity
Interosseous membrane
Fibula (shaft)
Tibia (shaft)
Lateral surface
Medial surface
Medial surface
Lateral surface
Anterior border
Tibiofibular syndesmosis
Medial malleolus
Lateral malleolus
Ankle mortise

A Anterior view.

Tibial plateau
Lateral condyle
Medial condyle
Tibiofibular joint
Intercondylar eminence
Head of fibula
Head of tibia
Neck of fibula
Soleal line
Interosseous membrane
Tibia (shaft)
Fibula (shaft)
Posterior surface
Medial malleolus
Lateral malleolar fossa
Lateral malleolus

B Posterior view.

305

— The **tarsal bones** consist of seven short bones of the foot (**Fig. 15.6A, B, C,** and **D**).

• The **talus** is the most superior tarsal bone.

  ○ The **body** articulates with the tibia and fibula at the ankle joint.

  ○ The **head**, which articulates with the navicular bone, is the highest part of the medial arch of the foot.

  ○ The inferior surface articulates with the calcaneus.

Fig. 15.6 ► **Bones of the right foot**

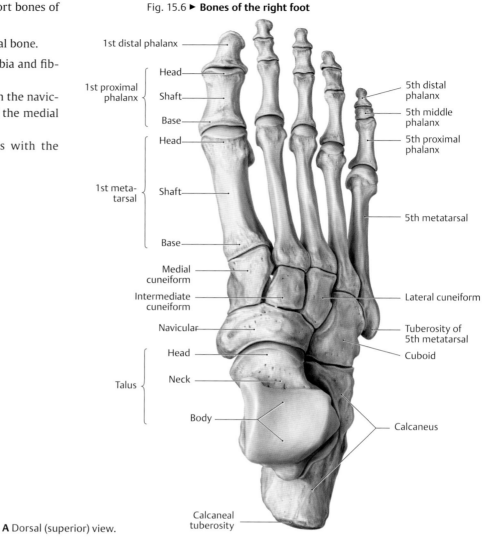

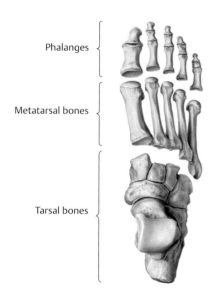

A Dorsal (superior) view.

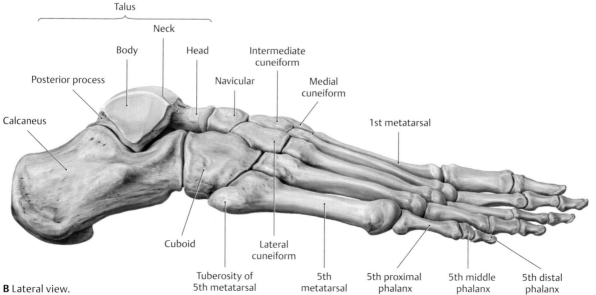

B Lateral view.

Fig. 15.6 ▶ **Bones of the right foot** (*continued*)

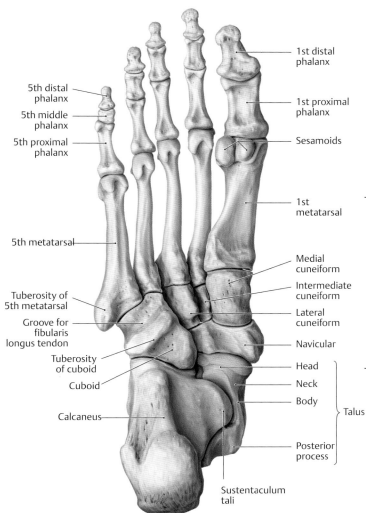

5th distal phalanx
5th middle phalanx
5th proximal phalanx
5th metatarsal
Tuberosity of 5th metatarsal
Groove for fibularis longus tendon
Tuberosity of cuboid
Cuboid
Calcaneus

1st distal phalanx
1st proximal phalanx
Sesamoids
1st metatarsal
Medial cuneiform
Intermediate cuneiform
Lateral cuneiform
Navicular
Head
Neck
Body
Posterior process
} Talus
Sustentaculum tali

C Plantar (inferior) view.

• The **calcaneus** is the large tarsal bone of the heel.
  ○ It articulates superiorly with the talus and anteriorly with the cuboid.
  ○ The **sustentaculum tali**, a medial process, forms part of the medial arch of the foot.
• The **navicular** lies anterior to the talus and forms part of the medial arch.
• The **cuboid** lies anterior to the calcaneus on the lateral side of the foot.
• The **medial**, **intermediate**, and **lateral cuneiform** bones lie anterior to the navicular and articulate distally with the metatarsal bones.
— The **metatarsal bones** consist of five long bones that are designated 1st (medial) through 5th (lateral).
  • Proximally, their **bases** articulate with the tarsal bones.
  • Distally, their **heads** articulate with the proximal phalanges.
  • The **shaft** connects the heads and bases.
  • Paired **sesamoid bones** are associated with the head of the 1st metatarsal.
  • A prominent tuberosity at the base of the 5th metatarsal is a site of attachment for muscles of the leg.
— The **phalanges** are small long bones of the toes.
  • The 2nd through 5th digits have a proximal, middle, and distal phalanx.
  • The 1st digit, the **hallux**, or great toe, has only a proximal and a distal phalanx.

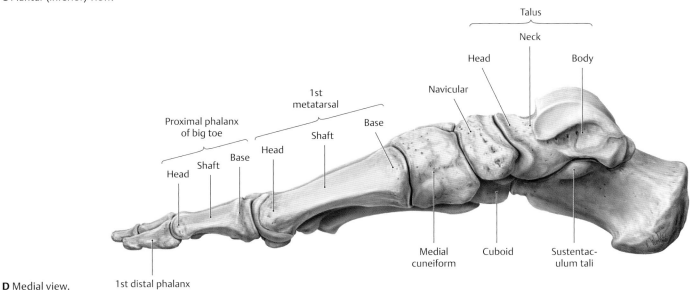

Talus
Neck
Head
Body
Navicular
1st metatarsal
Base
Shaft
Proximal phalanx of big toe
Shaft
Head
Base
Head
Head
Shaft
Base
Medial cuneiform
Cuboid
Sustentaculum tali
1st distal phalanx

D Medial view.

15.3 Fascia and Compartments of the Lower Limb

— Similar to the upper limb, the lower limb musculature is enclosed within a snug sleeve of deep fascia, which is continuous from the iliac crest to the sole of the foot but has regional designations.

- **Fascia lata** surrounds muscles of the thigh. Laterally, longitudinal fibers of the fascia lata form a tough band, the **iliotibial tract**, which extends from the iliac crest to the tibial tubercle (see **Fig. 16.28**).
- **Crural fascia** invests muscles of the leg, and at the ankle it forms the flexor and extensor retinacula.
- Fascia on the dorsum of the foot is thin, but on the sole it forms a thickened longitudinal band, the **plantar aponeurosis**.
- **Digital fibrous sheaths** are extensions of the plantar aponeurosis onto the toes, where they enclose the flexor tendons.

— The deep fascia creates compartments that separate the limb musculature. Muscles within each compartment are usually similar in function, innervation, and blood supply. Compartments of the lower limb (see **Fig. 16.35A and B**) include the following:

- **Anterior**, **medial**, and **posterior compartments** of the thigh
- **Anterior**, **lateral**, **superficial posterior**, and **deep posterior** compartments of the leg (crural compartments)
- **Medial**, **lateral**, **central**, and **interosseous compartments** on the sole of the foot
- **Dorsal compartment** on the dorsum of the foot

15.4 Neurovasculature of the Lower Limb

15.4a Arteries of the Lower Limb

Branches of the internal iliac artery in the pelvis and the femoral artery (a continuation of the external iliac artery) supply blood to the lower limb (**Fig. 15.7**).

— The branches of the internal iliac artery that supply the lower limb include

- the **superior gluteal** and **inferior gluteal arteries**, which exit the pelvis posteriorly through the greater sciatic foramen to supply the gluteal region; and
- the **obturator artery**, which exits the pelvis anteriorly through the obturator foramen to supply the medial thigh.

Fig. 15.7 ▶ **Course and branches of the femoral artery**

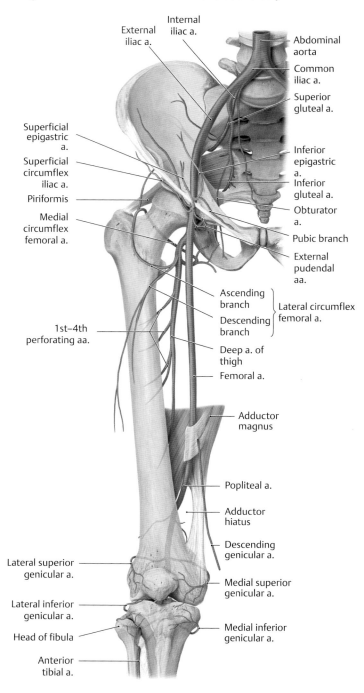

— The **femoral artery** enters the anterior thigh deep to the inguinal ligament enclosed within a **femoral sheath** (formed by extensions of the deep fascia of the abdomen). The artery descends along the anteromedial thigh between the anterior and medial muscular compartments and ends at the **adductor hiatus**, a gap in the tendon of the **adductor magnus** muscle. Its branches include

- the **superficial circumflex iliac** and **superficial epigastric arteries**, which supply the abdominal wall;
- the **superficial** and **deep external pudendal arteries**, which supply the inguinal region;
- the **descending genicular artery**, which contributes to the anastomosis around the knee; and
- the **deep artery of the thigh**, which is the primary blood supply to the thigh.

— The deep artery of the thigh (deep femoral artery, profunda femoris), the largest branch of the femoral artery, arises in the proximal thigh. Its branches include

- the **medial circumflex femoral artery**, which is the primary blood supply to the hip joint;
- the **lateral circumflex femoral artery**, which supplies the hip joint and contributes to the anastomosis around the knee joint; and
- the **1st through 3rd** (or 4th) **perforating arteries**, which supply muscles of the anterior, medial, and posterior muscles of the thigh.

— A **cruciate anastomosis** provides a collateral blood supply to structures around the hip. Contributions to the anastomosis include

- the medial and lateral circumflex femoral arteries,
- the 1st perforating artery, and
- the inferior gluteal artery.

Femoral neck fracture

Fractures of the femoral neck commonly occur following a low-energy impact in women over 60 years of age with osteoporosis. The distal fragment of bone is pulled upward by the quadriceps femoris, adductor, and hamstring muscles, causing shortening and lateral (external) rotation of the limb. Although an ample arterial anastomosis surrounds the hip joint, only the medial circumflex femoral artery supplies branches that enter the joint capsule and supply the femoral head. Tearing of those branches at the fracture site leads to avascular necrosis of the femoral head.

— The **popliteal artery** is the continuation of the femoral artery as it enters the **popliteal fossa**, a cavity posterior to the knee joint (**Fig. 15.8**).

- Five **genicular branches** run medially and laterally around the knee.
- **Anterior tibial** and **posterior tibial arteries**, the terminal branches of the popliteal artery, arise in the proximal part of the posterior leg compartment.

— A **genicular anastomosis** that supplies the knee joint receives contributions from

- the medial superior and inferior, lateral superior and inferior, and middle genicular arteries;
- the descending genicular artery from the thigh;
- the descending branch of the lateral circumflex artery; and
- the recurrent branches of anterior tibial and posterior tibial arteries.

Popliteal aneurysm

Aneurysms of the popliteal artery are the most common peripheral arterial aneurysm. They can be distinguished by a thrill (palpable pulse) and bruits (abnormal arterial sounds) overlying the popliteal fossa. Because the artery lies deep to the tibial nerve, an aneurysm may stretch the nerve or occlude its blood supply. Pain from nerve compression is referred to the skin overlying the medial aspect of the calf, ankle, and foot. Half of all popliteal aneurysms remain asymptomatic, and ruptures are rare, but symptomatic patients present with distal leg ischemia from acute embolization or thrombosis. Fifty percent of patients with a popliteal aneurysm have an aneurysm in the contralateral artery, and 25% have an aortic aneurysm.

Fig. 15.8 ▶ **Arteries of the knee and posterior leg**
Right leg, posterior view.

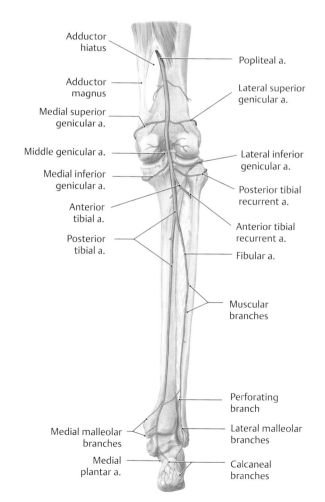

309

— The posterior tibial artery descends into the deep posterior leg compartment to supply muscles in the deep and superficial posterior compartments (see **Fig. 15.8**). Its branches include

- the **fibular artery**, which arises in the upper leg and descends within the posterior leg compartment; and
- the **medial plantar** and **lateral plantar arteries**, which arise as the terminal branches posterior to the medial malleolus (see **Fig. 15.9**).

— The fibular artery supplies muscles of the deep posterior compartment and, via small arteries that perforate the intermuscular septum, muscles of the lateral compartment. At the ankle it gives off

- a **perforating branch** that arises at the ankle and anastomoses with the anterior tibial artery and
- **malleolar branches** that contribute to an anastomosis around the ankle.

— Arteries of the sole arise from the posterior tibial artery and include (**Fig. 15.9**)

- the medial plantar artery, a small branch of the posterior tibial artery that supplies the medial part of the sole;
- the lateral plantar artery, the largest branch of the posterior tibial artery, which supplies the lateral side of the sole and curves medially to anastomose with the deep plantar artery;
- a **deep plantar arch**, which forms through the anastomosis of the deep plantar artery and lateral plantar artery; and

- four **plantar metatarsal arteries**, which arise from the deep plantar arch and their branches, the **common** and **proper plantar digital arteries**,

— The anterior tibial artery passes through an opening in the interosseous membrane to supply muscles of the anterior leg compartment (**Fig. 15.10**). Its branches are

- proximally, a **recurrent branch** to the knee and
- distally, the **dorsal pedal artery** as it emerges onto the dorsum of the foot.

Fig. 15.10 ▶ **Arteries of the anterior leg and foot**
Right leg, anterior view.

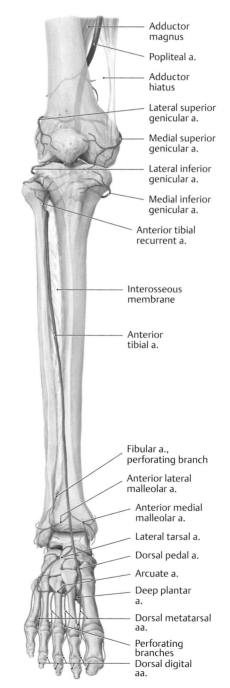

- Adductor magnus
- Popliteal a.
- Adductor hiatus
- Lateral superior genicular a.
- Medial superior genicular a.
- Lateral inferior genicular a.
- Medial inferior genicular a.
- Anterior tibial recurrent a.
- Interosseous membrane
- Anterior tibial a.
- Fibular a., perforating branch
- Anterior lateral malleolar a.
- Anterior medial malleolar a.
- Lateral tarsal a.
- Dorsal pedal a.
- Arcuate a.
- Deep plantar a.
- Dorsal metatarsal aa.
- Perforating branches
- Dorsal digital aa.

Fig. 15.9 ▶ **Arteries of the sole of the foot**
Right foot, plantar view.

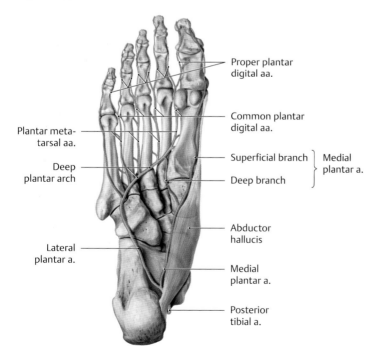

- Proper plantar digital aa.
- Common plantar digital aa.
- Plantar metatarsal aa.
- Superficial branch ⎫ Medial plantar a.
- Deep branch ⎭
- Deep plantar arch
- Abductor hallucis
- Lateral plantar a.
- Medial plantar a.
- Posterior tibial a.

Fig. 15.11 ▶ **Deep veins of the lower limb**
Right limb.

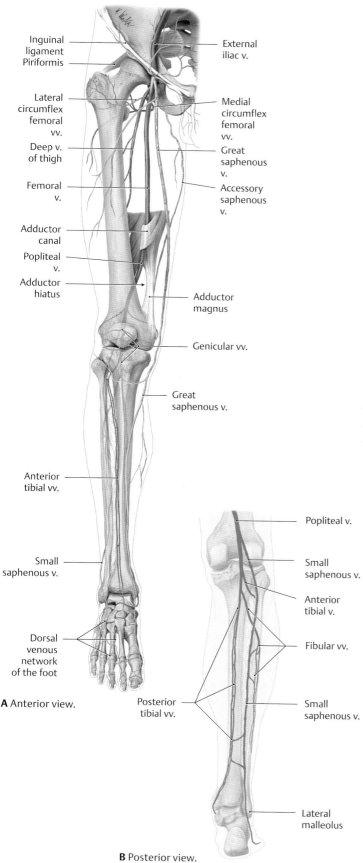

A Anterior view.

B Posterior view.

Labels (Figure A):
- Inguinal ligament
- Piriformis
- Lateral circumflex femoral vv.
- Deep v. of thigh
- Femoral v.
- Adductor canal
- Popliteal v.
- Adductor hiatus
- Anterior tibial vv.
- Small saphenous v.
- Dorsal venous network of the foot
- External iliac v.
- Medial circumflex femoral vv.
- Great saphenous v.
- Accessory saphenous v.
- Adductor magnus
- Genicular vv.
- Great saphenous v.
- Posterior tibial vv.

Labels (Figure B):
- Popliteal v.
- Small saphenous v.
- Anterior tibial v.
- Fibular vv.
- Small saphenous v.
- Lateral malleolus

— Arteries of the dorsum of the foot arise from the dorsal pedal artery and include

- the **lateral tarsal** and **arcuate arteries**, which form a loop on the dorsum of the foot;
- the **deep plantar artery**, which anastomoses with the lateral plantar artery on the sole; and
- the **dorsal metatarsal arteries** and their branches, the **dorsal digital arteries**, which arise from the arcuate artery or the dorsal pedal artery.

▎ **The dorsal pedal pulse**

The dorsal pedal artery is readily palpable on the dorsum of the foot as it runs toward the first web space lateral to the extensor hallucis tendon. Absence of the dorsal pedal pulse suggests arterial occlusion in the peripheral vasculature.

▎ **Lower limb ischemia**

Ischemia of the lower extremity is almost always related to atherosclerotic disease. Intermittent claudication is a symptom of chronic ischemic disease characterized by pain while walking, which intensifies over time and disappears at rest. Chronic disease has a benign course and, in the majority of patients, is treated conservatively. Acute ischemia has an abrupt onset from an embolitic or thrombolytic origin and usually requires aggressive treatment. The six signs (P signs) of acute ischemia are pain, pallor, pulselessness, paresthesia, paralysis, and poikilothermy.

15.4b Veins of the Lower Limb

The lower limb has both deep and superficial venous drainages, which anastomose through perforating veins. Veins of both systems have numerous valves along their length.

— Veins of the deep venous system travel with the major arteries and their branches and have similar names. As in the upper limb, these deep veins usually occur as paired accompanying veins in the distal part of the limb (**Fig. 15.11A** and **B**).

- The **femoral vein**, which drains the deep and superficial veins of the thigh and leg, passes under the inguinal ligament into the abdomen, where it becomes the external iliac vein.
- **Superior** and **inferior gluteal veins**, which drain the gluteal region, pass through the greater sciatic foramen to empty into the internal iliac vein of the pelvis.

— Superficial veins are located in the subcutaneous tissue and normally drain, via perforating veins, to the deep venous system (**Fig. 15.12A** and **B**).

- The largest superficial veins, the **great saphenous** and **small saphenous veins**, originate at the **dorsal venous arch** on the dorsum of the foot.
- The great saphenous vein arises from the medial side of the venous arch and passes superiorly, anterior to the medial malleolus and posteromedial to the knee. It drains into the femoral vein at the **saphenous opening**, an opening in the fascia lata in the upper thigh.
- The small saphenous vein arises from the lateral side of the venous arch, passes posterior to the lateral malleolus, and ascends the posterior leg. It drains into the **popliteal vein** behind the knee.

— The flow of blood from lower parts of the body must counter the downward force of gravity. In the lower limbs, venous return is assisted by

- the presence of valves in the veins,
- the pulsing of accompanying arteries, and
- the contraction of surrounding muscles.

■ Deep vein thromboses (DVT)

Thromboses (blood clots) in the deep veins of the leg result from stasis, the slowing or pooling of blood. This can result from prolonged inactivity (extended airplane travel, immobilization following surgery) or anatomic abnormalities such as laxity of the crural fascia. Thrombi from the legs can break off and travel to the heart and lungs, lodging in the pulmonary arterial tree as pulmonary emboli. Large clots can severely impair lung function and even cause death. Thrombophlebitis is the inflammation of a vein caused by thrombosis.

■ Varicose veins

Varicose disease of the superficial veins of the lower limb is the most common chronic venous disease. Degeneration of the wall of the vein leads to dilated, tortuous vessels and incompetent venous valves. Varices also develop when chronic occlusion of the deep veins causes a reversal of flow through the perforating veins. (Normal venous drainage flows from superficial to deep systems.) As the superficial veins dilate with increased volume, valve leaflets separate and become incompetent.

Fig. 15.12 ▶ **Superficial veins of the lower limb**
Right limb.

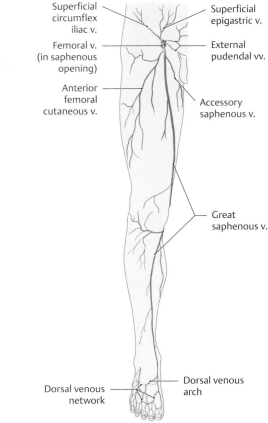

A Anterior view.

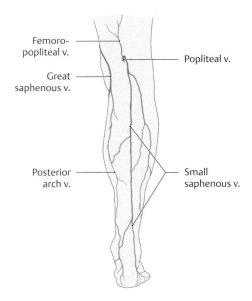

B Posterior view.

15.4c   Lymphatics of the Lower Limb

Lymph from the lower limb drains superiorly from the foot following the deep and superficial veins. Upward flow is facilitated by the contraction of surrounding muscles (**Fig. 15.13**).

— Lymph from deep tissues of the
  - gluteal region drains along the gluteal vessels to internal iliac nodes.
  - thigh drains to deep inguinal nodes.

— Lymph from superficial tissues of the gluteal region and thigh drain to superficial inguinal nodes.

— Lymph from the dorsum and sole of the lateral foot and lateral leg drains along the short saphenous vein to the **deep popliteal nodes** at the knee. These drain directly to deep inguinal nodes.

— Lymph from the dorsum and sole of the medial foot and the medial leg drains along the long saphenous vein to superficial inguinal nodes.

— Lymph from the thigh drains first to superficial inguinal nodes, which in turn drain to deep inguinal nodes.

— Deep inguinal nodes drain sequentially to external iliac, common iliac, and lumbar nodes.

Fig. 15.13 ▶ **Lymph nodes and drainage of the lower limbs**
Right limb, anterior view.

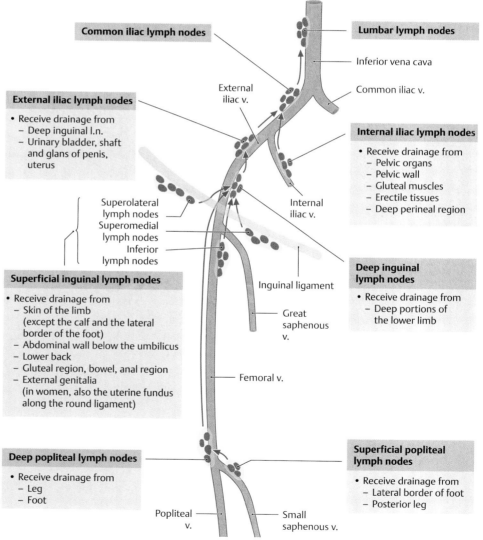

Table 15.1 ► **Nerves of the Lower Limb**		
Nerve	**Level**	**Area of Innervation**
Lumbar plexus		
Iliohypogastric n.	L1	Skin over upper lateral thigh and inguinal region
Ilioinguinal n.	L1	Skin over upper anterior thigh
Genitofemoral n.	L1–L2	Skin over upper thigh
Lateral femoral cutaneous n.	L2–L3	Skin of lateral thigh
Femoral n.	L2–L4	Iliopsoas, pectineus, sartorius, quadriceps femoris
—Anterior cutaneous n.		Skin of anterior and medial thigh
—Saphenous n.		Skin of medial leg and foot
Obturator n.	L2–L4	Obturator externus, adductor longus, adductor brevis, adductor magnus, gracilis, pectineus; skin of medial thigh
Sacral plexus		
Superior gluteal n.	L4–S1	Gluteus medius, gluteus minimus, tensor fascia latae
Inferior gluteal n.	L5–S2	Gluteus maximus
Direct branches	L5–S2	Piriformis, obturator internus, gemelli, quadratus femoris
Posterior femoral cutaneous n.	S1–S3	Skin of posterior thigh and inferior gluteal region
Tibial n.	L4–S3	Biceps femoris (long head), semimembranosus, semitendinosus, adductor magnus (medial part), gastrocnemius, soleus, popliteus, tibialis posterior, flexor digitorum longus, flexor hallucis longus
—Medial plantar n.		Abductor hallucis, flexor digitorum brevis, flexor hallucis brevis (medial head), 1st lumbrical; skin of medial sole, 1st–3rd digits, and half of 4th digit
—Lateral plantar n.		Quadratus plantae, flexor hallucis brevis (lateral head), abductor digiti minimi, flexor digiti minimi brevis, interossei, 2nd–4th lumbricals, adductor hallucis; skin of lateral sole, 5th digit, and half of 4th digit
Common fibular n.	L4–S2	Biceps femoris (short head)
—Superficial fibular n.		Fibularis longus and brevis; skin of dorsum of foot
—Deep fibular n.		Anterior tibialis, extensor hallucis longus and brevis, extensor digitorum longus and brevis, fibularis tertius; skin of web space between 1st and 2nd digits
Sural n. (tibial and common fibular nn. contributions)	S1	Skin of posterior and lateral leg and lateral foot

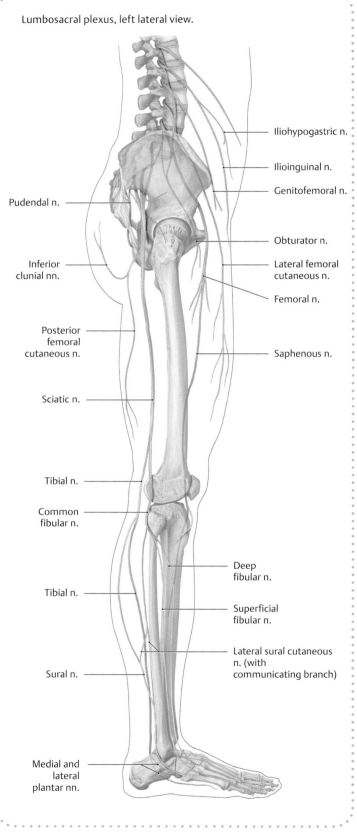

Lumbosacral plexus, left lateral view.

Iliohypogastric n.

Ilioinguinal n.

Genitofemoral n.

Pudendal n.

Obturator n.

Lateral femoral cutaneous n.

Femoral n.

Inferior clunial nn.

Posterior femoral cutaneous n.

Saphenous n.

Sciatic n.

Tibial n.

Common fibular n.

Deep fibular n.

Tibial n.

Superficial fibular n.

Sural n.

Lateral sural cutaneous n. (with communicating branch)

Medial and lateral plantar nn.

15.4d Nerves of the Lower Limb: Lumbosacral Plexus

The lumbar and sacral plexuses, often combined as the **lumbosacral plexus**, innervate the lower limb (**Table 15.1**; **Figs. 15.14, 15.15A** and **B**, and **15.16A** and **B**).

Nerves of the lumbar plexus enter the limb anteriorly to supply muscles of the anterior and medial thigh.

— The **iliohypogastric** (L1), **genital branch of the genitofemoral** (L1–L2), and **ilioinguinal** (L1) **nerves** are primarily nerves of the anterior abdominal wall and inguinal region. They also innervate small areas of skin over the upper lateral, anterior, and medial thigh, respectively.

— The **lateral femoral cutaneous nerve** (L2–L3), a sensory nerve that enters the lateral thigh anteromedial to the anterior superior iliac spine, innervates skin of the lateral thigh.

Fig 15.14 ▶ **Lumbosacral plexus**
Right side, anterior view.

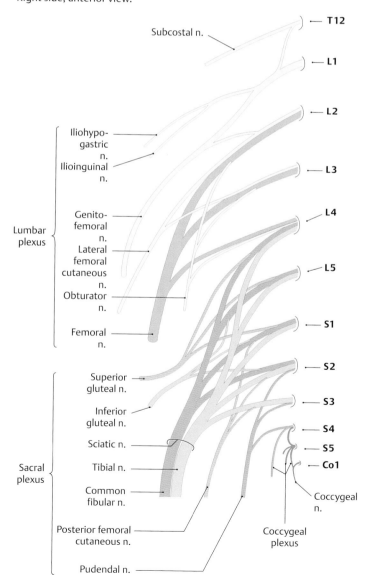

Fig. 15.15 ▶ **Cutaneous innervation of the lower limb**
Right limb.

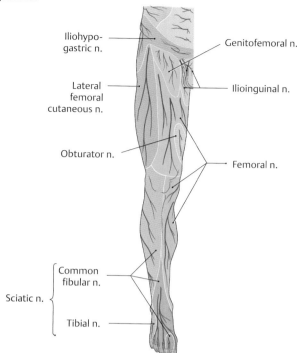

A Anterior view.

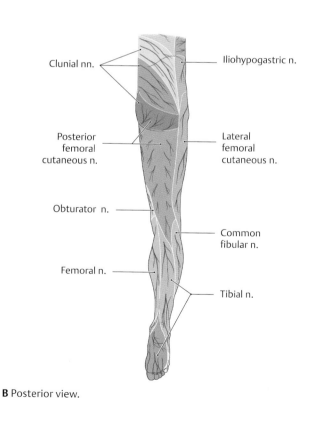

B Posterior view.

Fig. 15.16 ▶ **Dermatomes of the lower limb**
Right limb.

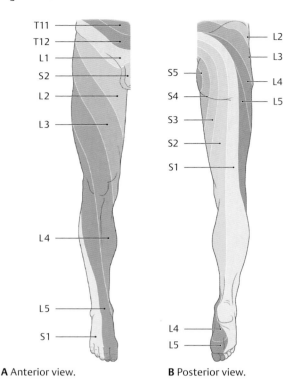

A Anterior view.   **B** Posterior view.

— The **femoral nerve** enters the anterior thigh through the retroinguinal space (deep to the inguinal ligament), lateral to the femoral artery.
   • It innervates muscles of the anterior compartment.
   • Its **saphenous branch** is a sensory nerve that descends inferiorly to innervate the skin of the medial leg and foot.

▌ Femoral nerve injury

Injuries of the femoral nerve can result in the following:
— Weakened flexion of the hip
— Loss of knee extension
— Loss of sensation on the medial side of the leg and foot
— Instability of the knee

— The **obturator nerve** (L2–L4) enters the medial thigh through the obturator foramen and innervates muscles of the medial compartment.

▌ Obturator nerve injury

Injury to the obturator nerve is most commonly associated with pelvic surgery or pelvic fractures and results in the following:
— Weakened adduction of the hip (e.g., inability to move the leg from the gas pedal to the brake)
— Weakened external rotation of the hip
— Loss of sensation over a palm-size area on the medial side of the thigh
— Instability of the pelvis; lateral swing of the limb with locomotion

The sacral plexus supplies muscles of the gluteal region, posterior thigh, and all muscular compartments of the leg and foot. Its branches enter the lower limb through the greater sciatic foramen in the gluteal region.

— The **superior gluteal nerve** (L4–S1) enters the gluteal region above the piriformis muscle and runs laterally between the deep gluteal muscles. It supplies the abductors of the hip joint in the gluteal region.

▌ Injury to the superior gluteal nerve and Trendelenburg test

When one foot is lifted off the floor, as happens during the gait cycle, abduction of the hip by the contralateral gluteus medius and gluteus minimus muscles (the supported side) maintains the pelvis in the horizontal position. With injury to the superior gluteal nerve, the loss of abduction on that side allows the pelvis on the opposite (unsupported) side to drop. This results in a characteristic "gluteal gait" in which the weight of the trunk is shifted toward the nerve-damaged side to maintain the center of gravity.
   The Trendelenburg test assesses the stability of the hip and its ability to support the pelvis when standing on one leg. The test is positive when the pelvis falls on the side of the unsupported leg, indicating an injury to the superior gluteal nerve and paralysis of the gluteus medius and gluteus minimus. Fractures of the greater trochanter (the site of distal attachment of the gluteus medius) or upward displacement of the greater trochanter will also result in a positive test.

— The **inferior gluteal nerve** (L5–S2) enters the gluteal region inferior to the piriformis muscle and innervates the large gluteus maximus muscle.
— The **posterior femoral cutaneous nerve** (L1–S3) is sensory to the thigh and posterior perineum. Its **inferior clunial branches** supply the inferior gluteal region.
— The **sciatic nerve** is made up of the **tibial** (L4–S3) and **common fibular** (L4–S2) **nerves**, which are bound together in a common sheath along their course in the posterior thigh. The two nerves diverge at the apex of the popliteal fossa.

▌ Sciatic nerve injury

The sciatic nerve can be injured by compression by the piriformis muscle, misplaced intramuscular injections in the gluteal region, pelvic fractures, or surgical procedures such as hip replacements. An injury in the gluteal region would affect muscles of the posterior thigh and all muscular compartments of the leg, the combined effects of damage to the tibial and common fibular nerves.

— The tibial nerve, the larger branch of the sciatic nerve, separates from the common fibular nerve and continues inferiorly through the popliteal fossa into the deep posterior leg compartment.

  • It innervates all of the muscles of the posterior thigh except the short head of the biceps femoris.
  • At the ankle, it passes posterior to the medial malleolus, where it terminates as the **medial plantar** and **lateral plantar nerves**.

▌ Tibial nerve injury

Tibial nerve injury is unusual because the nerve is well protected in the thigh and posterior leg. Injury in the gluteal region results in the following:
— Impaired extension of the hip
— Loss of flexion of the knee

In the popliteal fossa, it can be affected by aneurysms of the popliteal artery and knee trauma. These can cause the following:
— Loss of plantar flexion at the ankle
— Loss of plantar flexion, abduction, and adduction of the digits
— Loss of eversion of the foot
— Weakened inversion of the foot
— Loss of sensation on the posterolateral leg to the lateral malleolus, the sole and lateral side of the foot
— A shuffling gait with clawing of the toes

— The medial plantar nerve, comparable to the median nerve of the hand with small motor and large sensory components, is the largest branch of the tibial nerve.
  • It innervates plantar muscles on the medial side of the foot.
  • A superficial branch supplies a large area of skin on the medial side of the foot and the medial three and a half digits. It terminates as three **plantar digital nerves**.
— The lateral plantar nerve, the smaller branch of the tibial nerve, is comparable to the ulnar nerve of the hand.
  • It innervates the lateral plantar muscles and most deep muscles of the foot.
  • It innervates skin on the lateral sole and lateral one and a half digits and terminates as two **plantar digital nerves**.

— The common fibular nerve separates from the tibial nerve and, hugging the border of the biceps femoris muscle, passes laterally around the head of the fibula where it enters the lateral leg compartment.
  • In the thigh, it innervates the short head of the biceps femoris.
  • In the lateral leg compartment, it splits into its terminal branches, the **superficial fibular** and **deep fibular nerves**.

▌ Common fibular nerve injury

The common fibular nerve is the most vulnerable of the peripheral nerves due to its exposed location around the neck of the fibula. Injuries result in the following:
— Loss of eversion of the foot
— Loss of dorsiflexion at the ankle and digits
— Weakened inversion of the foot
— Loss of sensation over the lateral leg and dorsum of the foot
— Foot drop compensated by a high-stepping gait; instability on uneven surfaces

— The superficial fibular nerve innervates the muscles in the lateral leg compartment. At the midleg, its sensory component pierces the crural fascia and runs onto the dorsum of the foot.
— From its division from the superficial fibular nerve, the deep fibular nerve circles anteriorly to enter the anterior leg compartment. It descends along the interosseous membrane, innervating all muscles of the compartment. It emerges onto the foot with the dorsal pedal artery to innervate the skin on adjacent surfaces of the 1st and 2nd digits.

▌ Superficial and deep fibular nerve injury

Injury to the superficial fibular nerve only affects eversion of the foot and sensation over the lateral leg and most of the dorsum of the foot. Injury to the deep fibular has greater functional consequences, including the loss of all dorsiflexion. This results in footdrop and the compensating high-stepping gait.

— The **sural nerve** (S1), formed by communicating branches of the tibial and common fibular nerves on the surface of the posterior leg, runs posterior to the lateral malleolus at the ankle to innervate the skin of the lateral foot.

16 Functional Anatomy of the Lower Limb

The strong muscles and joints of the lower limb are adapted for bipedal locomotion and, in conjunction with the muscles of the trunk, maintain the body's center of gravity.

Schematics of lower limb muscles accompany the muscle tables (origin, attachment, innveration, and action) in the appropriate chapter sections. To see the muscles in situ, view the gallery of topographic images in Section 16.10 at the end of the chapter.

16.1 The Pelvic Girdle

The hip (coxal) bones and the sacrum form the pelvic girdle (bony pelvis), which is related anatomically and functionally to the pelvis and the lower limb (**Fig. 16.1A** and **B**). (See Section 10.2 for a discussion of the pelvic girdle.)

Fig. 16.1 ▶ **The hip bones and their relation to bones of the trunk**

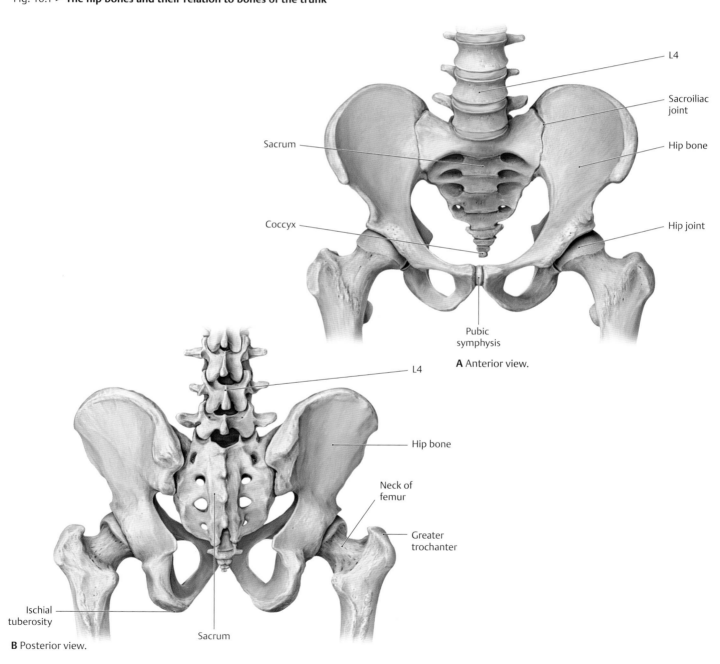

A Anterior view.

B Posterior view.

— Articulations at the sacroiliac joint and pubic symphysis, supported by strong sacroiliac, sacrotuberous, and sacrospinous ligaments, create a stable framework that
  • supports and encloses the pelvic viscera,
  • transfers the weight of the trunk to the lower limb, and
  • forms part of the hip joint and provides attachment sites for lower limb muscles.

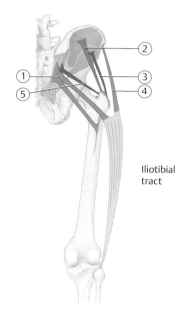

Iliotibial tract

16.2 The Gluteal Region

The gluteal region includes the buttock, which overlies the posterior part of the pelvic girdle, and the lateral hip region, which covers the hip joint and extends as far anteriorly as the anterior superior iliac spine.

— The muscular compartment of the gluteal region contains
  • muscles that laterally rotate, abduct, adduct, extend, and flex the hip joint (**Table 16.1**);
  • the superior gluteal, inferior gluteal, and sciatic nerves; and
  • the superior and inferior gluteal arteries and veins.

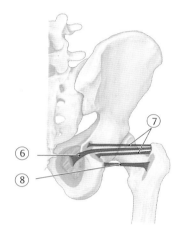

A Vertically oriented gluteal muscles, right side, posterior view.

B Horizontally oriented gluteal muscles, right side, posterior view.

Table 16.1 ▶ Gluteal Muscles

Muscle	Origin	Insertion	Innervation	Action
① Gluteus maximus	Sacrum (dorsal surface, lateral part), ilium (gluteal surface, posterior part), thoracolumbar fascia, sacrotuberous ligament	• Upper fibers: iliotibial tract • Lower fibers: gluteal tuberosity	Inferior gluteal n. (L5–S2)	• Entire muscle: extends and externally rotates the hip in sagittal and coronal planes • Upper fibers: abduction • Lower fibers: adduction
② Gluteus medius	Ilium (gluteal surface below the iliac crest between the anterior and posterior gluteal line)	Greater trochanter of the femur (lateral surface)	Superior gluteal n. (L4–S1)	• Entire muscle: abducts the hip, stabilizes the pelvis in the coronal plane • Anterior part: flexion and internal rotation • Posterior part: extension and external rotation
③ Gluteus minimus	Ilium (gluteal surface below the origin of the gluteus medius)	Greater trochanter of the femur (anterolateral surface)		
④ Tensor fasciae latae	Anterior superior iliac spine	Iliotibial tract		• Tenses the fascia lata • Hip joint: abduction, flexion, and internal rotation
⑤ Piriformis	Pelvic surface of the sacrum	Apex of the greater trochanter of the femur	Direct branches from the sacral plexus (S1–S2)	• External rotation, abduction, and extension of the hip joint • Stabilizes the hip joint
⑥ Obturator internus	Inner surface of the obturator membrane and its bony boundaries	Medial surface of the greater trochanter	Direct branches from the sacral plexus (L5–S1)	External rotation, adduction, and extension of the hip joint (also active in abduction, depending on the joint's position)
⑦ Gemelli	• Gemellus superior: ischial spine • Gemellus inferior: ischial tuberosity	Jointly with obturator internus tendon (medial surface, greater trochanter)		
⑧ Quadratus femoris	Lateral border of the ischial tuberosity	Intertrochanteric crest of the femur		External rotation and adduction of the hip joint

— Posteriorly, structures pass between the pelvis and the gluteal region through the greater sciatic foramen (**Fig. 16.2**). These structures include

- the piriformis muscle,
- the superior gluteal and inferior gluteal vessels,
- the superior gluteal and inferior gluteal nerves,
- the sciatic nerve,
- the pudendal nerve and internal pudendal vessels, and
- the posterior femoral cutaneous nerve.

— The lesser sciatic foramen, a passageway between the gluteal region and perineum, transmits

- the internal pudendal vessels,
- the pudendal nerve, and
- the tendon of the obturator internus muscle.

Intramuscular gluteal injections

Intramuscular injections are commonly given in the gluteal region. The injection site must be in the superior lateral quadrant or above the line connecting the posterior superior iliac spine and the top of the greater trochanter to avoid the large sciatic nerve and gluteal vascular structures.

Piriformis syndrome

The sciatic nerve normally passes into the gluteal region inferior to the piriformis muscle. Tightening or shortening of the muscle can compress and irritate the sciatic nerve, causing pain and paresthesia (tingling and numbness) in the buttocks and posterior thigh. In some cases the sciatic nerve, or its common fibular component, is compressed as it passes through the muscle. Piriformis syndrome should be distinguished from sciatica in which the pain and paresthesia result from compression of lumbar nerve roots by a herniated intervertebral disk.

16.3 The Hip Joint

The **hip joint** is a highly mobile, yet stable, ball-and-socket joint between the proximal femur and the acetabulum of the hip bone (**Fig. 16.3A** and **B**). Muscles crossing the joint, particularly in the gluteal region, provide additional stability as well as mobility.

— More than half of the large femoral head is seated in the bony acetabulum of the hip bone.

Fig. 16.2 ▶ **Sciatic foramina**
Right gluteal region.

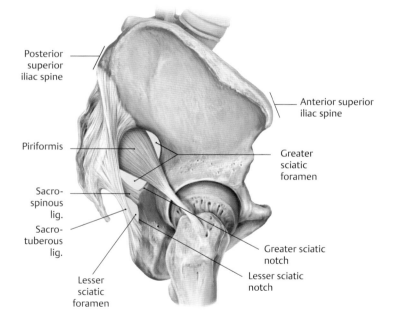

Fig. 16.3 ► **Right hip joint**
The head of the femur articulates with the acetabulum of the hip bone at the hip joint, a special type of spheroidal (ball-and-socket) joint. The roughly spherical femoral head (with an average radius of curvature of ~2.5 cm) is largely contained within the acetabulum.

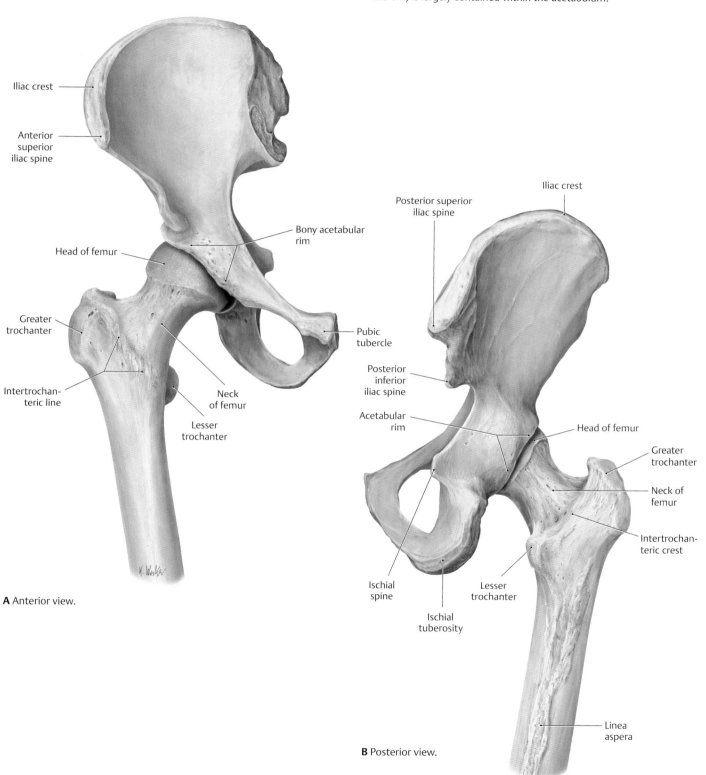

Iliac crest

Anterior superior iliac spine

Head of femur

Greater trochanter

Intertrochanteric line

Bony acetabular rim

Pubic tubercle

Neck of femur

Lesser trochanter

A Anterior view.

Posterior superior iliac spine

Iliac crest

Posterior inferior iliac spine

Acetabular rim

Head of femur

Greater trochanter

Neck of femur

Intertrochanteric crest

Ischial spine

Ischial tuberosity

Lesser trochanter

Linea aspera

B Posterior view.

— A strong fibrous capsule surrounds the hip joint (**Fig. 16.4A** and **B**).

- **Iliofemoral**, **pubofemoral**, and **ischiofemoral ligaments** are extracapsular ligaments that strengthen the capsule. The iliofemoral ligament is the strongest and most supportive of these.

— A fibrocartilaginous **acetabular labrum** attached to the acetabular rim deepens the joint (**Fig. 16.5**).

— A weak **ligament of the head of the femur** attaches to the acetabulum within the joint space but provides little support.

— Inferiorly, a **transverse ligament of the acetabulum** completes the circle of the C-shaped acetabular labrum.

— Muscles of the gluteal region and thigh move the hip joint (**Table 16.2**).

Fig. 16.4 ► **Ligaments of the hip joint and pelvic girdle**

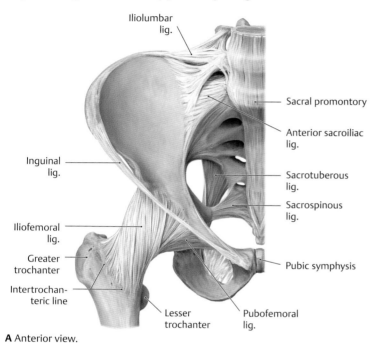

A Anterior view.

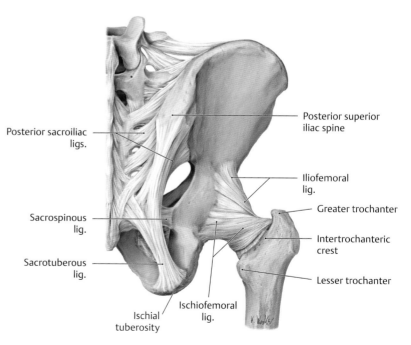

B Posterior view.

Fig. 16.5 ► **Joint capsule of the hip joint**
Lateral view. The capsule has been divided and the femoral head dislocated to expose the cut ligament of the head of the femur.

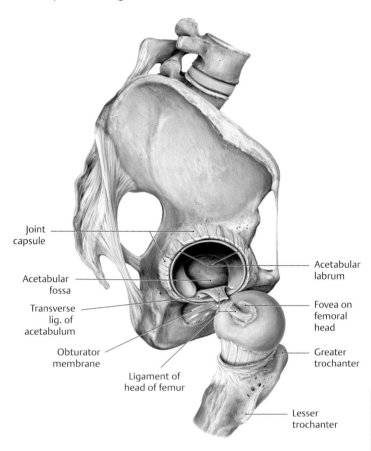

Joint capsule

Acetabular fossa

Transverse lig. of acetabulum

Obturator membrane

Ligament of head of femur

Acetabular labrum

Fovea on femoral head

Greater trochanter

Lesser trochanter

Table 16.2 ► **Movements of the Hip Joint**	
Action	**Muscle**
Flexion	Iliopsoas Tensor fascia latae Sartorius Rectus femoris Pectineus
Extension	Gluteus maximus Adductor magnus Biceps femoris, long head Semimembranosus Semitendinosus
Abduction	Gluteus medius Gluteus minimus Tensor fascia latae
Adduction	Adductor longus Adductor brevis Adductor magnus Pectineus Gracilis
Internal rotation	Gluteus medius Gluteus minimus Tensor fascia latae
External rotation	Gluteus maximus Quadratus femoris Piriformis Obturator externus Obturator internus

Acquired hip dislocation

Acquired hip dislocation usually occurs as a result of trauma that causes the femoral head to be displaced out of the acetabulum; anterior dislocations are rare, but posterior dislocations are common. Typically, in a head-on motor vehicle accident, the knees strike the dashboard, forcing the femoral head posteriorly through the joint capsule and onto the lateral surface of the ilium. The affected limb appears shortened and internally rotated. The sciatic nerve is particularly vulnerable to injury in these cases.

Congenital hip dislocation

Congenital hip dislocation (also known as hip dysplasia) is a common problem that occurs when the femoral head is not properly seated in the acetabulum. Hip abduction is impaired, and, since the femoral head sits higher than normal, the affected limb is shorter than the contralateral limb, resulting in a positive Trendelenburg test (see page 316, Injury to the superior gluteal nerve and trendelenburg test). In routine neonatal screenings, a dislocated hip will "click" when it is adducted and pushed posteriorly.

16.4 The Thigh

The thigh extends from the hip to the knee and contains the femur and thigh muscles.

16.4a Muscles of the Thigh

The powerful muscles of the thigh move the hip and knee joints and are separated into three compartments.

— The anterior thigh compartment contains

  • muscles that primarily flex the hip joint and extend the knee joint (**Table 16.3**);
  • the femoral nerve; and
  • branches of the femoral artery, the deep artery of the thigh, and their accompanying veins.

— The medial thigh compartment contains

  • muscles that primarily adduct, flex, and extend the hip joint (**Table 16.4**);
  • the obturator and femoral nerves; and
  • the obturator artery and vein and deep artery and vein of the thigh.

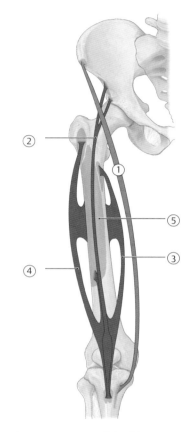

Thigh muscles, anterior compartment, right side.

Table 16.3 ▶ **Thigh Muscles, Anterior Compartment**				
Muscle		**Origin**	**Insertion**	**Innervation**	**Action**
① Sartorius		Anterior superior iliac spine	Medial to the tibial tuberosity (together with gracilis and semitendinosus)	Femoral n. (L2–L3)	• Hip joint: flexion, abduction, and external rotation • Knee joint: flexion and internal rotation
Quadriceps femoris*	② Rectus femoris	Anterior inferior iliac spine, acetabular roof of hip joint	Tibial tuberosity (via patellar ligament)	Femoral n. (L2–L4)	• Hip joint: flexion • Knee joint: extension
	③ Vastus medialis	Linea aspera (medial lip), intertrochanteric line (distal part)	Both sides of tuberosity on the medial and lateral condyles (via the medial and longitudinal patellar retinacula)		Knee joint: extension
	④ Vastus lateralis	Linea aspera (lateral lip), greater trochanter (lateral surface)			
	⑤ Vastus intermedius	Femoral shaft (anterior side)	Tibial tuberosity (via patellar ligament)		
	Articularis genus (distal fibers of vastus intermedius)	Anterior side of femoral shaft at level of the suprapatellar recess	Suprapatellar recess of knee joint capsule		Knee joint: extension; prevents entrapment of capsule
*The entire muscle inserts on the tibial tuberosity via the patellar ligament.				

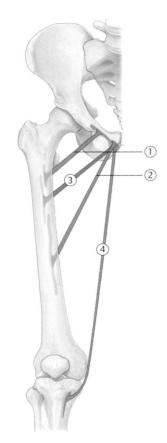

A Thigh muscles, medial compartment, superficial layer, anterior view.

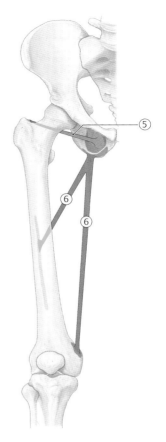

B Thigh muscles, medial compartment, deep layer, anterior view.

Table 16.4 ▶ **Thigh Muscles, Medial Compartment: Superficial and Deep Layers**				
Muscle	**Origin**	**Insertion**	**Innervation**	**Action**
Superficial layer				
① Pectineus	Pecten pubis	Femur (pectineal line and the proximal linea aspera)	Femoral n., obturator n. (L2–L3)	· Hip joint: adduction, external rotation, and slight flexion · Stabilizes the pelvis in the coronal and sagittal planes
② Adductor longus	Superior pubic ramus and anterior side of the symphysis	Femur (linea aspera, medial lip in the middle third of the femur)	Obturator n. (L2–L4)	· Hip joint: adduction and flexion (up to 70 degrees); extension (past 80 degrees of flexion) · Stabilizes the pelvis in the coronal and sagittal planes
③ Adductor brevis	Inferior pubic ramus			
④ Gracilis	Inferior pubic ramus below the symphysis	Tibia (medial border of the tuberosity, along with the tendons of sartorius and semitendinosus)	Obturator n. (L2–L3)	· Hip joint: adduction and flexion · Knee joint: flexion and internal rotation
Deep layer				
⑤ Obturator externus	Outer surface of the obturator membrane and its bony boundaries	Trochanteric fossa of the femur	Obturator n. (L3–L4)	· Hip joint: adduction and external rotation · Stabilizes the pelvis in the sagittal plane
⑥ Adductor magnus	Inferior pubic ramus, ischial ramus, and ischial tuberosity	· Deep part ("fleshy insertion"): medial lip of the linea spine	· Deep part: obturator n. (L2–L4)	· Hip joint: adduction, extension, and slight flexion (the tendinous insertion is also active in internal rotation) · Stabilizes the pelvis in the coronal and sagittal plane
		· Superficial part ("tendinous insertion"): adductor tubercle of the femur	· Superficial part: tibial n. (L4)	

— The posterior compartment contains
  • muscles that extend the hip joint and flex the knee joint (**Table 16.5**),
  • the sciatic nerve, and
  • branches of the deep artery and vein of the thigh.

■ Hamstring strains

Hamstring strains are tears of the hamstring muscles at their proximal attachment to the pelvic girdle. This is a common injury in individuals who participate in sports that involve sprinting with sudden starts and stops. Forced high kicks, especially with an extended knee, may avulse the muscle tendons from their origin at the ischial tuberosity. Symptoms include sudden, sharp pain in the back of the thigh during physical activity, a popping or tearing feeling in the muscle, swelling, muscle weakness, and an inability to bear weight on the affected leg.

— Three muscles of the thigh, the **sartorius**, **gracilis**, and **semitendinosus**, cross the knee medially and join to form the **pes anserinus**, a common tendon that overlies the **anserine bursa** inferomedial to the knee joint (see **Fig. 16.26**).

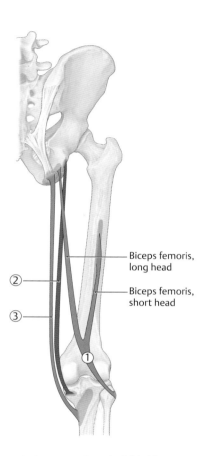

Biceps femoris, long head

②

Biceps femoris, short head

③

①

Thigh muscles, posterior compartment, right side.

Table 16.5 ▶ **Thigh Muscles, Posterior Compartment**				
Muscle	**Origin**	**Insertion**	**Innervation**	**Action**
① Biceps femoris	Long head: ischial tuberosity, sacrotuberous ligament (common head with semitendinosus)	Head of fibula	Tibial n. (L5–S2)	• Hip joint (long head): extends the hip, stabilizes the pelvis in the sagittal plane • Knee joint: flexion and external rotation
	Short head: lateral lip of the linea aspera in the middle third of the femur		Common fibular n. (L5–S2)	Knee joint: flexion and external rotation
② Semimembranosus	Ischial tuberosity	Medial tibial condyle, oblique popliteal ligament, popliteus fascia	Tibial n. (L5–S2)	• Hip joint: extends the hip, stabilizes the pelvis in the sagittal plane • Knee joint: flexion and internal rotation
③ Semitendinosus	Ischial tuberosity and sacrotuberous ligament (common head with long head of biceps femoris)	Medial to the tibial tuberosity in the pes anserinus (along with the tendons of gracilis and sartorius)		

16.4b Spaces of the Thigh

The femoral nerve, artery, and vein descend through narrow passages in the thigh that are created by the inguinal ligament and anterior and medial thigh muscles.

— Anteriorly, structures pass from the abdomen into the thigh through the **retroinguinal space**, deep to the inguinal ligament. The retroinguinal space is divided into a lateral muscular compartment and a medial vascular compartment (**Fig. 16.6**).

• The muscular compartment contains the femoral nerve and iliopsoas muscle.

• The vascular compartment contains the femoral vessels enclosed within the **femoral sheath**.

• The femoral sheath, formed by extensions of the transversalis and psoas fasciae, surrounds the femoral vessels as they pass under the inguinal ligament. Inferiorly, the sheath merges with the outer layer of the vessel walls (adventitia). Septa divide the sheath into compartments:

○ Lateral and central compartments contain the femoral artery and femoral vein, respectively.

○ A medial compartment within the sheath, the **femoral canal**, contains loose connective tissue, fat, and often a deep inguinal lymph node. The **femoral ring** defines the superior opening of the canal.

▮ Femoral hernias

Femoral hernias (usually of the small intestine) pass through the femoral ring and femoral canal and appear in the femoral triangle inferior and lateral to the pubic tubercle (below the inguinal ligament). They should be distinguished from inguinal hernias, which occur superior and lateral to the pubic tubercle (above the inguinal ligament).

Fig. 16.6 ► **Retroinguinal space: Muscular and vascular compartments**
Right inguinal region, anterior view.

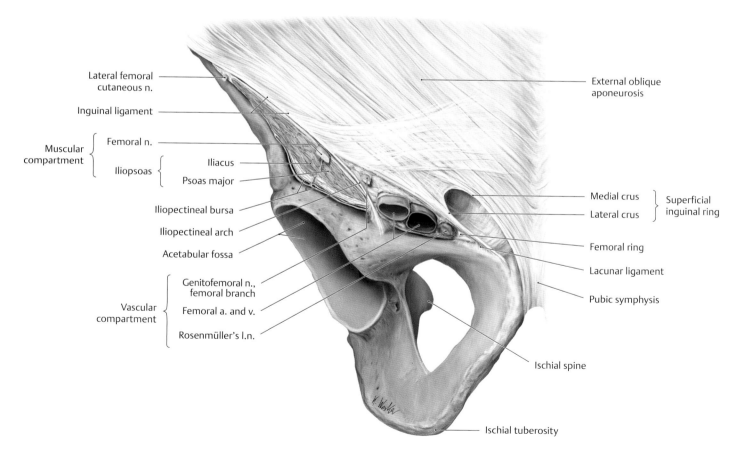

— The **femoral triangle** is an area of the anterior thigh (**Fig. 16.7**).

- It contains the femoral artery and vein and their branches and the terminal branches of the femoral nerve.
- Its boundaries are
  - superiorly, the inguinal ligament;
  - medially, the adductor longus muscle;
  - laterally, the sartorius muscle;
  - the floor, formed by the iliopsoas and pectineus muscles; and
  - the apex, formed by the inferior junction of the medial and lateral borders.

— The **adductor canal** is an intermuscular passage between the anterior and medial thigh muscles.

- It contains the femoral vessels and the saphenous branch of the femoral nerve.
- The canal begins at the inferior apex of the femoral triangle and ends at the **adductor hiatus**, an opening in the tendon of the adductor magnus muscle (see **Fig. 16.25B**).

Fig. 16.7 ▶ **Anterior thigh**
Right thigh, anterior view. *Revealed:* Femoral triangle. *Removed:* Skin, subcutaneous tissue, and fascia lata. *Partially transparent:* Sartorius.

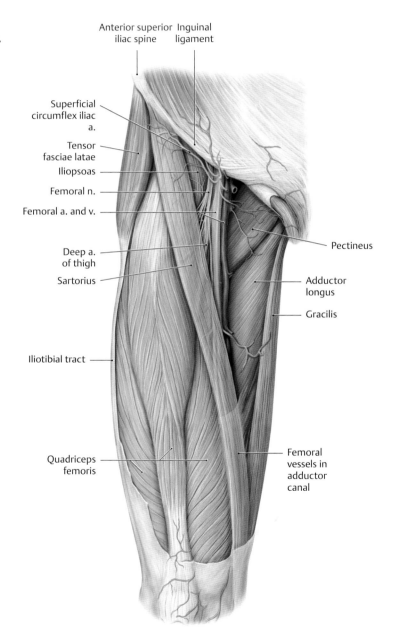

Anterior superior iliac spine

Inguinal ligament

Superficial circumflex iliac a.

Tensor fasciae latae

Iliopsoas

Femoral n.

Femoral a. and v.

Deep a. of thigh

Sartorius

Iliotibial tract

Quadriceps femoris

Pectineus

Adductor longus

Gracilis

Femoral vessels in adductor canal

16.5 The Knee and Popliteal Region

The popliteal region connects the thigh and leg. It contains the knee joint and the popliteal fossa and its contents.

16.5a The Knee Joint

The **knee joint** is a modified hinge joint that includes the medial and lateral articulations between the condyles of the femur and tibia, and the articulation between the femur and patella (**Fig. 16.8A** and **B**). Flexion and extension are the primary movements at the knee joint, but some rotation and sliding also occur.

— The patella articulates with the patellar surface of the femur between the medial and lateral condyles and protects the knee joint anteriorly. The patella is embedded in the tendon of the quadriceps femoris muscle, increasing the leverage of the muscle by holding the tendon away from the joint.

— Although the articular surfaces of the femur and tibia are extensive, there is little congruity between the bones, and stability depends chiefly on

- ligaments that connect the tibia and femur and
- muscles that surround the joint, most importantly the quadriceps femoris.

Fig. 16.8 ▶ **Right knee joint**

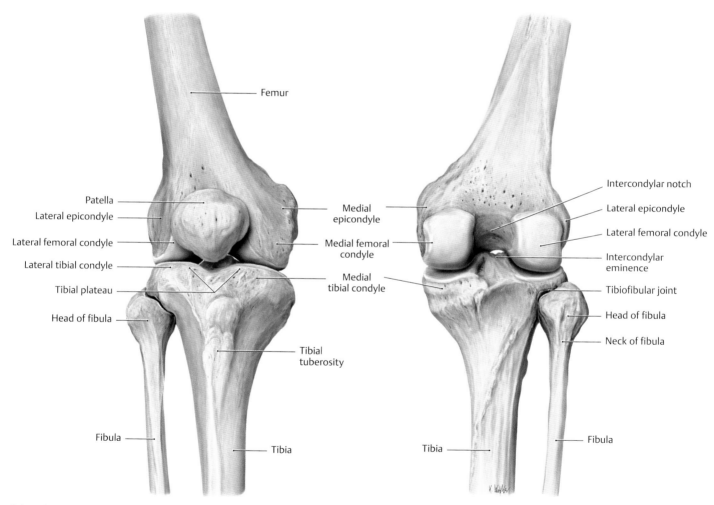

A Anterior view.

B Posterior view.

— The fibrous capsule of the knee joint is thin and incomplete and derives additional support from **patellar retinacula** (capsular ligaments that attach anteriorly to the quadriceps tendon), the patella, and **extracapsular ligaments** around the joint (**Fig. 16.9**).

Fig. 16.9 ▶ **Ligaments of the knee joint**
Right knee, anterior view.

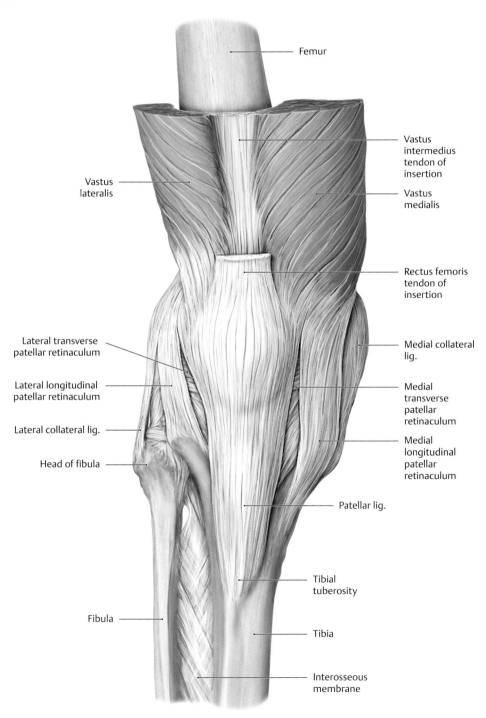

Femur

Vastus intermedius tendon of insertion

Vastus lateralis

Vastus medialis

Rectus femoris tendon of insertion

Lateral transverse patellar retinaculum

Medial collateral lig.

Lateral longitudinal patellar retinaculum

Medial transverse patellar retinaculum

Lateral collateral lig.

Head of fibula

Medial longitudinal patellar retinaculum

Patellar lig.

Tibial tuberosity

Fibula

Tibia

Interosseous membrane

— Extracapsular (external) ligaments support the fibrous capsule (**Figs. 16.10A** and **B** and **16.11**).

- The **patellar ligament**, the distal part of the quadriceps tendon that supports the knee joint anteriorly, extends from the patella to the tibial tuberosity.
- The two **collateral ligaments** limit rotation and prevent medial and lateral dislocation of the knee joint. They are tightest in extension and slacken during flexion.
    - The **lateral (fibular) collateral ligament** is cordlike and remains unattached to the joint capsule. It extends from the lateral epicondyle of the femur to the head of the fibula.
    - The **medial (tibial) collateral ligament** is flat and ribbonlike and is attached to the joint capsule and medial meniscus. It extends from the medial epicondyle of the femur to the medial condyle and anteromedial aspect of the tibia.

Patellar tendon reflex

The patellar tendon reflex is initiated by tapping the patellar tendon to elicit contraction of the quadriceps femoris muscle (extension of the knee). It tests the integrity of the L2–L4 spinal cord segments carried by the femoral nerve.

Fig. 16.10 ► **Collateral and patellar ligaments of the knee joint**
Right knee joint. Each knee joint has medial and lateral collateral ligaments. The medial collateral ligament is attached to both the capsule and the medial meniscus, whereas the lateral collateral ligament has no direct contact with either the capsule or the lateral meniscus. Both collateral ligaments are taut when the knee is in extension and stabilize the joint in the coronal plane.

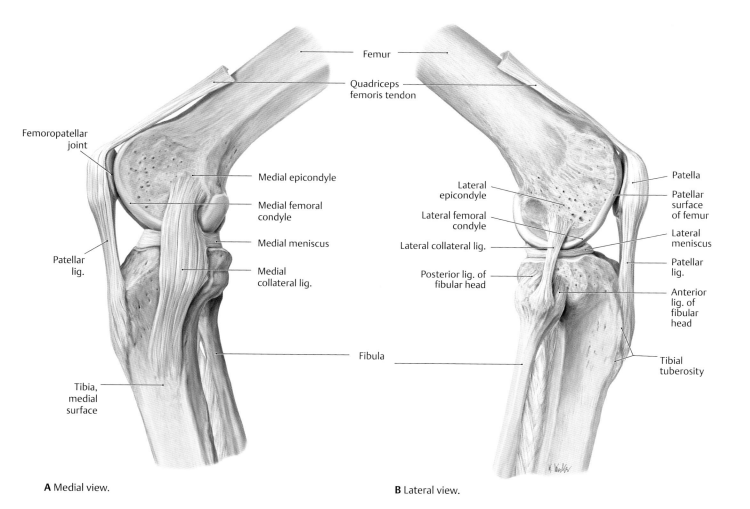

A Medial view.

B Lateral view.

- The **oblique popliteal ligament** is an expansion of the semimembranosus tendon, which supports the joint capsule posteriorly and laterally.
- The **arcuate popliteal ligament** extends from the fibular head to the posterior knee joint and reinforces the joint capsule posteriorly and laterally.

Fig. 16.11 ► **Capsule, ligaments, and periarticular bursae of the knee joint**
Right knee, posterior view.

— Intra-articular ligaments provide stability during movements of the joint (**Fig. 16.12A** and **B**).
  - Two **cruciate ligaments** are located within the joint capsule but lie external to the synovial layer. They provide stability in all positions, in addition to limiting rotation and preventing anterior and posterior dislocation of the joint.
    - The **anterior cruciate ligament** arises from the anterior intercondylar part of the tibia and extends posterolaterally to the medial aspect of the lateral femoral condyle.
    - The **posterior cruciate ligament** arises from the posterior intercondylar part of the tibia and extends anteromedially to the lateral aspect of the medial femoral condyle.
  - A **transverse ligament** connects the menisci to each other along their anterior edges.
  - A **posterior meniscofemoral ligament** joins the lateral meniscus to the posterior cruciate ligament and medial femoral condyle.

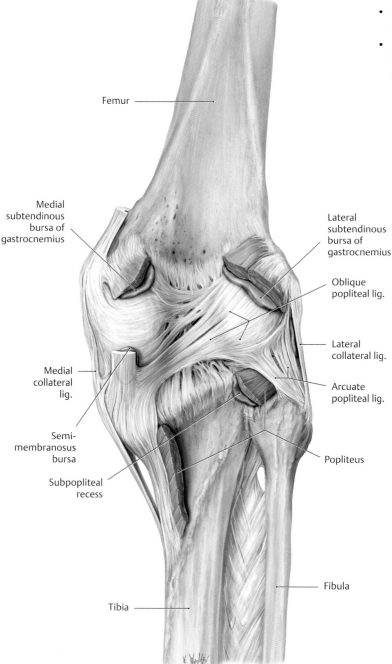

Fig. 16.12 ▶ **Cruciate and collateral ligaments of the knee joint**
Right knee. The cruciate ligaments keep the articular surfaces of the
femur and tibia in contact, while stabilizing the knee joint primarily in the
sagittal plane. Portions of the cruciate ligaments are taut in every joint
position.

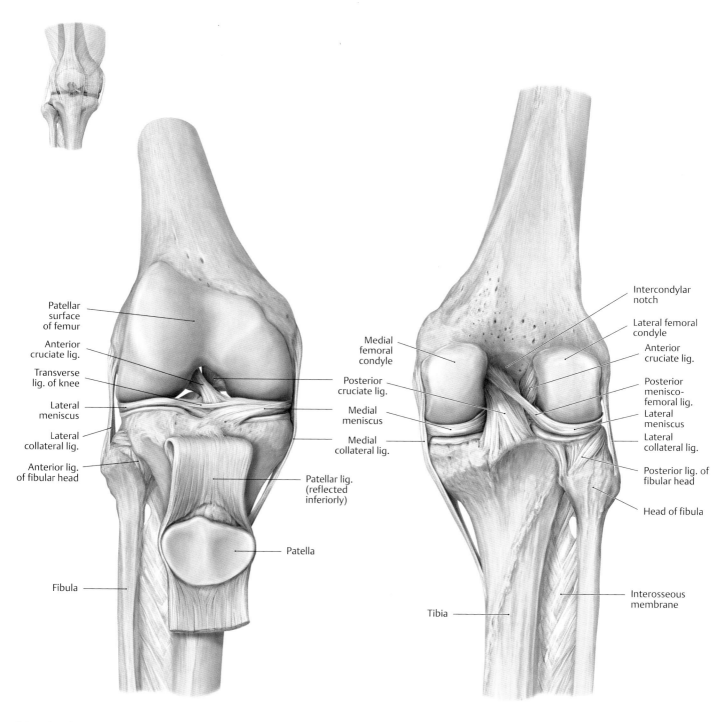

Patellar
surface
of femur

Anterior
cruciate lig.

Transverse
lig. of knee

Lateral
meniscus

Lateral
collateral lig.

Anterior lig.
of fibular head

Fibula

Posterior
cruciate lig.

Medial
meniscus

Medial
collateral lig.

Patellar lig.
(reflected
inferiorly)

Patella

Intercondylar
notch

Lateral femoral
condyle

Anterior
cruciate lig.

Posterior
menisco-
femoral lig.

Lateral
meniscus

Lateral
collateral lig.

Posterior lig. of
fibular head

Head of fibula

Medial
femoral
condyle

Medial
meniscus

Interosseous
membrane

Tibia

A Anterior view.

B Posterior view.

— **Menisci**, crescent-shaped fibrocartilaginous pads, deepen the articular surfaces of the tibial plateau (**Fig. 16.13**). Wedge-shaped in cross section, they are tallest at the outer rim, where they are attached to the joint capsule and the intercondylar ridge.

- The **medial meniscus** is C-shaped and relatively immobile due to its additional attachment to the tibial collateral ligament.
- The **lateral meniscus** is nearly circular and more mobile during flexion and extension of the joint than its medial counterpart.

— An extensive synovial layer lines the internal surface of the joint capsule. Its posterior aspect extends into the intercondylar space of the joint cavity and reflects around the intracapsular ligaments, dividing most of the joint space into medial and lateral parts (**Figs. 16.14** and **16.15**).

— At least 12 bursae are associated with the knee joint. The most important of these are

- the **suprapatellar bursa** (pouch), which lies deep to the quadriceps femoris tendon and communicates with the cavity of the knee joint;
- the **prepatellar bursa**, which is subcutaneous over the patella;
- the **superficial infrapatellar bursa**, which is subcutaneous over the patellar ligament;
- the **deep infrapatellar bursa**, which lies deep to the patellar ligament; and
- the **anserine bursa**, which lies between the pes anserinus and tibial collateral ligament.

— Muscles of the thigh and leg move the knee joint (**Table 16.6**).

Fig. 16.13 ▶ **Menisci in the knee joint**
Right tibial plateau with cruciate, patellar, and collateral ligaments divided, proximal view.

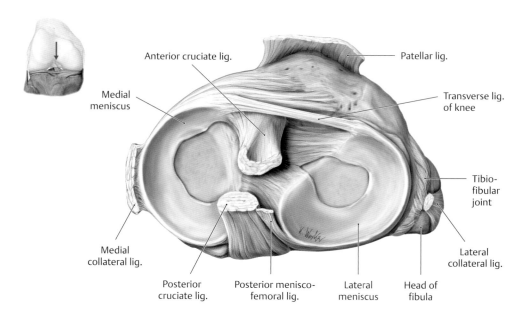

Anterior cruciate lig.

Medial meniscus

Patellar lig.

Transverse lig. of knee

Tibio-fibular joint

Medial collateral lig.

Lateral collateral lig.

Posterior cruciate lig.

Posterior menisco-femoral lig.

Lateral meniscus

Head of fibula

Genu varum and genu valgum

Although the femur lies diagonally within the thigh, the tibia is nearly vertical in the leg. This creates a Q angle at the knee between the long axes of the two bones. The angle varies with developmental stage and sex, but it can also be altered by disease. Normally, the head of the femur sits over the center of the knee joint, distributing weight evenly on the tibial plateau. In genu varum (bowleg), the Q angle is smaller than normal because the femur is more vertical. This increases the weight on the medial side of the knee, putting additional stress on the medial meniscus and medial (tibial) collateral ligament. When standing upright with feet and ankles together, the knees are wide apart. In genu valgum (knock knee), the Q angle is larger because the femur is more diagonal. Greater weight is put on the lateral side of the knee, stressing the lateral meniscus and lateral (fibular) collateral ligament. In the upright position, the knees touch, but the ankles do not.

Ligamentous injuries of the knee

Most knee injuries occur during physical activity and involve rupture or strain of the knee ligaments. A forceful blow to the lateral side of the knee can strain the medial collateral ligament and, because of their intimate relationship, tear the medial meniscus as well. A similar injury can result from excessive lateral rotation of the knee and is often accompanied by rupture of the anterior cruciate ligament (often called the "unhappy triad").

The Lachman test is used to demonstrate instability of the knee joint resulting from rupture of the cruciate ligaments. Excessive anterior translation of the free-hanging tibia from under the stabilized femur is a positive anterior drawer sign, indicating anterior cruciate rupture. Posterior displacement of the tibia is a positive posterior drawer sign, indicating rupture of the posterior cruciate ligament.

Fig. 16.14 ▶ **Joint cavity of the knee**
Right knee, lateral view. The joint cavity was demonstrated by injecting liquid plastic into the knee joint and later removing the capsule.

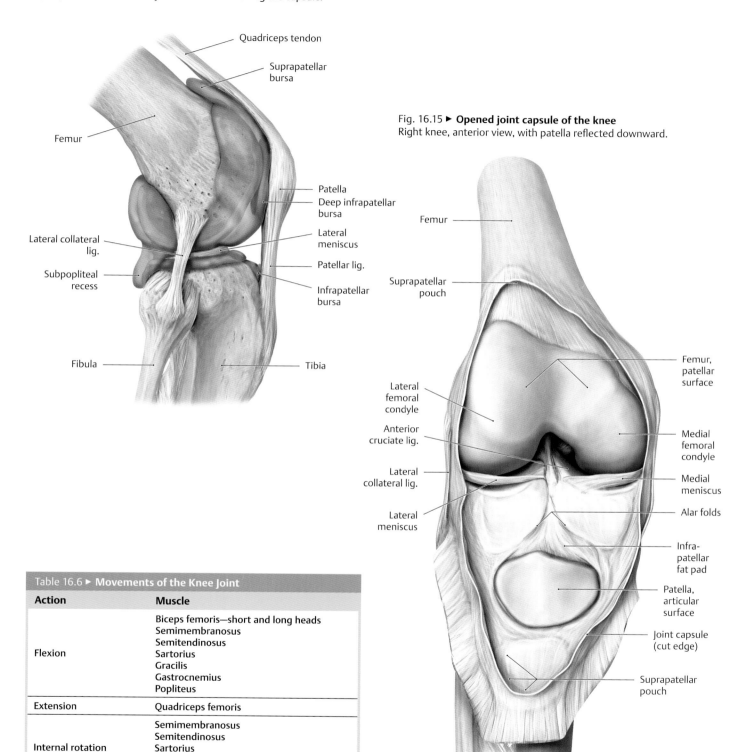

Fig. 16.15 ▶ **Opened joint capsule of the knee**
Right knee, anterior view, with patella reflected downward.

Table 16.6 ▶ Movements of the Knee Joint	
Action	**Muscle**
Flexion	Biceps femoris—short and long heads Semimembranosus Semitendinosus Sartorius Gracilis Gastrocnemius Popliteus
Extension	Quadriceps femoris
Internal rotation	Semimembranosus Semitendinosus Sartorius Gracilis Popliteus (of nonbearing leg)
External rotation	Biceps femoris

16.5b The Popliteal Fossa

The **popliteal fossa** is a diamond-shaped space posterior to the knee joint (**Fig. 16.16A** and **B**).

— Its muscular boundaries are
  • superomedially, the semimembranosus muscle;
  • superolaterally, the biceps femoris muscle; and
  • inferiorly, the medial and lateral heads of the gastrocnemius muscle.

— The contents of the fossa, which are embedded within popliteal fat, include
  • the popliteal artery and vein and their genicular branches,
  • popliteal lymph nodes, and
  • tibial and common fibular nerves.

— At the superior apex of the popliteal fossa, the sciatic nerve splits into its two terminal branches.
  • The tibial nerve descends into the posterior leg compartment with the popliteal vessels.
  • The common fibular nerve courses laterally along the edge of the biceps femoris muscle to enter the lateral leg compartment.

Popliteal (Baker's) cyst

Popliteal (Baker's) cysts, palpable fluid-filled synovial sacs that protrude into the popliteal fossa, are usually a consequence of chronic effusion of the knee joint. Often they result from a herniation of the bursae deep to the gastrocnemius or semimembranosus muscles. The sacs protrude through the fibrous layer of the joint capsule but maintain a communication with the synovial cavity. Some cysts may be asymptomatic, but others are painful and can impair flexion and extension of the knee joint.

Fig. 16.16 ▶ **Popliteal fossa**
Right leg, posterior view.

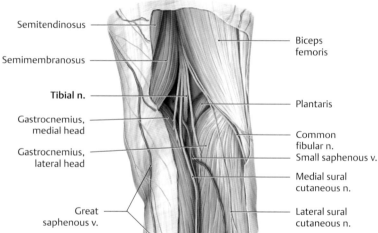

A Superficial neurovascular structures.

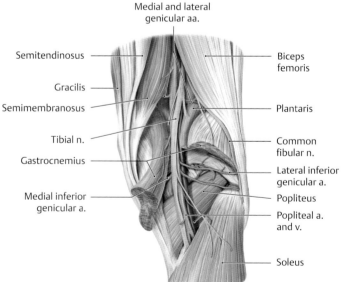

B Deep neurovascular structures.

16.6 The Leg

The leg extends from the knee to the ankle; it contains the tibia and fibula and the muscles of the leg (crural) compartments.

16.6a Tibiofibular Joints

The tibia and fibula are joined proximally at the knee and distally at the ankle. Unlike the extensive movement at the radioulnar joints in the forearm, only slight movement occurs at each tibiofibular joint, and no muscles are directly associated with them.

Fig. 16.17 ▶ **Ligaments of the ankle and foot**
Right foot.

— The proximal **tibiofibular joint** is a plane-type synovial joint between the fibular head and an articular facet of the lateral condyle of the tibia. **Anterior** and **posterior ligaments of the fibular head** secure the joint (see **Fig. 16.12A** and **B**).
— The distal **tibiofibular joint**, a compound fibrous joint, creates a mortise formed by the medial and lateral malleoli that cups the talus and stabilizes the ankle joint. Ligaments of the tibiofibular joint (**Fig. 16.17A** and **B**) include

- a deep **interosseous tibiofibular ligament**, the primary support of the joint, which is continuous with the interosseous membrane of the leg, and
- the external **anterior tibiofibular** and **posterior tibiofibular ligaments**.

— An interosseous membrane unites the shafts of the tibia and fibula and provides stability to the distal tibiofibular and ankle joints.

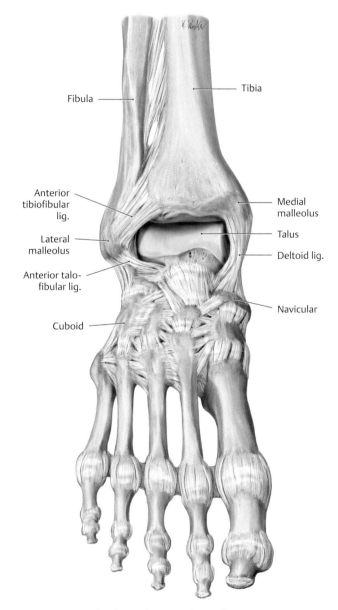

A Anterior view with talocrural joint in plantar flexion.

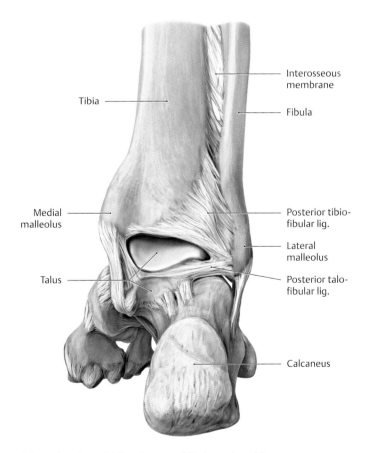

B Posterior view with foot in neutral (0-degree) position.

16.6b Muscles of the Leg

Muscles of the leg, which move the knee, ankle, and foot, are divided into four crural compartments.

— The anterior compartment contains

- muscles that dorsiflex the foot and toes and invert the foot (**Table 16.7**),
- the deep fibular nerve, and
- the anterior tibial artery and veins.

> ### Shin splints
>
> Shin splints result from chronic trauma of the tibialis anterior, usually incurred by overuse of the muscle during athletic activities. In what is considered a mild form of anterior compartment syndrome, small tears of the periosteum cause pain and swelling over the distal two thirds of the tibial shaft.

— The lateral compartment contains

- muscles that evert and plantar flex the foot (**Table 16.8**),
- the superficial fibular nerve, and
- the muscular branches of the fibular artery and veins from the posterior compartment.

— The superficial posterior compartment contains

- muscles that plantar flex the foot, two of which, the gastrocnemius and soleus, form the **triceps surae** and share a common tendon of insertion, the **calcaneal tendon** (**Table 16.9**);
- the tibial nerve; and
- the muscular branches of the posterior tibial artery and veins from the deep posterior compartment.

> ### Rupture of the calcaneal tendon
>
> Rupture of the calcaneal tendon tends to occur following sudden forced plantar flexion of the foot, unexpected dorsiflexion of the foot, or violent dorsiflexion of a plantar-flexed foot in people unaccustomed to exercise or who exercise intermittently. The rupture disables the gastrocnemius, soleus, and plantaris muscles, rendering the patient unable to plantar flex the foot.

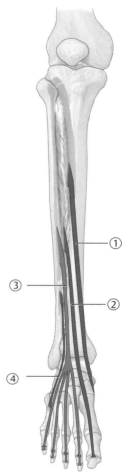

Leg muscles, anterior compartment
Right leg, anterior view.

Table 16.7 ▶ Leg Muscles, Anterior Compartment				
Muscle	**Origin**	**Insertion**	**Innervation**	**Action**
① Tibialis anterior	Tibia (upper two thirds of the lateral surface), interosseous membrane, superficial crural fascia (highest part)	Medial cuneiform (medial and plantar surface), first metatarsal (medial base)	Deep fibular n. (L4–L5)	• Talocrural joint: dorsiflexion • Subtalar joint: inversion (supination)
② Extensor hallucis longus	Fibula (middle third of the medial surface), interosseous membrane	1st toe (at the dorsal aponeurosis and the base of its distal phalanx)	Deep fibular n. (L5)	• Talocrural joint: dorsiflexion • Subtalar joint: active in both eversion and inversion (pronation/supination), depending on the initial position of the foot • Extends the MTP and IP joints of the big toe
③ Extensor digitorum longus	Fibula (head and anterior border), tibia (lateral condyle), interosseous membrane	2nd to 5th toes (at the dorsal aponeuroses and bases of the distal phalanges)	Deep fibular n. (L5–S1)	• Talocrural joint: dorsiflexion • Subtalar joint: eversion (pronation) • Extends the MTP and IP joints of the 2nd to 5th toes
④ Fibularis tertius	Distal fibula (anterior border)	5th metatarsal (base)	Deep fibular n. (L5–S1)	• Talocrural joint: dorsiflexion • Subtalar joint: eversion (pronation)
Abbreviations: IP, interphalangeal; MTP, metatarsophalangeal.				

Table 16.8 ▶ Leg Muscles, Lateral Compartment

Muscle	Origin	Insertion	Innervation	Action
① Fibularis longus	Fibula (head and proximal two thirds of the lateral surface, arising partly from the intermuscular septa)	Medial cuneiform (plantar side), 1st metatarsal (base)	Superficial fibular n. (L5–S1)	• Talocrural joint: plantar flexion • Subtalar joint: eversion (pronation) • Supports the transverse arch of the foot
② Fibularis brevis	Fibula (distal half of the lateral surface), intermuscular septa	5th metatarsal (tuberosity at the base, with an occasional division to the dorsal aponeurosis of the 5th toe)		• Talocrural joint: plantar flexion • Subtalar joint: eversion (pronation)

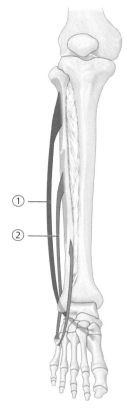

Leg muscles, lateral compartment
Right leg and foot, anterior view.

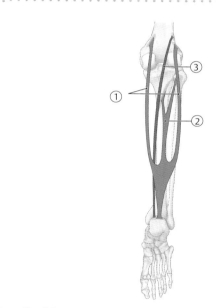

Superficial flexors, posterior compartment of leg
Right leg with foot in plantar flexion, posterior view,

Table 16.9 ▶ Leg Muscles, Posterior Compartment: Superficial Flexors

Muscle		Origin	Insertion	Innervation	Action
Triceps surae	① Gastrocnemius	Femur (medial and lateral epicondyles)	Calcaneal tuberosity via the Achilles' tendon	Tibial n. (S1–S2)	• Talocrural joint: plantar flexion • Knee joint: flexion (gastrocnemius)
	② Soleus	Fibula (head and neck, posterior surface), tibia (soleal line via a tendinous arch)			
③ Plantaris		Femur (lateral epicondyle, proximal to lateral head of gastrocnemius)			Negligible; may prevent compression of posterior leg musculature during knee flexion

— The deep posterior compartment contains

- muscles that plantar flex the foot and toes and invert the foot (**Table 16.10**) (only one muscle, the popliteus, crosses the knee and laterally rotates the femur),
- the tibial nerve, and
- the posterior tibial and fibular artery and veins.

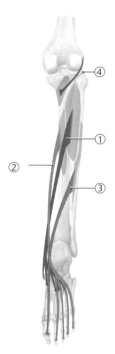

Deep flexors, posterior compartment of leg
Right leg with foot in plantar flexion, posterior view.

Compartment syndrome

Compartment syndrome is a condition that may follow burns, hemorrhage, complex fractures, or crush injuries. Swelling, infection, or bleeding into the compartment can increase intracompartmental pressure and, when high enough, compress the small vascular structures that supply the compartment contents. Nerves are particularly vulnerable to ischemia, and permanent loss of motor and sensory functions distal to the compartment can result. Symptoms include severe pain that is out of proportion to the injury, paresthesia (tingling and numbness), pallor of the skin, paralysis of muscles affected, and loss of distal pulses in the affected limb. Treatment is prompt surgery to decompress the compartment by making long cuts through the fascia (fasciotomy).

— Retinacula, thickened bands of the crural fascia, bind the tendons of the long extensor and flexor muscles as they cross the ankle (**Fig. 16.18A, B,** and **C**).

- **Superior extensor** and **inferior extensor retinacula** bind muscles of the anterior compartment.
- Medially, a **flexor retinaculum** binds muscles of the deep posterior compartment.
- **Superior fibular** and **inferior fibular retinacula** bind muscles of the lateral compartment.

— The **tarsal tunnel** is a passageway on the medial side of the ankle formed by the flexor retinaculum and its attachments to the medial malleolus and calcaneus. It transmits

- muscle tendons of the deep posterior compartment,
- posterior tibial artery and veins and their medial plantar and lateral plantar branches, and
- the tibial nerve and its medial plantar and lateral plantar branches.

Tarsal tunnel syndrome

Tarsal tunnel syndrome, similar to carpal tunnel syndrome of the hand, results from swelling of the synovial sheaths of the long flexor tendons within the tarsal tunnel. Compression of the tibial nerve can result in burning pain, numbness, and tingling that radiates to the heel.

Table 16.10 ▶ **Leg Muscles, Posterior Compartment: Deep Flexors**				
Muscle	**Origin**	**Insertion**	**Innervation**	**Action**
① Tibialis posterior	Interosseous membrane, adjacent borders of tibia and fibula	Navicular tuberosity; cuneiforms (medial, intermediate, and lateral); 2nd to 4th metatarsals (bases)	Tibial n. (L4–L5)	• Talocrural joint: plantar flexion • Subtalar joint: inversion (supination) • Supports the longitudinal and transverse arches
② Flexor digitorum longus	Tibia (middle third of posterior surface)	2nd to 5th distal phalanges (bases)	Tibial n. (L5–S2)	• Talocrural joint: plantar flexion • Subtalar joint: inversion (supination) • MTP and IP joints of the 2nd to 5th toes: plantar flexion
③ Flexor hallucis longus	Fibula (distal two thirds of posterior surface), adjacent interosseous membrane	1st distal phalanx (base)		• Talocrural joint: plantar flexion • Subtalar joint: inversion (supination) • MTP and IP joints of the 2nd to 5th toes: plantar flexion • Supports the medial longitudinal arch
④ Popliteus	Lateral femoral condyle, posterior horn of the lateral meniscus	Posterior tibial surface (above the origin at the soleus)	Tibial n. (L4–S1)	Knee joint: flexion and internal rotation (stabilizes the knee)

Abbreviations: IP, interphalangeal; MTP, metatarsophalangeal.

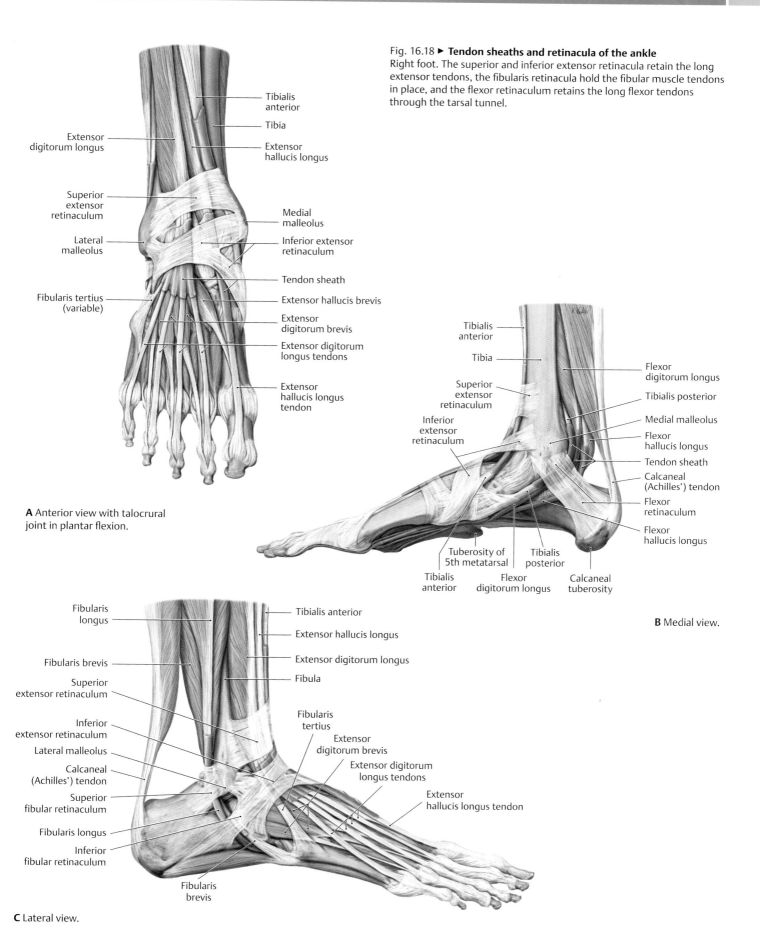

Tibialis anterior

Tibia

Extensor digitorum longus

Extensor hallucis longus

Superior extensor retinaculum

Medial malleolus

Lateral malleolus

Inferior extensor retinaculum

Tendon sheath

Fibularis tertius (variable)

Extensor hallucis brevis

Extensor digitorum brevis

Extensor digitorum longus tendons

Extensor hallucis longus tendon

Fig. 16.18 ► **Tendon sheaths and retinacula of the ankle**
Right foot. The superior and inferior extensor retinacula retain the long extensor tendons, the fibularis retinacula hold the fibular muscle tendons in place, and the flexor retinaculum retains the long flexor tendons through the tarsal tunnel.

Tibialis anterior

Tibia

Superior extensor retinaculum

Inferior extensor retinaculum

Flexor digitorum longus

Tibialis posterior

Medial malleolus

Flexor hallucis longus

Tendon sheath

Calcaneal (Achilles') tendon

Flexor retinaculum

Flexor hallucis longus

Tuberosity of 5th metatarsal

Tibialis posterior

Tibialis anterior

Flexor digitorum longus

Calcaneal tuberosity

A Anterior view with talocrural joint in plantar flexion.

B Medial view.

Fibularis longus

Fibularis brevis

Superior extensor retinaculum

Inferior extensor retinaculum

Lateral malleolus

Calcaneal (Achilles') tendon

Superior fibular retinaculum

Fibularis longus

Inferior fibular retinaculum

Fibularis brevis

Tibialis anterior

Extensor hallucis longus

Extensor digitorum longus

Fibula

Fibularis tertius

Extensor digitorum brevis

Extensor digitorum longus tendons

Extensor hallucis longus tendon

C Lateral view.

Fig. 16.19 ► **Joints of the foot**
Right foot with talocrural joint in plantar flexion, anterior view.

16.7 The Ankle (Talocrural) Joint

The weight of the body is transferred along the tibia of the leg, through the talus at the ankle joint, and onto the heel and ball of the foot. Strong bony and ligamentous supports stabilize the ankle and facilitate this transfer of weight.

The **ankle joint** includes articulations between the distal tibia and fibula and the talus (**Figs. 16.19** and **16.20**).

— At the ankle joint, the ankle mortise, which is formed by the distal tibiofibular joint, hugs the body of the talus. Tibiofibular ligaments that stabilize the ankle mortise also contribute to the stability of the ankle joint.
— The ankle joint is tighter and more stable with the foot in dorsiflexion, when the wider anterior part of the trochlea (of the talus) is wedged within the ankle mortise. Accordingly, the joint is looser and less stable in plantar flexion.

Fig. 16.20 ► **Talocrural and subtalar joints**
Right foot with foot in neutral (0-degree) position, posterior view.

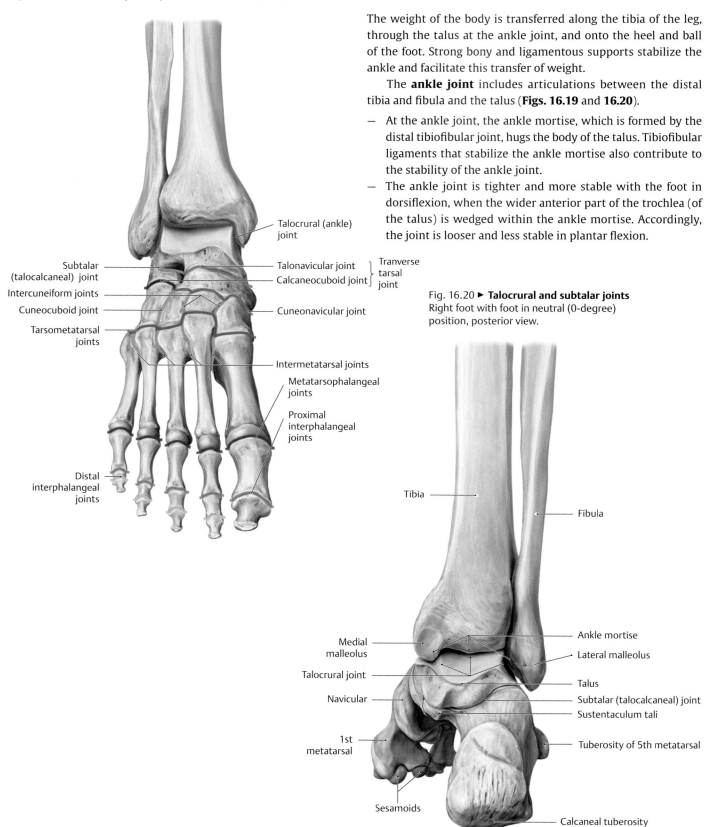

— Strong collateral talocrural ligaments connect the tibia and fibula to the tarsal bones and support the talocrural articulations (**Fig. 16.21A** and **B**).

- The medial **deltoid ligament** of the ankle extends from the medial malleolus of the tibia to the talus, calcaneus, and navicular. Its components are
  - the **anterior tibiotalar part**,
  - the **posterior tibiotalar part**,
  - the **tibiocalcaneal part**, and
  - the **tibionavicular part**.
- The **lateral ligament of the ankle** extends from the lateral malleolus of the fibula to the talus and calcaneus. Its parts are
  - the **anterior talofibular ligament**,
  - the **posterior talofibular ligament**, and
  - the **calcaneofibular ligament**.

Fig. 16.21 ▶ **Ligaments of the ankle and foot**
Right foot.

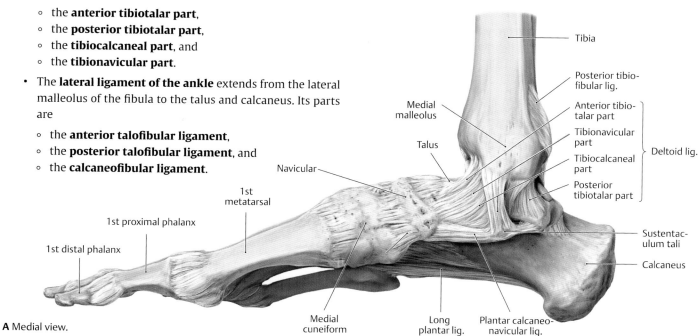

A Medial view.

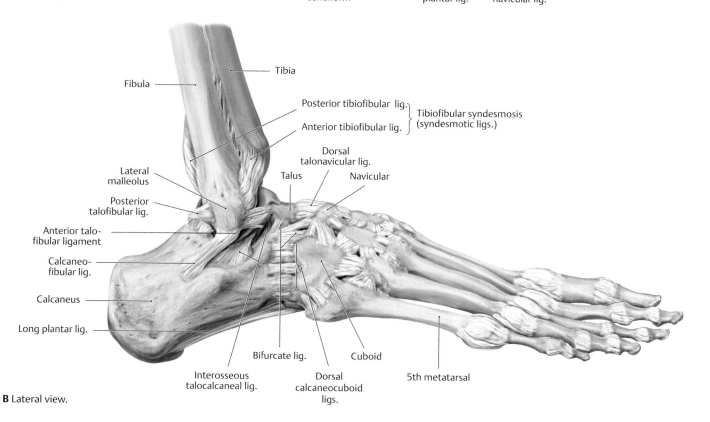

B Lateral view.

Ankle sprains

Ankle sprains (torn ligaments) are caused most often by forced inversion of the foot (e.g., walking on uneven ground). Damage to the lateral talocrural ligaments is correlated with the severity of the injury and proceeds from anterior to posterior: the anterior talofibular ligament is the most easily injured, followed by the calcaneofibular and the least frequently injured, the posterior talofibular ligament. Fracture of the lateral malleolus can also accompany inversion injuries.

- Movement at the ankle joint, provided by muscles of the leg, is limited primarily to dorsiflexion (extension) and plantar flexion (**Table 16.11**).

Table 16.11 ▶ Movements of the Ankle Joint	
Action	**Muscle**
Plantar flexion	Gastrocnemius Soleus Posterior tibialis Flexor digitorum longus Flexor hallucis longus
Dorsiflexion	Tibialis anterior Extensor hallucis longus Extensor digitorum longus Fibularis tertius

16.8 The Foot

The numerous joints of the foot create a flexible unit that effectively absorbs shock, distributes the weight of vertical loads, and participates in locomotion.

16.8a Joints of the Foot and Toes

Movements at the joints of the foot, particularly the intertarsal (subtalar and transverse tarsal), metatarsophalangeal, and interphalangeal joints, contribute to smooth locomotion and maintenance of balance (see **Figs. 16.19, 16.20,** and **16.21A** and **B**).

— The **subtalar joint** is an articulation between the inferior surface of the talus and underlying calcaneus (**Fig. 16.22**).

- It is a compound joint that has anterior and posterior compartments.
  - The anterior compartment contains the talocalcaneal component of the talocalcaneonavicular articulation.
  - The posterior compartment contains the posterior talocalcaneal articulation.

- A strong **interosseous talocalcaneal ligament** joins the bones and separates the anterior and posterior parts of the joint.
- This joint is the main articulation that allows inversion and eversion of the foot.

— The **transverse tarsal joint** is a compound joint that combines the talonavicular and calcaneocuboid articulations.

- Movement at this joint rotates the front of the foot relative to the heel, augmenting the inversion and eversion at the subtalar joint.
- This joint is a common site for surgical amputation of the foot.

— **The tarsometatarsal** and **intermetatarsal joints** are small and relatively immobile.

— **Metatarsophalangeal joints** are condyloid synovial joints between the heads of the metatarsals and base of the phalanges.

- Flexion, extension, and some abduction and adduction occur at this joint.

Fig. 16.22 ▶ Subtalar joint and ligaments
Right foot with opened subtalar joint, dorsal view. The subtalar joint consists of two distinct articulations separated by the interosseous talocalcaneal ligament: the posterior compartment (talocalcaneal joint) and the anterior compartment (talocalcaneonavicular joint).

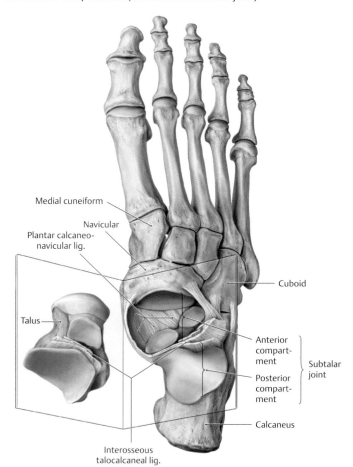

— **Interphalangeal joints** are hinge-type synovial joints that primarily allow flexion and extension of the toes, with some inversion and eversion of the foot.

- Digits 2 through 4 have **proximal interphalangeal (PIP)** and **distal interphalangeal (DIP) joints**.
- The great toe has only a single interphalangeal joint.

— Muscles of the leg and foot move the joints of the foot (**Table 16.12**).

Table 16.12 ▶ Movements of the Joints of the Foot	
Action	**Muscle**
Subtalar joint	
Inversion	Tibialis anterior Tibialis posterior
Eversion	Fibularis longus Fibularis brevis Fibularis tertius
Metatarsophalangeal and interphalangeal joints	
Flexion	Flexor hallucis longus Flexor hallucis brevis Flexor digitorum longus Flexor digitorum brevis Lumbricals Interossei
Extension	Extensor hallucis longus Extensor hallucis brevis Extensor digitorum longus Extensor digitorum brevis
Abduction	Abductor hallucis Abductor digiti minimi Dorsal interossei
Adduction	Adductor hallucis Plantar interossei

16.8b Arches of the Foot

The tarsal and metatarsal bones form flexible longitudinal and transverse arches on the sole of the foot.

— The arches function as a unit to
- distribute weight onto the heel and ball of the foot,
- act as shock absorbers during locomotion, and
- enhance the flexibility of the foot when planted on uneven surfaces.

— The longitudinal arch has medial and lateral parts (see **Fig. 15.6B** and **D**).

- The medial arch is the highest part of the longitudinal arch, formed by the talus, navicular, three cuneiforms, and medial metatarsals. The head of the talus is the keystone of the arch.
- The lateral arch is flatter than the medial arch and is formed by the calcaneus, cuboid, and lateral metatarsals.

— The transverse arch, formed by the cuboid, cuneiforms, and bases of the metatarsals, crosses the midfoot.

— The arches are supported by active and passive stabilizers (**Figs. 16.23** and **16.24**).

- The primary active stabilizers of the arches are muscles of the leg and foot:
  ◦ The tibialis posterior and fibularis longus of the leg
  ◦ The short flexors, abductors, and adductors of the foot

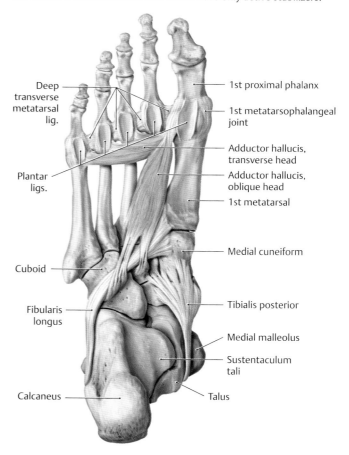

Fig. 16.23 ▶ Stabilizers of the transverse arch
Right foot, plantar view. The transverse pedal arch is supported by both active and passive stabilizing structures (muscles and ligaments, respectively). *Note:* The arch of the forefoot has only passive stabilizers, whereas the arches of the metatarsus and tarsus have only active stabilizers.

Deep transverse metatarsal lig.

Plantar ligs.

Cuboid

Fibularis longus

Calcaneus

1st proximal phalanx

1st metatarsophalangeal joint

Adductor hallucis, transverse head

Adductor hallucis, oblique head

1st metatarsal

Medial cuneiform

Tibialis posterior

Medial malleolus

Sustentaculum tali

Talus

Fig. 16.24 ▶ **Stabilizers of the longitudinal arch**
Right foot, medial view. Passive stabilizers (ligaments) of the longitudinal arch.

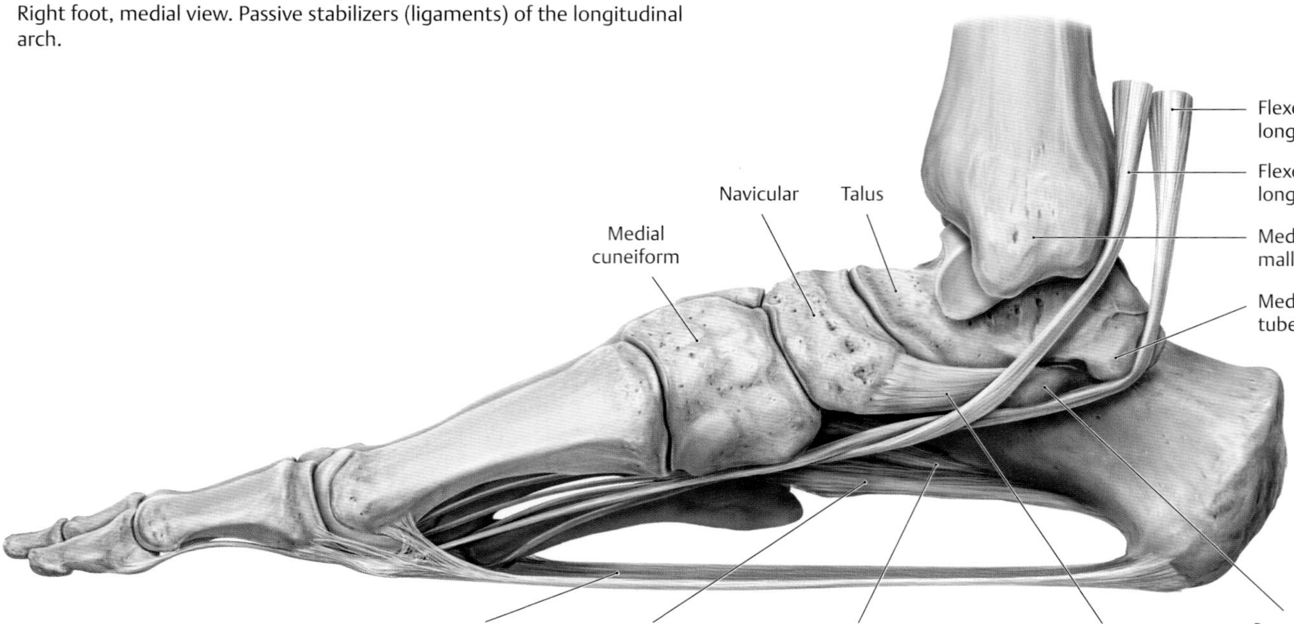

- The primary passive stabilizers of the arches are ligaments of the foot:
  - The plantar aponeurosis
  - The **plantar calcaneonavicular ligament** (spring ligament)
  - The **long plantar ligament**
  - The **plantar calcaneocuboid ligament** (short plantar ligament)

Pes planus

Pes planus, or flatfoot, is a condition in which both the active and the passive stabilizers of the medial longitudinal arch are lax or absent. Because the head of the talus is not supported, it can displace inferomedially, and the forefoot everts and abducts, putting increased stress on the plantar calcaneonavicular (spring) ligament. Pes planus commonly occurs in older individuals who stand for long periods. Flatfoot is normal in children younger than 3 years, but this resolves with maturity.

16.8c Dorsum of the Foot

— Surface anatomy on the dorsum of the foot reveals
  - skin that is thin and loose,
  - a superficial dorsal venous arch that is the origin of the great saphenous and small saphenous veins, and
  - tendons of extensor muscles of the anterior leg compartment.
— A **dorsal muscular compartment** of the foot contains two intrinsic muscles, the **extensor digitorum brevis** and the **extensor hallucis brevis**, which extend the toes (**Table 16.13**).

16.8d Sole of the Foot

— Surface anatomy on the sole of the foot reveals
  - tough, thickened skin, particularly on the heel, lateral side, and ball of the foot;
  - skin that is firmly attached to the underlying plantar aponeurosis; and
  - subcutaneous tissue divided by fibrous septa into fat-filled areas that act as shock absorbers, especially in the heel.
— The tough, longitudinal plantar aponeurosis (see **Fig. 16.32**)
  - attaches tightly to the skin of the sole,
  - originates at the calcaneus and is continuous distally with the fibrous digital sheaths that contain the flexor tendons of the toes,
  - protects the sole of the foot from injury, and
  - acts as a tie rod that supports the arches of the foot.
— The musculature of the sole is usually described as having four layers (**Tables 16.14** and **16.15**). However, as in the palm of the hand, the deep fascia separates the muscles of the sole into four fascial compartments:
  - The **medial compartment**, which contains the abductor and flexors of the 1st digit (hallux)
  - The **central compartment**, which contains the short and long flexors of the 2nd through 4th digits, the adductor hallucis, the lumbricals, and the quadratus plantae
  - The **lateral compartment**, which contains the abductor and flexor of the 5th digit
  - The **interosseous compartment**, which contains the interossei muscles

Table 16.13 ▶ Intrinsic Muscles of the Dorsum of the Foot

Muscle	Origin	Insertion	Innervation	Action
① Extensor digitorum brevis	Calcaneus (dorsal surface)	2nd to 4th toes (at dorsal aponeuroses and bases of the middle phalanges)	Deep fibular n. (L5–S1)	Extension of the MTP and PIP joints of the 2nd to 4th toes
② Extensor hallucis brevis		1st toe (at dorsal aponeurosis and proximal phalanx)		Extension of the MTP joints of the 1st toe

Abbreviations: MTP, metatarsophalangeal; PIP, proximal interphalangeal.

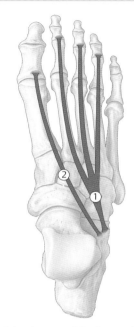

Intrinsic muscles of the dorsum of the foot, right foot, dorsal view.

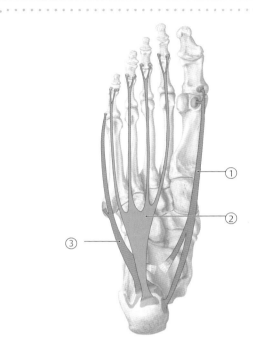

Superficial intrinsic muscles of the sole of the foot, right foot, first layer, plantar view.

Table 16.14 ▶ Superficial Intrinsic Muscles of the Sole of the Foot

Muscle	Origin	Insertion	Innervation	Action
① Abductor hallucis	Calcaneal tuberosity (medial process)	1st toe (base of proximal phalanx via the medial sesamoid)	Medial plantar n. (S1–S2)	• 1st MTP joint: flexion and abduction of the 1st toe • Supports the longitudinal arch
② Flexor digitorum brevis	Calcaneal tuberosity (medial tubercle), plantar aponeurosis	2nd to 5th toes (sides of middle phalanges)		• Flexes the MTP and PIP joints of the 2nd to 5th toes • Supports the longitudinal arch
③ Abductor digiti minimi		5th toe (base of proximal phalanx), 5th metatarsal (at tuberosity)	Lateral plantar n. (S1–S3)	• Flexes the MTP joint of the 5th toe • Abducts the 5th toe • Supports the longitudinal arch

Abbreviations: MTP, metatarsophalangeal; PIP, proximal interphalangeal.

Plantar fasciitis

Inflammation of the plantar aponeurosis is a common, and painful, affliction of runners that is characterized by tenderness on the sole, particularly on the calcaneus. Pain is usually greatest following rest and may dissipate with activity.

The plantar reflex

The plantar reflex tests the integrity of the L4–S2 nerve roots. It is performed by firmly stroking the lateral aspect of the sole from the heel and across the foot to the base of the big toe. In the normal individual, this elicits flexion of the toes. Extension of the big toe with flaring of the 2nd through 5th digits is called the Babinski sign, an abnormal response in adults, indicating brain damage. Because of the immaturity of their central nervous system, the Babinski sign is a normal response in young children (under 4 years).

Deep intrinsic muscles of the sole of the foot, right foot, plantar view.

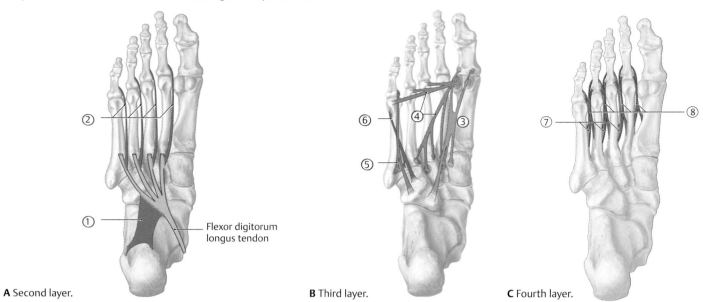

A Second layer.　　　　　　　　　　　　**B** Third layer.　　　　　　　　　　　　**C** Fourth layer.

Table 16.15 ▶ **Deep Intrinsic Muscles of the Sole**

Muscle	Origin	Insertion	Innervation	Action
① Quadratus plantae	Calcaneal tuberosity (medial and plantar borders on plantar side)	Flexor digitorum longus tendon (lateral border)	Lateral plantar n. (S1–S3)	Redirects and augments the pull of flexor digitorum longus
② Lumbricals (four muscles)	Flexor digitorum longus tendons (medial borders)	2nd to 5th toes (at dorsal aponeuroses)	1st lumbrical: medial plantar n. (S2–S3)	• Flexes the MTP joints of 2nd to 5th toes • Extension of IP joints of 2nd to 5th toes • Adducts 2nd to 5th toes toward the big toe
			2nd and 4th lumbrical: lateral plantar n. (S2–S3)	
③ Flexor hallucis brevis	Cuboid, lateral cuneiforms, and plantar calcaneocuboid ligament	1st toe (at base of proximal phalanx via medial and lateral sesamoids)	Medial head: medial plantar n. (S1–S2)	• Flexes the first MTP joint • Supports the longitudinal arch
			Lateral head: lateral plantar n. (S1–S2)	
④ Adductor hallucis	Oblique head: 2nd to 4th metatarsals (at bases)	1st proximal phalanx (at base, by a common tendon via the lateral sesamoid)	Lateral plantar n., deep branch (S2–S3)	• Flexes the first MTP joint • Adducts big toe • Transverse head: supports transverse arch • Oblique head: supports longitudinal arch
	Transverse head: MTPs of 3rd to 5th toes, deep transverse metatarsal ligament			
⑤ Flexor digiti minimi brevis	5th metatarsal (base), long plantar ligament	5th toe (base of proximal phalanx)	Lateral plantar n., superficial branch (S2–S3)	Flexes the MTP joint of the little toe
⑥ Opponens digiti minimi*	Long plantar ligament; fibularis longus (at plantar tendon sheath)	5th metatarsal		Pulls 5th metatarsal in plantar and medial direction
⑦ Plantar interossei (three muscles)	3rd to 5th metatarsals (medial border)	3rd to 5th toes (medial base of proximal phalanx)	Lateral plantar n. (S2–S3)	• Flexes the MTP joints of 3rd to 5th toes • Extension of IP joints of 3rd to 5th toes • Adducts 3rd to 5th toes toward 2nd toe
⑧ Dorsal interossei (four muscles)	1st to 5th metatarsals (by two heads on opposing sides)	1st interosseus: 2nd proximal phalanx (medial base)		• Flexes the MTP joints of 2nd to 4th toes • Extension of IP joints of 2nd to 4th toes • Abducts 3rd and 4th toes from 2nd toe
		2nd to 4th interossei: 2nd to 4th proximal phalanges (lateral base), 2nd to 4th toes (at dorsal aponeuroses)		

Abbreviations: IP, interphalangeal; MTP, metatarsophalangeal.
*May be absent.

16.9 The Gait Cycle

Gait is a complex activity that requires the coordinated action of muscles of the hip, thigh, and leg. **Table 16.16** is a summary of muscle action during the gait cycle.

— Gait is described in two phases: in normal walking, the stance phase makes up ~60%, and the swing phase makes up 40%.
— One cycle of gait consists of the action of one leg through each of the two phases.

Table 16.16 ▶ Muscle Action Sequence During the Gait Cycle	
Activity	**Active muscle groups**
Stance phase	
This phase begins with the heel strike;	Hip extensors Dorsiflexors
The foot begins to accept the weight of the body, and the pelvis is stabilized.	Hip adductors Knee extensors Plantar flexors
At midstance, the pelvis, knee, and ankle are stabilized.	Hip abductors Knee extensors Plantar flexors
This phase ends with the push off that includes "heel lift" and "toe off." Pelvis is stabilized.	Hip abductors Plantar flexors
Throughout the stance phase, the arches of the foot are preserved.	Long tendons of the foot Intrinsic muscles of the foot
Swing phase	
This phase begins with forward acceleration of the thigh.	Hip flexors
The foot needs to clear the ground as it swings forward.	Dorsiflexors
The thigh decelerates in preparation for landing.	Hip extensors
As the foot prepares for heel strike, the knee extends and positions the foot.	Knee extensor Dorsiflexors

16.10 Topographic Anatomy of Lower Limb Muscles

16.10a Thigh, Hip, and Gluteal Region

Fig. 16.25 ▶ **Muscles of the hip and thigh**
Right limb, anterior view. Muscle origins are shown in red, insertions in gray.

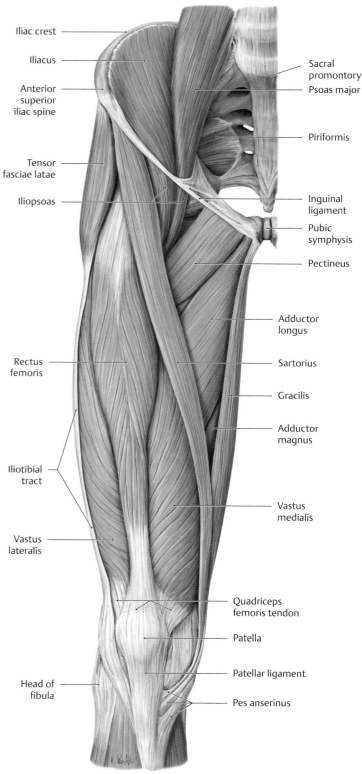

Iliac crest

Iliacus

Anterior superior iliac spine

Tensor fasciae latae

Iliopsoas

Rectus femoris

Iliotibial tract

Vastus lateralis

Head of fibula

Sacral promontory

Psoas major

Piriformis

Inguinal ligament

Pubic symphysis

Pectineus

Adductor longus

Sartorius

Gracilis

Adductor magnus

Vastus medialis

Quadriceps femoris tendon

Patella

Patellar ligament

Pes anserinus

A *Removed:* Fascia lata of the thigh (to the lateral iliotibial tract).

Fig. 16.25 ▸ **Muscles of the hip and thigh** (*continued*)

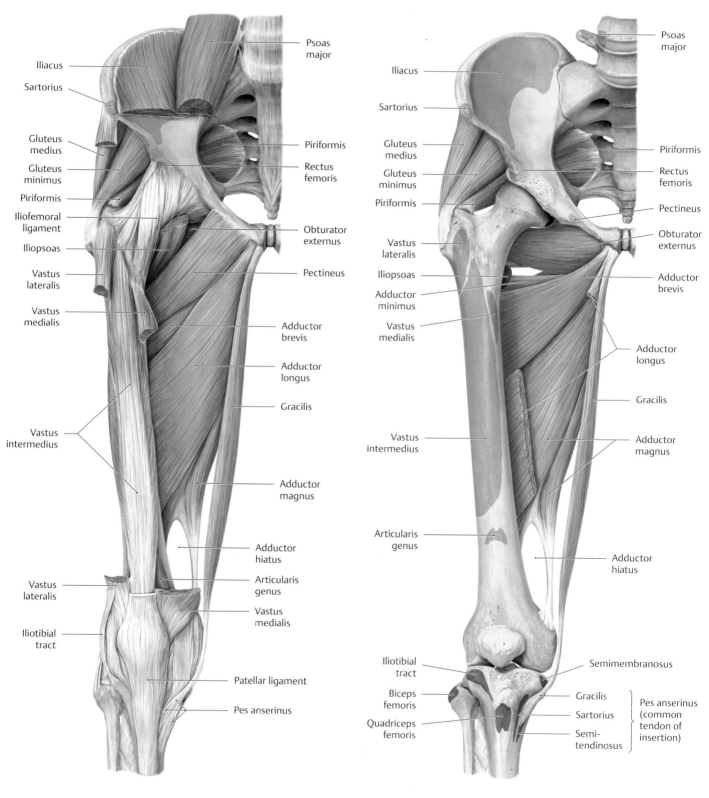

Iliacus
Sartorius
Gluteus medius
Gluteus minimus
Piriformis
Iliofemoral ligament
Iliopsoas
Vastus lateralis
Vastus medialis
Vastus intermedius
Vastus lateralis
Iliotibial tract

Psoas major
Piriformis
Rectus femoris
Obturator externus
Pectineus
Adductor brevis
Adductor longus
Gracilis
Adductor magnus
Adductor hiatus
Articularis genus
Vastus medialis
Patellar ligament
Pes anserinus

Iliacus
Sartorius
Gluteus medius
Gluteus minimus
Piriformis
Vastus lateralis
Iliopsoas
Adductor minimus
Vastus medialis
Vastus intermedius
Articularis genus
Iliotibial tract
Biceps femoris
Quadriceps femoris

Psoas major
Piriformis
Rectus femoris
Pectineus
Obturator externus
Adductor brevis
Adductor longus
Gracilis
Adductor magnus
Adductor hiatus
Semimembranosus
Gracilis
Sartorius
Semi-tendinosus
Pes anserinus (common tendon of insertion)

B *Removed:* Rectus femoris (completely), vastus lateralis, vastus medialis, iliopsoas, and tensor fasciae latae.

C *Removed:* Quadriceps femoris (rectus femoris, vastus lateralis, vastus medialis, vastus intermedius), iliopsoas, tensor fasciae latae, pectineus, and midportion of adductor longus.

351

Fig. 16.26 ▶ **Muscles of the hip, thigh, and gluteal region**
Midsagittal section, medial view.

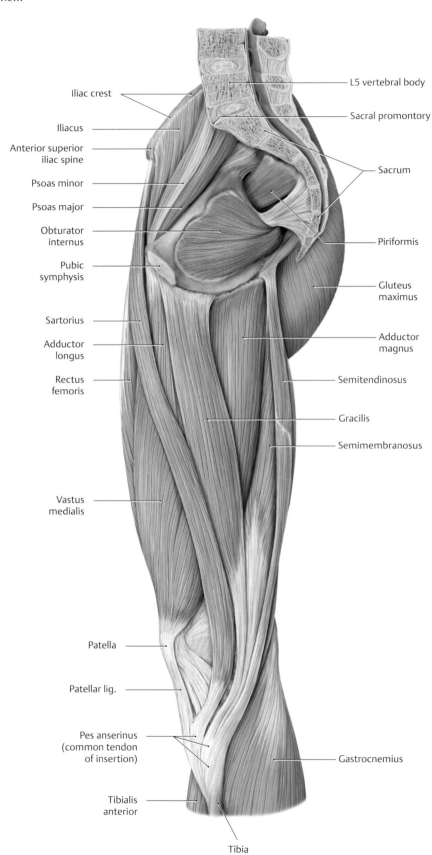

Iliac crest

Iliacus

Anterior superior
iliac spine

Psoas minor

Psoas major

Obturator
internus

Pubic
symphysis

Sartorius

Adductor
longus

Rectus
femoris

Vastus
medialis

Patella

Patellar lig.

Pes anserinus
(common tendon
of insertion)

Tibialis
anterior

L5 vertebral body

Sacral promontory

Sacrum

Piriformis

Gluteus
maximus

Adductor
magnus

Semitendinosus

Gracilis

Semimembranosus

Gastrocnemius

Tibia

Fig. 16.27 ▸ Muscles of the hip, thigh, and gluteal region
Right limb, posterior view.

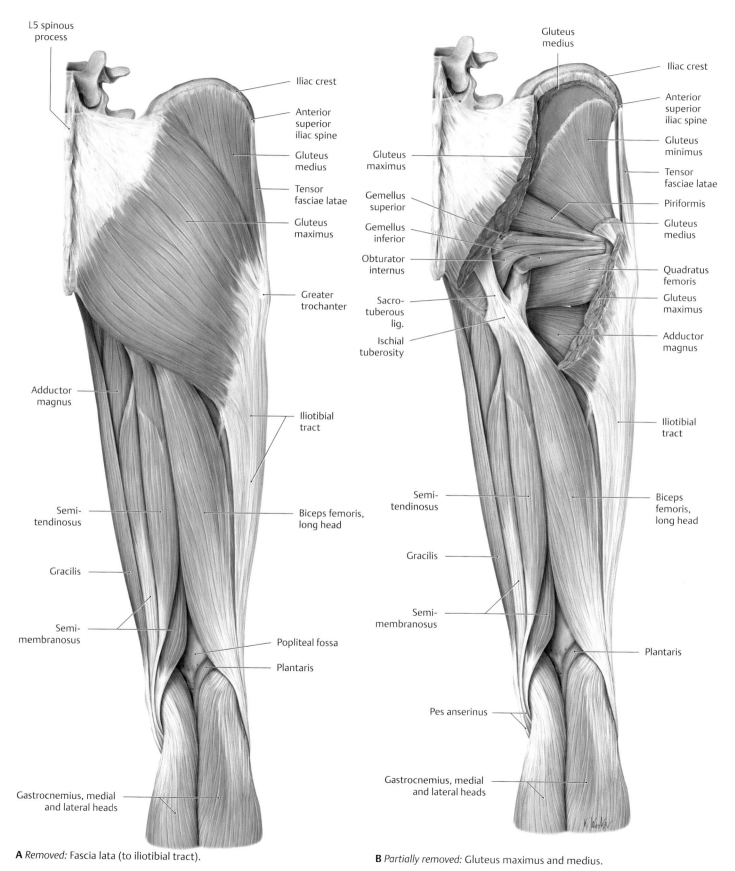

L5 spinous process

Iliac crest

Anterior superior iliac spine

Gluteus medius

Tensor fasciae latae

Gluteus maximus

Greater trochanter

Adductor magnus

Iliotibial tract

Semi-tendinosus

Biceps femoris, long head

Gracilis

Semi-membranosus

Popliteal fossa

Plantaris

Gastrocnemius, medial and lateral heads

Gluteus medius

Gluteus maximus

Gemellus superior

Gemellus inferior

Obturator internus

Sacro-tuberous lig.

Ischial tuberosity

Iliac crest

Anterior superior iliac spine

Gluteus minimus

Tensor fasciae latae

Piriformis

Gluteus medius

Quadratus femoris

Gluteus maximus

Adductor magnus

Iliotibial tract

Semi-tendinosus

Biceps femoris, long head

Gracilis

Semi-membranosus

Plantaris

Pes anserinus

Gastrocnemius, medial and lateral heads

A *Removed:* Fascia lata (to iliotibial tract).

B *Partially removed:* Gluteus maximus and medius.

Fig. 16.28 ▶ **Muscles of the hip, thigh, and gluteal region**
Lateral view. *Note:* The iliotibial tract (the thickened band of fascia lata)
functions as a tension band to reduce the bending loads on the proximal
femur.

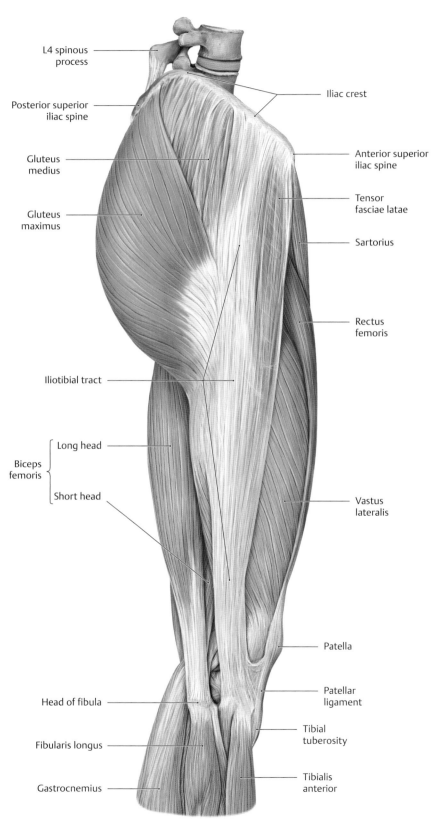

L4 spinous
process

Iliac crest

Posterior superior
iliac spine

Anterior superior
iliac spine

Gluteus
medius

Tensor
fasciae latae

Gluteus
maximus

Sartorius

Rectus
femoris

Iliotibial tract

Long head

Biceps
femoris

Short head

Vastus
lateralis

Patella

Patellar
ligament

Head of fibula

Tibial
tuberosity

Fibularis longus

Tibialis
anterior

Gastrocnemius

16.10b The Leg

Fig. 16.29 ▶ **Muscles of the leg**
Right leg, anterior view.

Fig. 16.30 ▶ **Muscles of the leg**
Right leg, lateral view.

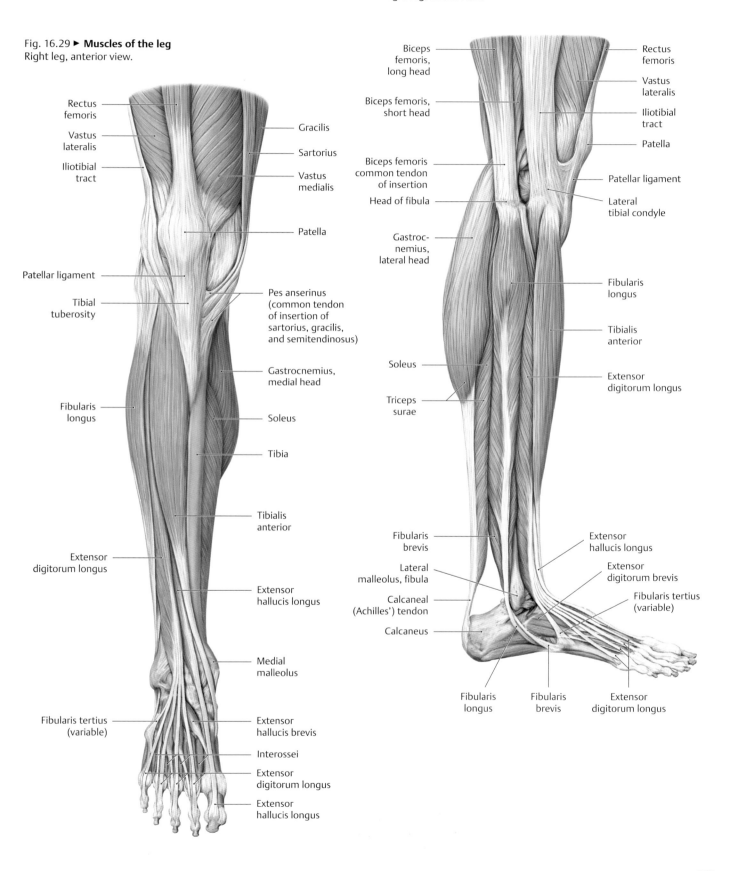

Labels (Fig. 16.29, anterior view):
- Rectus femoris
- Vastus lateralis
- Iliotibial tract
- Gracilis
- Sartorius
- Vastus medialis
- Patella
- Patellar ligament
- Tibial tuberosity
- Pes anserinus (common tendon of insertion of sartorius, gracilis, and semitendinosus)
- Gastrocnemius, medial head
- Fibularis longus
- Soleus
- Tibia
- Tibialis anterior
- Extensor digitorum longus
- Extensor hallucis longus
- Medial malleolus
- Fibularis tertius (variable)
- Extensor hallucis brevis
- Interossei
- Extensor digitorum longus
- Extensor hallucis longus

Labels (Fig. 16.30, lateral view):
- Biceps femoris, long head
- Biceps femoris, short head
- Biceps femoris common tendon of insertion
- Head of fibula
- Gastrocnemius, lateral head
- Soleus
- Triceps surae
- Fibularis brevis
- Lateral malleolus, fibula
- Calcaneal (Achilles') tendon
- Calcaneus
- Fibularis longus
- Fibularis brevis
- Extensor digitorum longus
- Rectus femoris
- Vastus lateralis
- Iliotibial tract
- Patella
- Patellar ligament
- Lateral tibial condyle
- Fibularis longus
- Tibialis anterior
- Extensor digitorum longus
- Extensor hallucis longus
- Extensor digitorum brevis
- Fibularis tertius (variable)

Fig. 16.31 ▶ **Muscles of the leg**
Right leg, posterior view. Muscle origins shown in red, insertions in gray.

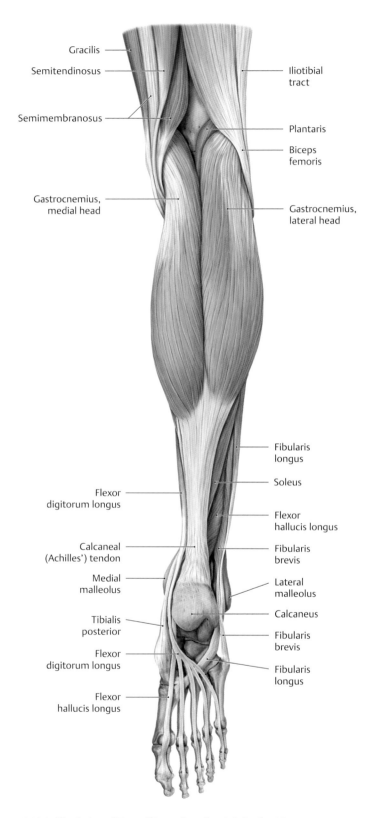

Gracilis

Semitendinosus

Semimembranosus

Gastrocnemius, medial head

Flexor digitorum longus

Calcaneal (Achilles') tendon

Medial malleolus

Tibialis posterior

Flexor digitorum longus

Flexor hallucis longus

Iliotibial tract

Plantaris

Biceps femoris

Gastrocnemius, lateral head

Fibularis longus

Soleus

Flexor hallucis longus

Fibularis brevis

Lateral malleolus

Calcaneus

Fibularis brevis

Fibularis longus

A *Note:* The bulge of the calf is produced mainly by the triceps surae (soleus and the two heads of the gastrocnemius).

Fig. 16.31 ▶ **Muscles of the leg** (*continued*)

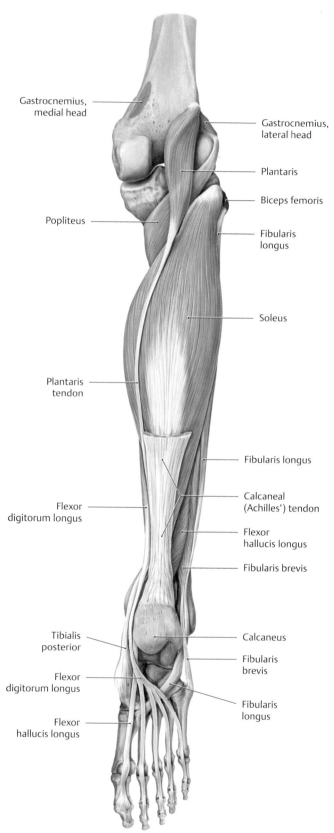

Gastrocnemius, medial head

Gastrocnemius, lateral head

Plantaris

Biceps femoris

Fibularis longus

Popliteus

Soleus

Plantaris tendon

Flexor digitorum longus

Fibularis longus

Calcaneal (Achilles') tendon

Flexor hallucis longus

Fibularis brevis

Tibialis posterior

Calcaneus

Flexor digitorum longus

Fibularis brevis

Flexor hallucis longus

Fibularis longus

B *Removed:* Gastrocnemius (both heads).

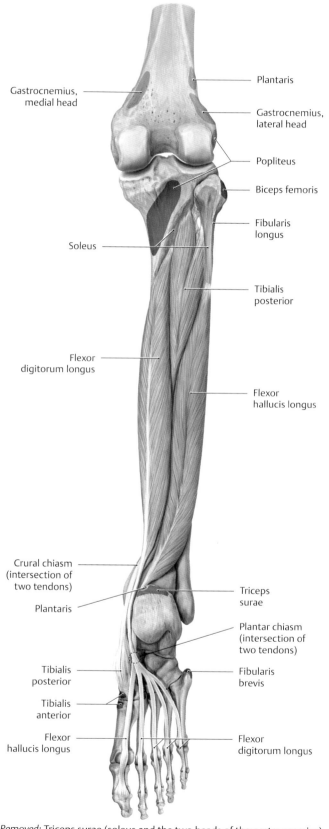

Plantaris

Gastrocnemius, medial head

Gastrocnemius, lateral head

Popliteus

Biceps femoris

Fibularis longus

Soleus

Tibialis posterior

Flexor digitorum longus

Flexor hallucis longus

Crural chiasm (intersection of two tendons)

Plantaris

Triceps surae

Plantar chiasm (intersection of two tendons)

Tibialis posterior

Fibularis brevis

Tibialis anterior

Flexor hallucis longus

Flexor digitorum longus

C *Removed:* Triceps surae (soleus and the two heads of the gastrocnemius), plantaris, popliteus, fibularis longus, and fibularis brevis muscles.

16.10c The Foot

Fig. 16.32 ► **Plantar aponeurosis**
Right foot, plantar view. The plantar aponeurosis is a tough aponeurotic sheet, thickest at the center, that blends with the dorsal fascia (not shown) at the borders of the foot.

Fig. 16.33 ►**Intrinsic muscles of the sole of the foot**
Right foot, plantar view.

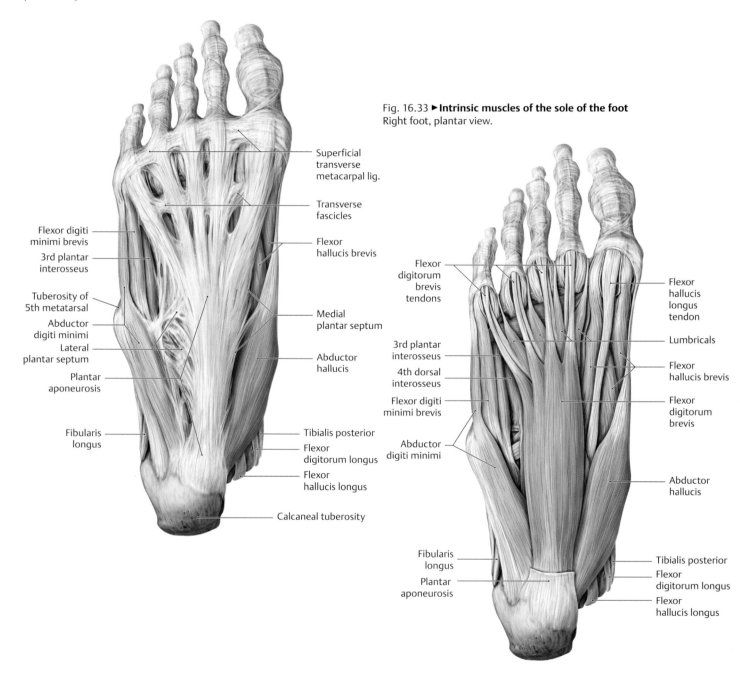

A Superficial (first) layer. *Removed:* Plantar aponeurosis, including the superficial transverse metacarpal ligament.

Fig. 16.33 ▶ **Intrinsic muscles of the sole of the foot** (*continued*)

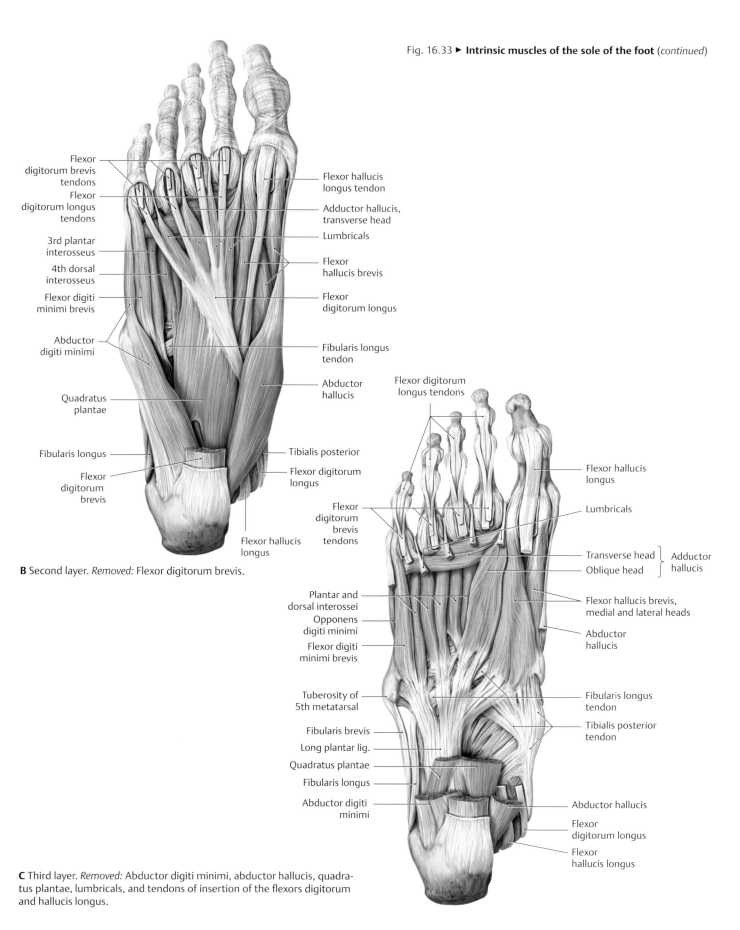

Flexor
digitorum brevis
tendons

Flexor
digitorum longus
tendons

3rd plantar
interosseus

4th dorsal
interosseus

Flexor digiti
minimi brevis

Abductor
digiti minimi

Quadratus
plantae

Fibularis longus

Flexor
digitorum
brevis

Flexor hallucis
longus tendon

Adductor hallucis,
transverse head

Lumbricals

Flexor
hallucis brevis

Flexor
digitorum longus

Fibularis longus
tendon

Abductor
hallucis

Tibialis posterior

Flexor digitorum
longus

Flexor hallucis
longus

B Second layer. *Removed:* Flexor digitorum brevis.

Flexor digitorum
longus tendons

Flexor
digitorum
brevis
tendons

Plantar and
dorsal interossei

Opponens
digiti minimi

Flexor digiti
minimi brevis

Tuberosity of
5th metatarsal

Fibularis brevis

Long plantar lig.

Quadratus plantae

Fibularis longus

Abductor digiti
minimi

Flexor hallucis
longus

Lumbricals

Transverse head } Adductor
Oblique head } hallucis

Flexor hallucis brevis,
medial and lateral heads

Abductor
hallucis

Fibularis longus
tendon

Tibialis posterior
tendon

Abductor hallucis

Flexor
digitorum longus

Flexor
hallucis longus

C Third layer. *Removed:* Abductor digiti minimi, abductor hallucis, quadratus plantae, lumbricals, and tendons of insertion of the flexors digitorum and hallucis longus.

16.10d Compartments

Fig. 16.34 ► **Windowed dissection**
Right limb, posterior view.

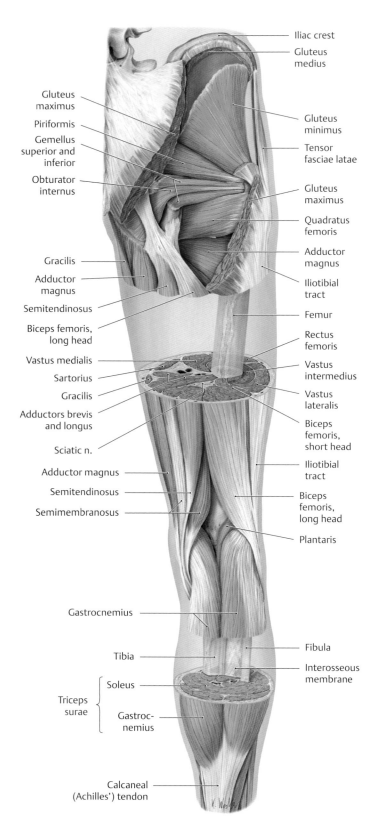

Iliac crest

Gluteus medius

Gluteus maximus

Piriformis

Gemellus superior and inferior

Obturator internus

Gluteus minimus

Tensor fasciae latae

Gluteus maximus

Quadratus femoris

Gracilis

Adductor magnus

Adductor magnus

Semitendinosus

Biceps femoris, long head

Iliotibial tract

Femur

Rectus femoris

Vastus medialis

Sartorius

Gracilis

Adductors brevis and longus

Sciatic n.

Vastus intermedius

Vastus lateralis

Biceps femoris, short head

Iliotibial tract

Adductor magnus

Semitendinosus

Semimembranosus

Biceps femoris, long head

Plantaris

Gastrocnemius

Tibia

Fibula

Interosseous membrane

Soleus

Triceps surae

Gastrocnemius

Calcaneal (Achilles') tendon

Fig. 16.35 ► **Transverse sections**
Right limb, proximal (superior) view.

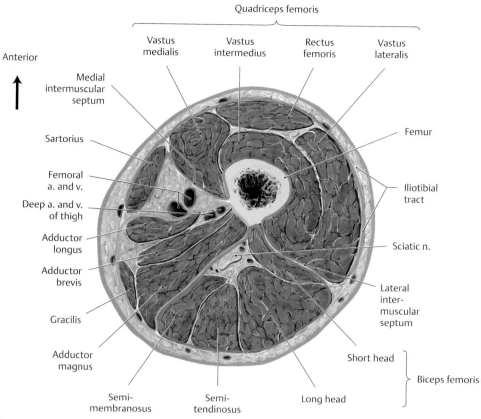

Quadriceps femoris

Anterior

Vastus medialis
Vastus intermedius
Rectus femoris
Vastus lateralis

Medial intermuscular septum

Sartorius

Femur

Femoral a. and v.

Iliotibial tract

Deep a. and v. of thigh

Adductor longus

Sciatic n.

Adductor brevis

Lateral inter-muscular septum

Gracilis

Adductor magnus

Short head

Biceps femoris

Semi-membranosus

Semi-tendinosus

Long head

A Thigh (plane of upper section in **Fig. 16.34**).
The anterior compartment is outlined in pink, the posterior compartment in green, and the medial compartment in orange.

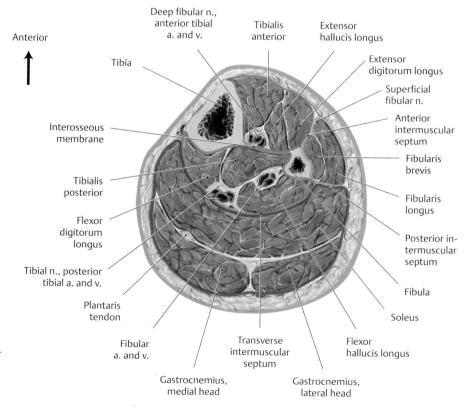

Anterior

Deep fibular n., anterior tibial a. and v.

Tibialis anterior

Extensor hallucis longus

Tibia

Extensor digitorum longus

Superficial fibular n.

Interosseous membrane

Anterior intermuscular septum

Tibialis posterior

Fibularis brevis

Flexor digitorum longus

Fibularis longus

Tibial n., posterior tibial a. and v.

Posterior in-termuscular septum

Plantaris tendon

Fibula

Soleus

Fibular a. and v.

Transverse intermuscular septum

Flexor hallucis longus

Gastrocnemius, medial head

Gastrocnemius, lateral head

B Leg (plane of lower section in **Fig. 16.34**).
The anterior compartment is outlined in pink, the lateral compartment in orange, the deep posterior compartment in green, and the superficial posterior compartment in blue.

Review Questions: Lower Limb

1. A young girl has recovered well from the severe injuries she sustained in a motor vehicle accident 9 months ago, but because of some lingering nerve problems, she still has difficulty walking. She is balanced during the midstance phase but has difficulty bringing her limb forward to initiate movement. What nerve seems to be affected?
   A. Superior gluteal
   B. Inferior gluteal
   C. Femoral
   D. Obturator
   E. Tibial

2. A young woman searching for driftwood walked several miles on the soft sandy beach of a Caribbean island. While walking on this uneven surface, the balance between inversion and eversion at her subtalar joint was maintained by the opposing actions of the fibularis longus and the
   A. fibularis brevis
   B. fibularis tertius
   C. soleus
   D. tibialis anterior
   E. extensor digitorum longus

3. Structures at the knee that are *not* attached to the joint capsule include the
   A. medial meniscus
   B. medial collateral ligament
   C. lateral collateral ligament
   D. patellar retinacula
   E. All of the above (A–D) are attached to the joint cavity.

4. A woman in her early 40s discovered a small lump at the top of her thigh that was later diagnosed as a femoral hernia. Where would this hernia be located?
   A. Retroinguinal space
   B. Femoral canal
   C. Femoral sheath
   D. Femoral ring
   E. All of the above

5. An elderly woman shopping with her daughter fell in the mall parking lot. After examining the woman, the paramedics who responded to the call noted that the limb was pulled upward, and the hip was rotated laterally. They confided to the daughter that it appeared that the woman had fractured her femoral neck. Which of the following muscles would be responsible for the lateral (external) rotation?
   A. Gluteus medius
   B. Tensor of the fascia lata
   C. Pectineus
   D. Vastus lateralis
   E. All of the above

6. The strongest and most supportive ligament of the hip joint is the
   A. transverse ligament of the acetabulum
   B. ligament of the head of the femur
   C. pubofemoral ligament
   D. ischiofemoral ligament
   E. iliofemoral ligament

7. A young man running on the beach severely lacerated his foot when he accidentally stepped into a pit with broken glass left by late-night partygoers. Surgery was required to remove the glass fragments and treat the lacerations. You opt to use regional anesthesia, injecting anesthetic near each of the nerves that cross the ankle. Where would you anesthetize the sural nerve?
   A. Anterior to the medial malleolus
   B. Posterior to the medial malleolus
   C. Posterior to the lateral malleolus
   D. Anterior to the lateral malleolus
   E. First web space

8. Sensation along the lateral side of the first toe is transmitted by branches of the
   A. saphenous nerve
   B. medial plantar nerve
   C. deep fibular nerve
   D. superficial fibular nerve
   E. lateral plantar nerve

9. Superficial veins of the lower limb
   A. lie deep to the fascia lata
   B. include the great saphenous vein that terminates at the popliteal vein
   C. include the small saphenous vein whose course runs anterior to the lateral malleolus
   D. drain to deep veins via perforating veins
   E. originate from the plantar venous arch on the sole

10. The dorsal pedal artery is a continuation of the
    A. posterior tibial artery
    B. fibular artery
    C. anterior tibial artery
    D. popliteal artery
    E. inferior medial genicular artery

11. The deep plantar arch of the foot is an anastomosis between the dorsal pedal artery and the following structure on the sole of the foot:
    A. Fibular artery
    B. Lateral plantar artery
    C. Plantar metatarsal arteries
    D. Plantar digital arteries
    E. Arcuate artery

12. An obese female patient suffers from peripheral edema (swelling of the legs) and large varicose veins in her leg. Which of the following might be coexisting symptoms related to her condition?
    A. Incompetent valves in the great saphenous vein
    B. Reversed flow in the perforating veins
    C. Deep vein thrombosis
    D. Thrombophlebitis
    E. All of the above

13. "Footdrop" occurs when the plantar flexor muscles are unopposed. This condition may be caused by damage to which of the following nerves?
    A. Superficial fibular
    B. Deep fibular
    C. Sural
    D. Tibial
    E. Medial plantar

14. As she was riding her bike home from her job as a camp counselor, Kristin was sideswiped by a large pickup trunk. She suffered multiple bruises, a fractured tibia, and a fractured pelvis. Several months later she still had an area of numbness on the medial side of her thigh and walked with a lateral swing to her gait. Which muscle was affected by her injury?
    A. Gluteus medius
    B. Gluteus maximus
    C. Semimembranosus
    D. Adductor longus
    E. Rectus femoris

15. In anatomy laboratory you have just dissected the gluteal region of your cadaver. You are surprised to discover that in your cadaver the lateral component of the sciatic nerve passes *through* the piriformis muscle instead of *inferior* to it. Being a dedicated student, you investigate this further and find this anomaly can cause a piriformis syndrome in which the nerve is compressed by contraction of the muscle. What symptom might this particular patient have experienced?
    A. Paresthesia (tingling) on the sole of the foot
    B. Loss of knee flexion
    C. Loss of knee extension
    D. Footdrop
    E. Sagging of the unsupported hip when walking

16. The adductor magnus muscle
    A. extends and adducts the hip joint
    B. is innervated by the femoral and obturator nerves
    C. inserts on the linea aspera of the femur and adductor tubercle of the tibia
    D. forms the anterior wall of the adductor canal
    E. originates from the superior pubic ramus

17. Which muscle(s) of the lower limb is/are capable of producing flexion at one joint and extension at a second joint?
    A. Semimembranosus
    B. Rectus femoris
    C. Lumbricals of foot
    D. Long head of biceps femoris
    E. All of the above (A–D)

18. During a street fight between two local gangs, one boy received a violent blow to the anterior knee that knocked him to the ground. In the emergency department, the physical exam of his knee revealed a positive posterior drawer sign. What structure appears to be injured?
    A. Anterior cruciate ligament
    B. Posterior cruciate ligament
    C. Patellar ligament
    D. Medial collateral ligament
    E. Lateral collateral ligament

19. A single woman looking for adventure signed up for a walking tour of the Scottish highlands. She was unprepared for the effort that it required but kept up with the more experienced walkers. After a few days she began to experience extreme tenderness in her anterior leg deep to the ridge of the tibia. The tour guide had seen this in previous clients and suggested that her pain was due to shin splints. Her pain originated from overuse of the
    A. extensor digitorum longus
    B. extensor digitorum brevis
    C. extensor hallucis longus
    D. fibularis tertius
    E. tibialis anterior

20. Which fibrous structure on the sole of the foot originates at the calcaneus and continues distally as digital fibrous sheaths?
    A. Plantar aponeurosis
    B. Plantar calcaneonavicular ligament
    C. Long plantar ligament
    D. Short plantar ligament
    E. Deltoid ligament

21. A man was on a hunting trip with friends when he was accidentally shot in the midthigh. He bled profusely from his femoral artery until his friends applied constant pressure over the wound and drove him to a local emergency clinic. Although examination of the wound site in surgery revealed a badly torn femoral artery, the man continued to have distal pulses in his leg. What vessel arises proximal to the injury site and can provide collateral blood supply to the distal limb?
    A. Medial circumflex femoral artery
    B. Lateral circumflex femoral artery
    C. Obturator artery
    D. Descending genicular artery
    E. Popliteal artery

22. An elderly woman slipped on a patch of ice in her driveway when she went to pick up the morning newspaper. Her neighbor witnessed the accident and called an ambulance. In the ER, X-rays revealed that she had fractured the neck of her femur. Her physician explained to her that avascular necrosis was a common complication of this injury in elderly women and convinced her to agree to a hip replacement. What vessel contributes most significantly to the blood supply of the hip joint?
    A. Obturator
    B. Superior gluteal
    C. Inferior gluteal
    D. Medial circumflex femoral
    E. Lateral circumflex femoral

23. Which of the following spaces contain the femoral nerve?
    A. Femoral sheath
    B. Adductor hiatus
    C. Popliteal fossa
    D. Femoral canal
    E. Retroinguinal space

24. The inferior gluteal nerve innervates the
    A. gluteus maximus
    B. gluteus medius
    C. gluteus minimus
    D. piriformis
    E. All of the above

25. Which of the following muscles insert on the iliotibial tract?
    A. Gluteus maximus
    B. Gluteus medius
    C. Gluteus minimus
    D. Quadratus femoris
    E. None of the above

26. Your 13-year-old son who studies martial arts is particularly flexible and is praised for his high kicks. After several weeks of training in preparation for an upcoming tournament, he complains of tenderness in his lower buttocks during practice and even when he sits on the hard stadium benches. As his pediatrician, how do you explain his problem?
    A. Inflammation of the ischial tuberosity
    B. Rupture of the obturator internus tendon from its insertion
    C. Compression of the sciatic nerve in the gluteal region
    D. Irritation of the tibial nerve in the thigh
    E. Irritation of the inferior gluteal nerve

27. Which of the following muscles are involved in knee flexion?
    A. Flexor hallucis longus
    B. Soleus
    C. Tibialis posterior
    D. Biceps femoris
    E. Rectus femoris

28. The lateral border of the femoral triangle is formed by the
    A. tensor fasciae latae
    B. femoral nerve
    C. sartorius
    D. adductor longus
    E. rectus femoris

29. An 18-year-old marathon runner finished fourth in the Detroit marathon but limped away from the finish line. He had been suffering from excruciating pain on the sole of his foot and immediately sought advice from the medical volunteers. Following a thorough exam, the EMTs explained that the muscle tendons running through his tarsal tunnel had swollen and were compressing the nerve that accompanies them. What bones form the wall of this tunnel?
    A. Navicular and talus
    B. Cuboid and calcaneus
    C. Talus and calcaneus
    D. Medial malleolus of the tibia and calcaneus
    E. Talus and base of the 1st metatarsal

30. An experienced 24-year-old backpacker has spent the last 4 months hiking the entire Appalachian trail. Although he has sturdy hiking boots, he often changes to the lightweight sneakers he brought as a backup. For the last few miles of the trek, he's been experiencing shooting pain along the side of his foot at the apex of his medial arch. What structure is probably the cause of the pain?

   A. Plantar calcaneonavicular (spring) ligament
   B. Deltoid ligament
   C. Posterior talofibular ligament
   D. Superior extensor retinaculm
   E. Tendon of fibularis longus

Answers and Explanations

1. **C** Forward movement at the beginning of the swing phase depends on the action of her hip flexors, particularly the rectus femoris, which is innervated by the femoral nerve (Sections 16.2, 16.4a, and 16.9).
   A The superior gluteal nerve innervates the abductors of the hip. Damage to this nerve would cause a sagging of the hip on the contralateral side just before the midstance.
   B The inferior gluteal nerve innervates the gluteus maximus. Injury to this nerve would affect the deceleration of the swing phase.
   D Injury to the obturator nerve, which innervates the adductors of the hip, would cause an outward swing of the limb but would not inhibit acceleration of the thigh.
   E The tibial nerve innervates the hamstring muscles of the posterior thigh, which are responsible for the deceleration at the end of the swing phase.

2. **D** The tibialis anterior and tibialis posterior are the strong inverters of the foot that counter the action of the fibularis longus and fibularis brevis (Section 16.8a).
   A The fibularis brevis, in the lateral crural compartment, inserts on the base of the 5th metatarsal, which allows it to evert the foot.
   B The fibularis tertius, a muscle of the anterior crural compartment, inserts on the base of the 5th metatarsal and everts the foot.
   C The soleus, in the posterior crural compartment, plantar flexes the foot.
   E The extensor digitorum, in the anterior crural compartment, everts the foot.

3. **C** The lateral (fibular) collateral ligament is an extracapsular ligament that extends from the lateral epicondyle of the femur to the head of the fibula and remains separate from the joint capsule of the knee (Section 16.5a).
   A The medial and lateral menisci attach along their outer rims to the joint capsule.
   B The medial (tibial) collateral ligament is a capsular ligament that extends from the medial epicondyle of the femur to the medial condyle and superior part of the medial tibia. It attaches to the joint capsule and to the medial meniscus.
   D The patellar retinacula are fibrous expansions of the tendons of the quadriceps femoris muscle. They form the joint capsule on either side of the patella.
   E Only the lateral (fibular) collateral ligament (C) is correct.

4. **E** A vascular compartment of the retroinguinal space contains the femoral sheath and the femoral canal. The femoral ring defines the upper edge of the femoral canal. A femoral hernia protrudes into the femoral canal (Section 16.4b).
   A The retroinguinal space contains the femoral canal, the site of the femoral hernia. B through D are also correct (E).
   B The femoral canal is a space within the femoral sheath that normally contains loose connective tissue, fat, and often a deep inguinal lymph node. A, C, and D are also correct (E).
   C The femoral sheath contains the femoral vessels and the femoral canal. A, B, and D are also correct (E).
   D The femoral ring defines the superior opening of the femoral canal. A, B, and C are also correct (E).

5. **C** The pectineus in the medial thigh compartment adducts and laterally rotates the hip (Sections 16.3 and 16.4a).
A The gluteus medius is an abductor of the hip.
B The tensor fascia lata abducts, flexes, and internally rotates the hip.
D The vastus lateralis extends the knee and has no influence over the hip joint.
E A, B, and D are incorrect.

6. **E** The iliofemoral ligament attaches proximally to the anterior inferior iliac spine and rim of the acetabulum and distally to the intertrochanteric line of the femur. It supports the hip joint during standing (Section 16.3).
A The transverse ligament completes the rim of the C-shaped acetabulum inferiorly.
B The ligament of the head of the femur attaches to the acetabulum within the joint but provides little support. A small artery runs within the ligament to the femoral head.
C The pubofemoral ligament runs laterally from the inferior aspect of the acetabular rim to merge with the iliofemoral ligament. It assists the iliofemoral ligament and limits abduction of the joint.
D The ischiofemoral ligament is the weakest of the three ligaments of the capsule. It arises from the ischial part of the acetabular rim and spirals anteriorly to insert on the femoral neck.

7. **C** The sural nerve innervates the lateral side of the foot and runs posterior to the lateral malleolus (Section 15.4d).
A The saphenous nerve runs anterior to the medial malleolus.
B The tibial nerve courses through the tarsal tunnel posterior to the medial malleolus.
D The superficial fibular nerve runs onto the dorsum of the foot anterior to the lateral malleolus.
E The deep fibular nerve accompanies the dorsal pedal artery onto the dorsum of the foot. It innervates the skin of the first web space.

8. **C** The deep fibular nerve, a branch of the common fibular nerve, supplies cutaneous innervation to the first web space, including the skin adjacent to the first and second digits. It also supplies motor innervation to the muscles of the anterior compartment of the leg (Section 15.4d).
A The saphenous nerve transmits sensation from the medial side of the foot.
B The medial plantar branch of the tibial nerve supplies cutaneous innervation to a large area of skin on the medial side of the foot and the medial three and a half digits.
D The superficial fibular nerve supplies cutaneous innervation to the dorsum of the foot.
E The lateral plantar branch supplies cutaneous innervation to the lateral foot and the lateral one and a half digits.

9. **D** Similar to superficial veins of the upper limb, superficial veins of the lower limb drain to deep veins via perforating veins (Section 15.4b).
A Superficial veins lie in the subcutaneous tissue, superficial to the deep fascia (fascia lata).
B The great saphenous vein pierces the fascia lata at the saphenous hiatus in the proximal thigh and terminates in the femoral vein.
C The small saphenous vein runs posterior to the lateral malleolus and superiorly to the popliteal fossa.
E The large superficial veins, the great and small saphenous veins, originate from the venous arch on the dorsum of the foot.

10. **C** The anterior tibial artery descends within the anterior crural compartment and emerges onto the dorsum of the foot as the dorsal pedal artery (Section 15.4a).
A The posterior tibial artery descends within posterior crural compartment and branches into the medial plantar and lateral plantar arteries that supply the sole of the foot.
B The fibular artery arises in the lateral part of the posterior leg and anastomoses with the anterior tibial artery to supply the ankle.
D The popliteal artery lies posterior to the knee. It gives rise to the genicular and tibial arteries.
E The inferior medial genicular artery is a branch of the popliteal artery and supplies blood to the patella and insertions of the sartorius, gracilis, and semitendinosus.

11. **B** The lateral plantar artery, similar to the ulnar artery in the hand, is the largest branch of the posterior tibial artery. It supplies the lateral side of the foot and forms the deep plantar arch with the dorsal pedal artery (Section 15.4a).
A The fibular artery supplies muscles in the posterior and lateral compartments of the leg and forms an anastomosis with the anterior tibial artery at the ankle, but it has no branches on the sole of the foot.
C The plantar metatarsal arteries arise from the deep plantar arch.
D Proper digital arteries arise from the plantar metatarsal arteries, which are branches of the deep plantar arch.
E The arcuate artery, a branch of the dorsal pedal artery, forms a loop on the dorsum of the foot and supplies the 2nd, 3rd, and 4th dorsal metatarsal arteries.

12. **E** Varicose, or dilated, veins can occur in conjunction with deep vein thromboses. When the deep veins are obstructed, the normal superficial-to-deep flow in the perforating veins reverses. With the increased volume, the superficial veins dilate, and their valves become incompetent. Thrombophlebitis, or venous inflammation, often occurs with thrombus formation (Section 15.4b).
A When venous valves are incompetent, upward flow is impeded, and blood pools in the veins. The resulting dilated veins are known as varicose veins. B through D are also correct (E).
B Superficial veins normally drain into the deep venous system through the perforating veins. If the deep veins are obstructed by thrombus, blood flows outward through the perforating veins into the superficial system, dilating the superficial veins. A, C, and D are also correct (E).
C When thrombus obstructs the deep veins of the leg, blood flows outward into the superficial veins, causing them to dilate. A, B, and D are also correct (E).
D Inflammation of veins can occur with thrombus formation. A through C are also correct (E).

13. **B** Footdrop is caused by an injury to the deep (or common) fibular nerve causing paralysis of the dorsiflexor muscles in the foot, leaving the plantar flexor muscles unopposed (Section 15.4d).
A Injury to the superficial fibular nerve will result in an inability to evert the foot and therefore an overall loss of balance and loss of sensation on the dorsum of the foot.
C Injury to the sural nerve will cause loss of sensation over the skin on the lateral side of the foot.
D Injury to the tibial nerve would cause paralysis of all of the muscles of the posterior thigh (except the short head of the biceps femoris) and posterior leg.
E Injury to the medial plantar nerve will cause paralysis of the muscles on the medial side of the foot and loss of sensation over a large area of skin on the medial side of the foot and the medial three and a half digits.

14. **D** A lateral swinging gait is caused by unopposed hip abduction, which occurs when the adductors are paralyzed. The obturator nerve innervates the adductor muscles of the thigh and can be injured by pelvic fractures. The area of numbness on the medial thigh also suggests an obturator nerve injury (Section 15.4d).
A The gluteus medius is an abductor of the hip. Injury to this muscle would result in a gluteal, or waddling, gait.
B The injury to the inferior gluteal nerve, which innervates the gluteus maximus, would impair extension of the hip but would not cause any sensory loss.
C Injury to the semimembranosus or its nerve, the tibial nerve, would impair hip extension, knee flexion, and sensation on the sole of the foot.
E Injury to the femoral nerve, which innervates the rectus femoris, would weaken flexion of the hip and extension of the knee. There would be a sensory loss from the anterior thigh and the medial side of the leg and foot.

15. **D** The common fibular nerve is the lateral component of the sciatic nerve. Compression will affect the dorsiflexors of the anterior leg compartment (through its deep fibular branch), resulting in footdrop (Sections 16.2 and 15.4d).
A Paresthesia on the sole of the foot would be a consequence of compression of the tibial nerve.
B The tibial nerve, the medial component of the sciatic nerve, innervates the hamstring muscles, which flex the knee. This action would remain intact.
C The knee extensors on the anterior thigh extend the knee and would not be affected by this anomaly.
E Sagging of the unsupported hip is characteristic of an injury to the superior gluteal nerve.

16. **A** The adductor magnus is the largest adductor of the hip but also works with the gluteus maximus to provide powerful extension of the hip joint (Section 16.4a).
B The adductor magnus has a dual innervation, the obturator and tibial nerves.
C The adductor magnus inserts entirely on the femur; the adductor tubercle is a feature on the distal femur.
D The adductor canal passes between the anterior and medial thigh compartments. The vastus medialis forms the anterior wall, and the adductor muscles form the posterior wall.
E The adductor magnus originates on the ischiopubic ramus, which includes the inferior pubic ramus and ischial ramus.

17. **E** Semimembranosus (A) produces flexion at the knee joint and extension at the hip joint. Rectus femoris (B) produces flexion at the hip joint and extension at the knee joint. The lumbricals of the foot (C) produce flexion of the metatarsophalangeal (MTP) joints of the 2nd to 5th toes and extension of the interphalangeal (IP) joints of the 2nd to 5th toes. The long head of the biceps femoris (D) produces extension of the hip joint and flexion of the knee joint (Sections 16.4a and 16.8c).
A Semimembranosus produces flexion at the knee joint and extension at the hip joint. B through D are also correct (E).
B Rectus femoris produces flexion at the hip joint and extension at the knee joint. A, C, and D are also correct (E).
C The lumbricals of the foot produce flexion of the MTP joints of the 2nd to 5th toes and extension of the IP joints of the 2nd to 5th toes. A, B, and D are also correct (E).
D The long head of the biceps femoris produces extension of the hip joint and flexion of the knee joint. A through C are also correct (E).

18. **B** The posterior displacement of the tibia is a positive posterior drawer sign that indicates an injury to the posterior cruciate ligament (Section 16.5a).

A Injury to the anterior cruciate ligament is recognized by the positive anterior drawer sign in which the tibia can be pulled anteriorly from under the femur.

C A positive drawer sign suggests anterior or posterior displacement of the tibia relative to the femur. Rupture of the patellar ligament destabilizes the knee joint but does not disrupt the alignment of the tibia and femur.

D Although the medial collateral ligament may be damaged by a forceful blow, it is not diagnosed by a posterior drawer sign.

E The lateral collateral ligament is unlikely to be damaged by a blow to the anterior knee and is not diagnosed by either anterior or posterior drawer signs.

19. **E** Shin splints are a result of inflammation of the tibialis anterior and small tears of the periosteum where the muscle attaches to the bone (Section 16.6b).

A The extensor digitorum originates from the head of the fibula, lateral condyle of the tibia, and interosseous membrane.

B The extensor digitorum brevis is an intrinsic muscle of the foot. It arises from the calcaneus.

C The extensor hallucis longus arises from the middle of the fibular shaft and the interosseous membrane.

D Fibularis tertius is a lateral muscle that arises from the distal fibula.

20. **A** The plantar aponeurosis is a thick fibrous band on the sole that is continuous with the deep fascia of the leg (Section 16.8c).

B The plantar calcaneonavicular ligament, or spring ligament, supports the head of the talus and maintains the medial side of the longitudinal arch of the foot.

C The long plantar ligament supports the lateral side of the longitudinal arch of the foot and extends from the calcaneus to the bases of the 1st, 2nd, and 3rd metatarsals.

D The short plantar ligament, or plantar calcaneocuboid ligament, supports the lateral arch of the foot.

E The deltoid ligament is a four-part ligament that supports the medial side of the ankle joint.

21. **B** The lateral circumflex femoral artery arises from the deep artery of the thigh in the proximal thigh. It supplies structures around the hip as well as a descending branch that anastomoses with the genicular arteries at the knee. Reverse flow in these branches could supply the popliteal artery and its branches in the leg (Section 15.4a).

A The medial circumflex femoral artery arises from the deep artery of the thigh and supplies the hip joint. It does not anastomose with the popliteal artery or other branches of the knee and leg.

C The obturator artery supplies the medial compartment of the thigh and does not anastomose with vessels of the leg.

D The descending genicular artery is a branch of the femoral artery, but it arises distal to the site of injury and therefore cannot provide collateral circulation.

E The popliteal artery anastomoses with the proximal femoral artery only through the lateral circumflex femoral artery.

22. **D** Although the medial and lateral circumflex femoral arteries and inferior gluteal artery anastomose around the hip, branches that supply the hip joint arise primarily from the medial circumflex femoral artery (Section 15.4a).

A The obturator artery supplies the medial thigh muscles and a small artery to the head of the femur. It is not a significant blood supply to the joint.

B The superior gluteal artery supplies muscles of the gluteal region but does not supply the hip joint.

C The inferior gluteal artery contributes to an anastomosis around the hip and primarily supplies muscles of the gluteal region.

E The lateral circumflex femoral artery anastomoses with the medial circumflex artery around the femoral neck, but it contributes less to the hip joint and more to the muscles of the lateral thigh.

23. **E** The femoral nerve enters the anterior thigh through the muscular compartment of the retroinguinal space. It branches immediately to innervate the muscles of the anterior thigh (Section 15.4d).

A The femoral sheath encloses only the femoral artery and vein.

B The femoral artery and vein pass through the adductor hiatus into the popliteal fossa.

C The popliteal fossa contains the tibial and common fibular nerves.

D The femoral canal lies medially within the femoral sheath and contains only loose connective tissue, fat, and lymph nodes.

24. A The inferior gluteal nerve innervates only the gluteus maximus muscle (Section 15.4d).
B The superior gluteal nerve innervates the gluteus medius and minimus and tensor of the fascia lata.
C The superior gluteal nerve innervates the gluteus medius and minimus and tensor of the fascia lata.
D The piriformis is innervated by the S1 and S2 branches of the sacral plexus.
E B, C, and D are incorrect

25. A The upper fibers of the gluteus maximus insert onto the iliotibial tract (Section 16.2).
B Gluteus medius inserts onto the lateral surface of the greater trochanter of the femur.
C Gluteus minimus inserts onto the anterolateral surface of the greater trochanter of the femur.
D Quadratus femoris inserts onto the intertrochanteric crest of the femur.
E Not applicable.

26. A The hamstring muscles originate at the ischial tuberosity and insert on the tibia and fibula. Repetitive stretching of these muscles over two joints (the flexed hip and extended knee) can irritate the site of origin (Section 16.4a).
B Pain from a tear at the insertion site of the obturator internus tendon would be focused over the greater trochanter of the femur.
C The sciatic nerve emerges from behind the piriformis muscle and can be compressed at this location. However, pain would reflect the sensory areas of the tibial and common fibular nerves, which include the anterolateral and posterior leg and the dorsum and lateral edge of the foot.
D Irritation of the tibial nerve would manifest as pain in the sole of the foot.
E The inferior gluteal nerve does not have a sensory component. Injury to the nerve would affect the gluteus maximus muscle and manifest as weakened extension and lateral rotation.

27. D The biceps femoris is one of the hamstring muscles (biceps femoris, semitendinosus, semimembranosus), which are the primary flexors of the knee (Section 16.4a).
A The flexor hallucis longus flexes the 1st digit and plantar flexes the foot.
B The soleus does not cross the knee joint and only plantar flexes the foot at the ankle.
C The tibialis posterior plantar flexes and inverts the foot.
E The rectus femoris extends the leg at the knee.

28. C The borders of the femoral triangle are the sartorius, adductor longus, and inguinal ligament (Section 16.4b).
A The tensor fasciae latae is the lateral boundary of the anterior thigh. The femoral triangle lies between the anterior and medial thigh compartments.
B The femoral nerve is one of the contents (lateral) of the femoral triangle but not a boundary.
D The adductor longus is the medial border of the triangle.
E The rectus femoris is lateral to the femoral triangle and lies inside the anterior compartment of the thigh.

29. D The tarsal tunnel is formed by the flexor retinaculum and its attachments to the calcaneus and medial malleolus of the tibia (Section 16.6b).
A The navicular and talus lie distal to the tarsal tunnel, and neither provide attachment for the flexor retinaculum, which forms the roof of the tunnel.
B The cuboid lies on the lateral side of the foot; the tarsal tunnel lies on the medial side of the ankle.
C The talus is not part of the tarsal tunnel.
E Neither the talus nor the 1st metatarsal is part of the tarsal tunnel.

30. A The plantar calcaneonavicular ligament supports the head of the talus, which forms the apex of the medial longitudinal arch (Section 16.8b).
B The deltoid ligament is the collateral ligament on the medial side of the ankle. It is not associated with the medial arch.
C The posterior talofibular ligament is part of the lateral ligament of the ankle and is not associated with the medial arch.
D The superior extensor retinaculum restrains the tendons on the dorsum of the foot (dorsiflexors).
E The tendon of the fibularis longus supports the transverse arch on the lateral side of the sole of the foot.

17 Overview of the Head and Neck

The head and neck region contains the brain, cranial meninges, cranial nerves, and sensory organs, as well as components of the respiratory, gastrointestinal, and endocrine systems. The skull encloses the brain, provides the bony framework for soft tissues of the head, and contains the nasal and oral cavities and bony orbits. The head and neck communicate with the thorax through the superior thoracic aperture and with the upper limb through the cervicoaxillary canal.

17.1 Bones of the Head: The Skull

The skull is made up of two parts: the large **neurocranium** and the smaller **viscerocranium** (**Fig. 17.1**).

— The neurocranium, which makes up the largest part of the skull, houses and protects the brain.
— The viscerocranium includes the lower jaw and the thin-walled bones of the facial skeleton.

17.1a The Neurocranium

The neurocranium is formed by eight bones: the frontal, occipital, sphenoid, and ethmoid bones and paired parietal and temporal bones. Four of these, the frontal, occipital, and two parietal bones, form the **calvaria**, or skullcap. These bones are composed of three layers: a dense **outer table**, a thin **inner table**, and a middle **diploë layer** (**Fig. 17.2A** and **B**).

Fig. 17.1 ▶ **Bones of the neurocranium and viscerocranium**
Left lateral view.

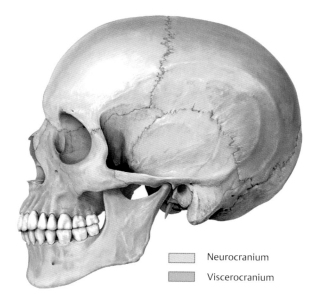

Neurocranium

Viscerocranium

Fig. 17.2 ▶ **Calvaria**

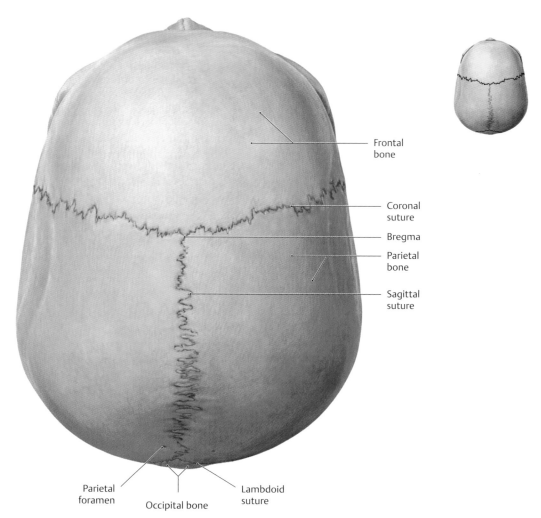

Frontal bone

Coronal suture

Bregma

Parietal bone

Sagittal suture

Parietal foramen

Occipital bone

Lambdoid suture

A External calvaria, superior view.

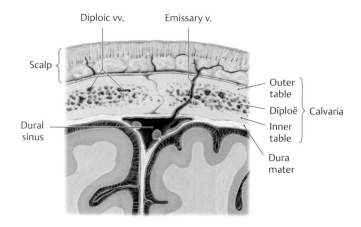

Diploic vv.

Emissary v.

Scalp

Dural sinus

Outer table

Diploë

Inner table

Dura mater

Calvaria

B Cross section of the calvaria.

— The **frontal bone** (**Figs. 17.3** and **17.4**) forms the forehead, the roof and superior rim of the orbit (eye socket), and the floor of the anterior cranial fossa (see Section 17.1d).

— The paired **parietal bones** (see **Figs. 17.2** and **17.3**) are flat bones that form the superolateral parts of the calvaria. Their internal surface has grooves for the middle meningeal arteries and the superior sagittal sinus.

Fig. 17.3 ▶ **Lateral skull**
Left lateral view.

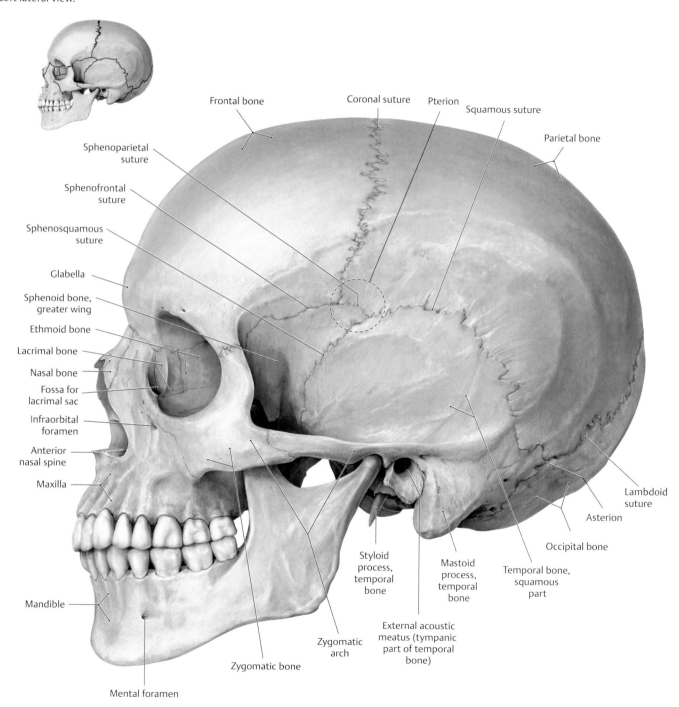

Fig. 17.4 ► **Anterior skull**
Anterior view.

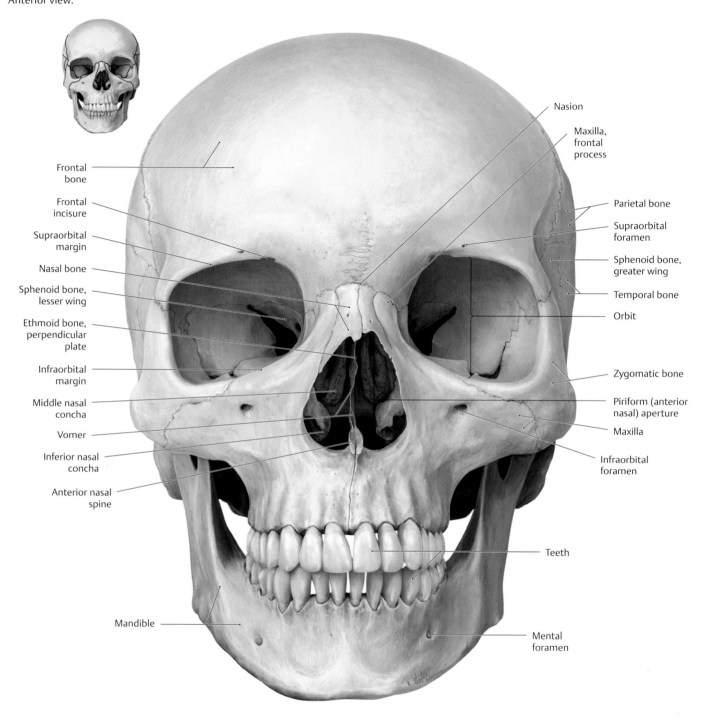

Frontal bone

Frontal incisure

Supraorbital margin

Nasal bone

Sphenoid bone, lesser wing

Ethmoid bone, perpendicular plate

Infraorbital margin

Middle nasal concha

Vomer

Inferior nasal concha

Anterior nasal spine

Mandible

Nasion

Maxilla, frontal process

Parietal bone

Supraorbital foramen

Sphenoid bone, greater wing

Temporal bone

Orbit

Zygomatic bone

Piriform (anterior nasal) aperture

Maxilla

Infraorbital foramen

Teeth

Mental foramen

— The **occipital bone** (**Figs. 17.5**, **17.6**, and **17.7**) forms the posterior cranial fossa of the skull base.

- A small anterior portion is called the **clivus**.
- Foramina (openings) include the large **foramen magnum**, the **jugular foramina**, and the **condylar canals**.
- Inferiorly, **occipital condyles** articulate with the first cervical vertebra.

- The internal surface has grooves for the sigmoid and transverse dural sinuses.
- The external surface is marked with **superior** and **inferior nuchal lines** and an **external occipital protuberance**.

— The paired **temporal bones** (see **Figs. 17.3**, **17.6**, and **17.7**) form part of the middle and posterior cranial fossae.

Fig. 17.5 ▶ **Posterior skull**
Posterior view.

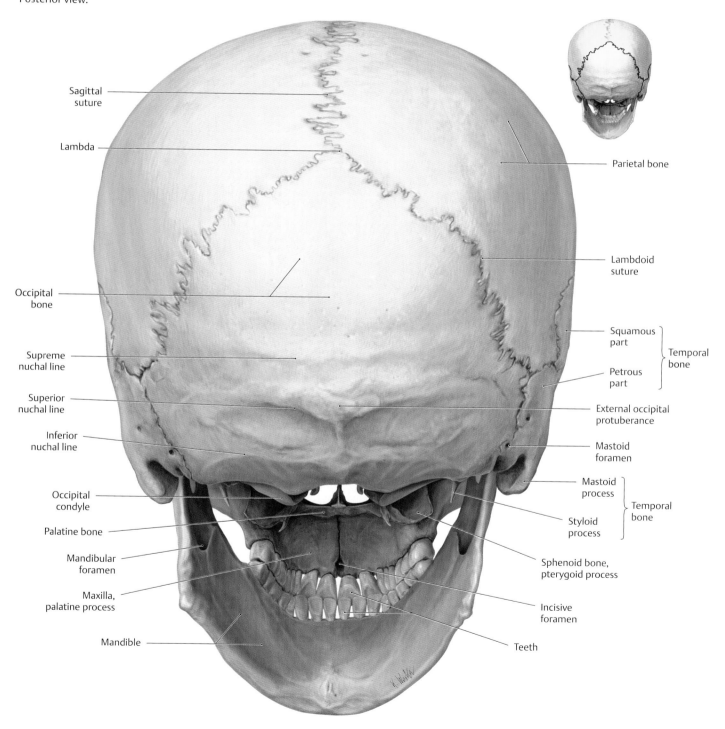

Sagittal suture

Lambda

Parietal bone

Lambdoid suture

Occipital bone

Squamous part

Temporal bone

Petrous part

Supreme nuchal line

Superior nuchal line

External occipital protuberance

Inferior nuchal line

Mastoid foramen

Mastoid process

Temporal bone

Occipital condyle

Styloid process

Palatine bone

Sphenoid bone, pterygoid process

Mandibular foramen

Maxilla, palatine process

Incisive foramen

Mandible

Teeth

Fig. 17.6 ▶ **Base of the skull: Exterior**
Inferior view.

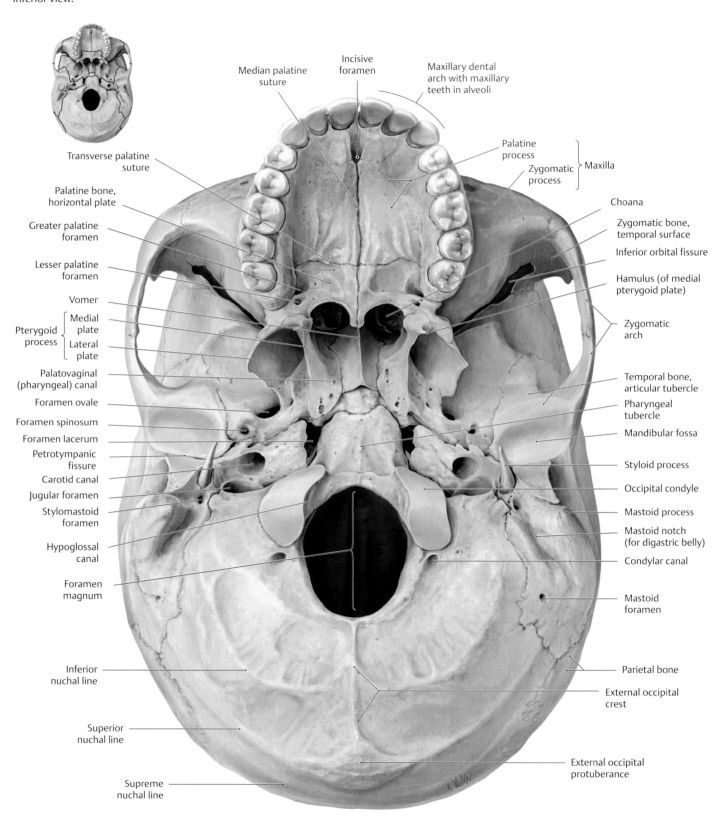

Incisive foramen

Median palatine suture

Maxillary dental arch with maxillary teeth in alveoli

Transverse palatine suture

Palatine bone, horizontal plate

Greater palatine foramen

Lesser palatine foramen

Vomer

Pterygoid process { Medial plate / Lateral plate }

Palatovaginal (pharyngeal) canal

Foramen ovale

Foramen spinosum

Foramen lacerum

Petrotympanic fissure

Carotid canal

Jugular foramen

Stylomastoid foramen

Hypoglossal canal

Foramen magnum

Inferior nuchal line

Superior nuchal line

Supreme nuchal line

Palatine process

Zygomatic process } Maxilla

Choana

Zygomatic bone, temporal surface

Inferior orbital fissure

Hamulus (of medial pterygoid plate)

Zygomatic arch

Temporal bone, articular tubercle

Pharyngeal tubercle

Mandibular fossa

Styloid process

Occipital condyle

Mastoid process

Mastoid notch (for digastric belly)

Condylar canal

Mastoid foramen

Parietal bone

External occipital crest

External occipital protuberance

- An outer **squamous part** forms the lateral skull, an inner **petrous part** encloses the middle and inner ear, and a **tympanic part** encloses the external auditory canal and tympanic membrane.

- Processes include a **mastoid process** composed of a mesh of **mastoid air cells**, the posterior part of the **zygomatic arch**, and a long, pointed **styloid process.**
- Foramina (openings) include an **internal acoustic meatus**, **external acoustic meatus**, **carotid canal**, and **stylomastoid foramen**.
- A **mandibular fossa** and **articular tubercle** articulate with the mandible.

Fig. 17.7 ▶ **Base of the skull: Interior**
Superior view.

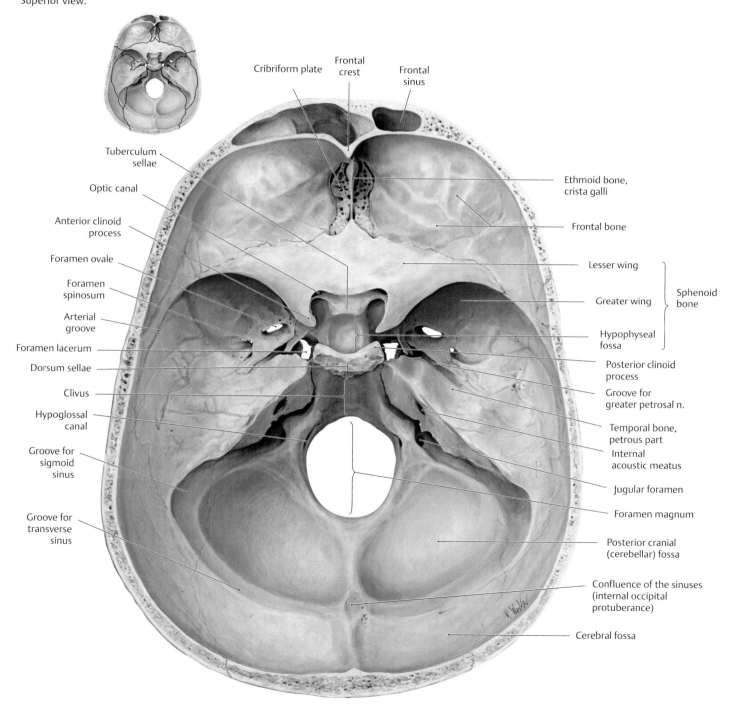

Cribriform plate

Frontal crest

Frontal sinus

Tuberculum sellae

Optic canal

Anterior clinoid process

Foramen ovale

Foramen spinosum

Arterial groove

Foramen lacerum

Dorsum sellae

Clivus

Hypoglossal canal

Groove for sigmoid sinus

Groove for transverse sinus

Ethmoid bone, crista galli

Frontal bone

Lesser wing

Greater wing

Sphenoid bone

Hypophyseal fossa

Posterior clinoid process

Groove for greater petrosal n.

Temporal bone, petrous part

Internal acoustic meatus

Jugular foramen

Foramen magnum

Posterior cranial (cerebellar) fossa

Confluence of the sinuses (internal occipital protuberance)

Cerebral fossa

— The **sphenoid bone** (**Fig. 17.8A** and **B**; see also **Figs. 17.6** and **17.7**) forms the posterior part of the orbit and the floor and lateral wall of the middle cranial fossa between the frontal and temporal bones.

- It has two **greater wings** that form parts of the middle cranial fossa and lateral walls of the skull.
- Two **lesser wings** form the posterior part of the anterior cranial fossa and end in **anterior clinoid processes**.
- The **sphenoid body** encloses the **sphenoid sinus**.

- A midline saddle-shaped formation, the **sella turcica**, contains the **hypophyseal fossa** and is limited anteriorly by the **tuberculum sellae** and posteriorly by the **dorsum sellae** and its **posterior clinoid processes**.
- Paired **pterygoid processes**, each with a **medial** and a **lateral pterygoid plate**, project inferiorly.
- Paired openings include the **optic canal**, **superior orbital fissure**, **foramen rotundum**, **foramen ovale**, and **foramen spinosum**.

Fig. 17.8 ► **Sphenoid bone**

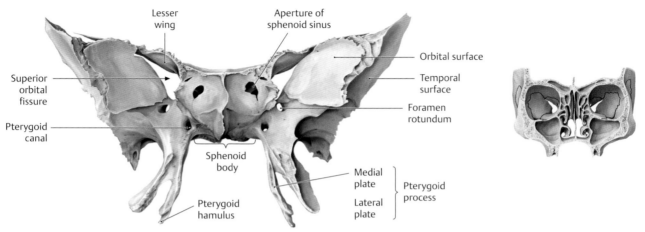

A Anterior view.

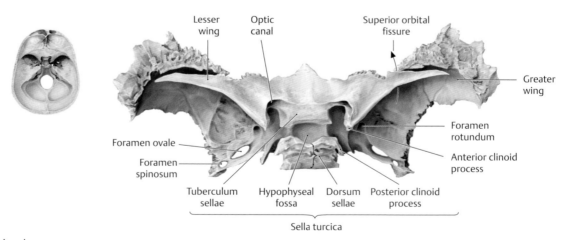

B Superior view.

— The **ethmoid bone** (**Fig. 17.9**; see also **Figs. 17.3** and **17.7**) forms part of the anterior cranial fossa, the medial walls of the orbits, and parts of the nasal septum and lateral nasal walls.

- The **cribriform plate** sits in the anterior cranial fossa above the nasal cavity.
- The **perpendicular plate** forms part of the nasal septum.
- Ethmoid processes include the **crista galli** superiorly and **superior** and **middle nasal concha** inferiorly on the lateral wall of the nasal cavity.
- Numerous thin-walled **ethmoid air cells** form the **ethmoid sinuses**.

17.1b The Viscerocranium

The **viscerocraniun**, or facial skeleton, is composed of 14 bones: the mandible and vomer, and the paired inferior nasal concha, maxillary, nasal, lacrimal, zygomatic, and palatine bones (see **Fig. 17.3**).

— Paired **maxillary bones** (maxilla) (see **Figs. 17.4**, **17.6**, and **17.9**) form the upper jaw, floors of the orbits, and parts of the nose and palate.

- The **maxillary dental arch** contains **alveoli** (sockets) for the upper teeth.
- **Palatine processes** form the anterior part of the palate, and **frontal processes** form part of the external nose.
- An **infraorbital foramen** opens onto the face.
- A large **maxillary sinus** within the maxilla sits below each orbit.

— The **mandible** (**Fig. 17.10**; see also **Fig. 17.3**) forms the lower jaw.

- A horizontal **body** connects posteriorly with a vertical **ramus** on each side.
- An **angle** forms on each side at the junction between the body and the ramus.
- The superior end of each ramus has an anterior **coronoid process** that is separated from the posterior **condylar process** by a **mandibular notch**.
- The **head** of the condylar process articulates with the mandibular fossa of the temporal bone.
- Foramina include a **mental foramen** externally and a **mandibular foramen** internally.
- The **mandibular dental arch** contains alveoli that house the lower teeth.

Fig. 17.9 ▶ **Bones of the orbit and nasal cavities**
Coronal section, anterior view.

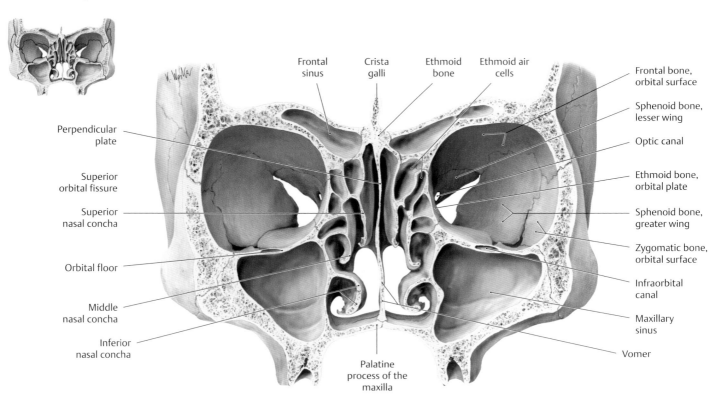

Fig. 17.10 ▶ **Mandible**
Oblique, left lateral view.

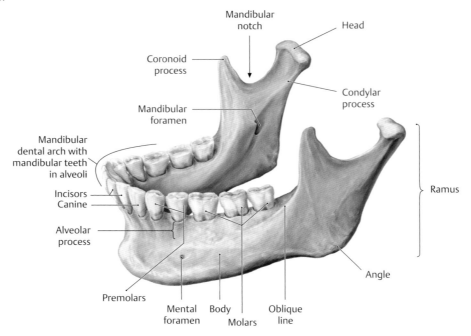

— Paired **nasal bones** (see **Fig. 17.4**) form the bridge of the nose.
— Paired **lacrimal bones** (see **Fig. 17.3**) form the anterior medial walls of the orbits and contain **fossae for the lacrimal sacs**.
— Paired **zygomatic bones** (see **Fig. 17.3**) form the bony prominences of the cheeks, anterior parts of the zygomatic arches, and lateral walls of the orbits.
— Paired **palatine bones** (see **Fig. 17.6**) have vertical parts that form the posterior lateral walls of the nasal cavity and **horizontal processes** that form the posterior parts of the palate.
— The **vomer** (see **Fig. 17.9**) forms the inferior and posterior part of nasal septum.
— Paired **inferior nasal conchae** (see **Fig. 17.9**) form the lowest scroll-like processes on the lateral walls of the nasal cavity.

17.1c Sutures of the Skull

— During development, the bones of the calvaria grow outward from their center toward adjacent bones; the bones eventually fuse to form fibrous joints called **sutures**.

— Although there are many smaller sutures, the major sutures of the calvaria (see **Figs. 17.2**, **17.3**, and **17.5**) are

  • the **sagittal suture** between the right and left parietal bones,
  • the **coronal suture** between the frontal and parietal bones,
  • the **lambdoid suture** between the occipital and parietal bones, and
  • the **squamous sutures** between the parietal and temporal bones.

— At birth, growth of the skull bones and formation of the sutures are incomplete. Large fibrous areas, known as **fontanelles**, remain between the bones and allow for continued growth of the brain. The largest of these, the **anterior fontanelle** at the junction of the frontal and parietal bones, closes between 18 and 24 months of age.

Craniosynostosis

Premature closure of the cranial sutures, a condition known as craniosynostosis, results in a variety of skull malformations, the shape of which depends on the suture involved. *Plagiocephaly*, the most common deformity, indicates premature closure of the coronal or lambdoid suture on one side and creates an asymmetrical appearance. *Scaphocephaly* is characterized by a long, narrow cranium produced by early closure of the sagittal suture. If untreated, craniosynostosis may lead to increased intracranial pressure, seizures, and delayed development of the skull and brain. Surgery is typically the recommended treatment to reduce the intracranial pressure and correct the deformities of the face and skull bones.

— Junctions of the sutures and other prominent points of the skull are useful for measuring growth of the skull and brain; determining race, gender, and age; and locating deep cranial structures (**Table 17.1**).

Landmark	Location of Point or Area
Nasion	Junction of frontonasal and internasal sutures
Glabella	Most anterior prominence of frontal bone at the top of the nose
Bregma	Junction of coronal and sagittal sutures
Pterion	Area encompassing junction of frontal, parietal, sphenoid, and temporal bones along the sphenoparietal suture
Vertex	Most superior point of the skull along the sagittal suture
Lambda	Junction of lambdoid and sagittal sutures
Asterion	Junction of sutures joining occipital, temporal, and parietal bones

Table 17.1 ▶ Landmarks of the Skull (see Figs. 17.2, 17.3, 17.4, and 17.5)

Skull fractures at the pterion

The thin bones that make up the pterion overlie the anterior branches of the middle meningeal artery, a branch of the maxillary artery that runs deep to the bone in the epidural space. Because of this relationship, skull fractures at the pterion can lead to a life-threatening epidural hemorrhage (see p. 398).

17.1d Cranial Fossae

— The floor of the cranial cavity is divided into three fossae, or spaces (**Fig. 17.11**; see also **Fig. 17.7**).

Fig. 17.11 ▶ **Cranial fossae**
Opened skull, superior view. The interior of the skull base consists of three successive fossae that become progressively deeper in the frontal-to-occipital direction.

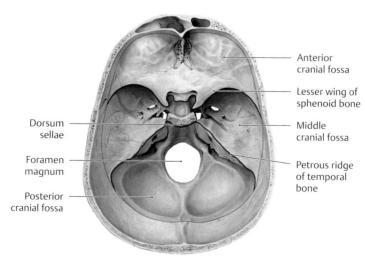

- The **anterior cranial fossa**, formed by the frontal and ethmoid bones and lesser wing of the sphenoid bone, contains the frontal lobe of the brain and the olfactory bulbs (see Section 18.2 for a description of the brain).
- The **middle cranial fossa**, formed by the greater and lesser wings of the sphenoid bone and squamous and petrous parts of the temporal bones, contains the temporal lobes of the brain, the optic chiasm, and the pituitary gland. The hypophyseal fossa separates the right and left halves of the middle cranial fossa.
- The **posterior cranial fossa**, formed primarily by the occipital bone and petrous parts of the temporal bones, contains the pons, medulla oblongata, and cerebellum of the brain. The medulla oblongata exits the skull through the foramen magnum located on the floor of the fossa, and grooves on the posterior and lateral walls accommodate the transverse and sigmoid dural venous sinuses.

— Foramina within the anterior, middle, and posterior fossae allow blood vessels and nerves to pass through the skull (**Fig. 17.12**).

(See Sections 17.3, 17.4, and 18.3 for arteries of the head, veins of the head, and cranial nerves, respectively.)

Fig. 17.12 ► **Neurovascular structures entering or exiting the cranial cavity**

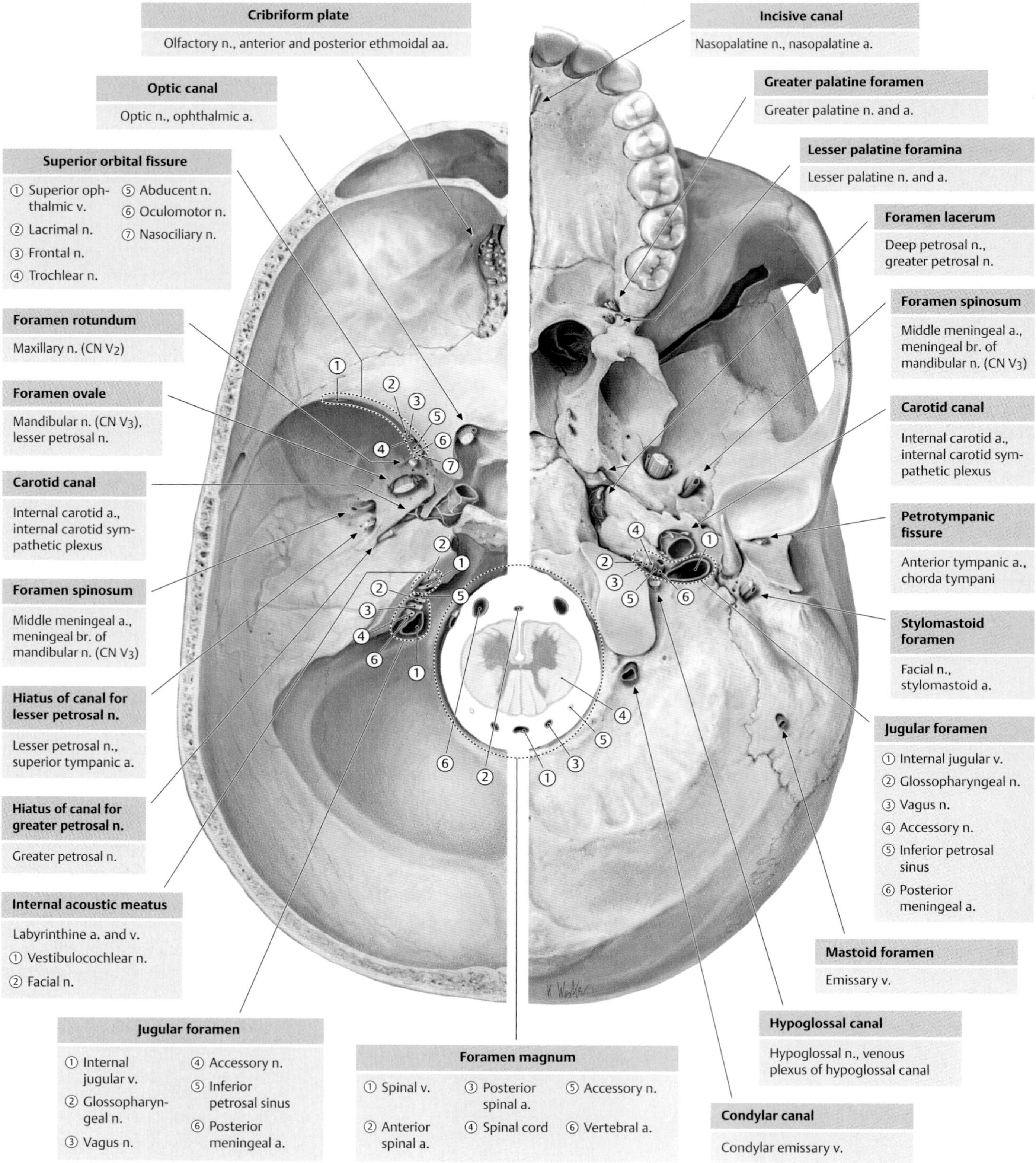

Cribriform plate

Olfactory n., anterior and posterior ethmoidal aa.

Incisive canal

Nasopalatine n., nasopalatine a.

Optic canal

Optic n., ophthalmic a.

Greater palatine foramen

Greater palatine n. and a.

Superior orbital fissure

① Superior oph-   ⑤ Abducent n.
thalmic v.   ⑥ Oculomotor n.
② Lacrimal n.   ⑦ Nasociliary n.
③ Frontal n.
④ Trochlear n.

Lesser palatine foramina

Lesser palatine n. and a.

Foramen lacerum

Deep petrosal n., greater petrosal n.

Foramen rotundum

Maxillary n. (CN V₂)

Foramen spinosum

Middle meningeal a., meningeal br. of mandibular n. (CN V₃)

Foramen ovale

Mandibular n. (CN V₃), lesser petrosal n.

Carotid canal

Internal carotid a., internal carotid sympathetic plexus

Carotid canal

Internal carotid a., internal carotid sympathetic plexus

Petrotympanic fissure

Anterior tympanic a., chorda tympani

Foramen spinosum

Middle meningeal a., meningeal br. of mandibular n. (CN V₃)

Stylomastoid foramen

Facial n., stylomastoid a.

Hiatus of canal for lesser petrosal n.

Lesser petrosal n., superior tympanic a.

Jugular foramen

① Internal jugular v.
② Glossopharyngeal n.
③ Vagus n.
④ Accessory n.
⑤ Inferior petrosal sinus
⑥ Posterior meningeal a.

Hiatus of canal for greater petrosal n.

Greater petrosal n.

Internal acoustic meatus

Labyrinthine a. and v.
① Vestibulocochlear n.
② Facial n.

Mastoid foramen

Emissary v.

Jugular foramen

① Internal jugular v.
② Glossopharyngeal n.
③ Vagus n.
④ Accessory n.
⑤ Inferior petrosal sinus
⑥ Posterior meningeal a.

Foramen magnum

① Spinal v.   ③ Posterior spinal a.   ⑤ Accessory n.
② Anterior spinal a.   ④ Spinal cord   ⑥ Vertebral a.

Hypoglossal canal

Hypoglossal n., venous plexus of hypoglossal canal

Condylar canal

Condylar emissary v.

A Cranial cavity (interior of skull base). Left side, superior view.

B Exterior of skull base. Left side, inferior view.

17.2 Bones of the Neck

Most bones of the neck are parts of the vertebral column, thoracic skeleton, or pectoral girdle (see **Fig. 1.7A**).

— The seven cervical vertebrae support the head on the vertebral column and provide attachment for neck muscles.
— The manubrium of the sternum forms the inferior midline boundary of the anterior neck.
— The clavicles form the lateral boundaries of the neck.
— The **hyoid bone**, a small U-shaped bone, lies anterior to the C3 vertebra in the neck (**Fig. 17.13**).

  • It has a **body** and paired **lesser** and **greater horns**.
  • The hyoid does not articulate directly with any other bones of the skeleton, but muscles and ligaments attach it to the mandible, styloid processes of the temporal bones, larynx, clavicles, sternum, and scapulae.

Fig. 17.13 ▶ **Hyoid bone**
The hyoid bone is suspended in the neck by muscles between the floor of the mouth and the larynx.

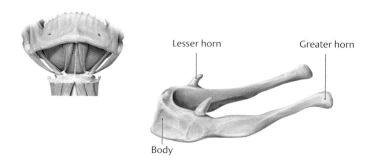

Lesser horn   Greater horn

Body

17.3 Arteries of the Head and Neck

Arteries of the head and neck are branches of the right and left **subclavian** and **common carotid arteries** (see **Fig. 3.4**).

— The brachiocephalic trunk arises from the aortic arch and divides behind the right sternoclavicular joint to form the right subclavian and right common carotid arteries.
— The left subclavian and left common carotid arteries are direct branches of the aortic arch in the superior mediastinum of the thorax.

17.3a The Subclavian Artery

The subclavian arteries enter the neck through the superior thoracic aperture and pass laterally between the anterior and middle scalene muscles. Two branches, the vertebral artery and the thyrocervical trunk, arise medial to the anterior scalene muscles on each side and supply structures in the head and neck (**Fig. 17.14**).

— The **vertebral artery** passes posteriorly in the neck to ascend through the transverse foramina of C1–C6 vertebrae and enters the foramen magnum at the base of the skull (see **Figs. 2.21B** and **18.12**).

  • In the neck, it contributes the single anterior spinal artery and paired posterior spinal arteries that supply the upper spinal cord.
  • In the skull, it gives off the **posteroinferior cerebellar arteries**.
  • It terminates by joining the contralateral vertebral artery to form a single **basilar artery**, which supplies the posterior circulation of the brain.

— The **thyrocervical trunk** is a short trunk that branches into four arteries:

  • The **inferior thyroid artery**, the largest branch, which turns medially to supply the larynx, trachea, esophagus, and thyroid and parathyroid glands
  • The **suprascapular** and **transverse cervical arteries**, which supply muscles of the back and scapular region
  • The **ascending cervical artery**, a small branch that supplies muscles in the neck

17.3b The Carotid Artery System

The carotid artery system supplies structures of the neck, face, skull, and brain and consists of paired common carotid, external carotid, and internal carotid arteries and their branches.

— The **common carotid artery** enters the neck from the thorax and ascends, with the internal jugular vein and vagus nerve, within a fascial sleeve, the **carotid sheath**.

383

Fig. 17.14 ► **Arteries of the neck**
Left lateral view. The structures of the neck are primarily supplied by the external carotid artery and subclavian artery.

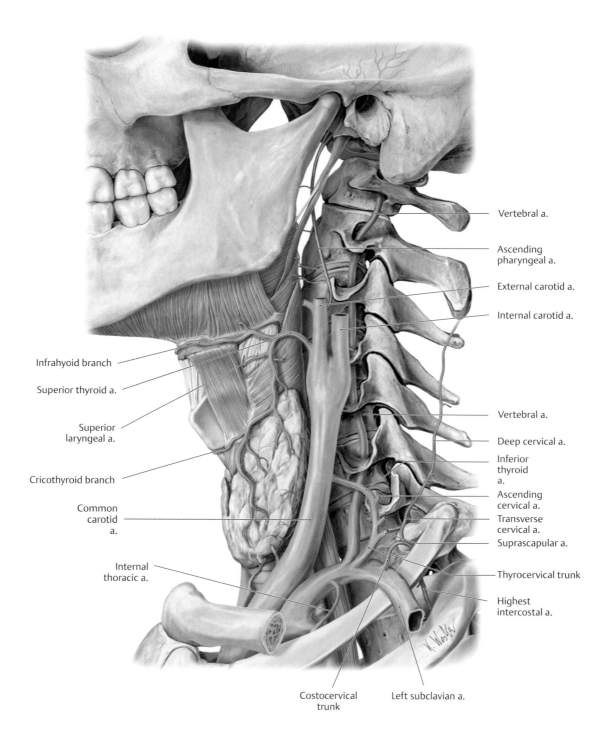

Vertebral a.

Ascending pharyngeal a.

External carotid a.

Internal carotid a.

Vertebral a.

Deep cervical a.

Inferior thyroid a.

Ascending cervical a.

Transverse cervical a.

Suprascapular a.

Thyrocervical trunk

Highest intercostal a.

Infrahyoid branch

Superior thyroid a.

Superior laryngeal a.

Cricothyroid branch

Common carotid a.

Internal thoracic a.

Costocervical trunk

Left subclavian a.

- Its only branches, the **external carotid** and **internal carotid arteries**, arise from its bifurcation at the C4 vertebral level (**Fig. 17.15**).

— The **external carotid artery** supplies most structures of the face and head except the brain and the orbits. Six branches arise from the external carotid artery in the neck before it passes behind the mandible and finally bifurcates into two terminal branches, the **maxillary** and **superficial temporal arteries**.

1. The **superior thyroid artery** supplies the thyroid gland and, through its **superior laryngeal artery**, the larynx.
2. The **lingual artery** supplies the posterior tongue and floor of the mouth.
3. The **facial artery** ascends deep to the submandibular gland, which it supplies, and crosses the mandible from below to enter the face. It passes lateral to the corners of the mouth

and terminates near the medial angle of the eye as the **angular artery**. The branches of the facial artery include

  o the **submental** and **tonsillar branches** in the neck and
  o the **superior** and **inferior labial arteries** and a **lateral nasal artery** on the face.

4. The **occipital artery** supplies branches to the posterior scalp.
5. The **ascending pharyngeal artery** sends branches to the pharynx, ear, and deep neck muscles.
6. The **posterior auricular artery** passes posteriorly to supply the scalp behind the ear.

— The maxillary artery arises posterior to the mandible and passes medially through the **infratemporal** and **pterygopalatine fossae** (see Sections 19.5 and 19.6). Branches from its three parts, the **mandibular, pterygoid**, and **pterygopalatine parts**, supply most structures of the face (**Table 17.2**; **Figs. 17.16A** and **B** and **17.17A** and **B**).

Fig. 17.15 ▶ **External carotid artery**
Left lateral view.

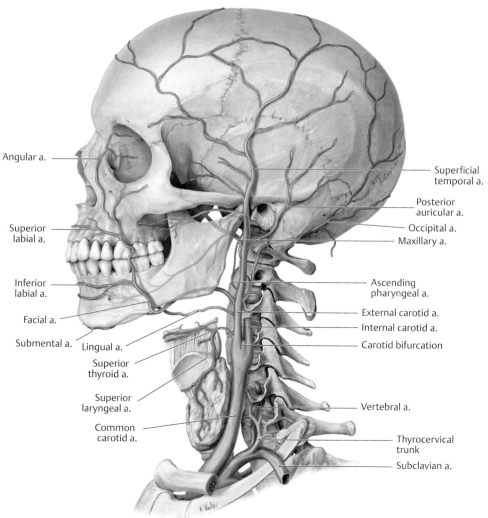

Table 17.2 ▶ Terminal Branches of the External Carotid Artery		
Artery	**Divisions and Distribution**	
Superficial temporal a.	Transverse facial a. (to soft tissues below the zygomatic arch); frontal branches; parietal branches; zygomatico-orbital a. (to lateral orbital wall)	
Maxillary a.	Mandibular part	Inferior alveolar a. (to mandible, teeth, gingiva); middle meningeal a.; deep auricular a. (to temporomandibular joint, external auditory canal); anterior tympanic a.
	Pterygoid part	Masseteric a.; deep temporal branches; pterygoid branches; buccal a.
	Pterygopalatine part	Posterior superior alveolar a. (to maxillary molars, maxillary sinus, gingiva); infraorbital a. (to maxillary alveoli)
		Descending palatine a. → Greater palatine a. (to hard palate)
		Descending palatine a. → Lesser palatine a. (to soft palate, palatine tonsil, pharyngeal wall)
		Sphenopalatine a. → Lateral posterior nasal aa. (to lateral wall of nasal cavity, conchae)
		Sphenopalatine a. → Posterior septal branches (to nasal septum)

Fig. 17.16 ▶ Maxillary artery
Left lateral view.

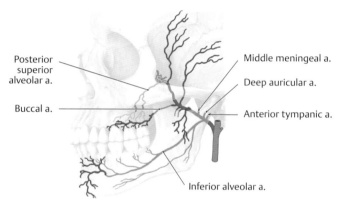

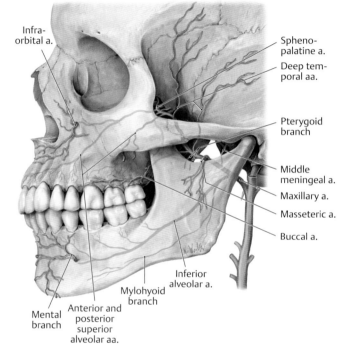

A Divisions of the maxillary artery: mandibular (blue), pterygoid (green), pterygopalatine (yellow).

B Course of the maxillary artery.

Fig. 17.17 ▶ Deep branches of the maxillary artery

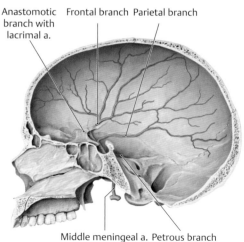

A Right middle meningeal artery. Opened skull, medial view.

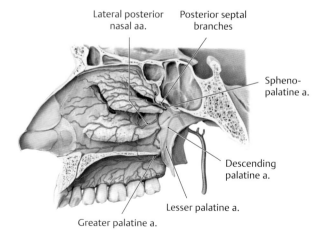

B Lateral wall of right nasal cavity and palate, medial view.

— The superficial temporal artery passes superiorly through the temporal region anterior to the ear and terminates as **frontal** and **parietal arteries** on the scalp. Its branches on the face (**Fig. 17.18**; see **Table 17.2**) include the following:

- The **transverse facial artery**, which supplies the parotid gland and duct and crosses anteriorly to supply the skin of the face
- The **zygomatico-orbital artery**, which supplies the lateral orbit
- The **middle temporal artery**, which supplies the temporal region

— The **internal carotid artery** is the continuation of the common carotid artery (**Fig. 17.19**).

- It is described in four parts:
  - A cervical part in the neck that has no branches
  - A petrous part that courses within the carotid canal of the temporal bone
  - A cavernous part that passes through (see **Figs. 18.5** and **18.6**) the **cavernous sinus** (a venous sinus lateral to the sella turcica)
  - A cerebral part that emerges into the middle cranial fossa posterior to the orbit

Fig. 17.18 ▶ **Superficial temporal artery**
Left lateral view.

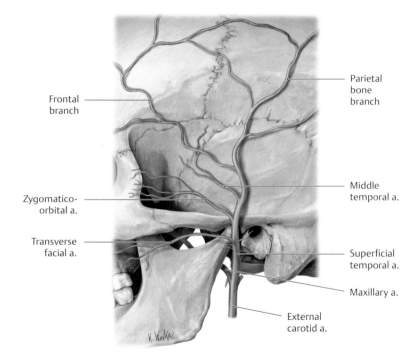

- Two receptors are located within the internal carotid artery near its origin.
  - The **carotid sinus**, a baroreceptor that responds to changes in arterial pressure, is noticeable as a small dilation near the origin of the internal carotid artery.
  - The **carotid body**, a small mass of tissue located near the carotid sinus, is a chemoreceptor that monitors blood oxygen levels. Stimulation of the carotid body initiates an increase in heart rate, respiration rate, and blood pressure.

- The **ophthalmic artery**, which arises within the skull as the first major branch of the internal carotid artery, passes through the optic canal to supply the orbital contents, including the retina of the eye through its **central retinal artery**.
  - Branches of the ophthalmic artery, the **supraorbital** and **supratrochlear arteries** to the anterior scalp and **ethmoidal arteries** to the nasal cavity, anastomose with branches of the external carotid artery.
- The **anterior** and **middle cerebral arteries** arise from the internal carotid artery to supply the anterior circulation of the brain (see Section 18.2c).

Fig. 17.19 ▶ **Internal carotid artery**
Left lateral view.

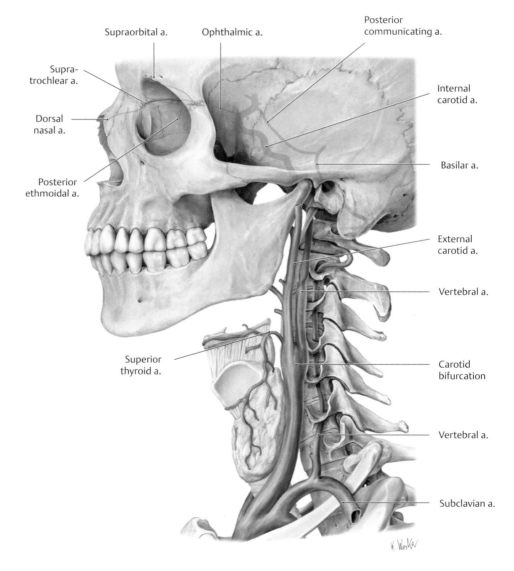

17.4 Veins of the Head and Neck

— Superficial and deep veins of the head and neck drain almost exclusively to the external and internal jugular veins, although some also communicate with the vertebral venous plexus of the vertebral column (**Fig. 17.20**).

— Superficial veins generally follow the course of the arteries, but the veins are usually more numerous, more variable, and more interconnected than the arteries.

— The most prominent superficial veins on each side of the head include

   • the **supratrochlear** and **supraorbital veins**, which drain to the angular vein;

   • the **angular vein**, which joins with the deep facial vein and continues inferiorly as the facial vein;

   • the **pterygoid venous plexus**, which drains areas supplied by the maxillary artery, including the orbit, nasal cavity, and oral cavity (it drains to the maxillary and deep facial veins);

   • the **deep facial vein**, which arises from the pterygoid venous plexus and drains to the facial vein;

   • the **facial vein**, which drains to the **internal jugular vein**;

   • the **superficial temporal** and **maxillary veins**, which join to form the retromandibular vein;

   • the **retromandibular vein**, which joins the **posterior auricular vein** to form the **external jugular vein**; and

   • the **occipital vein**, which drains to the external jugular vein.

Fig. 17.20 ▶ **Superficial veins of the head and neck** Left lateral view.

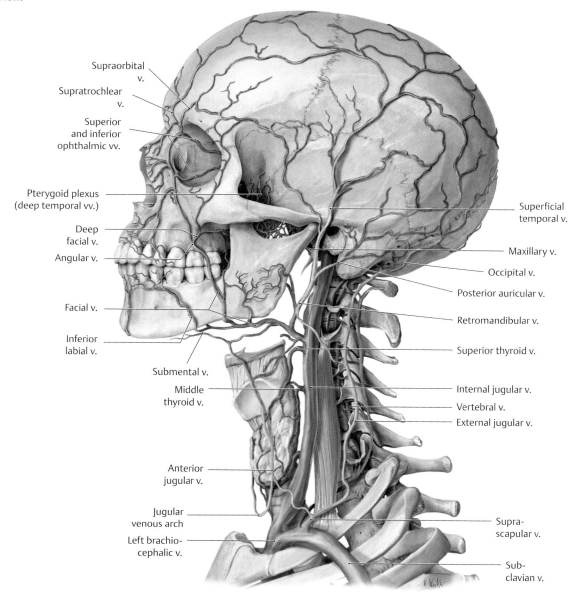

Labels, top to bottom, left side:
Supraorbital v.
Supratrochlear v.
Superior and inferior ophthalmic vv.
Pterygoid plexus (deep temporal vv.)
Deep facial v.
Angular v.
Facial v.
Inferior labial v.
Submental v.
Middle thyroid v.
Anterior jugular v.
Jugular venous arch
Left brachio-cephalic v.

Labels, top to bottom, right side:
Superficial temporal v.
Maxillary v.
Occipital v.
Posterior auricular v.
Retromandibular v.
Superior thyroid v.
Internal jugular v.
Vertebral v.
External jugular v.
Supra-scapular v.
Sub-clavian v.

— When present, right and left external jugular veins form posterior to the angle of the mandible by the union of the posterior auricular veins and the posterior division of the retromandibular veins.

- They cross the sternocleidomastoid muscle in the neck and drain into the subclavian vein.
- They drain the scalp and side of the face.
- Their tributaries include the retromandibular, posterior auricular, occipital, transverse cervical, suprascapular, and anterior jugular veins.

— A right and left **internal jugular vein** forms at the jugular foramen at the skull base and descends within the carotid sheath with the common carotid artery and vagus nerve.

- It joins the subclavian vein in the root of the neck to form the brachiocephalic vein. The junction of the internal jugular and subclavian veins is called the **jugulosubclavian junction**, or **venous angle**. The thoracic duct and right lymphatic duct terminate at this junction.
- It drains the brain, the anterior face and scalp, and the viscera and deep muscles of the neck.
- Its tributaries include the dural venous sinuses, facial vein, lingual vein, pharyngeal veins, and superior and middle thyroid veins.

— A small **anterior jugular vein** originates from superficial veins on each side near the hyoid bone.

- It descends to the base of the neck and terminates in the external jugular or subclavian vein.
- A **jugular venous arch** may connect the right and left anterior jugular veins at the base of the neck, above the sternum.

— Deep veins of the orbit and brain drain to **dural venous sinuses**, venous channels formed within the outer covering of the brain that have no arterial counterpart (see Section 18.1c). Dural venous sinuses drain eventually to the internal jugular vein.

17.5 Lymphatic Drainage of the Head and Neck

— Superficial lymph nodes of the head and neck extend along the external jugular vein.

- They receive lymph from local areas and drain to the deep cervical nodes.
- Superficial node groups include occipital, retroauricular, mastoid, parotid, anterior cervical, and lateral cervical nodes (**Fig. 17.21**; **Table 17.3**).

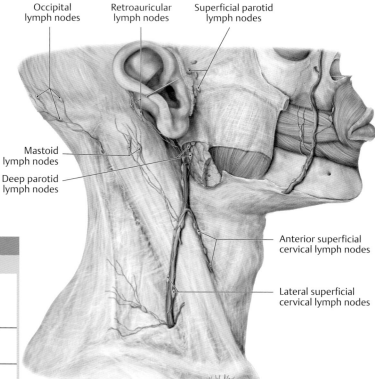

Fig. 17.21 ▶ **Superficial cervical lymph nodes**
Right lateral view.

Table 17.3 ▶ **Superficial Cervical Lymph Nodes**	
Lymph Nodes (l.n.)	**Drainage Region**
Retroauricular l.n.	Occiput
Occipital l.n.	
Mastoid l.n.	
Superficial parotid l.n.	Parotid–auricular region
Deep parotid l.n.	
Anterior superficial cervical l.n.	Sternocleidomastoid region
Lateral superficial cervical l.n.	

— Lymph from structures in the head and neck ultimately drains into **deep cervical lymph nodes** that lie along the internal jugular vein deep to the sternocleidomastoid muscle (**Fig. 17.22**; **Table 17.4**). There are two groups of deep cervical nodes:

- **Superior deep cervical nodes**, known as the jugulodigastric group, lie near the facial and internal jugular veins and posterior belly of the digastric muscle. Submandibular and submental nodes also drain to this group. Superior deep cervical nodes drain either to the inferior deep cervical nodes or directly to the jugular lymphatic trunks.
- **Inferior deep cervical nodes** are usually associated with the lower internal jugular vein, but some nodes also reside in the area around the subclavian vein and brachial plexus. Inferior deep cervical nodes drain directly to the jugular lymphatic trunks.

— Lymphatic vessels from the deep cervical nodes join to form **jugular lymphatic trunks**.

- On the right, these trunks drain directly or indirectly (via the right lymphatic duct) into the right jugulosubclavian junction (right venous angle).
- On the left, these trunks join the thoracic duct, which drains into the left jugulosubclavian junction (left venous angle).

17.6 Nerves of the Head and Neck

— Somatic nerves of the head and neck include the following:

- Spinal nerves C1 through C4, which innervate structures in the head and neck
  - ○ The **cervical plexus** is derived from anterior rami of cervical spinal nerves C1–C4 (see Section 21.3a).
  - ○ The **suboccipital**, **greater occipital**, and **third occipital nerves** are derived from posterior rami of cervical spinal nerves (see Section 19.1).
- Spinal nerves C5 through T1, whose anterior rami form the brachial plexus that innervates the upper limb (see Section 13.4d)
- Cranial nerves (CN I–CN XII), which arise from the brain (see Section 18.3)

— Autonomic nerves of the head and neck include

- parasympathetic nerves, which arise in association with four of the cranial nerves (CN III, VII, XI, and X) (see Section 18.3), and
- sympathetic nerves, which arise from the cervical sympathetic trunk (see Section 21.3c).

Fig. 17.22 ▶ **Deep cervical lymph nodes**
Right lateral view.

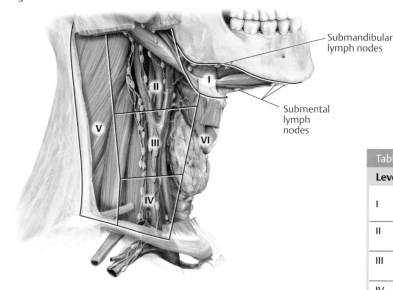

Submandibular lymph nodes

Submental lymph nodes

Table 17.4 ▶ **Deep Cervical Lymph Nodes**			
Level	**Lymph Nodes (l.n.)**		**Drainage Region**
I	Submental l.n.		Face
	Submandibular l.n.		
II	Lateral jugular l.n. group	Upper lateral group	Nuchal region, laryngo-tracheothyroidal region
III		Middle lateral group	
IV		Lower lateral group	
V	L.n. in posterior cervical triangle		Nuchal region
VI	Anterior cervical l.n.		Laryngo-tracheo-thyroidal region

18 Meninges, Brain, and Cranial Nerves

The cranial meninges continuous with the meninges of the spinal cord, as well as the 12 cranial nerves that arise from the brain, are essential parts of gross anatomy of the head and neck region and are discussed in detail in this unit. The study of the brain, however, is generally confined to the neuroanatomy curriculum, and only a brief overview is provided here.

18.1 The Meninges

The cranial meninges, coverings that protect the brain, consist of the external fibrous **dura mater**, the thin intermediate **arachnoid mater**, and the delicate inner **pia mater** (**Fig. 18.1**).

18.1a Dura mater

— The dura mater, or dura, a tough outer membrane surrounding the brain, is composed of a **periosteal layer** and a **meningeal layer**. The two layers are inseparable except where they enclose the venous sinuses that drain the brain (e.g., the superior sagittal sinus shown in **Fig. 18.3**).

  • The outer periosteal layer, formed by the periosteum of the skull, adheres tightly to the inner surface of the skull, particularly at the sutures. This layer ends at the foramen magnum and is not continuous with the dura around the spinal cord.

  • The inner meningeal layer, a strong membranous sheet that adheres to the inner surface of the periosteal layer, provides sheaths for the cranial nerves as they pass through the skull foramina. It is closely applied, although not attached, to the underlying **arachnoid mater** (see **Fig. 18.1**). It continues into the vertebral canal as dura of the spinal cord.

— The middle meningeal arteries, branches of the maxillary arteries, supply most of the dura, with contributions from the ophthalmic, occipital, and vertebral arteries. Veins accompany the arteries and drain into the pterygoid venous plexus.

— Branches of the trigeminal nerve (CN V) transmit sensation from the dura of the anterior and middle cranial fossa. Spinal nerves C1, C2, and C3 and small branches of the vagus nerve (CN X) innervate the dura of the posterior cranial fossa.

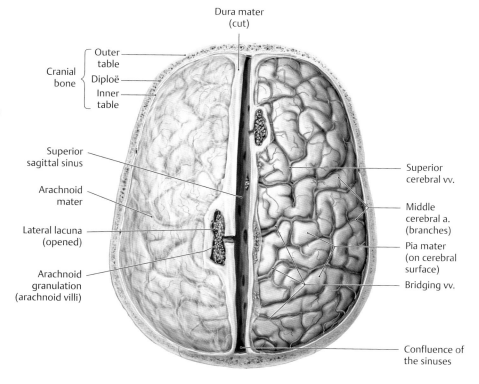

Fig. 18.1 ▶ **Layers of the meninges**
Opened cranium, superior view. *Left side:* Dura mater (outer layer) cut to reveal arachnoid mater (middle layer). *Right side:* Dura mater and arachnoid mater removed to reveal pia mater (inner layer) lining the surface of the brain. *Note:* Arachnoid granulations, sites for loss of cerebral spinal fluid into the venous blood, are protrusions of the arachnoid layer of the meninges into the venous sinus system.

Dura mater (cut)

Cranial bone
  Outer table
  Diploë
  Inner table

Superior sagittal sinus

Arachnoid mater

Lateral lacuna (opened)

Arachnoid granulation (arachnoid villi)

Superior cerebral vv.

Middle cerebral a. (branches)

Pia mater (on cerebral surface)

Bridging vv.

Confluence of the sinuses

18.1b Dural Partitions

Infoldings of the meningeal layer of the dura form incomplete membranous partitions that separate and support parts of the brain (**Fig. 18.2**).

— The **falx cerebri**, a vertical sickle-shaped partition separating the right and left cerebral hemispheres, is attached anteriorly to the crista galli and the inner crest of the frontal bone and is continuous posteriorly with the tentorium cerebelli. The inferior, free edge of the falx cerebri is unattached.
— The **tentorium cerebelli**, a horizontal continuation of the falx cerebri, separates the occipital lobes of the cerebrum from the cerebellar hemispheres in the posterior cranial fossae.

  • It is attached to the posterior clinoid processes and the petrous part of the temporal bones anteriorly and to the parietal and occipital bones posterolaterally.
  • A U-shaped **tentorial notch** separates the attachments to the petrous ridge on each side and connects the middle and posterior cranial fossae.

> **Tentorial herniation**
>
> Increased pressure within the middle cranial fossa created by a space-occupying lesion such as a tumor can squeeze the brain tissue and force part of the temporal lobe to herniate through the tentorial notch. Pressure on the adjacent brainstem can be fatal in this situation. The oculomotor nerve (CN III) can also be stretched or damaged, leading to fixed pupil dilation (loss of parasympathetic function) and a "down and out" gaze due to paralysis of most of the extraocular muscles.

— The **falx cerebelli**, a vertical partition separating the cerebellar hemispheres, is continuous superiorly with the tentorium cerebelli and is attached posteriorly to the occipital crest.
— The **diaphragma sellae**, a small dural fold attached to the anterior and posterior clinoid processes, forms a roof over the sella turcica, which encloses the hypophysis (pituitary gland).

18.1c Dural Venous Sinuses

Dural venous sinuses are valveless venous spaces that form as a result of the separation of the periosteal and meningeal layers of the dura. Most of the large veins of the brain, skull, orbit, and inner ear drain through the dural sinuses and into the internal jugular veins in the neck (**Figs. 18.3** and **18.4**; **Table 18.1**).

— The **confluence of sinuses** at the posterior edge of the tentorium cerebelli is a junction of the superior sagittal, straight, occipital, and transverse sinuses.
— The **superior sagittal sinus** runs in the attached superior border of the falx cerebri and ends in the confluence of sinuses.
— The **inferior sagittal sinus** runs in the free inferior edge of the falx cerebri and ends in the straight sinus.
— The **straight sinus** runs in the space formed by the union of the falx cerebri and tentorium cerebelli. It receives the inferior sagittal sinus and **great cerebral vein** and drains into the confluence of sinuses.
— The paired **transverse sinuses** run along the attached posterolateral margins of the tentorium cerebelli. Posteriorly, they join at the confluence of sinuses, and anteriorly they drain into the sigmoid sinuses, forming grooves in the occipital and parietal bones along their course.
— The paired **sigmoid sinuses** run in deep grooves of the occipital and temporal bones and drain into the internal jugular veins at the jugular foramen.
— The **occipital sinus** runs in the free edge of the falx cerebelli and ends in the confluence of sinuses.

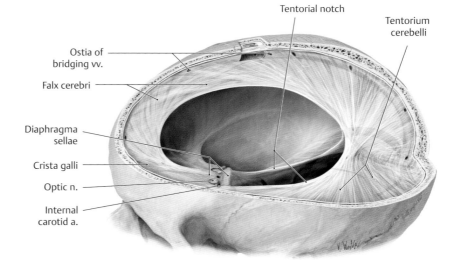

Fig. 18.2 ▶ Dural septa (folds)
Left anterior oblique view.

Tentorial notch
Tentorium cerebelli
Ostia of bridging vv.
Falx cerebri
Diaphragma sellae
Crista galli
Optic n.
Internal carotid a.

Fig. 18.3 ▶ Structure of a dural sinus
Superior sagittal sinus, coronal section, anterior view.

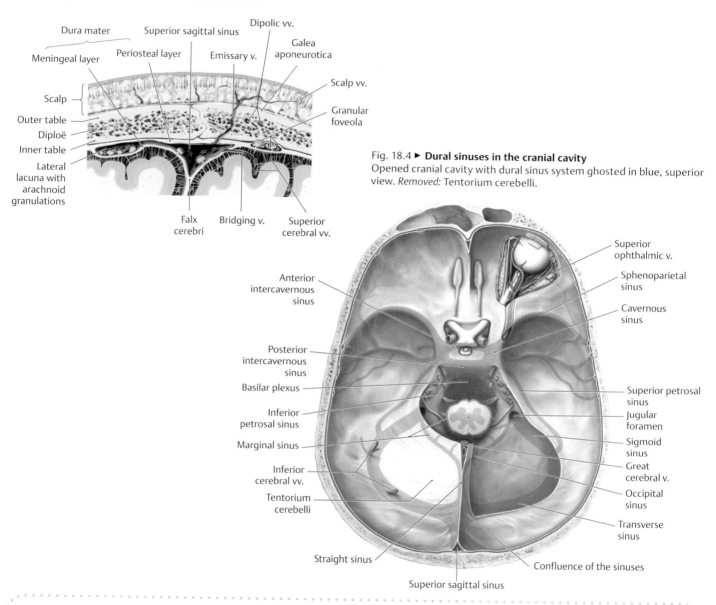

Dura mater
Meningeal layer
Periosteal layer
Superior sagittal sinus
Emissary v.
Dipolic vv.
Galea aponeurotica
Scalp vv.
Scalp
Outer table
Diploë
Inner table
Lateral lacuna with arachnoid granulations
Granular foveola
Falx cerebri
Bridging v.
Superior cerebral vv.

Fig. 18.4 ▶ Dural sinuses in the cranial cavity
Opened cranial cavity with dural sinus system ghosted in blue, superior view. *Removed:* Tentorium cerebelli.

Anterior intercavernous sinus
Posterior intercavernous sinus
Basilar plexus
Inferior petrosal sinus
Marginal sinus
Inferior cerebral vv.
Tentorium cerebelli
Straight sinus
Superior sagittal sinus
Superior ophthalmic v.
Sphenoparietal sinus
Cavernous sinus
Superior petrosal sinus
Jugular foramen
Sigmoid sinus
Great cerebral v.
Occipital sinus
Transverse sinus
Confluence of the sinuses

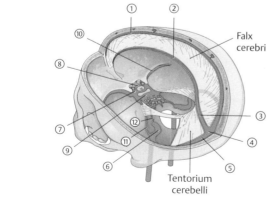

Falx cerebri
Tentorium cerebelli

Table 18.1 ▶ **Principal Dural Sinuses**		
Upper Group		**Lower Group**
① Superior sagittal sinus	⑦	Cavernous sinus
② Inferior sagittal sinus	⑧	Anterior intercavernous sinus
③ Straight sinus	⑨	Posterior intercavernous sinus
④ Confluence of the sinuses	⑩	Sphenoparietal sinus
⑤ Transverse sinus	⑪	Superior petrosal sinus
⑥ Sigmoid sinus	⑫	Inferior petrosal sinus

The occipital sinus is also included in the upper group.

- The paired **cavernous sinuses**, located on either side of the sella turcica, have characteristics that distinguish them from other dural sinuses (**Figs. 18.5** and **18.6**).
  - Each cavernous sinus contains a large plexus of thin-walled veins.
  - Several important structures are associated with each cavernous sinus:
    - Internal carotid artery, which is surrounded by the sympathetic internal carotid nerve plexus
    - Oculomotor nerve (CN III)
    - Trochlear nerve (CN IV)
    - Ophthalmic and maxillary divisions (CN V_1, V_2) of the trigeminal nerve
    - Abducent nerve (CN VI)
  - The cavernous sinuses receive the superior and inferior ophthalmic veins, the sphenoparietal sinuses, the superficial middle cerebral veins, and the central veins of the retina.

- The cavernous sinuses drain into the superior and inferior petrosal sinuses posteriorly and the pterygoid venous plexus inferiorly.
- Anterior and posterior **intercavernous sinuses** (see **Fig. 18.4**) connect the right and left cavernous sinuses.

Cavernous sinus thrombophlebitis

Cavernous sinus thrombophlebitis can occur secondary to thrombophlebitis of the facial vein. Although blood from the angle of the eye, lips, nose, and face usually drains inferiorly, it can also drain through the veins of the orbit to the cavernous sinus. Infections from the face, particularly from the *danger triangle of the face* (which extends from the bridge of the nose to the angles of the mouth) can spread infected thrombi to the cavernous sinus. This can affect the nerves that traverse the sinus (CN III, CN IV, CN V_1 and V_2, and CN VI) and result in acute meningitis.

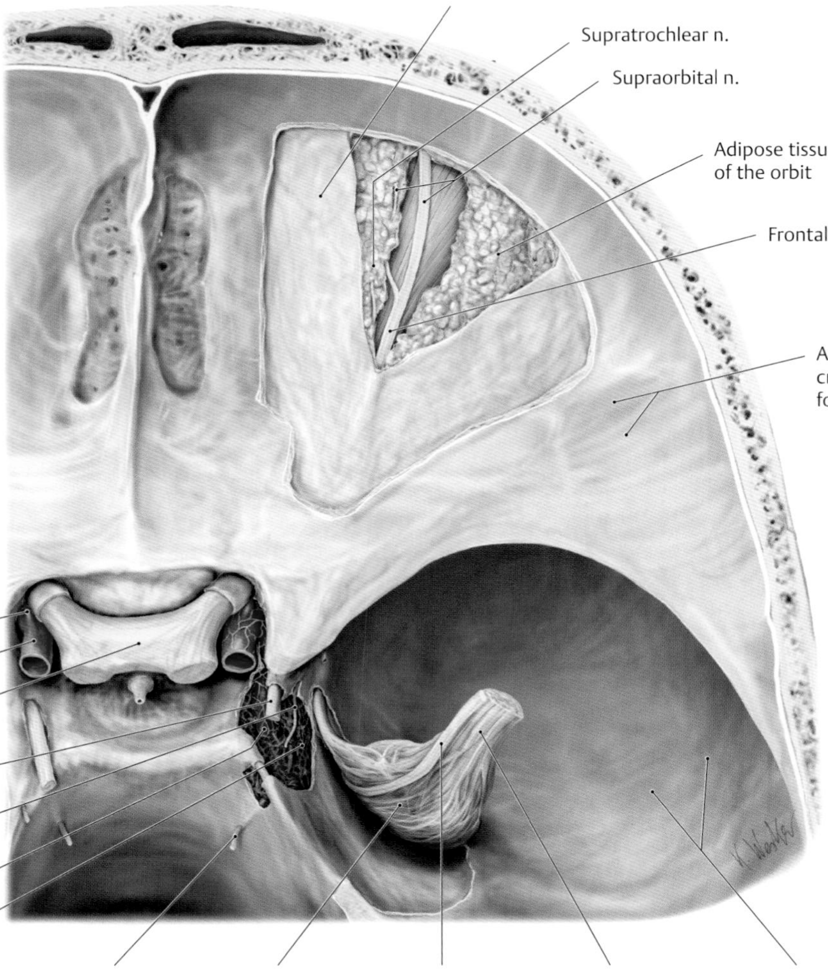

Fig. 18.5 ▶ Cavernous sinus and cranial nerves
Left anterior and middle cranial fossae, superior view. *Removed:* Lateral dural wall and roof of the cavernous sinus. The trigeminal ganglion is cut and retracted laterally following removal of its dural covering.

Fig. 18.6 ▶ **Cavernous sinus**
Middle cranial fossa, coronal section, anterior view.

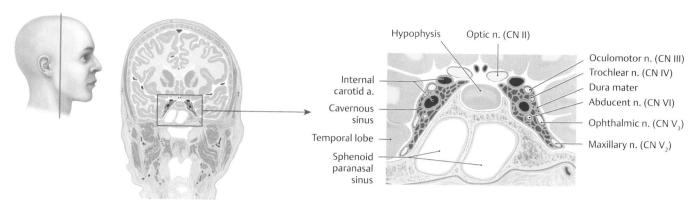

- Paired **superior petrosal sinuses**, which drain the cavernous sinuses, travel within the attached margins of the tentorium cerebelli along the top of the petrous part of the temporal bones and empty into the sigmoid sinuses.
- Paired **inferior petrosal sinuses** drain the cavernous sinuses, passing through a groove between the petrous part of the temporal bones and the basilar part of the occipital bone and emptying into the sigmoid sinuses at the origin of the internal jugular veins. The inferior petrosal sinuses communicate, through a **basilar plexus**, with the vertebral venous plexus.

18.1d Arachnoid Mater and Pia Mater (Fig. 18.7; see Figs. 18.1 and 18.3)

- **Arachnoid mater**, or **arachnoid**, is a thin, avascular, fibrous layer underlying the meningeal layer of the dura.

  • Cerebrospinal fluid presses the arachnoid against the dura, but the two layers are not attached. Weblike **arachnoid trabeculae** attach the arachnoid to the underlying **pia mater**.

Fig. 18.7 ▶ **Meningeal spaces**
Meninges, coronal section, anterior view.

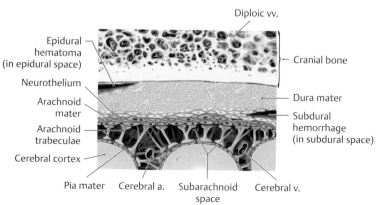

- • Delicate fingers of the arachnoid layer, the **arachnoid villi**, pierce the dura to allow the reabsorption of cerebrospinal fluid into the venous circulation and are especially numerous in the superior sagittal sinus. They form aggregations called **arachnoid granulations** that protrude into the largest dural venous sinuses and can push the dura ahead of them into the parietal bone, forming "pits."
- • Congregations of arachnoid granulations also occur in **lateral lacunae**, lateral expansions of the superior sagittal sinus.
- **Pia mater**, or pia, is a thin, highly vascular layer that adheres to the surface of the brain and closely follows its contours.

18.1e Meningeal Spaces

- The **epidural space** between the cranium and dura is not a natural space because the dura adheres to the skull. Meningeal vessels that supply the skull and dura travel in this space (see **Fig. 18.7**).
- The **subdural space** between the dura and arachnoid is a potential space, open only in pathological conditions such as a subdural hematoma. Superficial cerebral veins ("bridging veins") cross this space, connecting the venous circulation of the brain with the dural venous sinuses (see **Fig. 18.7**).
- The **subarachnoid space**, between the arachnoid and pia layers, contains cerebrospinal fluid, arteries, and veins (see **Fig. 18.7**).

  • **Subarachnoid cisterns** are spaces that form where the subarachnoid space enlarges around large infoldings of the brain. The largest of these include the **cerebellomedullary**, **pontomedullary**, **interpeduncular**, **chiasmatic**, **quadrigeminal**, and **ambient cisterns** (see Section 18.2b; see **Fig. 18.10**).

Extracerebral hemorrhage

Bleeding from vessels between the bony skull and the brain (extracerebral hemorrhage) increases intracranial pressure and can damage brain tissue. Three types of cerebral hemorrhages are distinguished based on their relationship to the meningeal layers.

Epidural hemorrhages commonly originate from a torn middle meningeal artery following a skull fracture at the pterion and result in bleeding into the epidural space. The hemorrhagic spread is usually limited by suture lines because the dura is attached to the skull at these points. As a result, the local accumulation of blood causes compression of the brain in that area.

Subdural hematomas result from tearing of the bridging veins as they traverse the gap between the dural sinus and cerebral cortex. The elderly are more susceptible to this type of hemorrhage because with brain shrinkage these veins bridge a larger gap and are more vulnerable to injury from head trauma. This condition may mimic a slowly evolving stroke with a fluctuating level of consciousness and localizing neurologic signs.

Most subarachnoid hemorrhages occur due to the rupture of aneurysms associated with vessels of the circle of Willis and most frequently with vessels of the anterior cerebral circulation. These hemorrhages into the subarachnoid space begin with a sudden, severe headache, neck stiffness, and drowsiness but can progress to severe consequences such as hemiplegia and coma.

18.2 The Brain

The brain, enclosed within the bony skull, is the largest part of the central nervous system. It communicates with the peripheral nervous system through the spinal cord and spinal nerves and through the 12 pairs of cranial nerves.

18.2a Regions of the Brain

The major regions of the brain are the cerebrum, diencephalon, brainstem (mesencephalon, pons, medulla oblongata), and cerebellum (**Fig. 18.8A, B,** and **C**).

— The **cerebrum** is the largest part of the brain and the center for integration within the central nervous system.
  • The falx cerebri lies in a **longitudinal fissure** between the **right** and **left cerebral hemispheres**.
  • Each cerebral hemisphere is further divided into **frontal**, **parietal**, **occipital**, and **temporal lobes** that occupy the anterior and middle cranial fossae.
  • Posteriorly, the cerebrum rests on the tentorium cerebelli.
  • The surface layer of the cerebrum forms **gyri** (folds) separated by **sulci** (grooves).
— The **diencephalon** forms the central core of the brain and consists of the **thalamus, hypophysis,** and **hypothalamus**.
— The **mesencephalon**, the most anterior part of the brainstem, passes through the tentorial notch between the middle and posterior cranial fossae.

  • It is associated with the oculomotor (CN III) and trochlear (CN IV) nerves.
— The **pons**, the middle part of the brainstem, lies in the anterior part of the posterior cranial fossa below the mesencephalon.
  • Several ascending and descending fiber tracts connect the pons to the cerebellum.
  • The pons is associated with the trigeminal (CN V), abducent (CN VI), and facial (CN VII) nerves.
— The **medulla oblongata**, the most posterior part of the brainstem, connects the brain and spinal cord.
  • It contains nuclei for the vestibulocochlear (CN VIII), glossopharyngeal (CN IX), vagus (CN X), and hypoglossal (XII) nerves.
— The **cerebellum**, which occupies most of the posterior cranial fossa, lies inferior to the cerebrum and is separated from it by the tentorium cerebelli.
  • It consists of paired hemispheres and a small middle section, the vermis.

18.2b Ventricular System and Cerebrospinal Fluid

The brain and spinal cord are suspended in cerebrospinal fluid (CSF). The buoyant environment created by the CSF reduces the pressure of the brain on the nerves and vessels on its inferior surface.

— CSF is produced in the **choroid plexuses**, vascular networks within four ventricles (spaces) of the brain. The first two of these ventricles are large and paired; the third and fourth are smaller and lie in the midline (**Fig. 18.9**).
  • The **1st** and **2nd (lateral) ventricles**, paired cavities that occupy a large portion of each cerebral hemisphere, communicate with the 3rd ventricle through the **interventricular foramina**.
  • The **3rd ventricle**, a slitlike space between the two halves of the diencephalon, communicates posteriorly with the 4th ventricle through a narrow passage, the **cerebral aqueduct**, which passes through the mesencephalon.
  • The **4th ventricle**, a pyramidally shaped space that extends from the pons to the medulla oblongata, is continuous with the spinal canal inferiorly and with the subarachnoid space through the **median** and **lateral apertures** in its roof.

Fig. 18.8 ▶ Adult brain
CN, cranial nerve.

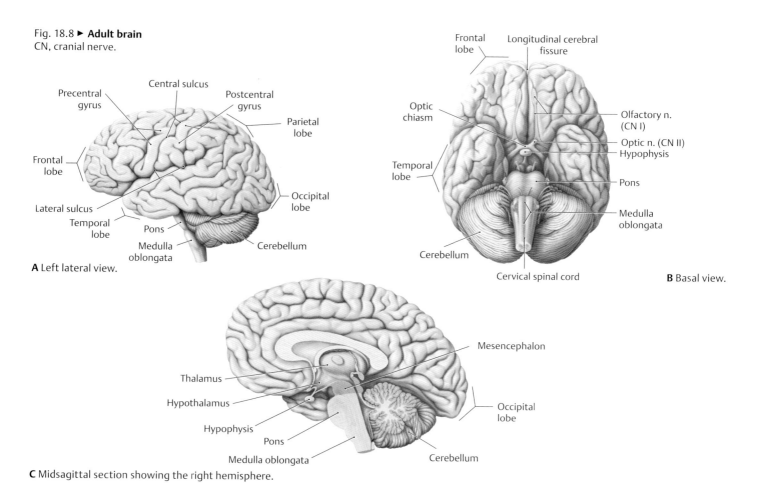

Precentral gyrus
Central sulcus
Postcentral gyrus
Parietal lobe
Frontal lobe
Occipital lobe
Lateral sulcus
Temporal lobe
Pons
Medulla oblongata
Cerebellum

A Left lateral view.

Frontal lobe
Longitudinal cerebral fissure
Optic chiasm
Olfactory n. (CN I)
Optic n. (CN II)
Hypophysis
Temporal lobe
Pons
Medulla oblongata
Cerebellum
Cervical spinal cord

B Basal view.

Mesencephalon
Thalamus
Hypothalamus
Occipital lobe
Hypophysis
Pons
Medulla oblongata
Cerebellum

C Midsagittal section showing the right hemisphere.

Fig. 18.9 ▶ Ventricular system in situ
Ventricular system with neighboring structures, left lateral view.

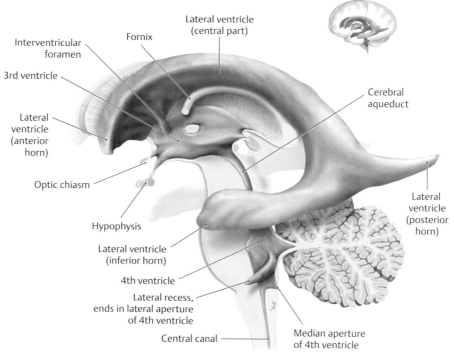

Interventricular foramen
Fornix
Lateral ventricle (central part)
3rd ventricle
Cerebral aqueduct
Lateral ventricle (anterior horn)
Optic chiasm
Lateral ventricle (posterior horn)
Hypophysis
Lateral ventricle (inferior horn)
4th ventricle
Lateral recess, ends in lateral aperture of 4th ventricle
Central canal
Median aperture of 4th ventricle

Fig. 18.10 ▶ **Circulation of cerebrospinal fluid (CSF)**

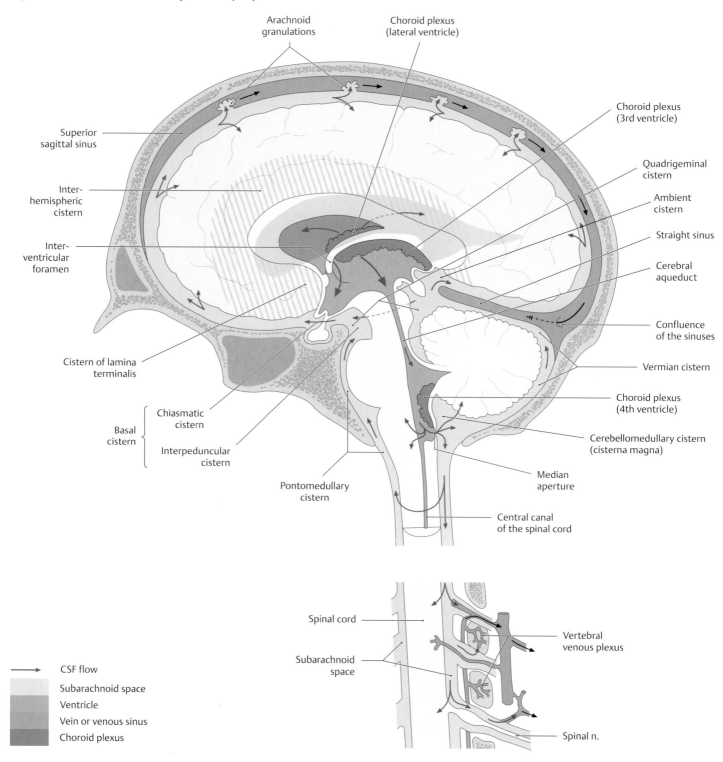

Arachnoid granulations

Choroid plexus (lateral ventricle)

Choroid plexus (3rd ventricle)

Superior sagittal sinus

Quadrigeminal cistern

Inter-hemispheric cistern

Ambient cistern

Straight sinus

Inter-ventricular foramen

Cerebral aqueduct

Confluence of the sinuses

Cistern of lamina terminalis

Vermian cistern

Basal cistern
- Chiasmatic cistern
- Interpeduncular cistern

Choroid plexus (4th ventricle)

Cerebellomedullary cistern (cisterna magna)

Pontomedullary cistern

Median aperture

Central canal of the spinal cord

Spinal cord

Vertebral venous plexus

Subarachnoid space

Spinal n.

→ CSF flow

Subarachnoid space

Ventricle

Vein or venous sinus

Choroid plexus

- CSF circulates through the ventricles and passes into the sub-arachnoid space and subarachnoid cisterns through the median and lateral apertures of the 4th ventricle. It flows superiorly through the fissures and sulci of the cerebrum and is reabsorbed into the venous circulation through the arachnoid granulations that protrude into the superior sagittal sinus (**Fig. 18.10**).

Hydrocephalus

Hydrocephalus, an excessive accumulation of cerebrospinal fluid (CSF) in the ventricles of the brain, can occur as a result of partial obstruction of the flow of CSF within the ventricular system, interference of CSF reabsorption into the venous circulation, or, in rare cases, overproduction of CSF. Excess CSF in the ventricles causes them to dilate and exert pressure on the surrounding cortex, causing the bones of the calvaria to separate, thus creating the characteristic increase in head size. Treatment involves the placement of a shunt between the ventricles and the abdomen, which allows CSF to drain to the peritoneal cavity, where it can be easily absorbed.

18.2c Arteries of the Brain

As a result of its high metabolic demand, the brain receives one sixth of the cardiac output and one fifth of the oxygen consumed by the body at rest. This blood supply, derived from the internal carotid and vertebral arteries, is divided into **anterior** and **posterior cerebral circulations** (**Fig. 18.11**), which unite on the ventral surface of the brain to form a **cerebral arterial circle** (of Willis) (**Fig. 18.12**).

- The internal carotid artery supplies the anterior cerebral circulation.
  - Its **petrous part** has a tortuous course as it enters the skull and follows the carotid canal horizontally and medially within the temporal bone. Small branches pass into the middle ear and pterygoid canal.
  - The **cavernous part** crosses over the foramen lacerum and runs anteriorly within the cavernous sinus. Small branches supply the meninges, hypophysis, and cranial nerves within the cavernous sinus.
  - The **cerebral part** in the middle cranial fossa gives off the ophthalmic artery (see **Fig. 20.8**) and immediately makes a U-turn to run posteriorly, where it divides into the anterior cerebral and middle cerebral arteries.
- The vertebral and basilar arteries supply the posterior cerebral circulation.
  - The vertebral artery enters the skull through the foramen magnum and supplies branches to the spinal cord and cerebellum before merging with the opposite vertebral artery to form a single basilar artery.
    - Intracranial branches of the vertebral artery include the posterior inferior cerebellar artery and the anterior and posterior spinal arteries.

Fig. 18.11 ▶ **Internal carotid artery**
Left lateral view.

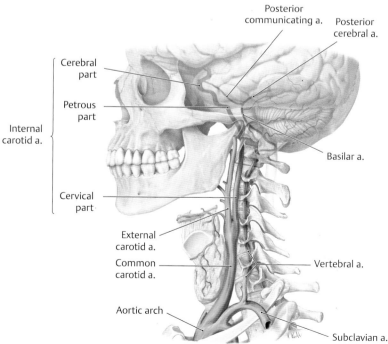

Fig. 18.12 ▶ **Arteries of the brain**
Inferior (basal) view.

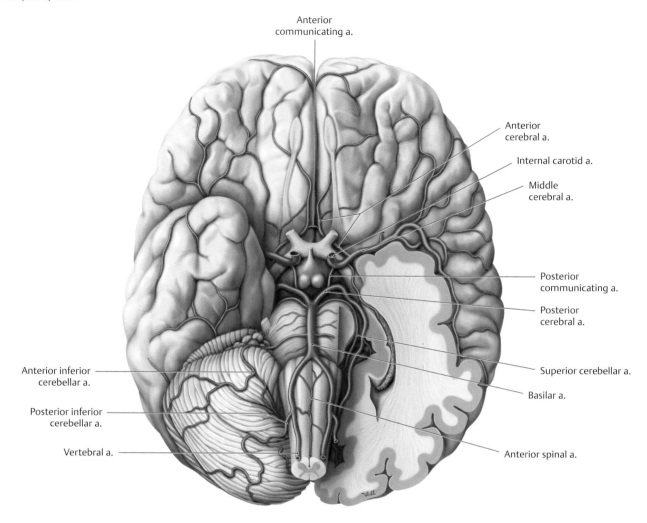

Anterior
communicating a.

Anterior
cerebral a.

Internal carotid a.

Middle
cerebral a.

Posterior
communicating a.

Posterior
cerebral a.

Superior cerebellar a.

Basilar a.

Anterior spinal a.

Anterior inferior
cerebellar a.

Posterior inferior
cerebellar a.

Vertebral a.

- The **basilar artery** ascends on the ventral surface of the brainstem, distributing branches to the brainstem, cerebellum, and cerebrum. It terminates as the right and left **posterior cerebral arteries**.
  - Major branches of the basilar artery are the **anterior inferior cerebellar artery** and the **superior cerebellar artery**.
- The **cerebral arterial circle** (of Willis), an important arterial anastomosis on the ventral surface of the brain, supplies the brain and connects the circulations of the internal carotid and vertebral arteries.
  - A small **anterior communicating artery** connects the two anterior cerebral arteries, linking the right and left anterior cerebral circulations.
  - A pair of **posterior communicating arteries** connects the internal carotid and posterior cerebral arteries on each side, completing the communication between the anterior and posterior cerebral circulations.

- The branches of the circle are
  - the anterior communicating arteries,
  - the anterior cerebral arteries,
  - the internal carotid arteries,
  - the posterior communicating arteries, and
  - the posterior cerebral arteries.
- The cerebral arteries that arise from the cerebral arterial circle provide the blood supply to the cerebral hemispheres (**Table 18.2**).

Table 18.2 ▶ **Distribution of the Cerebral Arteries**

Artery	Origin	Distribution
Anterior cerebral	Internal carotid artery	Frontal pole and medial and superior surfaces of the cerebral hemispheres
Middle cerebral	Internal carotid artery	Most of the lateral surface of the cerebral hemispheres
Posterior cerebral	Basilar artery	Occipital pole and inferior part of temporal lobe

Stroke

A stroke is the manifestation of a neurologic deficiency resulting from a cerebral vascular impairment. Ischemic strokes are usually caused by an embolus obstructing one of the major cerebral arteries. Although the vessels of the circle of Willis can provide collateral circulation to circumvent the obstruction, anastomoses between the vessels are often incomplete or of insufficient size to provide adequate flow. Hemorrhagic strokes are usually due to rupture of an aneurysm, most often a saccular, or berry, aneurysm that bleeds into the subarachnoid space. Symptoms occur shortly after the cerebral event and relate to the area of brain affected. They may include difficulty speaking, understanding language, or walking; vision problems; contralateral paralysis or numbness; and headache.

18.2d Veins of the Brain

Veins that drain the brain are thin-walled and valveless and usually drain into one of the dural venous sinuses (**Fig. 18.13A** and **B**).

— Superficial (external) veins that drain the cerebral hemispheres include

- the **superior cerebral veins**, which drain the supralateral and medial aspects. These "bridging veins" traverse the subdural space and drain into the superior sagittal sinus;
- the **middle cerebral veins**, which drain the lateral hemispheres and empty into the cavernous sinus and from there into the petrosal and transverse sinuses; and
- the **inferior cerebral veins**, which drain inferior aspects of the brain and join either the superior cerebral or the **basilar veins**.

— Basilar veins drain the small anterior cerebral veins and deep middle cerebral veins.

— **Internal cerebral veins** drain the 3rd and 4th ventricles and deep parts of the cerebrum. These unite to form the **great cerebral vein**.

— The great cerebral vein receives the basilar veins and merges with the inferior sagittal sinus to form the straight sinus.

— **Superior** and **inferior cerebellar veins** drain the cerebellum into adjacent dural sinuses or superficially into the great cerebral vein.

Fig. 18.13 ▶ **Cerebral veins**

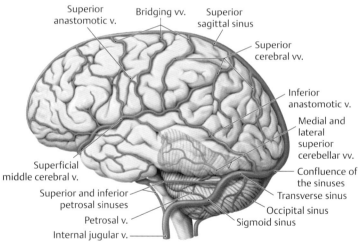

A Lateral view of the left hemisphere.

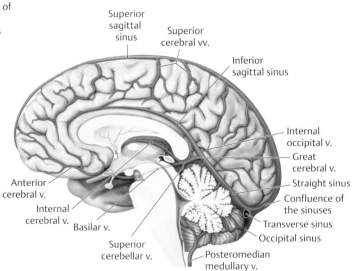

B Medial view of the right hemisphere.

Fig. 18.14 ► **Cranial nerves**
Inferior (basal) view. The 12 pairs of cranial nerves (CN) are numbered according to their emergence from the brainstem.

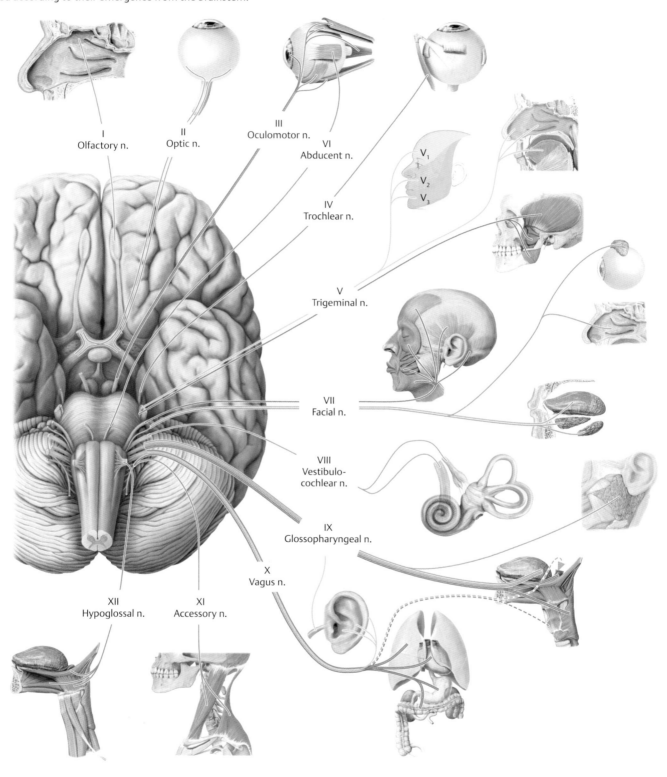

I
Olfactory n.

II
Optic n.

III
Oculomotor n.

VI
Abducent n.

IV
Trochlear n.

V_1
V_2
V_3

V
Trigeminal n.

VII
Facial n.

VIII
Vestibulo-
cochlear n.

IX
Glossopharyngeal n.

X
Vagus n.

XII
Hypoglossal n.

XI
Accessory n.

18.3 Cranial Nerves

The 12 cranial nerves arise from the brainstem (**Fig. 18.14**; **Table 18.3**). Like spinal nerves, cranial nerves can stimulate muscles or transmit sensation from a peripheral structure to the central nervous system. Some cranial nerves also carry fibers from the cranial portion of the parasympathetic nervous system. Seven types of nerve fibers are found (alone or in combination) in cranial nerves.

Table 18.3 ▶ Classification of Cranial Nerve Fibers	
Fiber Type	**Function**
General somatic motor	Innervate voluntary muscle
General visceral motor	Constitute the cranial component of the parasympathetic system, innervate involuntary muscles and glands
Special visceral motor (branchial motor)	Innervate muscles that developed from the primitive pharynx (pharyngeal arches)
General somatic sensory	Carry sensations such as touch, temperature, pain, and pressure
Special somatic sensory	Carry impulses from the eye for sight and from the ear for hearing and balance
General visceral sensory	Transmit information from viscera such as carotid bodies, the heart, esophagus, trachea, and gastrointestinal tract
Special visceral sensory	Transmit information regarding smell and taste

CN I, the **olfactory nerve**, carries special sensory fibers that transmit sensation of smell from the superior aspect of the lateral and septal walls of the nasal cavity (**Fig. 18.15**).

— Olfactory neurons pass through the cribriform plate of the ethmoid bone and synapse with secondary neurons in the **olfactory bulbs**.
  • The axons of these secondary neurons form the **olfactory tracts**.
  • The olfactory bulbs and tracts are extensions of the cerebral cortex.

CN II, the **optic nerve**, is a collection of special sensory nerve fibers that originate on the **retina** of the eye and converge at the **optic disc** at the back of the eyeball (**Fig. 18.16**; see also Section 20.1e).

— The nerve exits the orbit through the optic canal and joins the contralateral optic nerve to form the **optic chiasm**.
— The optic chiasm is a redistribution center where nerve fibers from the medial half of each optic nerve cross to the opposite side.
— Two **optic tracts** diverge from the chiasm. Each tract contains nerve fibers from the medial half of one eye and the lateral half of the other eye.

Fig. 18.15 ▶ Olfactory nerve (CN I)
Olfactory fibers, bulb, and tract. Portion of left nasal septum and lateral wall of right nasal cavity, left lateral view.

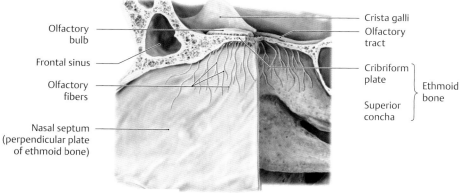

Fig. 18.16 ▶ Optic nerve (CN II)
Optic nerve in the left orbit, left lateral view.

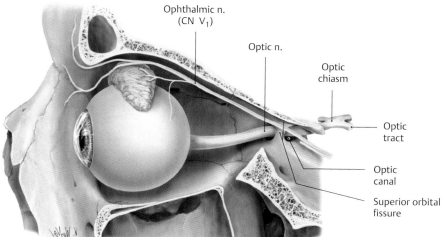

CN III, the **oculomotor nerve**; **CN IV**, the **trochlear nerve**; and **CN VI**, the **abducent nerve** innervate structures of the orbit (**Fig. 18.17**; see also Section 20.1e). They pass through the cavernous sinus before entering the orbit through the superior orbital fissure.

— The oculomotor nerve has somatic and visceral components.

  • General somatic motor fibers innervate four of the extraocular muscles (superior rectus, medial rectus, inferior rectus, and inferior oblique), which move the eyeball, and the levator palpebrae superioris muscle, which elevates the eyelid.

  • General visceral motor fibers carry preganglionic parasympathetic fibers that synapse in the **ciliary ganglion** and innervate the **pupillary sphincter muscle** (which constricts the pupil) and **ciliary body** (which changes the curvature of the lens of the eye) (see **Fig. 20.5**).

— The trochlear nerve carries general somatic motor fibers and innervates the superior oblique muscle, which turns the eye upward and outward.

— The abducent nerve carries general somatic motor fibers and innervates the lateral rectus muscle, which abducts the eye.

CN V, the **trigeminal nerve**, is the primary sensory nerve of the face (**Fig. 18.18**). Its small motor component innervates the muscles of mastication (chewing).

— The general somatic sensory neurons, which form the sensory root, synapse in the trigeminal ganglion located in a dural space on the petrous part of the temporal bone.

— A small motor root in the mandibular division (CN V$_3$) contains branchial motor fibers.

— Branches of the trigeminal nerve are associated with the parasympathetic ganglia of the head and distribute postganglionic parasympathetic fibers to their target organs.

— The trigeminal nerve has three divisions:

  1. The **ophthalmic division (CN V$_1$)** (see Section 20.1e)

  ○ contains only somatic sensory fibers;

  ○ passes through the cavernous sinus and superior orbital fissure into the orbit;

  ○ is associated with the **ciliary ganglion** (see Section 18.4);

  ○ distributes visceral motor fibers from the facial nerve (CN II) to the lacrimal gland via the lacrimal nerve;

  ○ innervates the orbit, the cornea, and the skin on the top of the nose, forehead, and scalp;

  ○ functions as the sensory component of the corneal reflex via the **nasociliary branch**; and

  ○ has **lacrimal**, **frontal**, and **nasociliary** branches.

Fig. 18.17 ▶ **Oculomotor (CN III), trochlear (IV), and abducent (VI) nerves**
Course of the nerves innervating the extraocular muscles, right orbit, lateral view.

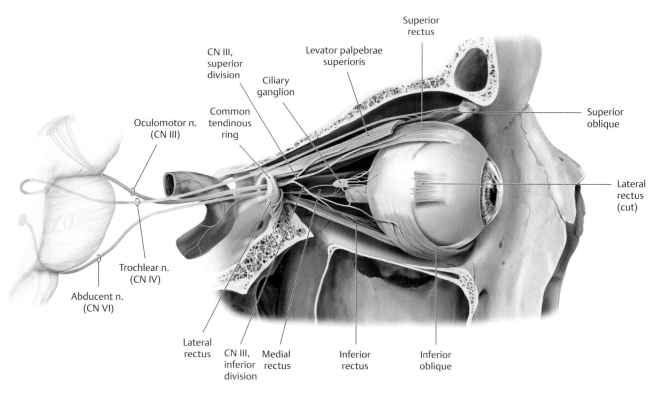

Fig. 18.18 ▸ Trigeminal nerve (CN V)
Course of the trigeminal nerve divisions.

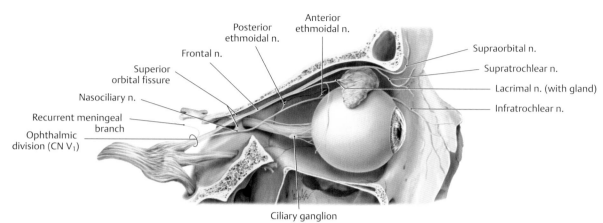

A Ophthalmic division (CN V1), partially opened right orbit.

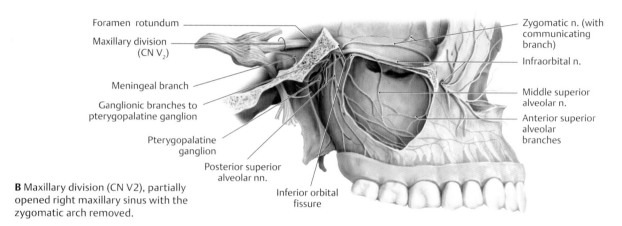

B Maxillary division (CN V2), partially opened right maxillary sinus with the zygomatic arch removed.

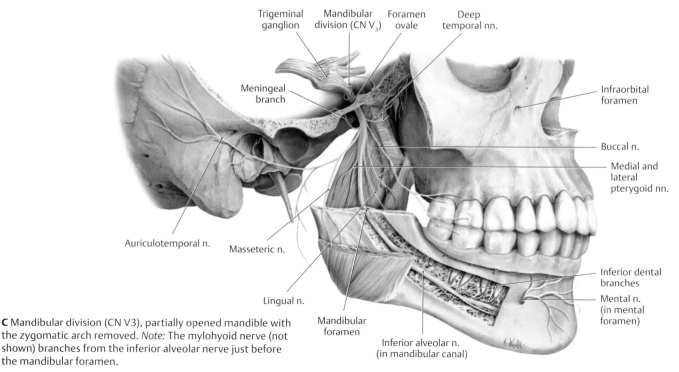

C Mandibular division (CN V3), partially opened mandible with the zygomatic arch removed. *Note:* The mylohyoid nerve (not shown) branches from the inferior alveolar nerve just before the mandibular foramen.

2. The **maxillary division (CN V₂)** (see Section 19.6)

   - contains only somatic sensory fibers;
   - travels through the cavernous sinus and the foramen rotundum to enter the **pterygopalatine fossa**;
   - is associated with the **pterygopalatine ganglion** (see Section 18.4);
   - innervates the skin of the midface (from the lower eyelid to the upper lip) and structures associated with the maxilla, such as the maxillary sinus, palate, nasal cavity, and maxillary teeth; and
   - has **infraorbital**, **zygomatic**, **greater** and **lesser palatine**, **superior alveolar**, and **nasopalatine** branches (see also **Fig. 19.18**).

3. The **mandibular division (CN V₃)** (see Section 19.4 and 19.5)

   - contains somatic sensory and branchial motor fibers;
   - passes through the foramen ovale into the **infratemporal fossa**;
   - is associated with the **otic** and **submandibular ganglia** (see Section 18.4);
   - distributes visceral motor fibers of the facial nerve (CN VII) to the submandibular and sublingual glands via the lingual nerve;
   - distributes visceral motor fibers of the glossopharyngeal nerve (CN IX) to the parotid gland via the auriculotemporal nerve;
   - has a sensory component that innervates skin over the lower jaw and lateral face and structures associated with the mandible, such as the lower teeth, **temporomandibular joint**, floor of the mouth, and anterior tongue;
   - has a motor component that innervates the **digastric** (anterior belly), **mylohyoid**, **tensor veli palatini**, and **tensor tympani muscles** and the **muscles of mastication** (see Sections 19.2, 19.8a, and 19.8b); and
   - has **meningeal**, **buccal**, **auriculotemporal**, **lingual**, **inferior alveolar**, and **muscular branches** (to muscles noted above).

Trigeminal neuralgia

Trigeminal neuralgia, a pathology of the sensory root of the trigeminal nerve (CN V), most commonly affects the maxillary division (CN V₂) and least frequently affects the ophthalmic division (CN V₁). The disorder is characterized by unilateral electric shock–like pain in the area supplied by the nerve. It usually lasts several seconds to several minutes. As the condition progresses, the pain may last longer, and there may be a shorter period between attacks. The pain may be initiated by touching a trigger point in the face by eating, talking, brushing teeth, or shaving. It is believed that trigeminal neuralgia is caused by the loss of myelin on the sensory root due to the pressure from an abnormal blood vessel. Surgery to destroy the nerve root or ganglion may be effective but may lead to permanent facial numbness.

CN VII, the **facial nerve**, is the primary motor nerve of the face but also has sensory and visceral components (**Figs. 18.19** and **18.20**). It contains a motor root that innervates the muscles of facial expression, and an intermediate nerve that carries special sensory (for taste) and visceral motor fibers (parasympathetic) and somatic sensory fibers. Both the motor root and the intermediate nerve pass through the internal acoustic meatus into the **facial canal** of the temporal bone, where three branches arise: the greater petrosal nerve, stapedial nerve, and chorda tympani.

— The motor root

   - exits the skull through the stylomastoid foramen and
   - contains branchial motor fibers, which
     - innervate the **stylohyoid**, **stapedius**, and **digastric** (posterior belly) **muscles** (see **Table 19.7**, **Figs. 19.21** and **20.12**, and Section 19.2) and
     - form the **parotid plexus within the parotid gland**, which innervates the **muscles of facial expression** (see Section 19.1). Branches of the parotid plexus include the posterior auricular, **temporal**, **zygomatic**, **buccal**, **marginal mandibular**, and **cervical branches**.

— The intermediate nerve contains the following:

   - The **greater petrosal nerve** (parasympathetic), which passes through the middle cranial fossa and combines with the **deep petrosal nerve** (sympathetic) to form the **nerve of the pterygoid canal** (see Section 19.6). The visceral motor (parasympathetic) fibers synapse in the pterygopalatine ganglion and are distributed to glands of the nasal mucosa and palate and to the lacrimal gland.
   - The **chorda tympani**, which passes through the middle ear cavity, exits through the stylomastoid foramen and travels with the lingual nerve of CN V₃. It carries
     - visceral motor fibers that synapse in the submandibular ganglion and supply the submandibular and sublingual salivary glands, and
     - special sensory fibers for taste from the anterior part of the tongue and palate.
   - General somatic sensory fibers, which transmit sensations from the external ear to the **geniculate ganglion**, the sensory ganglion of the facial nerve, located in the temporal bone.

Fig. 18.19 ▶ Course of the facial nerve
Visceral motor (parasympathetic) and special visceral sensory (taste)
fibers shown in black, right lateral view.

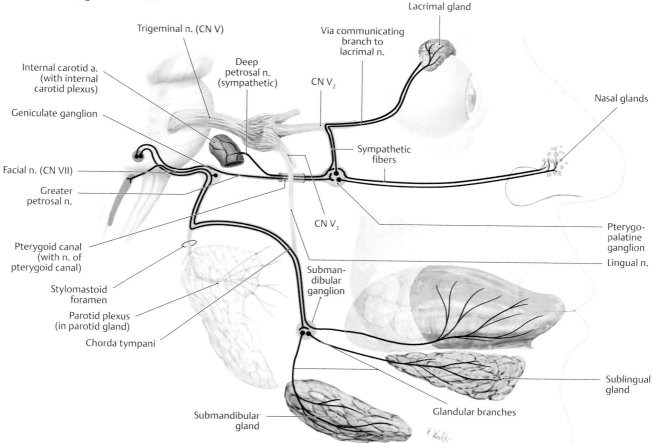

Fig. 18.20 ▶ Facial nerve (CN VII)
Branches of the facial nerve, right lateral view.

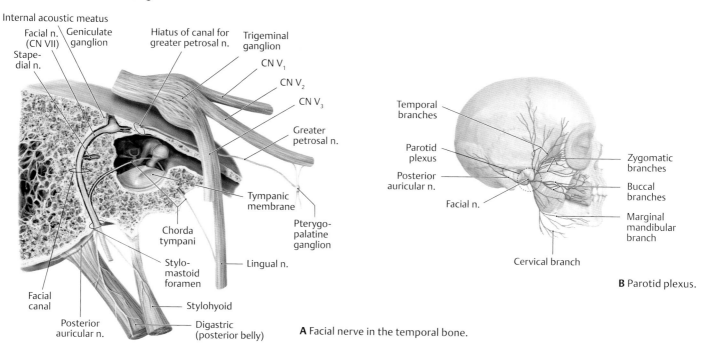

A Facial nerve in the temporal bone.

B Parotid plexus.

Fig. 18.21 ► **Vestibulocochlear nerve (CN VIII)**

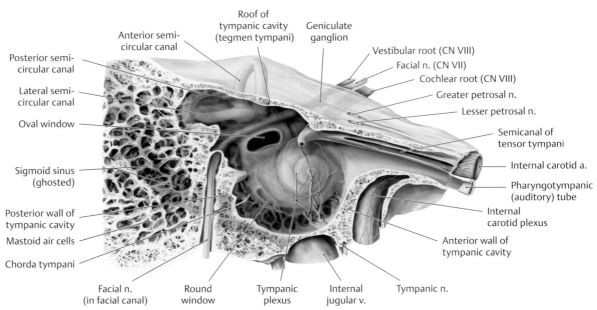

Anterior semi-
circular canal

Roof of
tympanic cavity
(tegmen tympani)

Geniculate
ganglion

Vestibular root (CN VIII)

Facial n. (CN VII)

Cochlear root (CN VIII)

Posterior semi-
circular canal

Greater petrosal n.

Lateral semi-
circular canal

Lesser petrosal n.

Oval window

Semicanal of
tensor tympani

Internal carotid a.

Sigmoid sinus
(ghosted)

Pharyngotympanic
(auditory) tube

Posterior wall of
tympanic cavity

Internal
carotid plexus

Mastoid air cells

Anterior wall of
tympanic cavity

Chorda tympani

Facial n.
(in facial canal)

Round
window

Tympanic
plexus

Internal
jugular v.

Tympanic n.

A Vestibulocochlear nerve in the temporal bone, medial
wall of the tympanic cavity, oblique sagittal section.

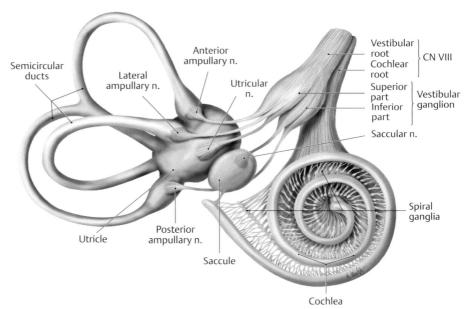

Semicircular
ducts

Anterior
ampullary n.

Vestibular
root
Cochlear
root

} CN VIII

Lateral
ampullary n.

Utricular
n.

Superior
part
Inferior
part

} Vestibular
ganglion

Saccular n.

Spiral
ganglia

Utricle

Posterior
ampullary n.

Saccule

Cochlea

B Vestibular and cochlear (spiral) ganglia.

Bell's palsy

Bell's palsy is paralysis of the facial muscles due to a lesion of the facial
nerve (CN VII). Symptoms usually begin suddenly and affect one side of the
face only. They include drooping of the corner of the mouth, eyebrow, and
lower eyelid and the inability to smile, whistle, blow out cheeks, wrinkle
the forehead, blink, or close the eyes forcefully. Taste is impaired on the
anterior two thirds of the tongue (due to involvement of the chorda tympani), decreased tear production leads to dry eyes (due to involvement of
the greater petrosal nerve), sensitivity to sounds is increased (due to paralysis of the stapedius), and the lower jaw and tongue deviate to the opposite side (due to paralysis of the posterior belly of the digastric muscle).

CN VIII, the **vestibulocochlear nerve**, is the sensory nerve
of hearing and balance. The nerve enters the temporal bone with
the facial nerve through the internal acoustic meatus.

— The two branches of the vestibulocochlear nerve carry special
   sensory fibers (**Fig. 18.21A** and **B**; see Section 20.2c):

   • The **cochlear root** supplies the **cochlea** and its **spiral or-
     gan**, the organ of hearing.

   • The **vestibular root**, which contains the **vestibular gan-
     glia**, supplies the **utricle**, **saccule**, and **semicircular ducts**,
     the organs of balance.

CN IX, the **glossopharyngeal nerve**, leaves the skull through the jugular foramen and contains special sensory (taste), visceral sensory, somatic motor, and visceral motor components (**Figs. 18.22, 18.23A and B**; **Table 18.4**).

— Somatic motor fibers innervate the **stylopharyngeus muscle**.
— Visceral motor fibers arise with the **tympanic nerve**, a branch of the glossopharyngeal nerve. Carrying sensory and visceral motor fibers, it runs through the **tympanic cavity** of the **middle ear** (see Section 20.2b), where it contributes to the **tympanic plexus**. It gives rise to the lesser petrosal nerve.

    ○ The **lesser petrosal nerve** passes through the middle cranial fossa and foramen ovale carrying visceral motor fibers that synapse in the otic ganglion. Postganglionic fibers travel with the auriculotemporal nerve (CN V$_3$) to innervate the parotid gland.
    ○ Sensory fibers of the tympanic plexus supply the tympanic cavity and **pharyngotympanic** (auditory) **tube**.

— Special sensory fibers transmit taste from the posterior third of the tongue.
— Visceral sensory fibers transmit information from the **tonsils**, **soft palate**, and posterior third of the tongue and, via the **branch to the carotid sinus**, from receptors in the carotid body and carotid sinus at the bifurcation of the common carotid artery.

Fig. 18.22 ► **Glossopharyngeal nerve (CN IX)**
Course of the glossopharyngeal nerve, left lateral view.

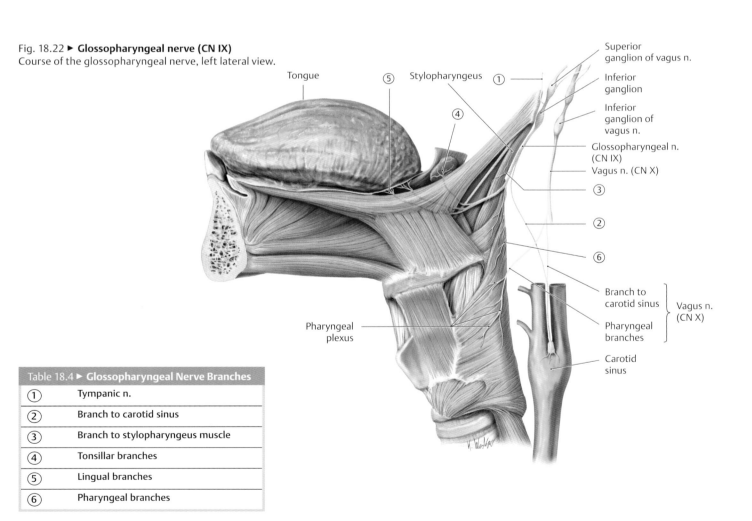

Table 18.4 ► Glossopharyngeal Nerve Branches	
①	Tympanic n.
②	Branch to carotid sinus
③	Branch to stylopharyngeus muscle
④	Tonsillar branches
⑤	Lingual branches
⑥	Pharyngeal branches

Fig. 18.23 ▸ **Branches of the glossopharyngeal nerve**

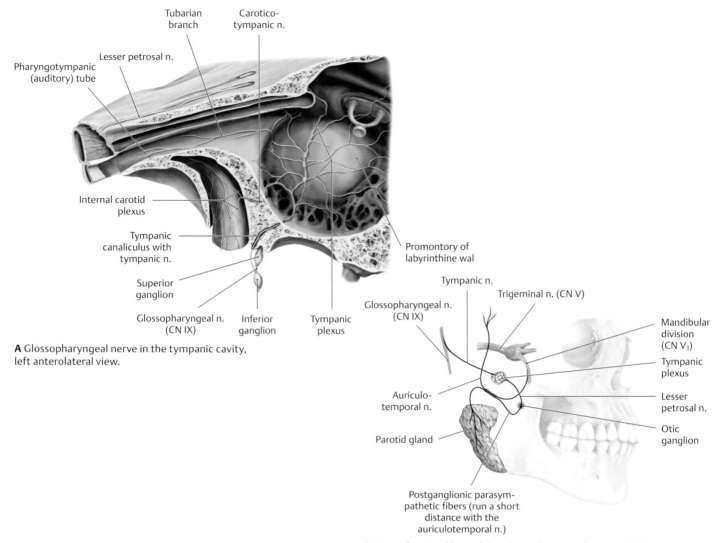

A Glossopharyngeal nerve in the tympanic cavity, left anterolateral view.

B Visceral motor fibers of the glossopharyngeal nerve, right lateral view.

CN X, the **vagus nerve**, has the most extensive distribution of the cranial nerves (**Fig. 18.24**; **Table 18.5**).

— Branchial motor fibers innervate the muscles of the soft palate (except tensor veli palatini), pharynx (except stylopharyngeus), and larynx, and the palatoglossus muscle of the tongue.

— Visceral motor fibers innervate smooth muscle and glands of the pharynx, larynx, thoracic organs, and abdominal foregut and midgut.

- General somatic sensory fibers transmit sensation from the dura in the posterior cranial fossa, the skin of the external ear, and the external auditory canal.
- Visceral sensory fibers transmit sensation from mucosa of the lower pharynx, the larynx, lungs and airway, the heart, the abdominal foregut and midgut, and the chemoreceptors of the aortic body and baroreceptors of the aortic arch.
- Special sensory fibers carry taste from the epiglottis.
- The vagus nerve has cervical, thoracic, and abdominal segments.
  - In the neck
    - each vagus nerve leaves the skull through the jugular foramen and descends within the carotid sheath of the neck, and

    - its branches are **pharyngeal branches**, the **superior laryngeal nerve**, **cervical cardiac** (parasympathetic) **branches**, and the **right recurrent laryngeal nerve** (which arises from the right vagus and recurs around the right subclavian artery).
  - In the thorax
    - the right and left vagus nerves enter the thorax posterior to the sternoclavicular joints and merge on the surface of the esophagus as the esophageal plexus (see Section 3.2d), and
    - their branches are the left recurrent laryngeal nerve (which arises from the left vagus and recurs around the arch of the aorta) and the thoracic cardiac and pulmonary branches (parasympathetic).
  - In the abdomen
    - right and left vagal trunks arise from the esophageal plexus and pass through the esophageal hiatus of the diaphragm as the anterior and posterior vagal trunks; and
    - their parasympathetic branches are distributed to organs of the foregut, midgut, and retroperitoneum.

Fig. 18.24 ▶ Vagus nerve (CN X)
Branches of the vagus nerve in the neck, anterior view.

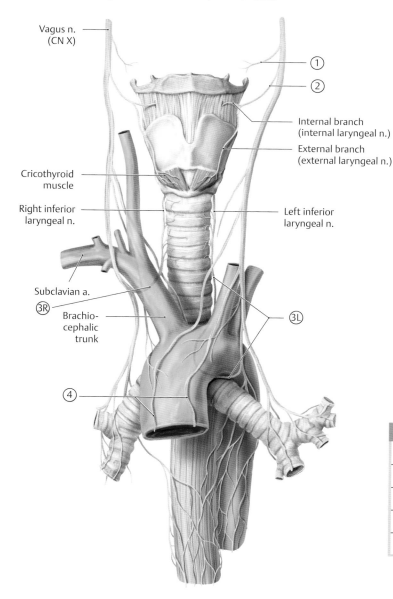

Vagus n. (CN X)

Cricothyroid muscle

Right inferior laryngeal n.

Subclavian a.
③R

Brachio-cephalic trunk

①

②

Internal branch (internal laryngeal n.)

External branch (external laryngeal n.)

Left inferior laryngeal n.

③L

④

Table 18.5 ▶ Vagus Nerve Branches in the Neck	
①	Pharyngeal branches
②	Superior laryngeal n.
③R	Right recurrent laryngeal n.
③L	Left recurrent laryngeal n.
④	Cervical cardiac branches

Fig. 18.25 ▶ **Accessory nerve (CN XI)**
Brainstem with the cerebellum removed, posterior view.

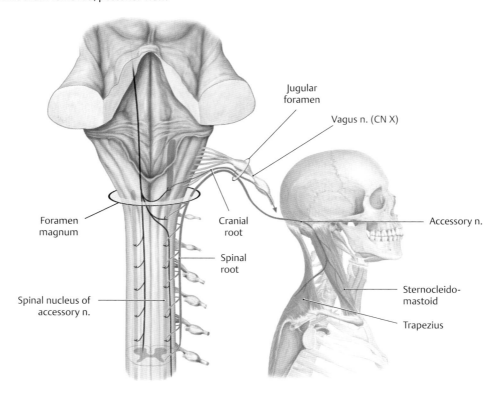

Fig. 18.26 ▶ **Hypoglossal nerve (CN XII)**
Brainstem with the cerebellum removed, posterior view. *Note:* C1, which
innervates the thyrohyoid and geniohyoid, runs briefly with the
hypoglossal nerve.

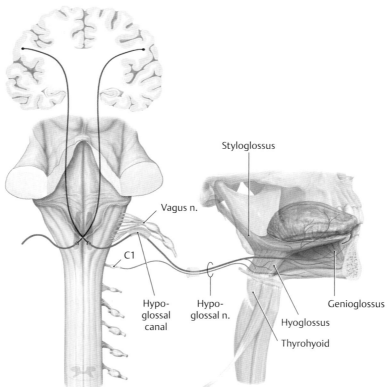

CN XI, the **accessory nerve**, contains general somatic motor fibers, which originate in a nucleus of the upper segments of the spinal cord (**Fig. 18.25**).

— The nerve emerges with the upper five or six cervical spinal nerves and ascends within the vertebral canal. It enters the skull through the foramen magnum and exits through the jugular foramen with the vagus and glossopharyngeal nerves.
— It innervates the sternocleidomastoid muscle in the neck and then crosses the lateral region of the neck to innervate the trapezius muscle.

CN XII, the **hypoglossal nerve**, contains only general somatic motor fibers (**Fig. 18.26**).

— The hypoglossal nerve leaves the skull through the hypoglossal canal and runs forward, medial to the angle of the mandible, to enter the oral cavity.
— It innervates all of the muscles of the tongue except the palatoglossus.

▌ Injury to the hypoglossal nerve

Injury to the hypoglossal nerve causes ipsilateral paralysis of half of the tongue. When the tongue is protruded, the tip deviates toward the paralyzed side because the action of the genioglossus muscle on the unaffected side is unopposed. Symptoms mainly manifest as slurring of speech. Over time, the tongue becomes weak and atrophies.

18.4 Autonomic Nerves of the Head

— Sympathetic nerves of the head arise as postganglionic fibers from the superior cervical ganglia (see Section 21.3c).

• The **internal carotid plexus** of sympathetic fibers surrounds the internal carotid artery and its branches within the skull. A similar **external carotid plexus** follows the branches of the external carotid artery on the face.
• Sympathetic fibers often travel with the parasympathetic nerves, but they do not synapse in the parasympathetic ganglia.

— The cranial portion of the parasympathetic (visceral motor) system is associated with the oculomotor (CN III), facial (CN VII), glossopharyngeal (CN IX), and vagus (CN X) nerves.

• Preganglionic parasympathetic fibers traveling with the oculomotor (CN III), facial (CN VII), and glossopharyngeal (CN IX) nerves synapse in the four parasympathetic ganglia of the head: the ciliary, pterygopalatine, submandibular, and otic ganglia (**Table 18.6**; see **Figs. 18.17, 18.19,** and **18.23B**).
• Parasympathetic nerves traveling with the vagus nerve (CN X) extend into the thorax and abdomen and synapse in ganglia of nerve plexuses in those regions.
• Parasympathetic ganglia of the head are usually attached to, or in close association with, a branch of the trigeminal nerve (CN V). The postganglionic parasympathetic fibers travel to their target organ by "piggybacking" on these trigeminal branches.

Table 18.6 ▶ Parasympathetic Ganglia of the Head			
Ganglion–Location	**Preganglionic Route**	**Postganglionic Route**	**Target Organs**
Ciliary–orbit	CN III–inferior branch	Short ciliary nn. CN V_1	Ciliary muscles and sphincter pupillae of iris
Pterygopalatine–pterygopalatine fossa	CN VII–greater petrosal n.	Zygomatic branch–CN V_2 Nasopalatine n., greater and lesser palatine nn.–CN V_2	Lacrimal gland Palatal and nasal glands
Submandibular–oral cavity	CN VII–chorda tympani	Lingual n.–CN V_3	Sublingual and submandibular glands
Otic–infratemporal fossa	CN IX–tympanic n. to lesser petrosal n.	Auriculotemporal n.–CN V_3	Parotid gland, buccal and lingual glands

19 Anterior and Lateral Regions of the Head

The anatomy of the head can be divided into smaller regions that lie anterior and lateral to the neurocranium and form the superficial and deep structures of the face. They include the scalp; the parotid region; the temporal, infratemporal, and pterygopalatine fossae; and the nasal and oral cavities.

19.1 The Scalp and Face

The **scalp** covers the neurocranium and extends from the superior nuchal lines of the occipital bone, which mark the superior limit of the neck, to the supraorbital ridge of the frontal bone. The face extends from the forehead to the chin and to the ears on either side.

— The scalp is composed of five layers:

- Skin
- Connective tissue containing the vessels of the scalp
- Aponeurosis of the **occipitofrontalis**, **temporoparietalis**, and **superior auricular** muscles
- Loose areolar tissue
- Periosteum of the skull

The first letter of each layer spells "**SCALP**."

— Muscles of facial expression lie in the loose connective tissue layer of the face and scalp. Their origin on bones of the face and insertion into the overlying skin allows them to create facial movements (**Fig. 19.1A and B; Tables 19.1 and 19.2**).
— Most arteries that supply the face and scalp are branches of the external carotid artery (see **Fig. 17.15**) and include the following:

- The superior and inferior labial arteries, the lateral nasal artery, and the angular branches of the facial artery, which supply the face between the eye and lower lip

- The mental branch of the inferior alveolar artery, which supplies the chin
- The superficial temporal, posterior auricular, and occipital arteries, which supply the lateral and posterior parts of the scalp
- The supratrochlear and supraorbital branches of the ophthalmic artery (a branch of the internal carotid artery), which supply the anterior scalp. These arteries anastomose with the angular artery on the face and form a connection between internal carotid and external carotid circulations (see **Fig. 20.8**).

— Superficial veins of the head drain the face and scalp. Most of these veins follow the arteries of similar name and territory but drain to the facial and retromandibular veins, which terminate in the internal and external jugular veins.
— Veins of the scalp have deep connections to (see **Fig. 18.3**)

- **diploic veins**, which run within the diplöe layer of the skull, and
- **emissary veins**, which drain through the skull from the dural venous sinuses.

Scalp infections

Infections of the scalp spread easily over the calvaria through the loose connective tissue layer. Spread into the posterior neck is inhibited by the attachment of the occipitofrontalis muscle to the occipital and temporal bones. Laterally, spread is inhibited beyond the zygomatic arches by the attachment of the epicranial aponeurosis to the zygomatic arches via the temporal fascia. Anteriorly, however, infections can spread to the eyelids and nose under the frontalis muscle. Additionally, emissary veins may carry infections intracranially to the dural sinuses and can result in meningitis.

Fig. 19.1 ▶ **Muscles of facial expression**

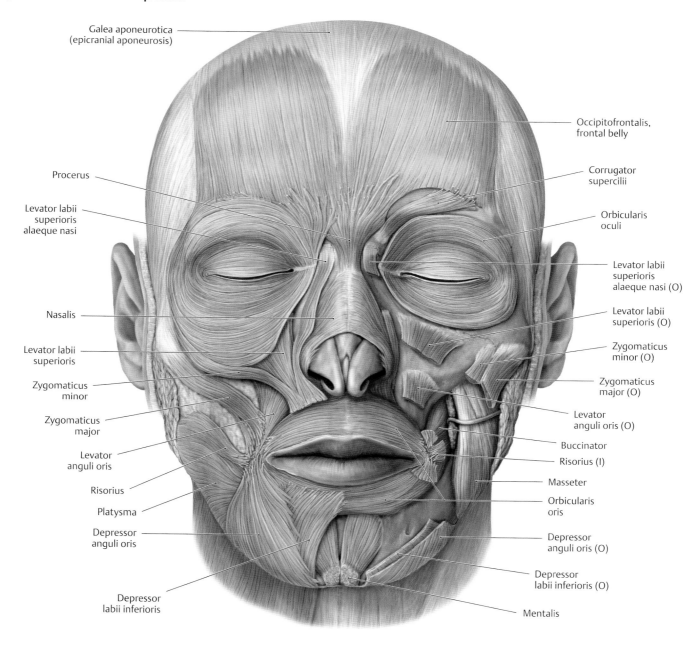

Galea aponeurotica
(epicranial aponeurosis)

Occipitofrontalis,
frontal belly

Procerus

Corrugator
supercilii

Levator labii
superioris
alaeque nasi

Orbicularis
oculi

Levator labii
superioris
alaeque nasi (O)

Nasalis

Levator labii
superioris (O)

Levator labii
superioris

Zygomaticus
minor (O)

Zygomaticus
minor

Zygomaticus
major (O)

Zygomaticus
major

Levator
anguli oris (O)

Levator
anguli oris

Buccinator

Risorius

Risorius (I)

Platysma

Masseter

Orbicularis
oris

Depressor
anguli oris

Depressor
anguli oris (O)

Depressor
labii inferioris (O)

Depressor
labii inferioris

Mentalis

A Anterior view. Muscle origins (O) and insertion (I) indicated on left
side of face.

Fig. 19.1 ▶ **Muscles of facial expression**
(*continued*)

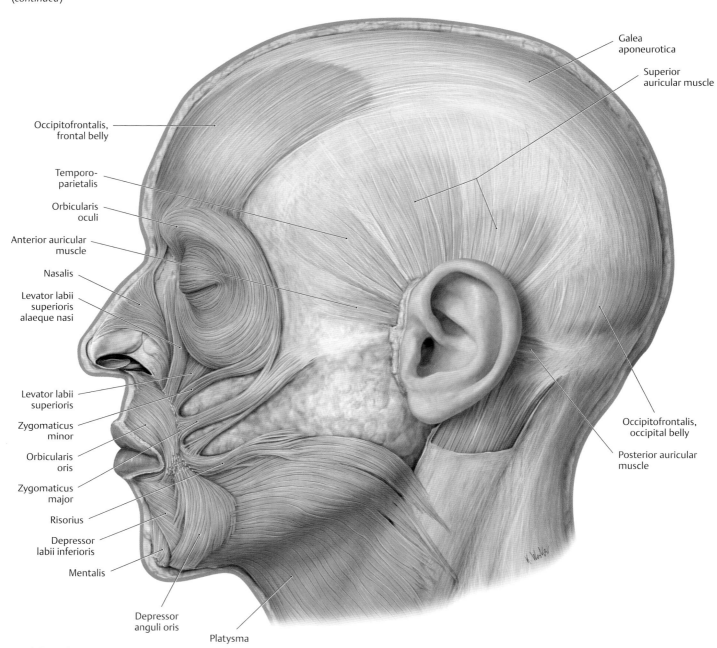

Galea
aponeurotica

Superior
auricular muscle

Occipitofrontalis,
frontal belly

Temporo-
parietalis

Orbicularis
oculi

Anterior auricular
muscle

Nasalis

Levator labii
superioris
alaeque nasi

Levator labii
superioris

Zygomaticus
minor

Orbicularis
oris

Zygomaticus
major

Risorius

Depressor
labii inferioris

Mentalis

Occipitofrontalis,
occipital belly

Posterior auricular
muscle

Depressor
anguli oris

Platysma

B Left lateral view.

Table 19.1 ► Muscles of Facial Expression: Forehead, Nose, and Ear

Muscle	Origin	Insertion*	Main Action(s)**
Calvaria			
Occipitofrontalis (frontal belly)	Epicranial aponeurosis	Skin and subcutaneous tissue of eyebrows and forehead	Elevates eyebrows, wrinkles skin of forehead
Palpebral fissure and nose			
Procerus	Nasal bone, lateral nasal cartilage (upper part)	Skin of lower forehead between eyebrows	Pulls medial angle of eyebrows inferiorly, producing transverse wrinkles over bridge of nose
Orbicularis oculi	Medial orbital margin, medial palpebral ligament; lacrimal bone	Skin around margin of orbit, superior and inferior tarsal plates	Acts as orbital sphincter (closes eyelids) • Palpebral portion gently closes • Orbital portion tightly closes (as in winking)
Nasalis	Maxilla (superior region of canine ridge)	Nasal cartilages	Flares nostrils by drawing ala (side) of nose toward nasal septum
Levator labii superioris alaeque nasi	Maxilla (frontal process)	Alar cartilage of nose and upper lip	Elevates upper lip, opens nostril
Ear			
Anterior auricular muscles	Temporal fascia (anterior portion)	Helix of the ear	Pull ear superiorly and anteriorly
Superior auricular muscles	Epicranial aponeurosis on side of head	Upper portion of auricle	Elevate ear
Posterior auricular muscles	Mastoid process	Convexity of concha of ear	Pull ear superiorly and posteriorly

* There are no bony insertions for the muscles of facial expression.
** All muscles of facial expression are innervated by the facial nerve (CN VII) via temporal, zygomatic, buccal, mandibular, or cervical branches arising from the parotid plexus.

Table 19.2 ► Muscles of Facial Expression: Mouth and Neck

Muscle	Origin	Insertion*	Main Action(s)**
Mouth			
Zygomaticus major	Zygomatic bone (lateral surface, posterior part)	Skin at corner of the mouth	Pulls corner of mouth superiorly and laterally
Zygomaticus minor		Upper lip just medial to corner of the mouth	Pulls upper lip superiorly
Levator labii superioris alaeque nasi	Maxilla (frontal process)	Alar cartilage of nose and upper lip	Elevates upper lip, opens nostril
Levator labii superioris	Maxilla (frontal process) and infraorbital region	Skin of upper lip, alar cartilages of nose	Elevates upper lip, dilates nostril, raises angle of the mouth
Depressor labii inferioris	Mandible (anterior portion of oblique line)	Lower lip at midline; blends with muscle from opposite side	Pulls lower lip inferiorly and laterally
Levator anguli oris	Maxilla (below infraorbital foramen)	Skin at corner of the mouth	Raises angle of mouth, helps form nasolabial furrow
Depressor anguli oris	Mandible (oblique line below canine, premolar, and first molar teeth)	Skin at corner of the mouth; blends with orbicularis oris	Pulls angle of mouth inferiorly and laterally
Buccinator	Mandible, alveolar processes of maxilla and mandible, pterygomandibular raphe	Angle of mouth, orbicularis oris	Presses cheek against molar teeth, working with tongue to keep food between occlusal surfaces and out of oral vestibule; expels air from oral cavity/resists distension when blowing. *Unilateral:* Draws mouth to one side
Orbicularis oris	Deep surface of skinSuperiorly: maxilla (median plane) Inferiorly: mandible	Mucous membrane of lips	Acts as oral sphincter • Compresses and protrudes lips (e.g., when whistling, sucking, and kissing) • Resists distension (when blowing)
Risorius	Fascia over masseter	Skin of corner of the mouth	Retracts corner of mouth as in grimacing
Mentalis	Mandible (incisive fossa)	Skin of chin	Elevates and protrudes lower lip
Neck			
Platysma	Skin over lower neck and upper lateral thorax	Mandible (inferior border), skin over lower face, angle of mouth	Depresses and wrinkles skin of lower face and mouth; tenses skin of neck; aids in forced depression of the mandible

* There are no bony insertions for the muscles of facial expression.
** All muscles of facial expression are innervated by the facial nerve (CN VII) via temporal, zygomatic, buccal, mandibular, or cervical branches arising from its parotid plexus.

— Primary sensory nerves of the face and scalp (**Fig. 19.2A** and **B**) include

- the **supraorbital** and **supratrochlear nerves** (CN V_1);
- the infraorbital nerve and **zygomaticotemporal** and **zygomaticofacial nerves** (V_2);
- the auriculotemporal, buccal, and mental (a branch of the inferior alveolar nerve) nerves (V_3);
- the **great auricular** and **lesser occipital nerve**, which are anterior rami of C2 and C3 via the cervical plexus; and
- the **greater occipital** and **third occipital nerves**, which are posterior rami of C2 and C3, respectively.

— Motor nerves of the face and scalp (see **Figs. 19.2B** and **18.18C**) include

- the temporal, zygomatic, buccal, and marginal mandibular branches of the facial nerve (CN VII), which innervate muscles of the face;
- the temporal and posterior auricular branches of the facial nerve, which innervate muscles of the scalp; and
- the muscular branches of the mandibular division of the trigeminal nerve (CN V_3), which innervate the muscles of mastication.

Fig. 19.2 ▶ **Cutaneous innervation of the face**

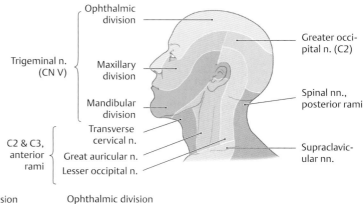

A Cutaneous innervation of the head and neck, left lateral view. The occiput and nuchal regions are supplied by the dorsal rami (blue) of the spinal nerves (the greater occipital nerve is the dorsal ramus of C2).

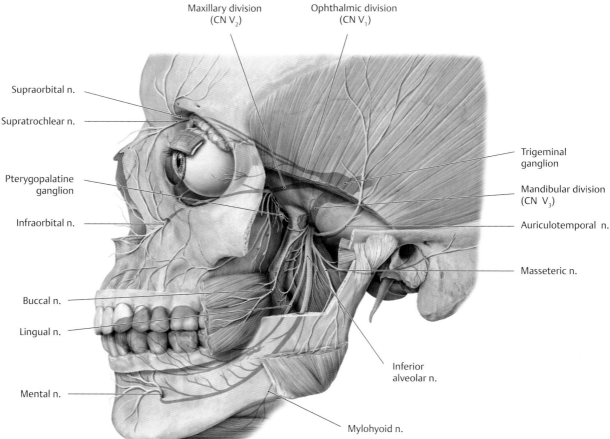

B Divisions of the trigeminal nerve, left lateral view.

19.2 The Temporomandibular Joint and Muscles of Mastication

— The **temporomandibular joint** (TMJ), which joins the mandible to the skull, is a synovial articulation between the head of the mandible and the mandibular fossa and articular tubercle of the temporal bone (**Figs. 19.3** and **19.4A** and **B**).

- An articular disk divides the joint cavity into a separate upper part for gliding movement and a lower part for hinge movement.
- The **lateral ligament** strengthens the fibrous capsule that surrounds the joint.
- **Sphenomandibular** and **stylomandibular ligaments** support the joint during chewing.

Fig. 19.3 ▶ **Temporomandibular joint**
The head of the mandible articulates with the mandibular fossa in the temporomandibular joint. Temporomandibular joint, sagittal section, left lateral view.

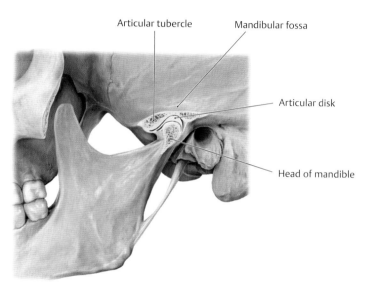

Fig. 19.4 ▶ **Ligaments of the temporomandibular joint**

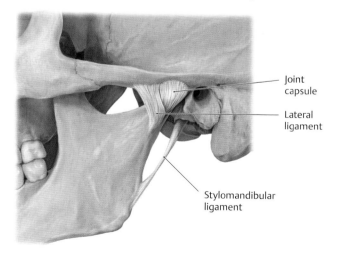

A Lateral view of the left temporomandibular joint.

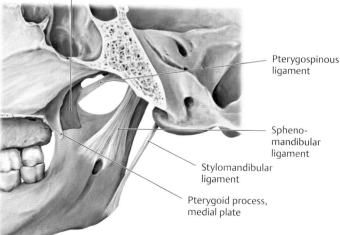

B Medial view of the right temporomandibular joint.

— Muscles of mastication, which include the **masseter, temporalis, lateral pterygoid, and medial pterygoid muscles,** act at the temporomandibular joint to move the mandible during chewing (**Figs. 19.5, 19.6,** and **19.7**; **Table 19.3**). They reside in the parotid region and in the temporal and infratemporal fossae.

▌ Dislocation of the temporomandibular joint

In some individuals yawning (or other activities in which the mouth opens very widely) may cause the condyle of the mandible to slide in front of the anterior tubercle, where it locks the mandible in the protruded position. The ligaments supporting the joint become stretched, which causes severe spasm (trismus) of the masseter, medial pterygoid, and temporalis muscles.

Fig. 19.5 ▶ **Masseter and temporalis muscles**
Left lateral view.

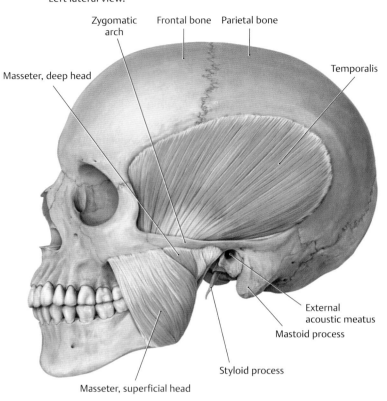

Fig. 19.6 ▶ **Lateral pterygoid muscle**
Left lateral view. *Removed:* Coronoid process of mandible.

Fig. 19.7 ▶ **Medial pterygoid muscles**
Oblique posterior view. *Revealed:* Muscular sling formed by the masseter and medial pterygoid muscles that embed the mandible.

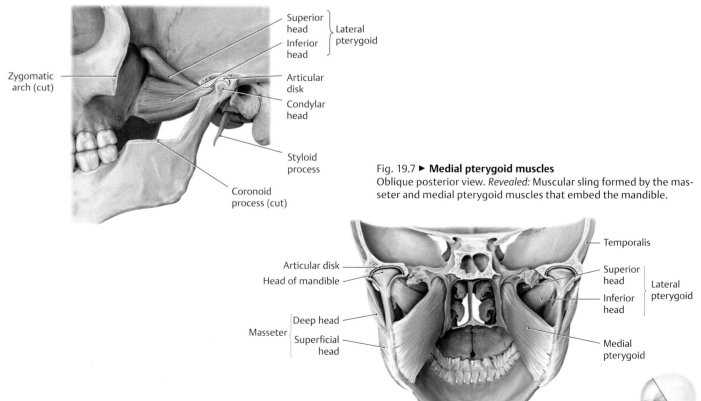

Muscle		Origin	Insertion	Innervation	Action
Masseter		Superficial head: zygomatic arch (anterior two thirds)	Mandibular angle (masseteric tuberosity)	Mandibular n. (CN V₃) via masseteric n.	Elevates (adducts) and protrudes mandible
		Deep part: zygomatic arch (posterior one third)			
Temporalis		Temporal fossa (inferior temporal line)	Coronoid process of mandible (apex and medial surface)	Mandibular n. (CN V₃) via deep temporal nn.	*Vertical fibers:* elevate (adduct) mandible *Horizontal fibers:* retract (retrude) mandible *Unilateral:* lateral movement of mandible (chewing)
Lateral pterygoid	Superior head	Greater wing of sphenoid bone (infratemporal crest)	Temporomandibular joint (articular disk)	Mandibular n. (CN V₃) via lateral pterygoid n.	*Bilateral:* protrudes mandible (pulls articular disk forward) *Unilateral:* lateral movements of mandible (chewing)
	Inferior head	Lateral pterygoid plate (lateral surface)	Mandible (condylar process)		
Medial pterygoid	Superficial head	Maxilla (tuberosity)	Pterygoid tuberosity on medial surface of the mandibular angle	Mandibular n. (CN V₃) via medial pterygoid n.	Elevates (adducts) mandible
	Deep head	Medial surface of lateral pterygoid plate and pterygoid fossa			

Table 19.3 ▸ Muscles of Mastication

19.3 Parotid Region

The parotid region lies superficial to the ramus of the mandible and includes the parotid gland and its surrounding structures (**Figs. 19.8** and **19.9**).

— The **parotid gland**, the largest of the three salivary glands, lies anterior to the ear on the lateral side of the face.

- A superficial part of the gland lies on the masseter muscle.
- A deep part of the gland curves around the posterior edge of the ramus of the mandible.
- A tough parotid fascia derived from the deep cervical fascia encloses the gland.
- Secretomotor (parasympathetic) fibers to the parotid gland arise with the glossopharyngeal nerve (CN IX) and synapse in the otic ganglion. Postganglionic fibers hitchhike on the auriculotemporal nerve of CN V₃.

— The **parotid duct** crosses the masseter muscle superficially to pierce the buccinator muscle and enter the mouth, where it opens opposite the second upper molar tooth.

Fig. 19.8 ▸ Parotid gland
Left lateral view. *Note:* The parotid duct penetrates the buccinator muscle to open opposite the second upper molar.

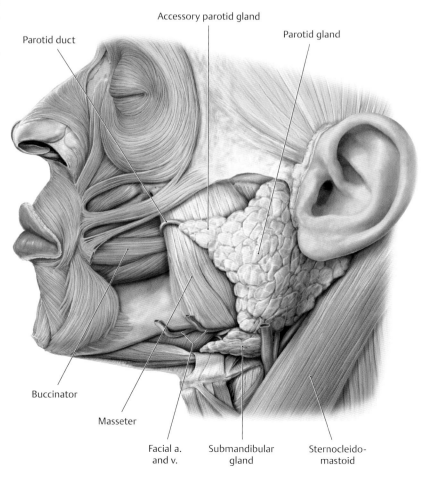

Accessory parotid gland

Parotid gland

Parotid duct

Buccinator

Masseter

Facial a. and v.

Submandibular gland

Sternocleido-mastoid

— The parotid plexus, formed by the facial nerve (CN VII), is embedded within the parotid gland and gives rise to five branches that supply muscles of the face: the temporal, zygomatic, buccal, marginal mandibular, and cervical branches (see **Fig. 18.20B**).

— Structures traversing, or embedded within, the parotid gland include

- the parotid plexus of the facial nerve (CN VII);
- the retromandibular vein, formed by the superficial temporal and maxillary veins;
- the external carotid artery and the origin of its terminal branches, the superficial temporal and maxillary arteries; and
- the parotid lymph nodes, which drain the parotid gland, the external ear, the forehead, and the temporal region.

Fig. 19.9 ▶ **Parotid region**
Left lateral view. *Removed:* Parotid gland, sternocleidomastoid, and veins of the head. *Revealed:* Parotid bed and carotid triangle.

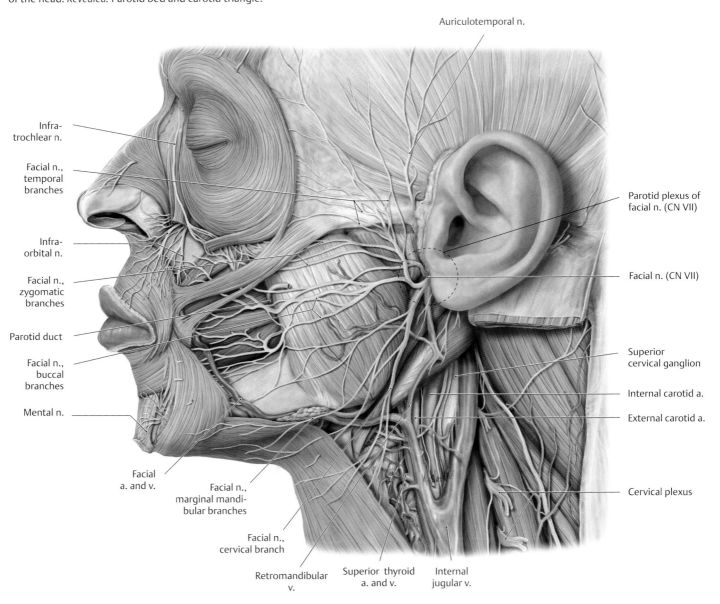

19.4 Temporal Fossa

The temporal fossa lies superior and medial to the parotid region and covers the lateral aspect of the head (**Fig. 19.10**, see also **Fig. 17.3**).

— The boundaries of the temporal fossa are

- anteriorly, the frontal process of the zygomatic bone and zygomatic process of the frontal bone;
- laterally, the zygomatic arch;
- medially, the frontal bone, parietal bone, greater wing of the sphenoid bone, and squamous part of the temporal bone; and

- inferiorly, the infratemporal fossa.

— The temporal fossa contains
- the temporalis muscle and **temporal fascia**,
- the superficial temporal artery and vein,
- the **deep temporal branches** of the maxillary artery, and
- the **deep temporal nerves** and auriculotemporal nerve of the mandibular division of the trigeminal nerve (CN V$_3$).

Fig. 19.10 ▶ **Temporal and infratemporal fossae**
Left lateral view. *Removed:* Ramus of mandible. *Note:* The mylohyoid nerve branches from the inferior alveolar nerve just before the mandibular foramen.

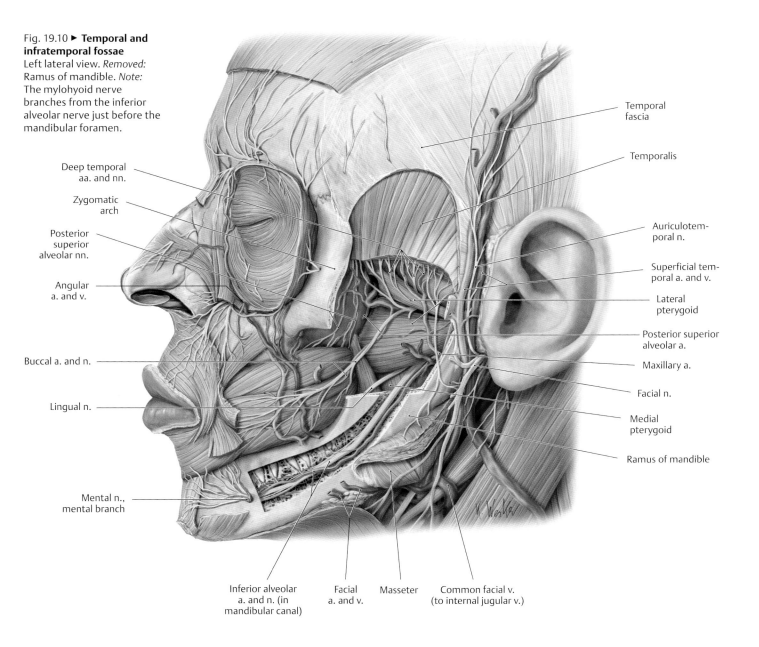

Deep temporal aa. and nn.

Zygomatic arch

Posterior superior alveolar nn.

Angular a. and v.

Buccal a. and n.

Lingual n.

Mental n., mental branch

Temporal fascia

Temporalis

Auriculotemporal n.

Superficial temporal a. and v.

Lateral pterygoid

Posterior superior alveolar a.

Maxillary a.

Facial n.

Medial pterygoid

Ramus of mandible

Inferior alveolar a. and n. (in mandibular canal)

Facial a. and v.

Masseter

Common facial v. (to internal jugular v.)

19.5 Infratemporal Fossa

The infratemporal fossa lies deep to the ramus of the mandible and is continuous superiorly with the temporal fossa (**Fig. 19.11**; see also **Figs. 17.3, 17.6,** and **19.10**).

— The bony boundaries of the infratemporal region are

  • anteriorly, the posterior wall of the maxilla;
  • posteriorly, the mandibular fossa of the temporal bone;
  • medially, the lateral pterygoid plate of the sphenoid bone;
  • laterally the ramus of the mandible; and
  • superiorly, the temporal bone and greater wing of the sphenoid bone.

— The infratemporal fossa communicates with the orbit anteriorly, the pterygopalatine fossa medially, and the middle cranial fossa superiorly.

— The contents of the infratemporal fossa include

  • the temporomandibular joint,
  • the medial and lateral pterygoid muscles and the inferior part of the temporalis muscle,
  • the maxillary artery and its branches (**Table 19.4**),
  • the pterygoid venous plexus,
  • the mandibular division of the trigeminal nerve (CN V$_3$) and its branches,
  • the otic ganglion, and
  • the chorda tympani of the facial nerve (CN VII).

Fig. 19.11 ▶ **Infratemporal fossa: Deep dissection**
Left lateral view. *Removed:* Lateral pterygoid muscle (both heads).
Revealed: Deep infratemporal fossa and mandibular nerve as it enters the mandibular canal via the foramen ovale in the roof of the fossa.

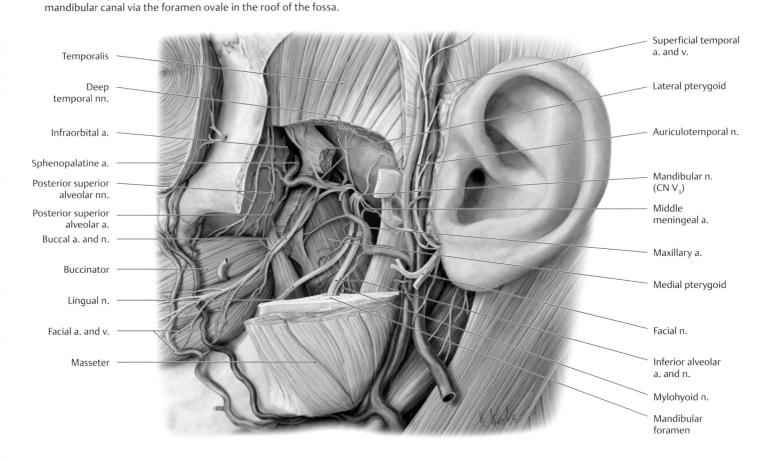

Temporalis

Deep temporal nn.

Infraorbital a.

Sphenopalatine a.

Posterior superior alveolar nn.

Posterior superior alveolar a.

Buccal a. and n.

Buccinator

Lingual n.

Facial a. and v.

Masseter

Superficial temporal a. and v.

Lateral pterygoid

Auriculotemporal n.

Mandibular n. (CN V$_3$)

Middle meningeal a.

Maxillary a.

Medial pterygoid

Facial n.

Inferior alveolar a. and n.

Mylohyoid n.

Mandibular foramen

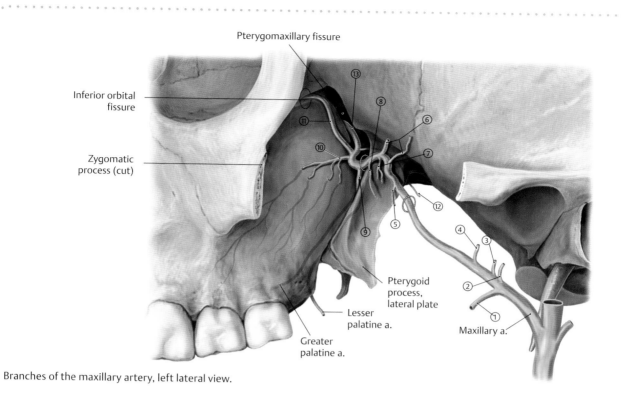

Branches of the maxillary artery, left lateral view.

Table 19.4 ▶ Branches of the Maxillary Artery

Part	Artery		Distribution
Mandibular part (between the origin and the first circle around artery)	① Inferior alveolar a.		Mandible, teeth, gingiva
	② Anterior tympanic a.		Tympanic cavity
	③ Deep auricular a.		Temporomandibular joint, external auditory canal
	④ Middle meningeal a.		Calvaria, dura, anterior and middle cranial fossae
Pterygoid part (between circles around the artery)	⑤ Masseteric a.		Masseter muscle
	⑥ Deep temporal aa.		Temporalis muscle
	⑦ Pterygoid branches		Pterygoid muscles
	⑧ Buccal a.		Buccal mucosa
Pterygopalatine part (from second circle through the pterygomaxillary fissure)	⑨ Descending palatine a.	Greater palatine a.	Hard palate
		Lesser palatine a.	Soft palate, palatine tonsil, pharyngeal wall
	⑩ Posterior superior alveolar a.		Maxillary molars, maxillary sinus, gingiva
	⑪ Infraorbital a.		Maxillary alveoli
	⑫ A. of pterygoid canal		
	⑬ Sphenopalatine a.	Lateral posterior nasal aa.	Lateral wall of nasal cavity, choanae
		Posterior septal branches	Nasal septum

— The mandibular nerve (CN V$_3$), the nerve of the infratemporal fossa and the only division of the trigeminal nerve that carries general sensory and somatic motor fibers, distributes postganglionic parasympathetic (visceral motor) fibers that arise from the otic and submandibular ganglia (**Fig. 19.12, Table 19.5;** see **Fig. 18.18C**).

19.6 Pterygopalatine Fossa

The **pterygopalatine fossa**, a narrow space located medial to the infratemporal fossa, is an important distribution center for branches of the maxillary division of the trigeminal nerve (CN V$_2$) and the accompanying branches of the maxillary artery.

— The bony boundaries of the pterygopalatine fossa are (see **Fig. 20.1B**)
  - superiorly, the apex of the orbit;
  - anteriorly, the maxillary sinus;
  - posteriorly, the lateral pterygoid plate of the sphenoid bone;
  - laterally, the pterygomaxillary fissure; and
  - medially, the vertical plate of the palatine bone.

— Contents of the pterygopalatine fossa include
  - the pterygopalatine part of the maxillary artery, its branches, and its accompanying veins;
  - the nerve of the pterygoid canal;
  - the pterygopalatine ganglion; and
  - the maxillary division of the trigeminal nerve (CN V$_2$) and its branches.

— The pterygopalatine fossa communicates anteriorly with the orbit, medially with the nasal cavity and palate, and posteriorly with the middle cranial fossa and base of the skull (**Table 19.6**).

— The maxillary artery passes from the infratemporal fossa to the pterygopalatine fossa through the **pterygomaxillary fissure** (see **Table 19.4**). Its branches accompany the branches of the maxillary nerve (CN V$_2$) to supply the nose, palate, and pharynx.

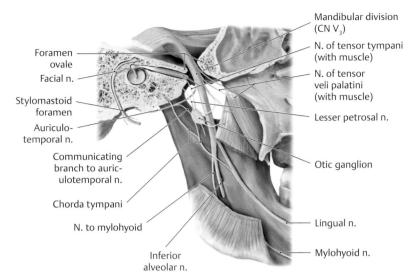

Fig. 19.12 ▶ **Mandibular nerve (CN V$_3$) in the infratemporal fossa** Medial view.

— The **nerve of the pterygoid canal**, which enters the pterygopalatine fossa from the middle cranial fossa, is an autonomic nerve that carries
  - preganglionic parasympathetic fibers from the **greater petrosal nerve**, a branch of the facial nerve (CN VII); and
  - postganglionic sympathetic fibers from the **deep petrosal nerve**, which arises from the internal carotid plexus.

— The pterygopalatine ganglion receives general sensory fibers from the maxillary nerve (CN V$_2$) and parasympathetic and sympathetic fibers from the nerve of the pterygoid canal. Only the parasympathetic fibers synapse in the ganglion; general sensory and sympathetic fibers pass through the ganglion but do not synapse there (**Table 19.7**).

Table 19.5 ▶ **Nerves of the Infratemporal Fossa**		
Nerve	**Nerve Fibers**	**Distribution**
Muscular branches (CN V$_3$)	Branchial motor	Muscles of mastication; mylohyoid; tensor tympani; tensor veli palatini; anterior belly of digastric
Auriculotemporal (CN V$_3$)	General sensory	Auricle, temporal region, and temporomandibular joint
	Visceral motor from glossopharyngeal n. (CN IX)	Parotid gland
Inferior alveolar (CN V$_3$)	General sensory	Mandibular teeth; mental branch supplies skin of lower lip and chin
Lingual (CN V$_3$)	General sensory	Anterior two thirds of tongue, floor of mouth
Buccal (CN V$_3$)	General sensory	Skin and mucous membrane of cheek
Meningeal (CN V$_3$)	General sensory	Dura of middle cranial fossa
Chorda tympani (CN VII)	Special sensory taste	Anterior two thirds of tongue
	Visceral motor	Submandibular and sublingual glands via submandibular ganglion and lingual n. (CN V$_3$).

Table 19.6 ► Passage of Neurovascular Structures into the Pterygopalatine Fossa

Origin of Structures	Passageway	Transmitted Nerves	Transmitted Vessels
Orbit	Inferior orbital fissure	① Infraorbital n.	Infraorbital a. (and accompanying vv.)
		② Zygomatic n.	Inferior ophthalmic v.
		③ Orbital branches (from CN V₂)	
Middle cranial fossa	Foramen rotundum	④ Maxillary n. (CN V₂)	
Base of skull	Pterygoid canal	⑤ N. of pterygoid canal (greater and deep petrosal nn.)	A. of pterygoid canal (with accompanying vv.)
Palate	Greater palatine canal	⑥ Greater palatine n.	Descending palatine a.
			Greater palatine a.
	Lesser palatine canals	⑦ Lesser palatine nn.	Lesser palatine aa. (terminal branches of descending palatine a.)
Nasal cavity	Sphenopalatine foramen	⑧ Medial and lateral posterior superior and posterior inferior nasal branches (from nasopalatine n., CN V₂)	Sphenopalatine a. (with accompanying vv.)

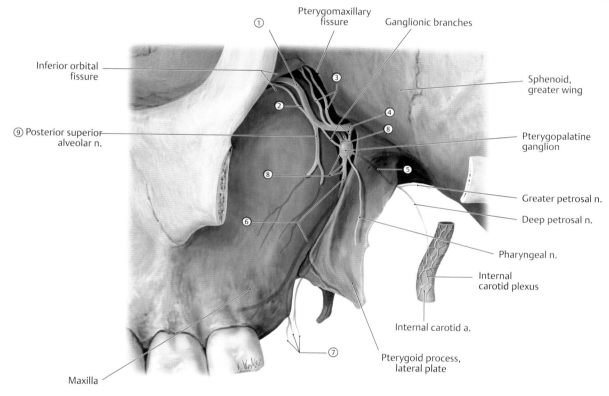

Pterygomaxillary fissure
Ganglionic branches
Inferior orbital fissure
①
③
②
④
⑧
Sphenoid, greater wing
⑨ Posterior superior alveolar n.
Pterygopalatine ganglion
⑧
⑤
Greater petrosal n.
⑥
Deep petrosal n.
Pharyngeal n.
Internal carotid plexus
Internal carotid a.
⑦
Maxilla
Pterygoid process, lateral plate

Table 19.7 ► Nerves of the Pterygopalatine Fossa

Nerve	Motor Innervation	Sensory Distribution
① Infraorbital n. (CN V₂)		Skin of the midface, maxillary sinus, teeth, and gingiva
② Zygomatic n. (CN V₂)–communicating branch from zygomaticotemporal n.	Visceral motor (postganglionic) to lacrimal gland	Skin of lateral cheek, temple
③ Orbital branches (CN V₂)		Orbit, ethmoid and sphenoid sinuses
④ Maxillary (CN V₂)		
⑤ N. of the pterygoid canal (CN VII)	Visceral motor (preganglionic) to glands of the nasal mucosa, and palate; lacrimal gland	
⑥ Greater palatine n. (CN V₂)		Hard palate
⑦ Lesser palatine n. (CN V₂)		Soft palate, palatine tonsil
⑧ Medial and lateral posterior superior and inferior nasal nn. (CN V₂)		Nasal septum, upper lateral nasal wall, ethmoid sinuses
⑨ Superior alveolar n. (CN V₂)		Maxillary sinus, cheeks, gingiva, maxillary molars

— The maxillary division of the trigeminal nerve (CN V$_2$)

- passes from the middle cranial fossa to the pterygopalatine fossa through the **foramen rotundum**;
- suspends the pterygopalatine ganglion by two small **ganglionic nerves**, which transmit general sensory fibers of the maxillary nerve;
- distributes postganglionic parasympathetic (secretomotor) and sympathetic (vasoconstrictive) fibers to the lacrimal, nasal, palatial, and pharyngeal glands; and
- distributes general sensory fibers to the midface, maxillary sinus, maxillary teeth, nasal cavity, palate, and superior pharynx.

19.7 Nasal Cavity

The **nasal cavity** is located in the middle of the face between the orbits and maxillary sinuses and above the oral cavity.

19.7a Structure of the Nasal Cavity

The nose has an external portion and paired internal nasal cavities that are separated by a nasal septum (**Figs. 19.13A** and **B** and **19.14A** and **B**).

Fig. 19.13 ▶ **Skeleton of the nose**
The skeleton of the nose is composed of an upper bony portion and a lower cartilaginous portion. The proximal portions of the nostrils (alae) are composed of connective tissue with small embedded pieces of cartilage.

— The external nose consists of

- anteriorly, the **alar** and **lateral nasal cartilages**, which form the nasal **ala** and **crura** surrounding the nostrils and the **apex**, or tip of the nose; and
- posteriorly, the frontal, maxillary, and nasal bones, which form the **root**, or bridge, of the nose.

— The nasal cavities are pyramidally shaped spaces that communicate anteriorly with the outside through the **nares** (nostrils) and posteriorly with the nasopharynx through the **choanae**.

— The lateral walls of the nasal cavities are formed by the superior and middle nasal conchae of the ethmoid bone; the inferior nasal conchae; and the maxillary, palatine, lacrimal, and nasal bones.

- The superior, middle, and inferior nasal conchae are scroll-like bony processes that project into the nasal cavity.
- The **superior**, **middle**, and **inferior nasal meatuses** are recesses below the respective nasal conchae.

— The nasal septum forms the medial wall of each nasal cavity and consists of the vomer, the perpendicular plate of the ethmoid bone, and the septal cartilage.

— The **hard palate**, consisting of the maxilla and palatine bones, forms the floor of the nasal cavities and separates them from the oral cavity (see Section 19.8b and **Figs. 19.19** and **19.20**).

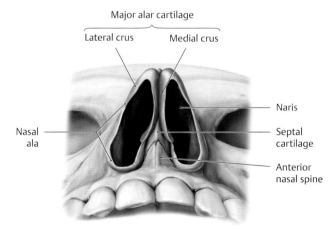

Glabella

Nasal bone

Frontal process of maxilla

Lateral nasal cartilage

Major alar cartilage

Minor alar cartilages

Major alar cartilage

Lateral crus   Medial crus

Nasal ala

Naris

Septal cartilage

Anterior nasal spine

A Left lateral view.

B Inferior view.

Fig. 19.14 ▶ **Bones of the nasal cavity**

The left and right nasal cavities are flanked by lateral walls and separated by the nasal septum. Air enters the nasal cavity through the anterior nasal aperture and travels through three passages: the superior, middle, and inferior meatuses (*arrows*). These passages are separated by the superior, middle, and inferior conchae. Air leaves the nose through the choanae, entering the nasopharynx.

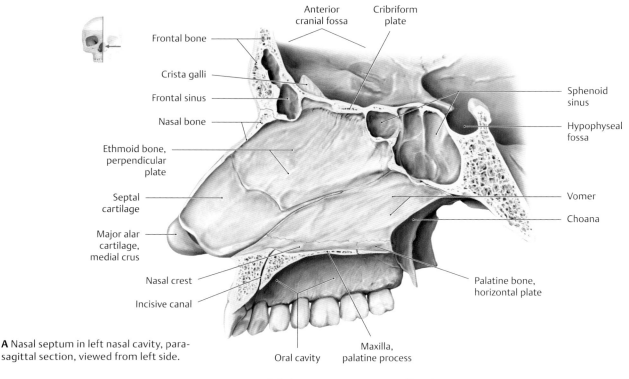

Frontal bone
Anterior cranial fossa
Cribriform plate
Crista galli
Frontal sinus
Nasal bone
Ethmoid bone, perpendicular plate
Septal cartilage
Major alar cartilage, medial crus
Nasal crest
Incisive canal
Sphenoid sinus
Hypophyseal fossa
Vomer
Choana
Palatine bone, horizontal plate
Oral cavity
Maxilla, palatine process

A Nasal septum in left nasal cavity, parasagittal section, viewed from left side.

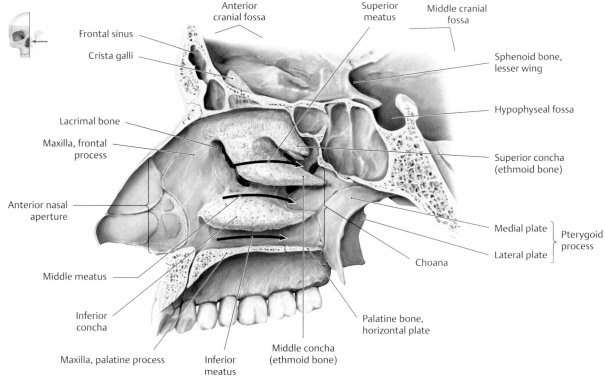

Anterior cranial fossa
Superior meatus
Middle cranial fossa
Frontal sinus
Crista galli
Sphenoid bone, lesser wing
Lacrimal bone
Maxilla, frontal process
Hypophyseal fossa
Superior concha (ethmoid bone)
Anterior nasal aperture
Medial plate
Lateral plate
Pterygoid process
Middle meatus
Choana
Inferior concha
Palatine bone, horizontal plate
Maxilla, palatine process
Inferior meatus
Middle concha (ethmoid bone)

B Lateral wall of the right nasal cavity, sagittal section, medial view. *Removed:* Nasal septum. *Note:* The superior and middle conchae are parts of the ethmoid bone, whereas the inferior nasal conchae is a separate bone. Arrows indicate the direction of airflow through the nasal conchae.

Fig. 19.15 ▶ **Location of the paranasal sinuses**
The paranasal sinuses (frontal, ethmoid, maxillary, and sphenoid) are air-filled cavities that reduce the weight of the skull.

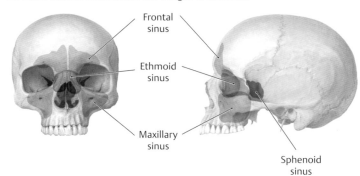

A Anterior view.   **B** Left lateral view.

Fig. 19.16 ▶ **Paranasal sinuses**
Openings of the paranasal sinuses and nasolacrimal duct. Right nasal cavity, sagittal section, medial view. Mucosal secretions from the sinuses and nasolacrimal duct drain the nose.

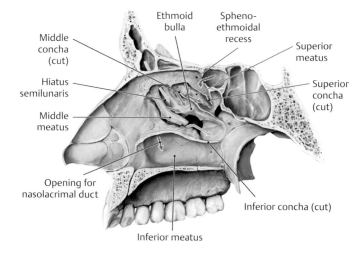

Table 19.8 ▶ Opening of Nasal Structures into the Nose	
Nasal Passage	**Sinuses/Duct**
Sphenoethmoid recess	Sphenoid sinus (blue)
Superior meatus	Posterior ethmoid sinus (green)
Middle meatus	Anterior and middle ethmoid sinus (green)
	Frontal sinus (yellow)
	Maxillary sinus (orange)
Inferior meatus	Nasolacrimal duct (red)

— **Paranasal sinuses** are air-filled cavities within bones of the skull that communicate with the nasal cavities (**Figs. 19.15A** and **B** and **Fig. 19.16**; **Table 19.8**).

- Paired **frontal sinuses**, which are usually asymmetrical, lie above the root of the nose and drain into the middle meatus through a **frontonasal duct** into the **hiatus semilunaris**.
- **Sphenoid sinuses**, which form within the body of the sphenoid bone, lie between the right and left cavernous sinuses and drain into the **sphenoethmoidal recess** in the posterosuperior part of the nasal cavities above the superior concha.
- **Ethmoid sinuses** comprise the medial wall of the orbit and are formed by numerous thin-walled ethmoid air cells. They lie between the orbits above the nasal cavities and drain into the superior and middle meatuses.
- Paired **maxillary sinuses**, the largest of the paranasal sinuses, lie on either side of the nasal cavities, inferior to the orbits, and drain into the middle meatuses.

███████   Infection of the maxillary sinuses

Infections arising in the nasal cavity may spread to any of the paranasal sinuses, but the maxillary sinuses are the most commonly affected. Mucus builds up within the maxillary sinuses and is unable to drain because their ostia are located high on the superomedial walls. The ostia are also commonly obstructed by inflammation of the mucous membranes of the sinuses (maxillary sinusitis). Maxillary sinusitis usually follows the common cold or influenza virus but may also arise from the spread of infections from posterior maxillary teeth.

— A **nasolacrimal duct** drains tears from the medial corner of each eye and empties into the inferior meatus on each side.

19.7b Neurovasculature of the Nasal Cavity

— The external carotid artery via its maxillary and facial branches, and the internal carotid artery via its ophthalmic branch, supply the nasal cavity. The area of overlap between the external and internal circulations is referred to as Kiesselbach's area (**Fig. 19.17A** and **B**).

- Branches of the maxillary artery include
  - the lateral posterior nasal and posterior septal arteries, branches of the sphenopalatine artery; and
  - the greater palatine artery, a branch of the descending palatine artery.
- Branches of the facial artery include the lateral nasal artery and a septal artery, a branch of the superior labial artery.
- Branches of the ophthalmic artery include anterior and posterior ethmoidal arteries.

— Veins that drain the nasal cavity form a submucosal venous plexus that drains into the ophthalmic, facial, and sphenopalatine veins.

Epistaxis

Bleeding, or epistaxis, of the highly vascular nasal mucosa is a common consequence of nasal trauma, and even minor trauma can disrupt the veins in the vestibule. Most bleeding originates from the arteries of Kiesselbach's area in the anterior third of the nasal cavity. These include the sphenopalatine, greater palatine, anterior ethmoidal, and superior labial arteries.

— The olfactory nerve (CN I) and the ophthalmic (CN V_1) and maxillary (CN V_2) divisions of the trigeminal nerve innervate the nose (**Fig. 19.18A** and **B**).

- Olfactory nerves, which are responsible for smell, arise from the olfactory epithelium in the roof of the nasal cavity. They pass through the cribriform plate and end in the olfactory bulbs.
- Infratrochlear and anterior ethmoid branches of CN V_1 and the infraorbital branch of CN V_2 innervate the external nose.
- The anterior and posterior ethmoidal branches of CN V_1 innervate the external nose and the mucosa of the anterosuperior nasal cavity through internal, external, medial, and lateral nasal branches.
- The posterior nasal branches of the nasopalatine nerve on the septum and nasal branches of the greater palatine nerve on the lateral walls (both branches of CN V_2) innervate the mucosa of the posteroinferior nasal cavity.

Fig. 19.17 ▶ **Arteries of the nasal cavity**

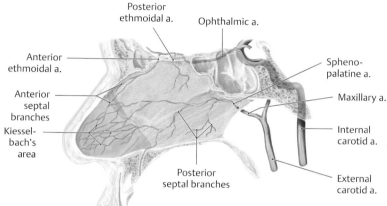

A Arteries of the nasal septum, left lateral view.

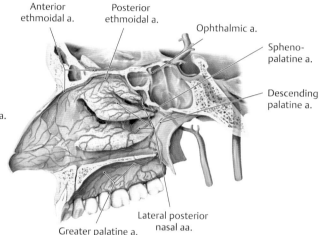

B Arteries of the right lateral nasal wall, medial view.

Fig. 19.18 ▶ **Nerves of the nasal cavity**

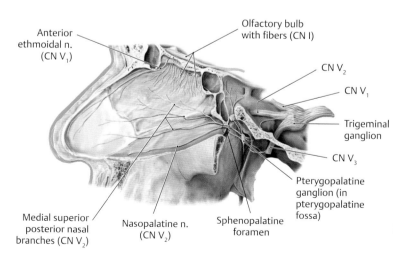

A Nerves of the nasal septum, left lateral view.

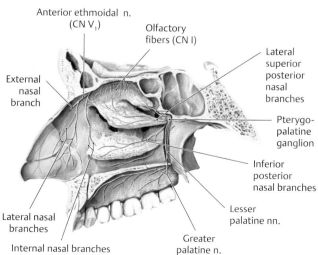

B Nerves of the right lateral nasal wall, medial view.

433

19.8 Oral Region

The oral cavity, located below the nasal cavity and anterior to the pharynx, is bounded superiorly by the palate, inferiorly by the tongue and muscular floor, anteriorly by the lips, posteriorly by the uvula, and laterally by the cheeks (**Fig. 19.19**).

19.8a Lips, Cheeks, Gingiva, Teeth, and Oral Cavity

— The **lips** frame the mouth and surround the **oral fissure**, the opening into the oral cavity.

• The lips contain the sphincter-like obicularis oris muscle and superior and inferior labial muscles. Externally, they are covered by skin; internally, they are covered by the mucous membrane of the oral cavity.

• The **philtrum**, an external midline depression on the upper lip, extends superiorly to the nasal septum.

• **Labial frenula** are midline folds of mucous membrane that attach the inner surfaces of the upper and lower lips to the gums.

Cleft lip

Cleft lip is a congenital defect that occurs early in embryonic life when the maxillary prominence and the median nasal prominence fail to fuse. It is seen in ~1:1000 live births and is more common in males than females. The cleft may be unilateral or bilateral and is described as complete when it extends into the nose and incomplete when it appears as a notch in the lip. Corrective surgery is usually performed when the infant is around 10 weeks old.

Fig. 19.19 ▶ **Oral cavity and pharynx**
Midsagittal section, left lateral view.

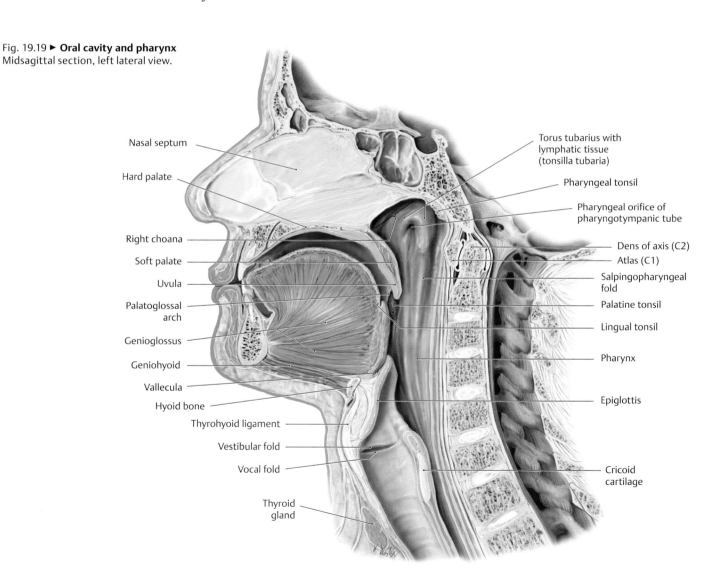

Nasal septum

Hard palate

Right choana

Soft palate

Uvula

Palatoglossal arch

Genioglossus

Geniohyoid

Vallecula

Hyoid bone

Thyrohyoid ligament

Vestibular fold

Vocal fold

Thyroid gland

Torus tubarius with lymphatic tissue (tonsilla tubaria)

Pharyngeal tonsil

Pharyngeal orifice of pharyngotympanic tube

Dens of axis (C2)

Atlas (C1)

Salpingopharyngeal fold

Palatine tonsil

Lingual tonsil

Pharynx

Epiglottis

Cricoid cartilage

— The **cheeks**, continuous with the lips, form the walls of the mouth and the **buccal region** of the face.

- The buccinator muscle, innervated by the buccal branch of the facial nerve (CN VII), forms the moveable wall of the cheek.
- Buccal fat pads, encapsulated cushions of fat that lie superficial to the buccinator muscles, are proportionately large in infants and reduced in adults.
- The zygomatic bone and zygomatic arch form the "cheek bone."

— Teeth are anchored in **alveoli** (sockets) of the **maxillary** and **mandibular dental arches** (see **Figs. 17.6** and **17.10**).

- Children have 20 deciduous teeth, which are replaced at predictable intervals between ages 7 and 25 years.
- Adult have 32 teeth, consisting of incisors, canines, premolars, and molars.

— The **gingivae**, or gums, made of fibrous tissue covered by the mucous membrane of the oral cavity, are firmly attached to the maxilla and mandible.

— The oral cavity, or mouth, is divided into two regions: the **oral vestibule** and the **oral cavity proper** (**Fig. 19.20**).

- The oral vestibule is the narrow space between the lips and cheeks and the dental arches of the maxilla and mandible.
- The oral cavity proper is the space bounded anteriorly and laterally by the upper and lower dental arches. Superiorly, the **palate** forms the roof, and inferiorly, the tongue rests on a muscular floor.

— The oral cavity connects posteriorly to the pharynx through a narrow space, the **faucial isthmus**.

Fig. 19.20 ▶ **Divisions of the oral cavity**
Anterior view.

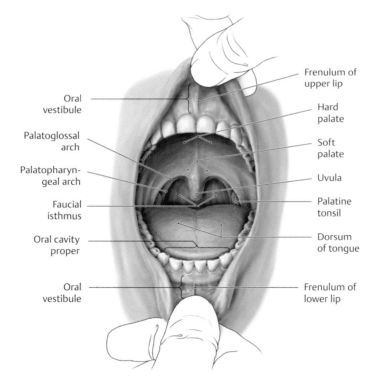

Oral vestibule	Frenulum of upper lip
	Hard palate
Palatoglossal arch	Soft palate
Palatopharyngeal arch	Uvula
Faucial isthmus	Palatine tonsil
Oral cavity proper	Dorsum of tongue
Oral vestibule	Frenulum of lower lip

- Muscles that form the floor of the mouth, the **suprahyoid muscles**, are attached to the hyoid bone in the neck (**Fig. 19.21A** and **B**; **Table 19.9**). They have a complex innervation with contributions from the trigeminal and facial nerves and the C1 spinal nerve via the hypoglossal nerve.
- The lingual, facial, and maxillary branches of the external carotid artery supply the lips, cheeks, floor of the mouth, and upper and lower teeth.

Fig. 19.21 ▶ **Muscles of the oral floor: Suprahyoid muscles**

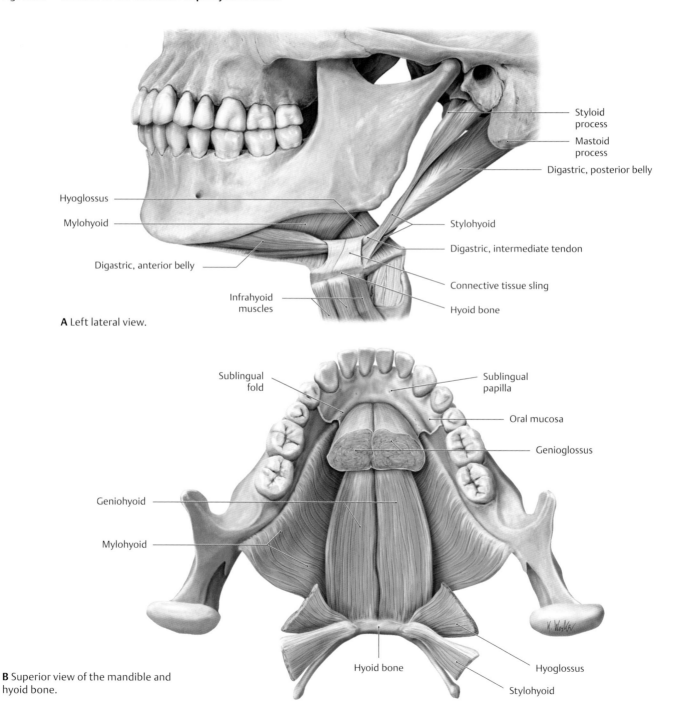

Styloid process

Mastoid process

Digastric, posterior belly

Hyoglossus

Mylohyoid

Stylohyoid

Digastric, intermediate tendon

Digastric, anterior belly

Connective tissue sling

Infrahyoid muscles

Hyoid bone

A Left lateral view.

Sublingual fold

Sublingual papilla

Oral mucosa

Genioglossus

Geniohyoid

Mylohyoid

Hyoid bone

Hyoglossus

Stylohyoid

B Superior view of the mandible and hyoid bone.

Table 19.9 ▶ Suprahyoid Muscles

Muscle		Origin	Insertion		Innervation	Action
Digastric	Anterior belly	Mandible (digastric fossa)	Via an intermediate tendon with a fibrous loop		Mylohyoid n. (from CN V$_3$)	Elevates hyoid bone (during swallowing), assists in opening mandible
	Posterior belly	Temporal bone (mastoid notch, medial to mastoid process)			Facial n. (CN VII)	
Stylohyoid		Temporal bone (styloid process)	Via a split tendon			
Mylohyoid		Mandible (mylohyoid line)	Hyoid bone (body)	Via median tendon of insertion (mylohyoid raphe)	Mylohyoid n. (from CN V$_3$)	Tightens and elevates oral floor, draws hyoid bone forward (during swallowing), assists in opening mandible and moving it side to side (mastication)
Geniohyoid		Mandible (inferior mental spine)		Body of hyoid bone	Anterior ramus of C1 via hypoglossal n. (CN XII)	Draws hyoid bone forward (during swallowing), assists in opening mandible
Hyoglossus		Hyoid bone (superior border of greater cornu)	Sides of tongue		Hypoglossal n. (CN XII)	Depresses the tongue

— The trigeminal nerve (CN V) transmits sensation from the mouth.

- The superior alveolar branch of the maxillary division (CN V$_2$) innervates the upper teeth.
- Inferior alveolar, lingual, and buccal branches of the mandibular division (CN V$_3$) innervate the cheek, lower teeth, and floor of the mouth.

— Visceral motor fibers carried by the chorda tympani (CN VII) synapse in the submandibular ganglion in the floor of the mouth. Postganglionic fibers travel via the lingual nerve to innervate the submandibular and sublingual glands.

19.8b The Palate

The palate forms the roof of the oral cavity and the floor of the nasal cavity and separates the oral cavity from the pharynx posteriorly.

— Nasal mucosa covers the superior surface, and oral mucosa, densely packed with mucus-secreting palatine glands, covers the inferior surface.

— The palate has anterior and posterior regions.

- The **hard palate**, formed by the palatine processes of the maxillary bones and the horizontal processes of the palatine bones, makes up the anterior two thirds of the palate (see **Fig. 17.6**).
- The **soft palate**, the posterior third of the palate, has an anterior aponeurotic part that is attached to the hard palate and a posterior muscular part with an unattached posterior margin that ends in a conical projection, the **uvula** (see **Fig. 19.19**).

▮ Cleft palate

Cleft palate is a congenital defect that occurs early in embryonic life when the lateral palatine processes fail to fuse with each other, with the nasal septum, and/or with the median palatine processes. It is seen in ~1:2500 live births and is more common in females than males. The cleft (a fissure or opening) is described as complete when it involves the soft and hard palate and incomplete when it appears as a "hole" in the roof of the mouth (usually in the soft palate). In each case the uvula is usually also split. The cleft connects the oral cavity directly to the nasal cavity. Initial treatment involves the use of a prosthetic device called a palatal obturator to seal the cleft until corrective surgery is performed when the infant is between 6 and 12 months old.

— During swallowing, muscles of the soft palate can tense and elevate it against the posterior pharyngeal wall to prevent food from passing into the nasal cavity. They can also draw the palate downward against the tongue to prevent food from entering the pharynx (**Fig. 19.22**; **Table 19.10**). Muscles of the soft palate include the **tensor veli palatini, levator veli palatini, musculus uvulae, palatoglossus,** and **palatopharyngeus**.

— The paired **palatoglossal** and **palatopharyngeal arches**, formed by the **palatoglossus** and **palatopharyngeus muscles**, anchor the soft palate to the tongue and pharynx (see **Fig. 19.20**).

— Greater palatine, lesser palatine, and sphenopalatine branches of the maxillary artery supply the palate (**Fig. 19.23**, see also **Fig. 19.17B**).

— The greater palatine, lesser palatine, and nasopalatine branches of the maxillary division (CN V_2) carry sensory innervation from the palate.

Fig. 19.22 ▶ **Muscles of the soft palate**
Inferior view. The soft palate forms the posterior boundary of the oral cavity, separating it from the oropharynx.

19.8c The Tongue

The tongue is a muscular organ that is involved in speech, taste, and manipulation of food during the initial phase of swallowing. Two thirds of the tongue lies in the oral cavity; the remainder forms the anterior wall of the oropharynx, the part of the pharynx posterior to the oral cavity.

— The tongue has three parts (**Fig. 19.24**):
  • the **root**, the attached posterior portion;
  • the **body**, the largest portion, between the root and apex; and
  • the **apex**, the anterior tip.

— The **sulcus terminalis**, a groove on the dorsum of the tongue, divides the anterior two thirds of the tongue from the posterior third. A small pit at the center of the groove, the **foramen cecum**, marks the embryonic origin of the thyroid gland.

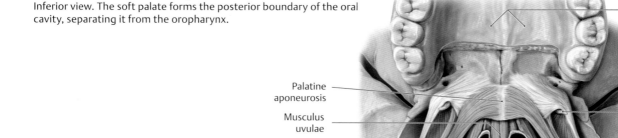

Palatine aponeurosis — Musculus uvulae — Uvula — Oropharynx (isthmus) — Hard palate — Pterygoid hamulus — Tensor veli palatini — Levator veli palatini

Table 19.10 ▶ **Muscles of the Soft Palate**				
Muscle	**Origin**	**Insertion**	**Innervation**	**Action**
Tensor veli palatini	Medial pterygoid plate (scaphoid fossa); sphenoid bone (spine); cartilage of pharyngotympanic tube	Palatine aponeurosis	Medial pterygoid n. (CN V_3 via otic ganglion)	Tightens soft palate; opens inlet to pharyngotympanic tube (during swallowing, yawning)
Levator veli palatini	Cartilage of pharyngotympanic tube; temporal bone (petrous part)		Accessory n. (CN XI, cranial part) via pharyngeal plexus (vagus n., CN X)	Raises soft palate to horizontal position
Musculus uvulae	Uvula (mucosa)	Palatine aponeurosis; posterior nasal spine		Shortens and raises uvula
Palatoglossus	Tongue (side)			Elevates tongue (posterior portion); pulls soft palate onto tongue
Palatopharyngeus		Palatine aponeurosis		Tightens soft palate; during swallowing pulls pharyngeal walls superiorly, anteriorly, and medially

Fig. 19.23 ► **Neurovasculature of the hard palate**
Inferior view. The hard palate receives sensory innervation primarily from terminal branches of the maxillary division of the trigeminal nerve (CN V₂). The arteries of the hard palate arise from the maxillary artery.

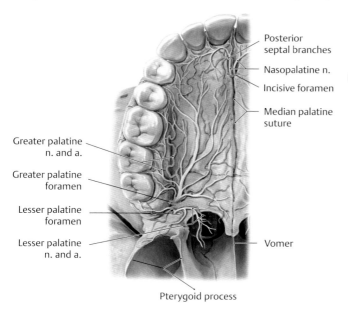

Fig. 19.24 ► **Structure of the tongue**
Superior view. The V-shaped sulcus terminalis divides the tongue into an anterior (oral, presulcal) and a posterior (pharyngeal, postsulcal) part.

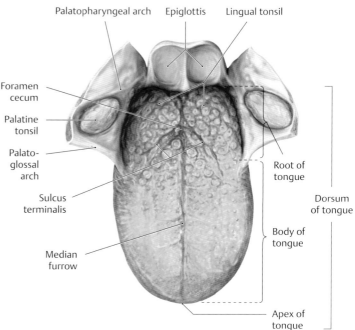

— Numerous lingual papillae, many containing taste buds, give the mucosa of the anterior two thirds of the tongue its rough texture.

- **Vallate papillae**, the largest of the lingual papillae, are arranged in a row directly anterior to the sulcus terminalis.
- **Foliate papillae** are found on the small lateral folds of the lingual mucosa and are not well developed.
- **Filiform papillae** contain afferent nerve endings that are sensitive to touch but not to taste. These are highly keratinized and facilitate rasplike licking activity.
- **Fungiform papillae** are most numerous at the apex and margins of the tongue.

— The **lingual tonsil** is a collection of lymphoid nodules distributed over the mucosa of the posterior part of the tongue. Lingual tonsils have crypts that are flushed by glands below them.
— The **frenulum of the tongue**, a midline mucosal fold, attaches the inferior surface of the tongue to the floor of the oral cavity and restricts its movement.
— Extrinsic muscles of the tongue, which originate outside the tongue and are responsible primarily for tongue movements, include the genioglossus, hyoglossus, palatoglossus, and styloglossus muscles (**Fig. 19.25**).

Fig. 19.25 ► **Extrinsic muscles of the tongue**
Left lateral view.

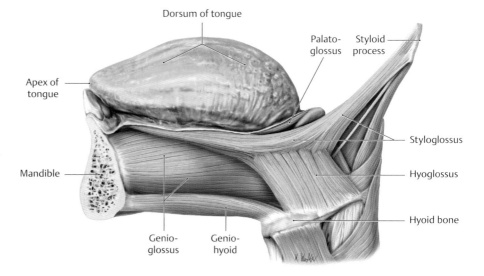

- Intrinsic muscles of the tongue have no bony attachments and are responsible for changing the shape of the tongue. They include the superior and inferior longitudinal muscles and the transverse and vertical muscles.
- All extrinsic and intrinsic muscles of the tongue, except the palatoglossus, are innervated by the hypoglossal nerve (CN XII). The palatoglossus is innervated by the vagus nerve (CN X).
- The lingual arteries, branches of the external carotid arteries, supply the tongue. The lingual veins accompany the arteries and drain into the internal jugular vein.
- Lymph from the tongue ultimately drains to deep cervical and jugular nodes in the neck, although the drainage from the various parts of the tongue follows four different pathways (**Fig. 19.26A** and **B**; **Table 19.11**). These drainage routes can be clinically important in the metastasis of lingual tumors.
- The five cranial nerves (trigeminal, facial, glossopharyngeal, vagus, and hypoglossal) that innervate the tongue carry motor, general sensory, and special sensory fibers (**Table 19.12**; **Fig. 19.27**).

Fig. 19.26 ▶ **Lymphatic drainage of the tongue and oral floor**
Lymph flows to the submental and submandibular lymph nodes of the tongue and oral floor, which ultimately drain into the jugular lymph nodes along the internal jugular vein. Because the lymph nodes receive drainage from both the ipsilateral and contralateral sides (B), tumor cells may become widely disseminated in this region (e.g., metastatic squamous cell carcinoma, especially on the lateral border of the tongue, frequently metastasizes to the opposite side).

19.8d Salivary Glands

Three pairs of salivary glands, the parotid, sublingual, and submandibular, produce and secrete saliva into the mouth (**Fig. 19.28**; see **Fig. 19.8**).

- The **sublingual gland**, the smallest of the three glands, lies deep to the mucosa of the floor of the mouth, forming the **sublingual folds**, onto which it secretes saliva through numerous small ducts.
- The **submandibular gland** has a superficial part located in the neck and a deep part located in the floor of the mouth, which connect around the posterior border of the mylohyoid muscle. The **submandibular (Wharton's) duct** opens via the **sublingual papilla** at the base of the lingual frenulum.
- The parotid gland, the largest of the three glands, is located in the parotid region on the lateral side of the head, anterior to the ear. The parotid duct opens into the vestibule of the mouth at the parotid papilla located adjacent to the second maxillary molar (see Section 19.3).

Table 19.11 ▶ Lymphatic Drainage of the Tongue		
Area of the Tongue	**Drainage Pattern**	**Primary Nodes**
Root	Bilaterally	Superior deep cervical
Medial part of the body	Bilaterally	Inferior deep cervical
Lateral parts of the body	Ipsilaterally	Submandibular
Apex and frenulum	Midline—bilaterally Sides—ipsilaterally	Submental

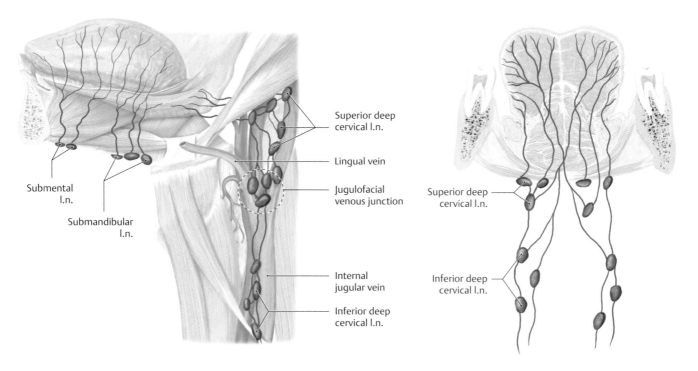

Submental l.n.

Submandibular l.n.

Superior deep cervical l.n.

Lingual vein

Jugulofacial venous junction

Internal jugular vein

Inferior deep cervical l.n.

Superior deep cervical l.n.

Inferior deep cervical l.n.

A Left lateral view.

B Anterior view.

Table 19.12 ▶ Innervation of the Tongue

Nerve	Nerve Fibers	Distribution
Lingual nerve (CN V₃)	General sensory	Anterior two thirds of the tongue
Chorda tympani (CN VII)	Special sensory	Anterior two thirds of the tongue
Glossopharyngeal nerve (CN IX)	General sensory and special sensory	Posterior third of the tongue
Vagus nerve (CN X)	General sensory and special sensory	Root of the tongue
Hypoglossal nerve (CN XII)	Somatic motor	Muscles of the tongue, except the palatoglossus, which is innervated by the vagus nerve (CN X)

- The facial, lingual, maxillary, and superficial temporal arteries supply the salivary glands. Veins of similar names accompany the arteries and drain into the retromandibular vein.
- The sublingual and submandibular glands receive parasympathetic secretomotor fibers via the chorda tympani (a branch of CN VII) and submandibular ganglion.
- The parotid gland receives secretomotor (parasympathetic) fibers of the glossopharyngeal nerve (CN IX) that synapse in the otic ganglion.
- Sympathetic innervation to the glands arises from the superior cervical ganglion and follows the branches of the external carotid artery.

Fig. 19.27 ▶ **Somatosensory and taste innervation of the tongue** Anterior view.

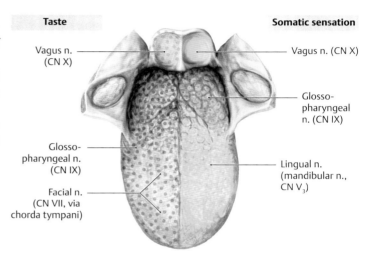

Fig. 19.28 ▶ **Salivary glands**
Submandibular and sublingual glands, superior view with tongue removed.

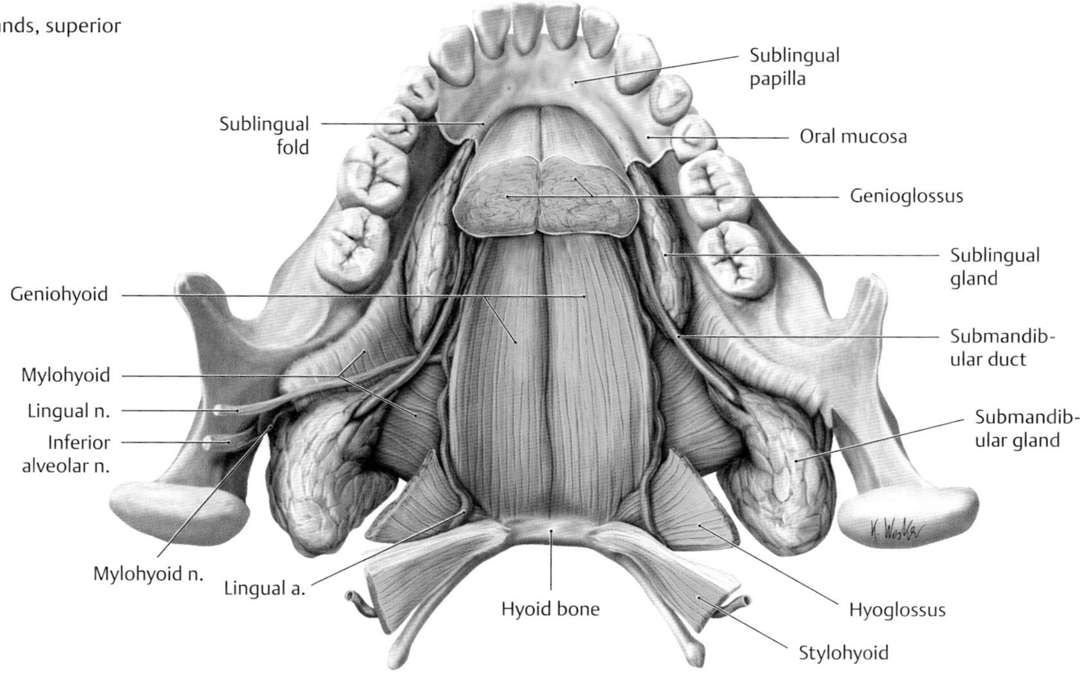

20 The Eye and Ear

The eye, the organ of vision, and the ear, which contains the organs for hearing and balance, are anatomically the most complex of the sense organs. The eyes, enclosed within the bony orbits, are prominent features of the face. The ears have superficial and deep components that are related to the temporal bones on the sides of the head.

20.1 The Eye

The anatomy of the eye includes the bony orbit, the eyelids and lacrimal apparatus, the eyeball, and six extraocular muscles.

20.1a The Bony Orbit

The paired **orbits** lie on either side of the superior part of the nasal cavity, above the maxillary sinuses and below the anterior cranial fossae. These cavities are shaped like quadrangular pyramids with the apex directed posteriorly and the base opening onto the face (**Fig. 20.1A** and **B**).

— Seven bones of the skull form the bony orbit.
  - The frontal bone forms the roof.
  - The maxilla forms the floor.
  - The ethmoid, lacrimal, nasal, and sphenoid bones form the medial wall.
  - The zygomatic and sphenoid bones form the lateral wall.
— Numerous openings allow nerves and vessels to pass between the orbit and the middle cranial fossa, the nasal cavity, the pterygopalatine fossa, and the face (**Table 20.1**).
— The eyeball occupies the anterior part of the orbit, accompanied by six extraocular muscles, ophthalmic vessels, and five cranial nerves (optic, oculomotor, trochlear, trigeminal, and abducent). Periorbital fat supports and surrounds these structures.

Table 20.1 ▶ Openings in the Orbit for Neurovascular Structures

Opening*	Nerves	Vessels
Optic canal	Optic n. (CN II)	Ophthalmic a.
Superior orbital fissure	Oculomotor n. (CN III) Trochlear n. (CN IV) Abducent n. (CN VI) Trigeminal n., ophthalmic division (CN V_1) • Lacrimal n. • Frontal n. • Nasociliary n.	Superior ophthalmic v.
Inferior orbital fissure	Infraorbital n. (CN V_2) Zygomatic n. (CN V_2)	Infraorbital a. and v., inferior ophthalmic v.
Infraorbital canal	Infraorbital n. (CN V_2), a., and v.	
Supraorbital foramen	Supraorbital n. (lateral branch)	Supraorbital a.
Frontal incisure	Supraorbital n. (medial branch)	Supratrochlear a.
Anterior ethmoidal foramen	Anterior ethmoidal n., a., and v.	
Posterior ethmoidal foramen	Posterior ethmoidal n., a., and v.	

* The nasolacrimal canal transmits the nasolacrimal duct.

Fig. 20.1 ▶ Bones of the orbit

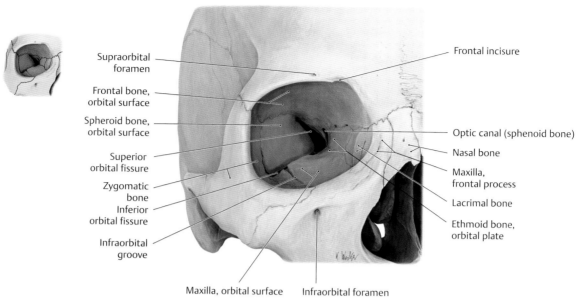

Supraorbital foramen

Frontal bone, orbital surface

Spheroid bone, orbital surface

Superior orbital fissure

Zygomatic bone

Inferior orbital fissure

Infraorbital groove

Maxilla, orbital surface

Infraorbital foramen

Frontal incisure

Optic canal (sphenoid bone)

Nasal bone

Maxilla, frontal process

Lacrimal bone

Ethmoid bone, orbital plate

A Anterior view.

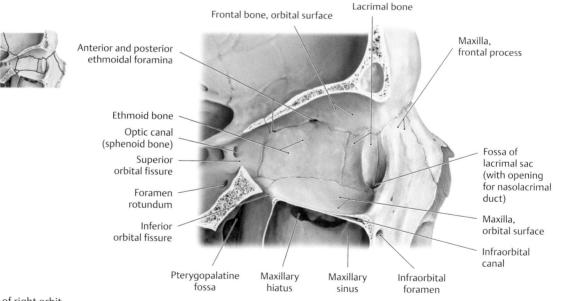

Frontal bone, orbital surface

Lacrimal bone

Anterior and posterior ethmoidal foramina

Maxilla, frontal process

Ethmoid bone

Optic canal (sphenoid bone)

Superior orbital fissure

Foramen rotundum

Inferior orbital fissure

Fossa of lacrimal sac (with opening for nasolacrimal duct)

Maxilla, orbital surface

Infraorbital canal

Pterygopalatine fossa

Maxillary hiatus

Maxillary sinus

Infraorbital foramen

B Lateral view of right orbit.

20.1b Eyelids and Lacrimal Apparatus (Figs. 20.2 and 20.3)

The upper and lower **eyelids** are moveable folds of skin that protect the eyeball from injury, irritation, and light.

— The eyelids are covered externally by skin and internally by the **palpebral conjunctiva**, a thin inner membrane that reflects onto the anterior eyeball as the **bulbar conjunctiva**. When the eyes are closed, the palpebral and bulbar conjunctivae form the **conjunctival sac**.

— **Tarsal plates** or **tarsus**, bands of dense connective tissue that provide support for both the upper and lower eyelids, are attached to **medial** and **lateral palpebral ligaments**, which connect to the medial and lateral margins of the orbit, respectively. Tarsal glands within the tarsal plates lubricate the edges of the eyelids to prevent them from sticking together.

— The **orbicularis oculi muscle** (see **Fig. 19.1**), innervated by the facial nerve (CN VII), closes the eye in a sphincter-like fashion. The **levator palpebrae superioris muscle**, innervated by the oculomotor nerve (CN III) and attached to the superior tarsal plate, opens the eye by lifting the upper eyelid.

— An **orbital septum**, which connects the tarsal plates to the margins of the orbit, holds the orbital fat within the orbit and helps to limit the spread of infection to and from the orbit.

Fig. 20.2 ▶ **Eyelids and conjunctiva**
Sagittal section through the anterior orbital cavity.

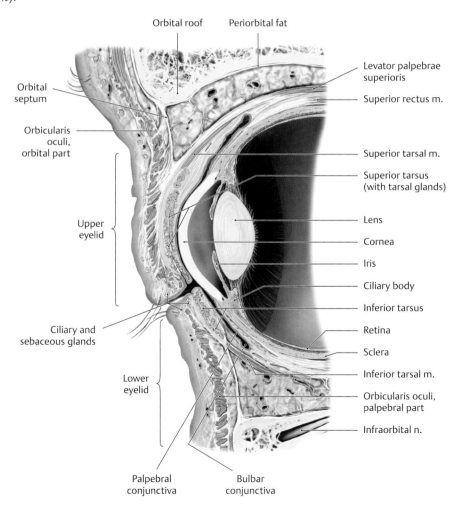

Orbital roof Periorbital fat

Levator palpebrae superioris

Orbital septum

Superior rectus m.

Orbicularis oculi, orbital part

Superior tarsal m.

Superior tarsus (with tarsal glands)

Upper eyelid

Lens

Cornea

Iris

Ciliary body

Inferior tarsus

Ciliary and sebaceous glands

Retina

Sclera

Inferior tarsal m.

Lower eyelid

Orbicularis oculi, palpebral part

Infraorbital n.

Palpebral conjunctiva

Bulbar conjunctiva

The **lacrimal apparatus** produces and drains tears that cleanse and lubricate the outer surface of the eye.

- The **lacrimal gland**, which produces and secretes tears, resides in the lacrimal fossa in the supralateral aspect of the orbit. Secretomotor parasympathetic fibers from the facial nerve (CN VII) stimulate the gland (see **Fig. 18.19**).

- Blinking of the eye sweeps the tears across the eye toward the medial angle, where they drain via **superior** and **inferior puncta** (openings) into **lacrimal canaliculi** and the **lacrimal sac**, the dilated superior part of the nasolacrimal duct.

- The **nasolacrimal duct** is a membranous structure that begins in the medial angle of the eye and terminates in the inferior meatus of the nasal cavity. Tears drain into the nasal cavity via this duct.

Fig. 20.3 ► **Lacrimal apparatus**
Right eye, anterior view. *Removed:* Orbital septum (partial). *Divided:* Levator palpebrae superioris (tendon of insertion).

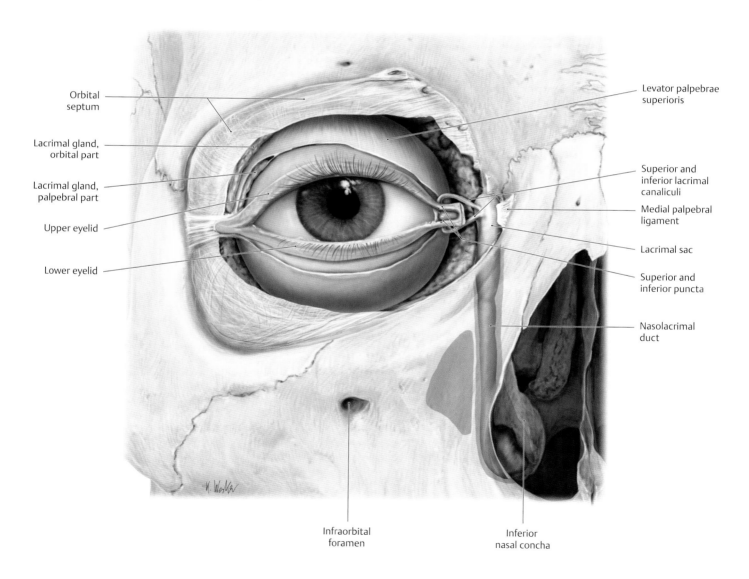

20.1c The Eyeball

The eyeball, the organ of vision, has three concentric layers that form its outer walls: the sclera, the choroid, and the retina (**Fig. 20.4**).

— The **sclera**, the white part of the eye, forms the posterior five sixths of the outer fibrous layer of the eye; the **cornea**, the transparent part of the sclera, forms the anterior sixth. This outer layer is largely avascular but provides structure to the eyeball.

— The **choroid**, the middle vascular layer, provides oxygen and nutrients to the underlying retina (**Fig. 20.5**).

• The **ciliary body** connects the choroid with the circumference of the iris. Short, smooth muscle fibers, **zonular fibers**, which attach the ciliary body to the lens, control the thickness and refractive power of the lens and therefore the focus of the eye.

• The **iris**, an adjustable muscular diaphragm, surrounds a central aperture, the **pupil**.

  ○ The **pupillary sphincter muscle** of the iris responds to parasympathetic stimulation to constrict the pupil.

  ○ The **pupillary dilator muscle** of the iris responds to sympathetic stimulation to dilate the pupil.

Fig. 20.4 ▶ **Structure of the eyeball**
Transverse section through the right eyeball, superior view.

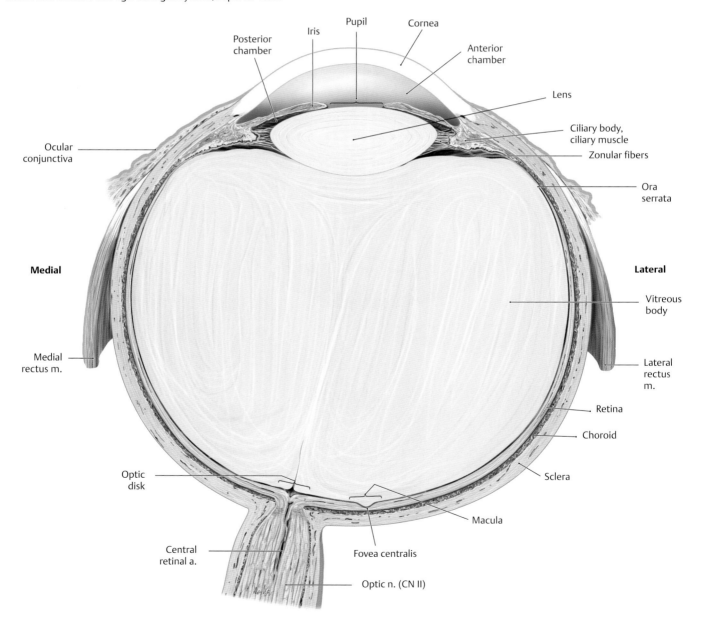

Fig. 20.5 ▶ Cornea, iris, and lens
Transverse section through the anterior segment of the eye, anterosuperior view.

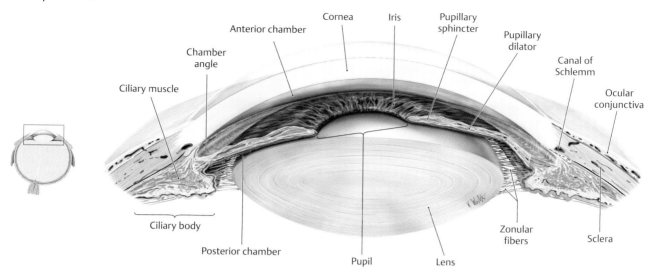

— The **retina**, the inner sensory layer, has a posterior **optic part** that is sensitive to light and a **nonvisual part** that continues anteriorly over the ciliary body and iris.

- The **optic disc**, a point on the retina where the optic nerve exits the eyeball, lacks photoreceptors and therefore is insensitive to light and is known as the **blind spot**.
- The **macula** of the retina, a spot lateral to the optic disk, is an area of intense visual acuity.
- The **fovea centralis**, a depression in the macula, is the area of greatest visual acuity.

— Light passes through four refractive media before focusing on the retina of the eye:

1. The cornea, the primary refractive medium for light entering the eye
2. The **aqueous humor**, a watery solution that fills the **anterior** and **posterior chambers** of the eye that lie anterior to the lens and ciliary body. The balance between its production and drainage determines the intraocular pressure.
3. The **lens**, a transparent biconcave disk that focuses objects on the retina by changing its thickness. In the process of **accommodation**, which is mediated by parasympathetic stimulation, the ciliary muscle contracts, causing the lens to thicken and bring near objects into focus.
4. The **vitreous body**, a jelly-like substance that fills the chamber of the eye posterior to the lens.

Corneal reflex

A positive corneal reflex is the bilateral contraction of the orbicularis oculi muscles (a blink) when the cornea is touched or exposed to bright light. The afferent limb is the nasociliary nerve of the ophthalmic division of the trigeminal nerve (CN V1); the efferent limb is the facial nerve (CN VII). The reflex protects the eye from foreign bodies and bright light.

Pupillary light reflex

The pupillary light reflex is rapid constriction (miosis) of both pupils (via the constrictor pupillae muscle) in response to shining a light into the eye. The afferent limb of the reflex is the optic nerve (CN II). The efferent limb is the parasympathetic fibers of the oculomotor nerve (CN III). Both pupils constrict because each retina sends fibers into the optic tracts of both sides. If the parasympathetic fibers are interrupted, both pupils dilate (mydriasis) as a result of the unopposed sympathetic outflow to the dilator pupillae muscle. This reflex mediates papillary aperture variation and is therefore one of the means by which the eye adapts to changes in light intensity.

Presbyopia and cataracts

The lens of the eye undergoes age-related changes that affect vision in the older patient. The loss of elasticity of the lens, and the subsequent loss of accommodation, diminishes a patient's ability to focus on near objects, a condition known as presbyopia. Opacities of the lens or its capsule, known as cataracts, allow less light to reach the retina, resulting in blurred, cloudy vision. Treatment involves surgical removal of the affected lens and replacement with a plastic lens implant.

Glaucoma

Glaucoma refers to a group of eye diseases that involve increased intraocular pressure and atrophy of the optic nerve. In primary open-angle glaucoma, the most common form, venous channels in the angle between the cornea and the iris that allow drainage of the aqueous humor from the anterior and posterior chambers are blocked. The subsequent buildup of aqueous humor results in raised intraocular pressure and eventual damage to the optic nerve. This leads to a gradual loss of peripheral vision that progresses to tunnel vision. Pressure on the retina can lead to blindness.

20.1d Extraocular Muscles

— The six extraocular muscles that control the movement of the eyeball (**Fig. 20.6A** and **B**; **Table 20.2**) include

  • four rectus muscles, the **superior rectus**, **medial rectus**, **inferior rectus**, and **lateral rectus**, that originate from a **common tendinous ring** at the apex of the orbit; and

  • two oblique muscles, the **superior oblique** that arises near the apex and reflects back via the trochlea to attach to the eyeball, and the **inferior oblique** that arises from the medial aspect of the orbital floor.

Fig. 20.6 ▶ **Extraocular muscles**
Right eye.

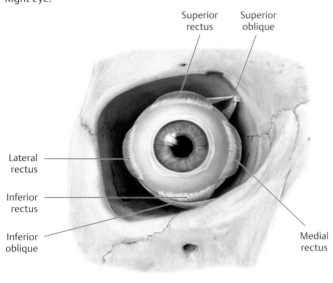

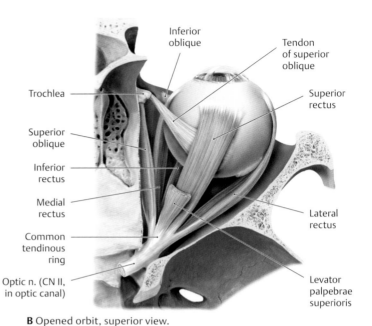

A Anterior view.

B Opened orbit, superior view.

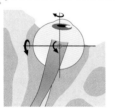
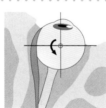
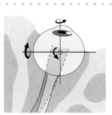
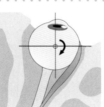
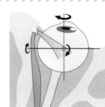
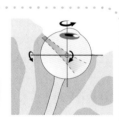

A Superior rectus. **B** Medial rectus. **C** Inferior rectus. **D** Lateral rectus. **E** Superior oblique. **F** Inferior oblique.

Table 20.2 ▶ **Actions of the Extraocular Muscles**

Muscle	Origin	Insertion	Action*			Innervation
			Vertical Axis (red)	Horizontal Axis (black)	Anteroposterior Axis (blue)	
Superior rectus	Common tendinous ring (common annular tendon)	Sclera of the eye	Elevates	Adducts	Rotates medially	Oculomotor n. (CN III), superior branch
Medial rectus			–	Adducts	–	Oculomotor n. (CN III), inferior branch
Inferior rectus			Depresses	Adducts	Rotates laterally	
Lateral rectus			–	Abducts	–	Abducent n. (CN VI)
Superior oblique	Sphenoid bone+		Depresses	Abducts	Rotates medially	Trochlear n. (CN IV)
Inferior oblique	Medial orbital margin		Elevates	Abducts	Rotates laterally	Oculomotor n. (CN III), inferior branch

* Starting from gaze directed anteriorly.
+ The tendon of insertion of the superior oblique passes through a tendinous loop (trochlea) attached to the superomedial orbital margin.

— The muscles allow six cardinal directions of gaze, which are the normal movements of the eyeball tested during clinical evaluation of ocular mobility (**Fig. 20.7A** and **B**).

Fig. 20.7 ▶ **Testing the extraocular muscles**

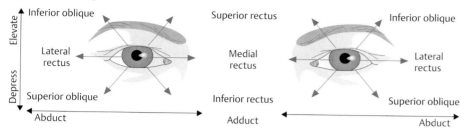

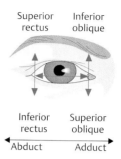

A Starting with the eyes directed anteriorly, movement to any of the cardinal directions of gaze (*arrows*) requires activation of two extraocular muscles, each of which is innervated by a different cranial nerve, thus testing the function of those pairs of muscles.

B Starting with the eyes adducted or abducted, elevating or lowering the eyes activates only the oblique or rectus muscles, respectively, allowing for the testing of the function of individual muscles.

20.1e Neurovasculature of the Orbit

— The ophthalmic artery supplies most structures of the orbit. One of its branches, the **central retinal artery**, runs within the optic nerve and is the sole arterial supply to the retina through its terminal branches (**Fig. 20.8**).

• The ophthalmic artery anastomoses with the facial artery through its supratrochlear branch and with the maxillary artery through its anterior and posterior ethmoidal and middle meningeal branches.

Fig. 20.8 ▶ **Arteries of the orbit**
Right orbit, superior view. *Opened:* optic canal and orbital roof.

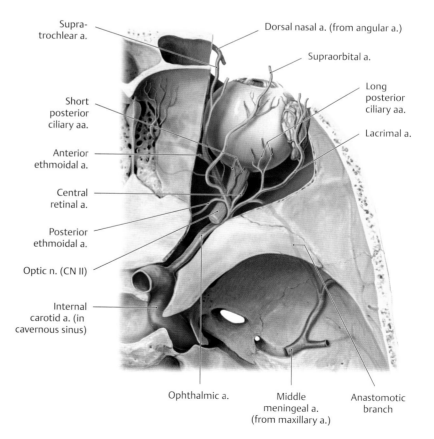

— The **superior** and **inferior ophthalmic veins**, which drain structures in the orbit, primarily drain into the cavernous sinus but also communicate with the facial vein and pterygoid venous plexus (**Fig. 20.9**).

— Six cranial nerves (optic, oculomotor, trochlear, trigeminal, abducent, and facial) innervate structures in the orbit (**Table 20.3**; **Fig. 20.10**).

• The optic nerve (CN I) transmits images from the retina.

• The oculomotor nerve (CN III), trochlear nerve (CN IV), and abducent nerve (CN VI) innervate the extraocular muscles.

• The ophthalmic division of the trigeminal nerve (CN V$_1$) carries general sensory fibers from structures in the orbit and distributes postganglionic autonomic fibers to target organs of the orbit and face.

• The facial nerve (CN VII) provides secretomotor (parasympathetic) innervation to the lacrimal gland.

Oculomotor nerve injury

The oculomotor nerve innervates most of the extraocular muscles. With paralysis of these muscles, the eye is directed downward and outward because of the unopposed action of the lateral rectus (innervated by the abducent nerve) and superior oblique (innervated by the trochlear nerve). The dilator pupillae is also unopposed, so the pupil remains fully dilated. Paralysis of the levator palpebrae superior allows the superior eyelid to droop.

— Autonomic innervation of structures in the orbit includes the following:

• Sympathetic fibers from the carotid plexus innervate the ciliary body and pupillary dilator muscle (responsible for pupil dilation).

• Parasympathetic fibers from the oculomotor nerve (CN III) synapse in the ciliary ganglion and travel via the short ciliary nerves to innervate the ciliary body and pupillary sphincter muscles (responsible for pupil constriction).

• Parasympathetic fibers from the facial nerve (CN VII) synapse in the pterygopalatine ganglion and travel via the zygomatic nerve (CN V$_2$) to innervate the lacrimal gland (responsible for tear secretion).

Horner's syndrome

Horner's syndrome is a kaleidoscope of symptoms resulting from disruption of the cervical sympathetic trunk in the neck. The absence of sympathetic innervation is manifested on the affected side of the face as pupillary constriction (miosis), a sunken eye (enophthalmos), drooping of the upper eyelid (ptosis), loss of sweating (anhydrosis), and vasodilation.

Fig. 20.9 ▶ **Veins of the orbit**
Right orbit, lateral view. *Removed:* lateral orbital wall. *Opened:* maxillary sinus.

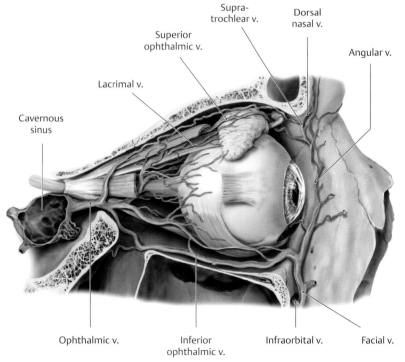

Table 20.3 ► Nerves of the Orbit

Nerve	Nerve Fibers	Distribution
Optic (CN II)	Special sensory for vision	Retina
Oculomotor (CN III)	Somatic motor	Muscles of the orbit, except the lateral rectus and superior oblique muscles
	Parasympathetic: synapse in ciliary ganglion; post-synaptic fibers travel with nasociliary n. (CN V_1)	Pupilary sphincter muscle and ciliary body
Trochlear (CN IV)	Somatic motor	Superior oblique muscle
Ophthalmic (CN V_1)		
Lacrimal	General sensory	Lacrimal gland, upper lateral eyeball
Frontal		
- Supratrochlear	General sensory	Anterior scalp
- Supraorbital	General sensory	Anterior scalp
Short ciliary	General sensory	Ciliary body and iris
	Parasympathetic (CN III) and sympathetic	
Nasociliary		
- Anterior and posterior ethmoidal	General sensory	Nasal cavity, ethmoid and sphenoid sinuses
- Infratrochlear	General sensory	External nose, conjunctiva, lacrimal sac
- Long ciliary	General sensory	Iris and cornea
	Sympathetic (carotid plexus)	Pupil dilator
Abducent (CN VI)	Somatic motor	Lateral rectus muscle
Facial (CN VII)	Parasympathetic: synapse in pterygopalatine ganglion; postsynaptic fibers travel with zygomatic n. (CN V_2)	Lacrimal gland

Fig. 20.10 ► **Innervation of the orbit**
Right orbit, lateral view. *Removed:* Temporal bony wall.

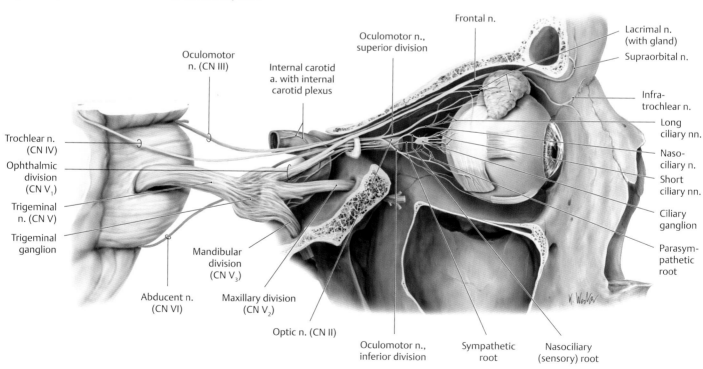

20.2 The Ear

The ear, which contains the organs for hearing and equilibrium, is divided into external, middle, and internal parts (**Fig. 20.11**).

20.2a The External Ear

The external ear collects and conducts sound.

— The **auricle**, the visible external part of the ear, has a skeleton composed of elastic cartilage that is covered by skin.

— The **external acoustic meatus** (external auditory canal), a canal that extends 2 to 3 cm from the auricle to the tympanic membrane, conducts sound waves toward the middle ear. The outer third of the canal is cartilaginous, and the inner two thirds are formed by the temporal bone. Ceruminous and sebaceous glands in the subcutaneous tissue lining the cartilaginous part secrete earwax.

— The **tympanic membrane**, a thin, transparent membrane, separates the external and middle ear.

  • Skin covers the tympanic membrane externally, and a mucous membrane lines it internally.

  • The concave outer surface of the membrane has a central conelike depression, the **umbo**.

• A thin, superior portion of the membrane, the **flaccid part** (pars flaccida), is distinct from the rest of the membrane, the **tense part** (pars tensa).

— Posterior auricular and anterior auricular arteries, branches of the superficial temporal artery, supply the external ear.

— Sensation from the external ear is transmitted by

  • the great auricular nerve (cervical plexus) from the auricle;

  • the auriculotemporal nerve, a branch of CN V$_3$, from the auricle and external surface of the tympanic membrane;

  • the auricular branch of the vagus nerve (CN X) from the external surface of the tympanic membrane; and

  • the glossopharyngeal nerve (CN IX) from the internal surface of the tympanic membrane.

Fig. 20.11 ▶ **Ear**
Coronal section through the right ear, anterior view.

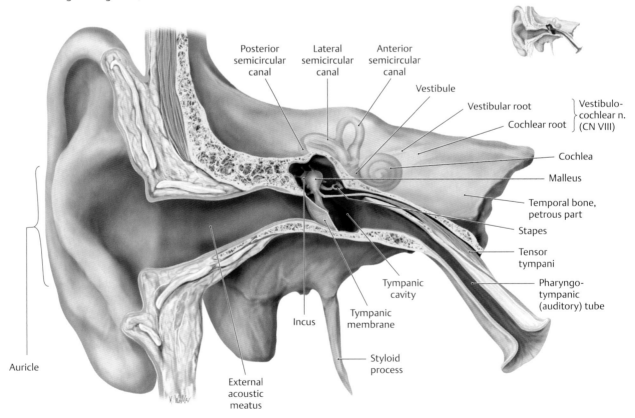

20.2b The Middle Ear

- The middle ear, also known as the **tympanic cavity**, is an air-filled chamber housed in the petrous portion of the temporal bone (**Figs. 20.12** and **20.13**).
  - Anteriorly, a **pharyngotympanic tube**, which connects the tympanic cavity to the nasopharynx, helps equalize pressure in the middle ear.
  - Posteriorly, the **aditus** (inlet) to the **mastoid antrum** (a cavity in the mastoid process of the temporal bone) connects the tympanic cavity to the bony meshwork of **mastoid air cells**.
  - A thin bony plate, the **tegmen tympani**, forms the roof of the tympanic cavity and separates it from the middle cranial fossa.
  - The medial wall, which separates the tympanic cavity from the internal ear, has a **promontory**, covered by the tympanic nerve plexus, and two openings, the **oval** and **round windows** (see **Fig. 20.15**).

- The **auditory ossicles**, the **malleus**, **incus**, and **stapes** bones of the middle ear, articulate with each other through synovial joints and form a bony chain between the tympanic membrane and the oval window of the internal ear.
  - The handle of the malleus is embedded in the tympanic membrane, and its head articulates with the incus.
  - The **incus** articulates with the malleus and stapes.
  - The head of the **stapes** articulates with the incus, and its base fits into the oval window of the bony labyrinth of the inner ear.

Fig. 20.12 ▶ **Tympanic cavity**
Right tympanic cavity, anterior view. *Removed:* Anterior wall.

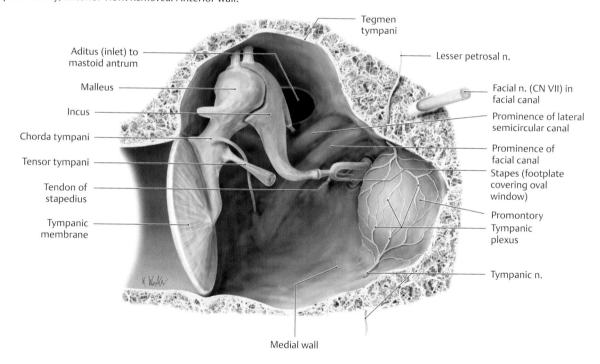

Fig. 20.13 ▶ **Muscles and neurovascular relations in the tympanic cavity**
Right middle ear, lateral view.

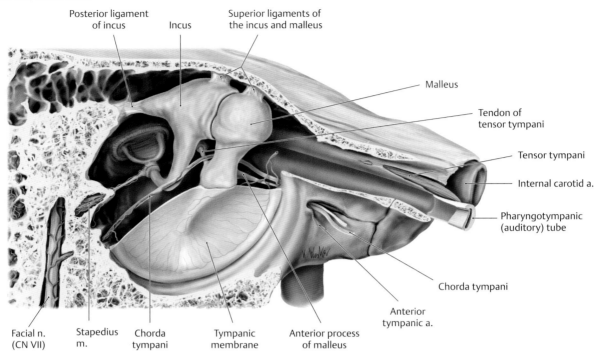

Posterior ligament of incus · Incus · Superior ligaments of the incus and malleus · Malleus · Tendon of tensor tympani · Tensor tympani · Internal carotid a. · Pharyngotympanic (auditory) tube · Chorda tympani · Anterior tympanic a. · Anterior process of malleus · Tympanic membrane · Chorda tympani · Stapedius m. · Facial n. (CN VII)

— Muscles of the middle ear dampen the movements of the auditory ossicles, thereby lessening the sound transmitted from the external ear.

  • The **tensor tympani**, which is innervated by a branch of the mandibular nerve (CN V₃), lessens the damage from loud sounds by tensing the tympanic membrane.

  • The **stapedius**, which is innervated by a branch of the facial nerve (CN VII), dampens the vibrations of the stapes on the oval window.

— The ascending pharyngeal, maxillary, and posterior auricular branches of the external carotid artery and a small branch of the internal carotid artery supply the middle ear.

— The chorda tympani, a branch of the facial nerve (CN VII), has no branches in the middle ear but passes between the malleus and incus to exit the cavity through a small opening in the temporal bone.

— The glossopharyngeal nerve (CN IX) transmits sensation from the tympanic cavity and pharyngotympanic tube. Preganglionic parasympathetic fibers carried in the tympanic nerve (a branch of the glossopharyngeal nerve) synapse in the otic ganglion. The postganglionic fibers join with sympathetic fibers of the internal carotid plexus to form the tympanic plexus (see **Fig. 18.22**).

Otitis media

Otitis media is an infection of the middle ear that occurs commonly in children often following an upper respiratory tract infection. Fluid that accumulates in the middle ear can temporarily diminish hearing, and inflammation of the lining of the tympanic cavity can block the pharyngotympanic tube.

Hyperacusis

The stapedius muscle protects the delicate inner ear by modifying the vibrations of very loud sounds as they are transmitted through the middle ear to the stapes. Paralysis of the muscle resulting from a lesion of the facial nerve causes an extreme sensitivity to sound, a condition known as hyperacusis.

20.2c The Internal Ear

— The internal ear, which contains the organ for hearing, the auditory apparatus, and the organ for balance, the vestibular apparatus, is encased within the petrous part of the temporal bone and consists of (**Figs. 20.14** and **20.15**) the following:

- A bony **otic capsule**, which forms the walls of the bony labyrinth
- A **bony labyrinth**, a series of chambers and canals within the otic capsule containing the fluid **perilymph**. It includes the **cochlea**, the **vestibule**, and the **semicircular canals**.
- A **membranous labyrinth**, a series of sacs and ducts suspended within the bony labyrinth, and filled with a fluid, **endolymph**. The membranous labyrinth is made up of
  - the **cochlear duct** contained within the cochlea,
  - the **utricle** and **saccule** contained within the vestibule, and
  - the **semicircular ducts** contained within the semicircular canals.

Fig. 20.14 ▶ Projection of the otic capsule of the inner ear onto the skull
Petrous part of the temporal bone, superior view.

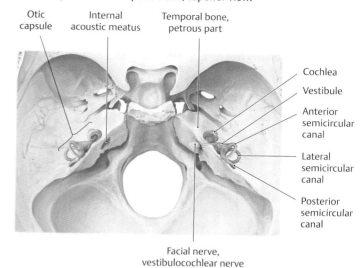

Fig. 20.15 ▶ Schematic of the inner ear
Right lateral view. The inner ear is embedded within the petrous part of the temporal bone. It is composed of a membranous labyrinth filled with endolymph floating within a similarly shaped bony labyrinth filled with perilymph.

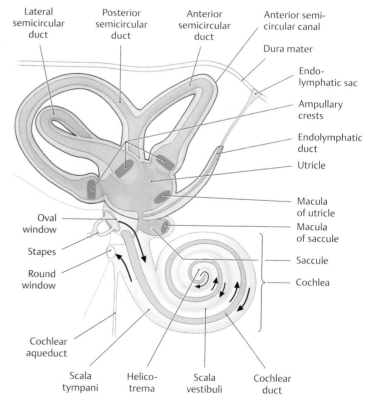

— The auditory apparatus consists of the following:

- The **cochlea**, a space within the bony labyrinth that includes the bony **cochlear** (spiral) **canal**, which makes 2.5 turns around its axis, the **modiolus** (**Fig. 20.16A**). The basal turn of the cochlea forms the promontory on the medial wall of the middle ear and contains the round window, which is closed by a membrane.
- The **cochlear duct**, part of the membranous labyrinth, which is a blind-ended duct filled with endolymph and suspended within the cochlear canal (**Fig. 20.16B**):
    - The cochlear duct divides the cochlear canal into two channels, the **scala vestibuli** and **scala tympani**, which are continuous with each other at the helicotrema, a space at the apex of the canal.
    - At the base of the cochlea, the scala vestibuli lies against the oval window, and the scala tympani lies against the round window.
- The **spiral organ** (of Corti), which contains the sensory receptors for hearing, and is embedded in the **basement membrane** on the floor of the cochlear duct

— The sequence of sound transmission through the ear involves (**Fig. 20.17**) the following:

1. Transmission of sound waves from the external ear and external acoustic meatus to the tympanic membrane of the middle ear. The waves vibrate the auditory ossicles and, in turn, the oval window that is attached to the base of the stapes.
2. Transmission of vibrations of the oval window to the perilymph of the scala vestibuli, which creates pressure waves that displace the basement membrane and spiral organ of the cochlear duct. Nerve endings in the spiral organ transmit impulses to the brain along the cochlear nerve.
3. Transmission of the pressure waves of the perilymph from the scala vestibuli along the scala tympani to the round window, with dissipation into the tympanic cavity.

Fig. 20.16 ▶ **Auditory apparatus**

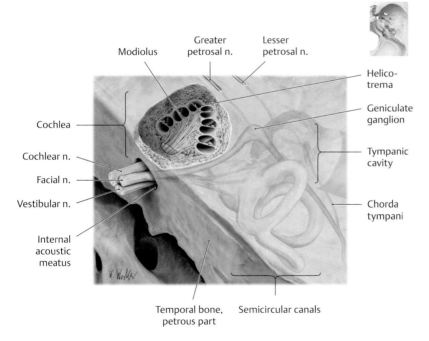

A Location of the cochlea. Superior view of the petrous part of the temporal bone with the cochlea sectioned transversely.

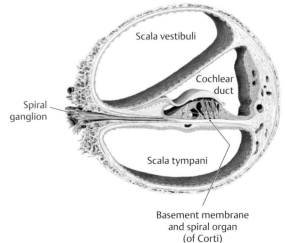

B Compartments of the cochlear canal, cross section.

Fig. 20.17 ▶ **Propagation of sound waves by the ossicular chain**

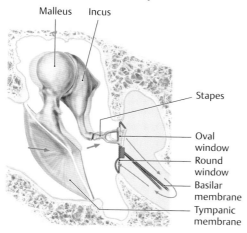

Malleus   Incus

Stapes

Oval window

Round window

Basilar membrane

Tympanic membrane

— The vestibular apparatus consists of the following (see **Fig. 20.15**):

- The vestibule of the bony labyrinth that communicates with the cochlea and semicircular canals

  o A small extension, the **vestibular aqueduct**, communicates with the posterior cranial fossa and contains the **endolymphatic sac**, a membranous storage space for excess endolymph.

- The utricle and saccule, part of the membranous labyrinth, which lie within the vestibule

  o The utricle communicates with the semicircular ducts; the saccule communicates with the cochlear duct.

  o Both the uticle and saccule contain specialized sensory fields called **maculae**, which occupy different positions in space and are sensitive to movement of the endolymph in the horizontal and vertical planes.

- Three semicircular canals of the bony labyrinth, which are arranged perpendicular to one another and communicate with the vestibule. Each canal has a swelling at one end, the **bony ampulla**.

- Three semicircular ducts, parts of the membranous labyrinth contained within the semicircular canals, that communicate with the utricle

  o An **ampulla** at one end of each semicircular duct contains the **ampullary crest**, an area of sensory epithelium. The ampullary crests respond to motion of the endolymph within the ducts caused by rotation of the head.

— The membranous labyrinth receives its blood supply from the internal auditory artery, a branch of the basilar artery via its anterior inferior cerebellar artery.

— The **vestibular** and **cochlear nerves** within the internal acoustic meatus form the vestibulocochlear nerve (CN VIII) (see **Fig. 18.21**)

- The vestibular nerve innervates organs of the vestibular apparatus: the maculae of the utricle and saccule and the ampullary crests of the semicircular canals. Neuron cell bodies lie within the vestibular ganglion in the internal acoustic meatus.

- The cochlear nerve innervates the spiral organ (of Corti) in the cochlea. Neuron cell bodies lie in the spiral ganglion of the cochlea at the modiolus.

Meniere's disease

Meniere's disease is an inner ear disorder resulting from blockage of the cochlear duct. Recurring episodes are characterized by tinnitus (ringing or buzzing in the ear), vertigo (the illusion of movement), and hearing loss. The hearing loss may fluctuate in intensity and from ear to ear but eventually becomes permanent.

Vertigo, tinnitus, and hearing loss

Trauma to the ear can cause three types of symptoms: vertigo, tinnitus, and hearing loss. Vertigo refers to the illusion of movement, or dizziness, and results from injury to the semicircular canals. Tinnitus refers to a ringing in the ears and is a disorder involving the cochlear duct. Causes of hearing loss can be either peripheral or centrally located. Conductive hearing loss occurs when there is impaired transmission of sound waves through the auditory canal to the auditory ossicles. Sensorineural hearing loss occurs when there is damage to the pathway between the cochlea and the brain.

21 The Neck

The neck extends from the base of the skull to the clavicles and manubrium. It contains vital neurovascular structures that supply the head, the thorax, and the upper limb. The neck also contains viscera of the gastrointestinal, respiratory, and endocrine systems.

21.1 Deep Fascia of the Neck

Layers of **deep cervical fascia** surround and compartmentalize the structures of the neck (**Table 21.1**).

— The investing (superficial) **layer of the deep fascia** of the neck, a thin layer that lies deep to the skin, surrounds the entire neck but splits to enclose the sternocleidomastoid and trapezius muscles and contains cutaneous nerves, superficial vessels, and superficial lymphatics of the neck.

— The **pretracheal fascia** in the anterior neck has a muscular lamina (layer) that encloses the infrahyoid muscles and a visceral lamina that encloses the viscera of the anterior neck.

— The **prevertebral fascia** surrounds the vertebral column and the deep neck muscles and is continuous with the **nuchal fascia** posteriorly.

— The **carotid sheath**, a condensation of the pretracheal, prevertebral, and investing fasciae, forms a narrow cylindrical tube that encloses the neurovascular bundle of the neck: the internal jugular vein, common carotid artery, and vagus nerve.

— The **retropharyngeal space**, a potential space between the visceral layer of the pretracheal fascia and the prevertebral fascia, extends from the base of the skull superiorly to the superior mediastinum inferiorly.

Table 21.1 ▶ Deep Cervical Fascia

The deep cervical fascia is divided into four layers that enclose the structures of the neck.

Layer	Type of Fascia	Description
① Investing (superficial) layer	Muscular	Envelopes entire neck; splits to enclose sternocleidomastoid and trapezius muscles
Pretracheal layer	② Muscular	Encloses infrahyoid muscles
	③ Visceral	Surrounds thyroid gland, larynx, trachea, pharynx, and esophagus
④ Prevertebral layer	Muscular	Surrounds cervical vertebral column and associated muscles
⑤ Carotid sheath	Neurovascular	Encloses common carotid artery, internal jugular vein, and vagus nerve

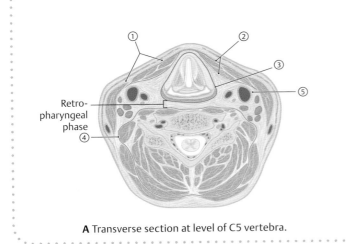

A Transverse section at level of C5 vertebra.

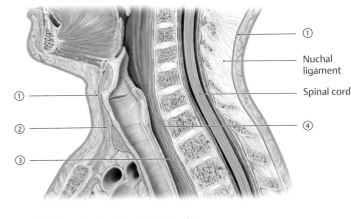

B Midsagittal section, left lateral view.

21.2 Muscles of the Neck

— Three muscles form the most superficial muscular layer of the neck (**Fig. 21.1**; **Table 21.2**):

- The **platysma**, a muscle of facial expression, and therefore a subcutaneous muscle, that extends onto the anterolateral surfaces of the neck
- The **sternocleidomastoid muscle**, a visible landmark that divides the neck into anterior and lateral cervical regions
- The trapezius, a muscle of the shoulder girdle that extends onto the neck and forms the posterior border of the lateral cervical region

Congenital torticollis

Congenital torticollis (wryneck) is a condition in which one of the sternocleidomastoid muscles (SCM) is abnormally short, causing the head to tilt to one side with the chin pointing upward to the opposite side. This shortening is thought to be the result of trauma at birth (tears or stretching of the SCM) causing bleeding and swelling within the muscle and subsequent scar tissue formation.

Fig. 21.1 ▶ Superficial musculature of the neck
Left lateral view.

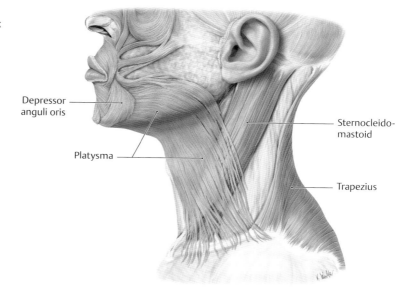

Depressor anguli oris

Platysma

Sternocleido-mastoid

Trapezius

Table 21.2 ▶ Superficial Neck Muscles					
Muscle		**Origin**	**Insertion**	**Innervation**	**Action**
Platysma		Skin over lower neck and upper lateral thorax	Mandible (inferior border), skin over lower face and angle of mouth	Cervical branch of facial n. (CN VII)	Depresses and wrinkles skin of lower face and mouth, tenses skin of neck, aids forced depression of mandible
Sternocleidomastoid	Sternal head	Sternum (manubrium)	Temporal bone (mastoid process), occipital bone (superior nuchal line)	*Motor*: accessory n. (CN XI) *Pain and proprioception*: cervical plexus (C2, C3)	*Unilateral*: Tilts head to same side, rotates head to opposite side *Bilateral*: Extends head, aids in respiration when head is fixed
	Clavicular head	Clavicle (medial one third)			
Trapezius	Descending part	Occipital bone, spinous processes of C1–C7	Clavicle (lateral one third)		Draws scapula obliquely upward, rotates glenoid cavity superiorly

— Muscles attached to the hyoid bone lie between the superficial and deep neck muscles.

- Suprahyoid muscles, the **digastric**, **stylohyoid**, **mylohyoid**, **geniohyoid**, and **hyoglossus**, form the floor of the mouth and elevate the hyoid and larynx during swallowing and phonation (see **Table 19.9**).
- **Infrahyoid muscles** in the neck, **omohyoid**, **sternohyoid**, **sternothyroid**, and **thyrohyoid**, depress the hyoid and larynx during swallowing and phonation (**Fig. 21.2**; **Table 21.3**).

— The deep muscles of the neck lie deep to the prevertebral fascia and include the prevertebral and scalene muscles (**Fig. 21.3**; **Table 21.4**).

Fig. 21.2 ▶ **Suprahyoid and infrahyoid muscles**
Anterior view. The sternohyoid has been cut on the right side.
See **Table 19.9** for the suprahyoid muscles.

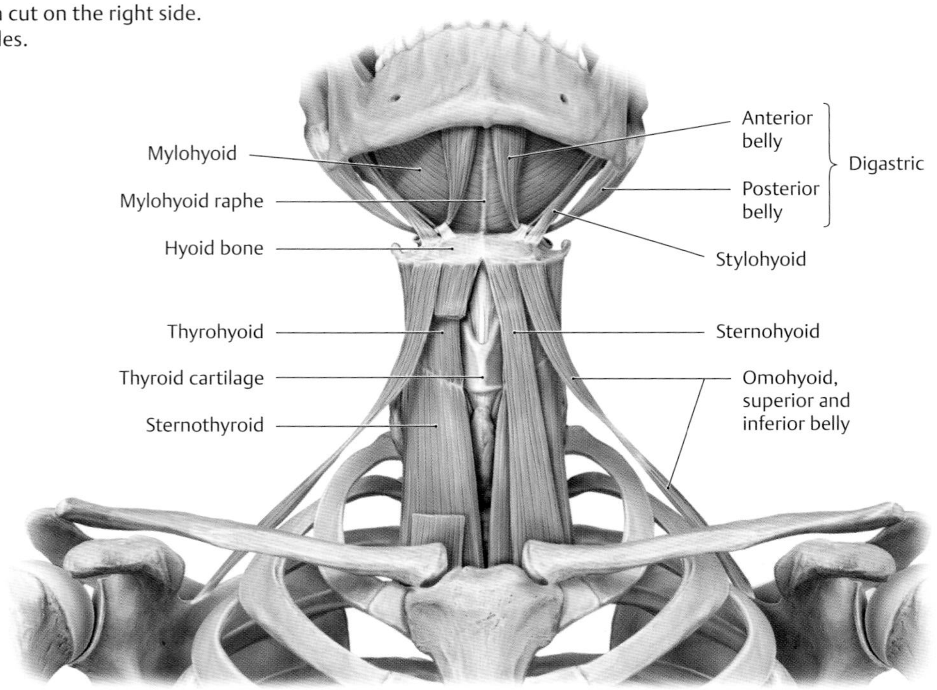

Table 21.3 ▶ Infrahyoid Muscles				
Muscle	**Origin**	**Insertion**	**Innervation**	**Action**
Omohyoid	Scapula (superior border)	Hyoid bone (body)	Ansa cervicalis of cervical plexus (C1–C3)	Depresses (fixes) hyoid, draws larynx and hyoid down for phonation and terminal phases of swallowing*
Sternohyoid	Manubrium and sternoclavicular joint (posterior surface)			
Sternothyroid	Manubrium (posterior surface)	Thyroid cartilage (oblique line)	Ansa cervicalis (C2–C3)	
Thyrohyoid	Thyroid cartilage (oblique line)	Hyoid bone (body)	C1 via hypoglossal n. (CN XII)	Depresses and fixes hyoid, raises the larynx during swallowing

* The omohyoid also tenses the cervical fascia (with an intermediate tendon).

Fig. 21.3 ► Deep muscles of the neck

Prevertebral and scalene muscles, anterior view. *Removed:* Longus capitis and anterior scalene.

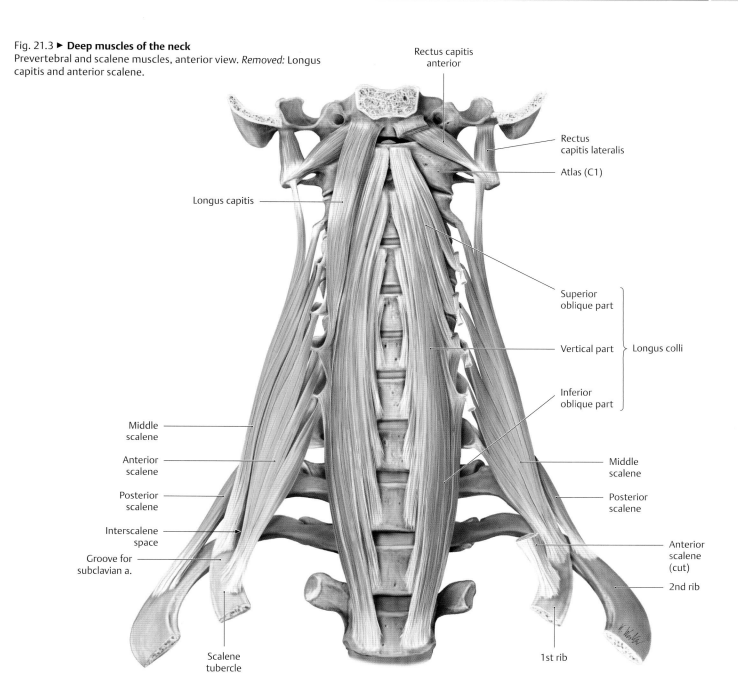

Labels: Rectus capitis anterior · Rectus capitis lateralis · Atlas (C1) · Longus capitis · Superior oblique part · Vertical part · Inferior oblique part · Longus colli · Middle scalene · Anterior scalene · Posterior scalene · Interscalene space · Groove for subclavian a. · Scalene tubercle · Middle scalene · Posterior scalene · Anterior scalene (cut) · 2nd rib · 1st rib

Table 21.4 ► Deep Muscles of the Neck

Muscles	Origin	Insertion	Innervation	Action
Prevertebral				
Longus capitis Longus colli Rectus capitis anterior Rectus capitis lateralis	Cervical and upper thoracic vertebrae	Cervical vertebrae and basilar part of occipital bone	Anterior rami of C1–C6 (cervical plexus)	Flex the head and cervical spine
Scalene				
Anterior scalene Middle scalene Posterior scalene	Cervical vertebrae	1st and 2nd ribs	Anterior rami of C3–C8	Flex the cervical spine and elevate the ribs during inspiration

Fig. 21.4 ▶ **Deep lateral cervical region**
Right lateral view with sternocleidomastoid
windowed.

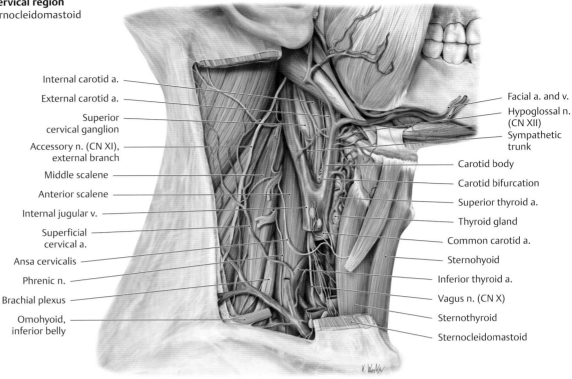

Internal carotid a.
External carotid a.
Superior cervical ganglion
Accessory n. (CN XI), external branch
Middle scalene
Anterior scalene
Internal jugular v.
Superficial cervical a.
Ansa cervicalis
Phrenic n.
Brachial plexus
Omohyoid, inferior belly

Facial a. and v.
Hypoglossal n. (CN XII)
Sympathetic trunk
Carotid body
Carotid bifurcation
Superior thyroid a.
Thyroid gland
Common carotid a.
Sternohyoid
Inferior thyroid a.
Vagus n. (CN X)
Sternothyroid
Sternocleidomastoid

Table 21.5 ▶ Branches of the Spinal Nerves in the Neck

Posterior (Dorsal) Ramus

	Nerve	Sensory function	Motor function
C1	Suboccipital n.	No C1 dermatome	Innervate intrinsic nuchal muscles
C2	Greater occipital n.	Innervate C2 dermatome	
C3	3rd occipital n.	Innervate C3 dermatome	

Anterior (Ventral) Ramus

	Sensory branches	Sensory function	Motor branches	Motor function
C1	—	—	Form ansa cervicalis (motor part of cervical plexus)	Innervate infrahyoid muscles (except thyrohyoid)
C2	Lesser occipital n.	Form sensory part of cervical plexus, innervate anterior and lateral neck		
C2–C3	Great auricular n.			
	Transverse cervical n.			
C3–C4	Supraclavicular nn.		Contribute to phrenic n.*	Innervate diaphragm and pericardium*

* The anterior roots of C3–C5 combine to form the phrenic nerve.

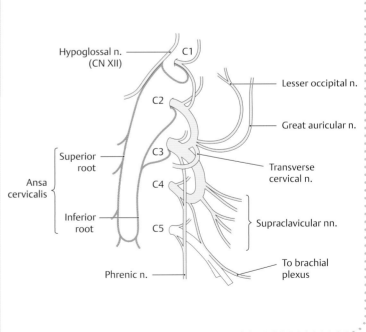

Hypoglossal n. (CN XII)
C1
Lesser occipital n.
C2
Great auricular n.
Superior root
C3
Transverse cervical n.
Ansa cervicalis
C4
Supraclavicular nn.
Inferior root
C5
Phrenic n.
To brachial plexus

21.3 Nerves of the Neck

Nerves of the neck include cervical and thoracic spinal nerves, nerves from the cervical sympathetic trunk, and cranial nerves (**Fig. 21.4**).

21.3a Cervical Nerves

The C1–C4 spinal nerves supply the regions of the neck (**Table 21.5**).

— Posterior rami of cervical spinal nerves C1 through C3 form three nerves that provide motor and cutaneous innervation to the posterior neck and scalp: the **suboccipital** (C1), **greater occipital** (C2), and **3rd occipital nerves** (C3) (**Fig. 21.5**).

— Anterior rami of C1–C4 cervical spinal nerves form the **cervical plexus**, which has sensory and motor components.

• The sensory nerves of the plexus, the **lesser occipital** (C1), **great auricular** (C2–C3), **transverse cervical** (C2–C3), and **supraclavicular nerves** (C3–C4), innervate the skin of the anterior and lateral neck and lateral scalp. They emerge from behind the midpoint of the posterior border of the sternocleidomastoid muscle, a location known as the **nerve point of the neck** (or Erb's point) (**Fig. 21.6**).

Fig. 21.6 ▶ **Sensory innervation of the anterolateral neck**
Sensory branches of the cervical plexus, left lateral view.

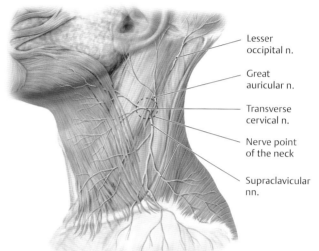

Fig. 21.5 ▶ **Innervation of the nuchal region**
Posterior view.

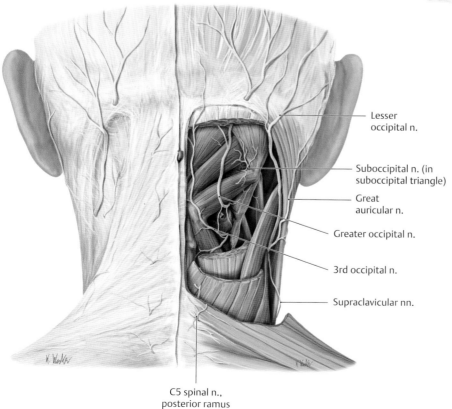

463

- The **ansa cervicalis** (C1–C3), the motor part of the plexus, which has a superior and inferior root, innervates all of the infrahyoid muscles except the thyrohyoid and usually lies anterior to the internal jugular vein (**Fig. 21.7**).

— The phrenic nerve, which arises from anterior rami of C3–C5 spinal nerves, descends on the surface of the anterior scalene muscle and enters the thorax, where it supplies the diaphragm with sensory and motor innervation.

21.3b Brachial Plexus

The brachial plexus, which innervates the upper limb, forms from the anterior rami of C5–T1. It emerges through the **interscalene groove** (the space between the anterior and middle scalene muscles) in the lateral region of the neck before continuing into the axilla (see Section 13.4d).

21.3c The Cervical Sympathetic Trunk

The cervical sympathetic trunk, a continuation of the thoracic sympathetic trunk, extends into the neck to the level of the C1 vertebra, where it lies anterolateral to the vertebral column and posterior to the carotid sheath.

— The cervical sympathetic trunk receives no white rami communicantes from cervical spinal nerves. The preganglionic fibers that synapse in the cervical ganglia originate in thoracic spinal nerves and ascend in the sympathetic trunk to the cervical region.

— Postganglionic fibers from the cervical sympathetic ganglia are distributed along three routes:
  - Via gray rami communicantes to join cervical spinal nerves
  - Via cervical cardiac (cardiopulmonary) nerves to the cardiac plexus in the thorax
  - Via sympathetic nerve plexuses surrounding vessels (periarterial plexuses), especially along the external carotid, internal carotid, and vertebral arteries, to supply structures of the head and neck

— The cervical sympathetic trunk has superior, middle, and inferior ganglia.
  - The **superior cervical ganglion** lies anterior to C1 vertebra and posterior to the internal carotid artery. Its branches include
    - the **superior cervical sympathetic cardiac nerve**,
    - branches to the **pharyngeal nerve plexus**,
    - an **internal carotid nerve** that forms the **internal carotid plexus**, and
    - an **external carotid nerve** that forms the **external carotid plexus**.
    - gray rami communicantes to anterior rami of C1–C4 spinal nerves.

Fig. 21.7 ► **Motor innervation of the anterolateral neck**
Left lateral view.

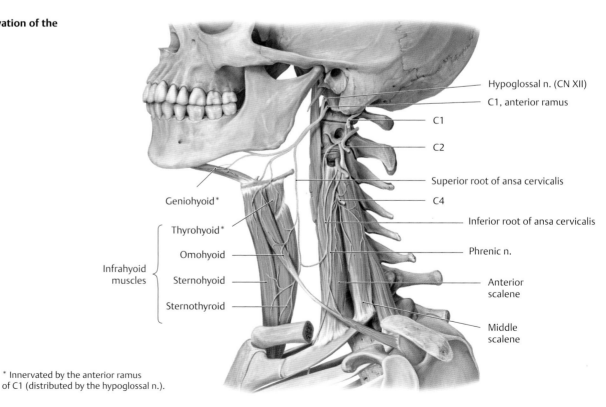

Hypoglossal n. (CN XII)
C1, anterior ramus
C1
C2
Superior root of ansa cervicalis
C4
Inferior root of ansa cervicalis
Phrenic n.
Anterior scalene
Middle scalene

Geniohyoid*
Thyrohyoid*
Omohyoid
Infrahyoid muscles
Sternohyoid
Sternothyroid

* Innervated by the anterior ramus of C1 (distributed by the hypoglossal n.).

- The **middle cervical ganglion** lies at the level of the C6 vertebra and gives off the **middle cervical sympathetic cardiac nerve**, which joins the cardiac plexus in the thorax, and gray rami communicantes to anterior rami of C5 and C6 spinal nerves.
- The **inferior cervical ganglion** usually combines with the most superior thoracic ganglion (T1) to form the **stellate ganglion**, which lies anterior to the transverse process of the C7 vertebra. It gives off the **inferior cervical sympathetic cardiac nerve**, which descends into the thorax, and gray rami communicantes to anterior rami of C7 and C8 spinal nerves.

21.3d Cranial Nerves in the Neck

Four of the cranial nerves are found in the neck.

— The glossopharyngeal nerve (CN IX) sends branches to the tongue and pharynx in the head and descends into the neck to innervate the carotid body and carotid sinus (see **Fig. 18.22**). It innervates one muscle, the stylopharyngeus.

— The vagus nerve (CN X) descends within the carotid sheath in the neck before entering the thorax. Its branches to cervical structures arise from both thoracic and cervical parts of the nerve (see **Fig. 18.24**).

- A **superior laryngeal nerve** arises from the cervical part of each vagus nerve and innervates the upper larynx through its internal and external branches.
- The **right recurrent laryngeal nerve** arises from the inferior cervical part of the right vagus nerve and recurs around the subclavian artery in the neck.
- The **left recurrent laryngeal nerve** arises from the thoracic part of the left vagus nerve. It recurs around the arch of the aorta and ascends in the neck between the trachea and esophagus.

- Cervical **cardiac nerves** carry visceral motor (presynaptic parasympathetic) fibers and visceral sensory fibers to the cardiac plexus.

— The spinal accessory nerve (CN XI), which is derived from roots of the upper cervical spinal cord segments, enters the skull through the foramen magnum. After exiting the skull through the jugular foramen, it innervates the sternocleidomastoid muscle, then crosses the lateral region of the neck to innervate the trapezius muscle (see **Fig. 18.25**).

- The cranial root joins the vagus nerve.
- The spinal root innervates the sternocleidomastoid muscle, then crosses the lateral region of the neck to innervate the trapezius muscle.

— The hypoglossal nerve (CN XII), which exits the skull through the hypoglossal canal and courses anteriorly to the submandibular region, enters the oral cavity to innervate muscles of the tongue.

- Along its course, fibers from C1 join the hypoglossal nerve briefly, eventually diverging from it to innervate the geniohyoid and thyrohyoid muscles and to form the superior root of the ansa cervicalis (see **Fig. 21.7**).

21.4 The Pharynx

The **pharynx**, a fibromuscular tube that forms part of the upper airway and the upper digestive tract, transmits air from the nasal cavity to the trachea and food from the oral cavity to the esophagus.

21.4a Regions of the Pharynx

The pharynx, which extends from the base of the skull to the inferior aspect of the larynx (cricoid cartilage), is divided into three regions (**Figs. 21.8** and **21.9**; see also **Fig. 19.19**): the nasopharynx, the oropharynx, and the laryngopharynx.

— The **nasopharynx**, the uppermost part of the pharynx, lies posterior to the nasal cavity and above the soft palate. Anteriorly, the nasopharynx communicates with the nasal cavity through the paired choanae.
  • The orifices (openings) of the pharyngotympanic tubes are located on the lateral pharyngeal wall. Above the orifice, the cartilaginous part of the tube protrudes into the pharynx to form a bulge, the **torus tubarius**.
  • A **salpingopharyngeal fold**, formed by the **salpingopharyngeus muscle** deep to the mucosa, extends inferiorly from the torus tubarius.

— The **oropharynx**, which lies posterior to the oral cavity, extends superiorly to the soft palate and inferiorly to the top of the larynx. The posterior tongue forms the anterior boundary.
  • Two arches, the anterior palatoglossal arch (fold) and the posterior palatopharyngeal arch (fold), formed by the palatoglossus and palatopharyngeal muscles, respectively, separate the oropharynx from the oral cavity (see **Fig. 19.20**). Both muscles are innervated by the vagus nerve (CN X).
  • The palatine tonsil lies between these arches in the tonsillar fossa.
  • A median fold of mucosa divides the space between the base of the tongue and the epiglottis. The spaces on either side of the fold are called **valleculae**.

Fig. 21.8 ► **Regions of the pharynx**
Midsagittal section, left lateral view. The blue arrow indicates flow of air and the red arrow, passage of food.

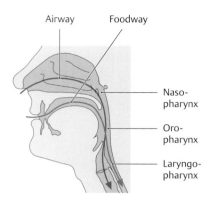

— The **laryngopharynx**, which lies posterior to the larynx, extends from the epiglottis to the inferior border of the cricoid cartilage, where it narrows and is continuous with the esophagus.
  • The laryngopharynx communicates with the larynx through the **laryngeal inlet**.
  • **Aryepiglottic folds** separate the laryngeal inlet from mucus-lined fossae on the lateral walls of the pharynx called **piriform recesses**.

Fig. 21.9 ▶ **Pharynx**
Posterior view of opened pharynx.

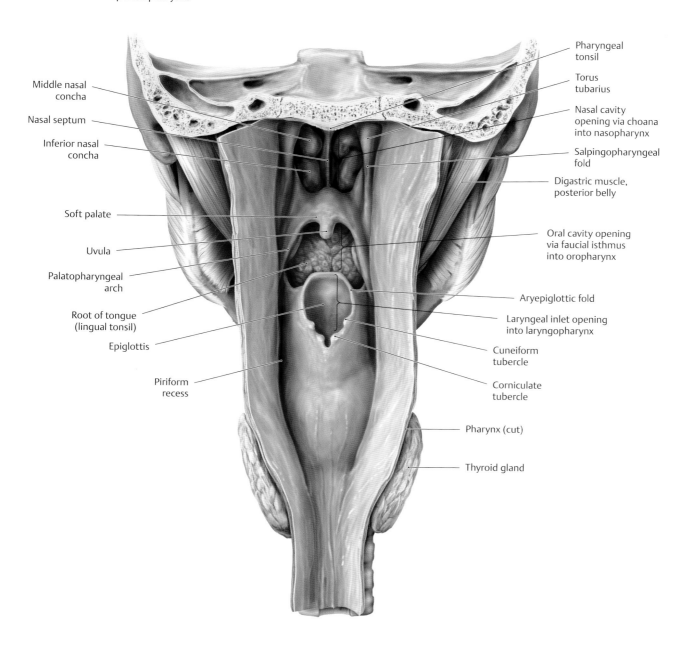

Middle nasal concha

Nasal septum

Inferior nasal concha

Soft palate

Uvula

Palatopharyngeal arch

Root of tongue (lingual tonsil)

Epiglottis

Piriform recess

Pharyngeal tonsil

Torus tubarius

Nasal cavity opening via choana into nasopharynx

Salpingopharyngeal fold

Digastric muscle, posterior belly

Oral cavity opening via faucial isthmus into oropharynx

Aryepiglottic fold

Laryngeal inlet opening into laryngopharynx

Cuneiform tubercle

Corniculate tubercle

Pharynx (cut)

Thyroid gland

Fig. 21.10 ▶ **Pharyngeal muscles**
Posterior view.

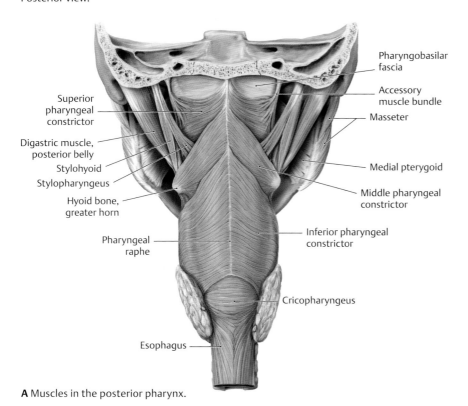

Pharyngobasilar
fascia

Accessory
muscle bundle

Masseter

Medial pterygoid

Middle pharyngeal
constrictor

Inferior pharyngeal
constrictor

Cricopharyngeus

Superior
pharyngeal
constrictor

Digastric muscle,
posterior belly

Stylohyoid

Stylopharyngeus

Hyoid bone,
greater horn

Pharyngeal
raphe

Esophagus

A Muscles in the posterior pharynx.

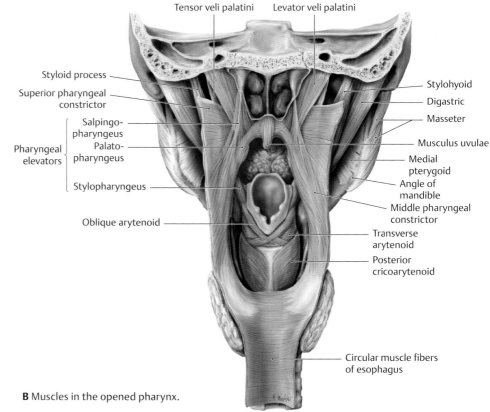

Tensor veli palatini   Levator veli palatini

Styloid process

Superior pharyngeal
constrictor

Pharyngeal
elevators

Salpingo-
pharyngeus

Palato-
pharyngeus

Stylopharyngeus

Oblique arytenoid

Stylohyoid

Digastric

Masseter

Musculus uvulae

Medial
pterygoid

Angle of
mandible

Middle pharyngeal
constrictor

Transverse
arytenoid

Posterior
cricoarytenoid

Circular muscle fibers
of esophagus

B Muscles in the opened pharynx.

21.4b Muscles of the Pharynx

An outer circular layer and inner longitudinal layer of skeletal muscles form the walls of the pharynx (**Fig. 21.10A and B**; **Table 21.6**). Pharyngeal muscles function during swallowing.

— Circular superior, middle, and inferior pharyngeal constrictor muscles propel a bolus of food downward through the oropharynx and laryngopharynx.

— Longitudinal muscles, the salpingopharyngeus and palatopharyngeus innervated by the vagus nerve (CN X) and pharyngeal plexus, and the stylopharyngeus innervated by the glossopharyngeal nerve (CN IX), elevate the soft palate to prevent food from entering the nasopharynx.

21.4c Tonsils

— **Tonsils**, masses of lymphoid tissue found in the mucosal lining of the pharynx, form an incomplete circular ring called the **pharyngeal lymphatic ring** (Waldeyer's ring) around the superior part of the pharynx (**Fig. 21.11**). They include

- **pharyngeal tonsils** (also known as adenoids) in the mucous membrane of the roof and posterior wall of the pharynx,
- **tubal tonsils** near the orifices of the pharyngotympanic tube,
- **palatine tonsils** in the fossae between the palatoglossal and palatopharyngeal arches, and
- **lingual tonsils** on the posterior one third of the dorsum of the tongue.

— Tonsillar lymphatic vessels drain to the jugulodigastric node near the angle of the mandible before draining to the deep cervical lymph nodes.

Tonsillectomy

During a tonsillectomy, the palatine tonsils are removed from the tonsillar bed along with their accompanying fascia. The glossopharyngeal nerve, which lies on the lateral wall of the pharynx, is vulnerable to injury during the procedure and may result in loss of sensation and taste from the posterior one third of the tongue. Bleeding may occur from the large external palatine vein or from the tonsillar branches of the facial, ascending pharyngeal, maxillary, and lingual arteries. The internal carotid artery may also be vulnerable because it runs just lateral to the tonsil.

Fig. 21.11 ▶ **Tonsils: Waldeyer's ring**
Posterior view of the opened pharynx.

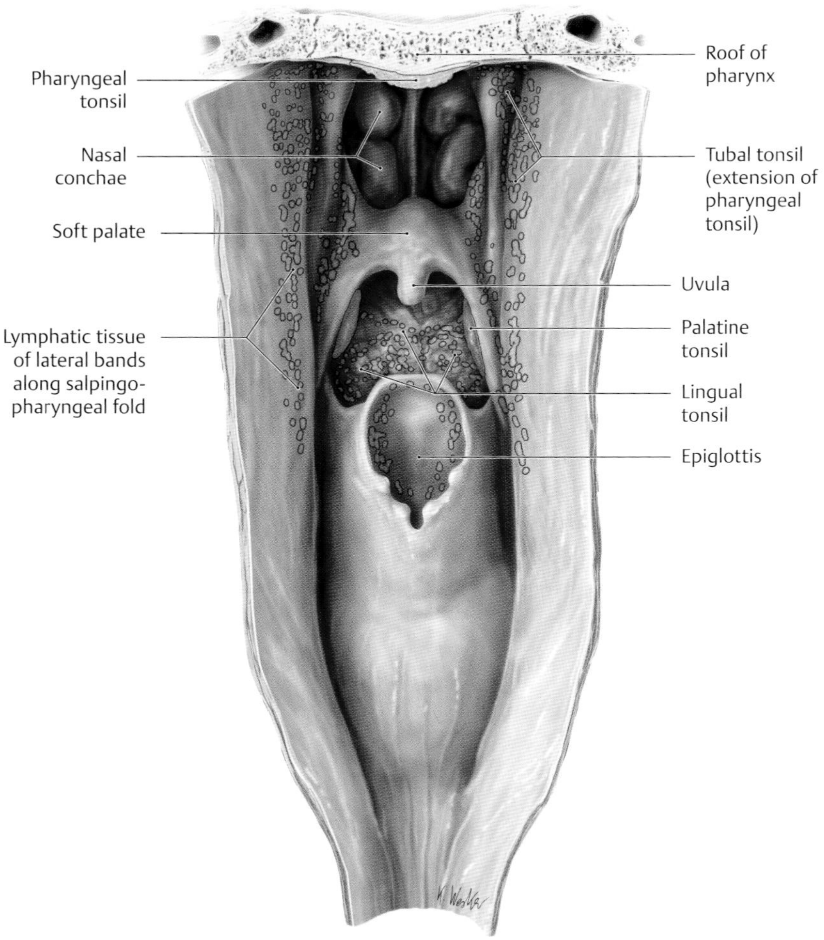

Table 21.6 ▶ **Muscles of the Pharynx**

Muscles	Innervation	Action
Longitudinal muscles		
Salpingopharyngeus	Pharyngeal plexus–CN X	Elevates pharynx
Palatopharyngeus		Elevates pharynx and larynx
Stylopharyngeus	CN IX	Elevates pharynx
Circular muscles		
Superior constrictor	Pharyngeal plexus–CN X	Constricts pharynx
Middle constrictor		
Inferior constrictor	Pharyngeal plexus, superior laryngeal (external br.), recurrent laryngeal nn.–CN X	

21.4d Neurovasculature of the Pharynx

- Direct and indirect branches of the external carotid artery supply the pharynx. These include the facial, lingual, ascending palatine, descending palatine, and ascending pharyngeal arteries (see **Fig. 17.14**).
- Venous drainage of the pharynx passes through the pharyngeal venous plexus to the internal jugular vein (see **Fig. 17.20**).
- Sensory innervation of the pharynx varies by region.
  - The maxillary nerve (CN V_2) innervates the nasopharynx.
  - The glossopharyngeal nerve (CN IX) innervates the oropharynx.
  - The vagus nerve (CN X) via its internal laryngeal branch innervates the laryngopharynx.

> **▬▬ Gag reflex**
>
> The gag reflex is a reflexive contraction of the pharyngeal muscles that protects the airway by preventing accidental ingestion and aspiration. It is elicited by touching the soft palate or back of the tongue. The glossopharyngeal nerve (CN IX) is the afferent limb, and the vagus nerve (CN X) serves as the efferent limb of the reflex.

21.5 Esophagus

The esophagus is a muscular tube that connects the pharynx in the neck to the stomach in the abdomen (see Section 5.6 and **Fig. 21.10A** and **B**).

- The cervical esophagus begins at the C6 vertebral level, which corresponds to the inferior border of the cricoid cartilage. The cervical esophagus is posterior to the trachea, anterior to the cervical vertebrae, and continuous with the laryngopharynx superiorly.
- At the pharyngoesophageal junction, the **cricopharyngeus**, the lowest part of the inferior pharyngeal constrictor, forms the superior esophageal sphincter.
- The inferior thyroid arteries, branches of the subclavian arteries via the thyrocervical trunks, supply the cervical part of the esophagus. Veins of similar name accompany the arteries.
- Lymphatic vessels from the cervical esophagus drain to paratracheal and deep cervical nodes.
- The recurrent laryngeal nerves, branches of the vagus nerve (CN X), and vasomotor fibers from the cervical sympathetic trunk innervate the esophagus in the neck.

21.6 Larynx and Trachea

The larynx, part of the upper airway, is responsible for sound production. It communicates superiorly with the pharynx and inferiorly with the trachea and lies anterior to the C3–C6 vertebrae. The trachea, the upper part of the tracheobronchial tree, descends into the thorax, where it is continuous with the bronchi of the lungs.

21.6a Laryngeal Skeleton

Three single cartilages and two sets of paired cartilages form the laryngeal skeleton (**Figs. 21.12**, **21.13**, and **21.15B** and **D**). All except the epiglottis (elastic cartilage) are formed of hyaline cartilage.

- The **thyroid cartilage**, the largest of the nine cartilages, has two **laminae** that join at the midline to form a **laryngeal prominence** (Adam's apple). The **superior horn** of the thyroid cartilage attaches to the hyoid bone, and the **inferior horn** articulates with the cricoid cartilage at the **cricothyroid joint**.
- The **cricoid cartilage**, the only part of the laryngeal skeleton to form a complete ring around the airway, articulates superiorly with the thyroid cartilage and is attached inferiorly to the first tracheal ring. The anterior part of the cricoid cartilage, the **arch**, is short, and the **lamina**, its posterior part, is tall.
- The **epiglottis**, a leaf-shaped cartilage that forms the anterior wall of the laryngeal inlet at the root of the tongue, is attached inferiorly to the thyroid cartilage and anteriorly to the hyoid bone.
- The paired pyramidal **arytenoid cartilages**, which articulate with the superior border of the cricoid lamina, have an apex that articulates with the tiny **corniculate cartilages** and a **vocal process** that attaches to the thyroid cartilage through the **vocal ligaments**.
- The small paired corniculate and **cuneiform cartilages** appear as tubercles within the **aryepiglottic fold**. Although the corniculate cartilages articulate with the arytenoids, the cuneiform cartilages do not articulate with the other cartilages.

Fig. 21.12 ▶ **Structure of the larynx**

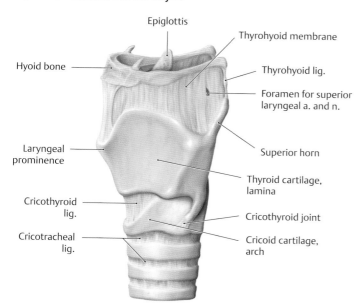

A Left anterior oblique view.

Epiglottis
Thyrohyoid membrane
Hyoid bone
Thyrohyoid lig.
Foramen for superior laryngeal a. and n.
Superior horn
Laryngeal prominence
Thyroid cartilage, lamina
Cricothyroid lig.
Cricothyroid joint
Cricotracheal lig.
Cricoid cartilage, arch

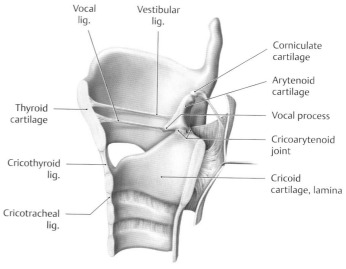

B Sagittal section viewed from the left medial aspect. *Removed*: Hyoid bone and thyrohyoid ligament. The arytenoid cartilage alters the position of the vocal folds during phonation.

Vocal lig.
Vestibular lig.
Corniculate cartilage
Arytenoid cartilage
Thyroid cartilage
Vocal process
Cricoarytenoid joint
Cricothyroid lig.
Cricoid cartilage, lamina
Cricotracheal lig.

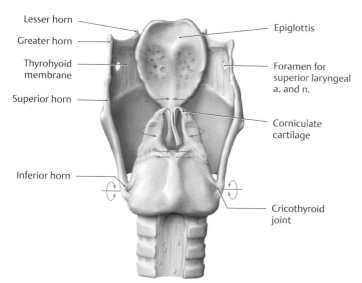

C Posterior view. Arrows indicate the direction of movement in the various joints.

Lesser horn
Greater horn
Thyrohyoid membrane
Superior horn
Inferior horn
Epiglottis
Foramen for superior laryngeal a. and n.
Corniculate cartilage
Cricothyroid joint

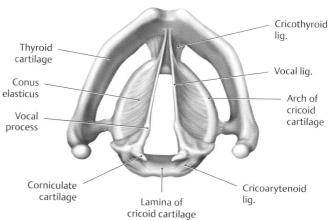

D Superior view of thyrohyoid, cricoid, and corniculate cartilages.

Thyroid cartilage
Cricothyroid lig.
Vocal lig.
Conus elasticus
Arch of cricoid cartilage
Vocal process
Corniculate cartilage
Cricoarytenoid lig.
Lamina of cricoid cartilage

21.6b Membranes and Ligaments of the Larynx

Membranes of the larynx connect the laryngeal cartilages to each other and to the hyoid bone and trachea (**Figs. 21.13** and **21.14**; see also **Fig. 21.12A** and **B**).

— The **thyrohyoid membrane** attaches the thyroid cartilage to the hyoid bone superiorly.

— The **cricotracheal ligament** attaches the cricoid cartilage to the first tracheal ring inferiorly.

— The **quadrangular membrane** extends posteriorly from the lateral border of the epiglottis to the arytenoid cartilage on each side.

   • The superior free margin of this membrane forms the **aryepiglottic ligament**, which, when covered by mucosa, is known as the **aryepiglottic fold**.

   • The inferior free margin is the **vestibular ligament**, which, when covered by mucosa, is known as the **vestibular fold** or false vocal cord.

— The **cricothyroid membrane** connects the cricoid and thyroid cartilages and extends superiorly deep to the thyroid cartilage as the **conus elasticus** (see **Figs. 21.12D** and **21.15C**).

— The free superior border of the conus elasticus forms the **vocal ligament**, which extends from the midpoint of the thyroid cartilage to the vocal processes of the arytenoid cartilage. The vocal ligament and the **vocalis muscle** form the **vocal fold** or **vocal cord**.

■ Tracheostomy and cricothyroidotomy

When the upper airway is obstructed, airway access can be reestablished using two different approaches. Tracheostomy is a surgical procedure in which a tracheostomy tube is inserted through an incision in the proximal trachea. This procedure is generally used for long-term management of the airway. Cricothyroidotomy is a related procedure in which an incision is made in the cricothyroid membrane. This procedure, usually performed in emergency situations, is less technically difficult than tracheostomy and has fewer complications.

21.6c Laryngeal Cavity

The laryngeal cavity begins at the laryngeal inlet and extends to the inferior border of the cricoid cartilage (see **Figs. 21.13** and **21.14**).

— The vestibular and vocal folds define spaces within the laryngeal cavity.

   • The **supraglottic space** (laryngeal vestibule) or supraglottic space, lies above the vestibular folds.

   • The **rima vestibuli** is the aperture between the two vestibular folds.

   • The **laryngeal ventricles** are recesses of the laryngeal cavity between the vestibular and vocal folds.

   • **Laryngeal saccules** are the blind ends of the laryngeal ventricles.

   • The **rima glottidis** is the aperture between the two vocal folds.

   • The **subglottic space** (infraglottic cavity) is the inferior part of the laryngeal cavity, which lies below the vocal folds and extends to the inferior border of the cricoid cartilage.

— Sound is produced as air passes through the laryngeal cavity between the vocal folds. Variations in sound arise from changes in the position, tension, and length of these folds.

— The vestibular folds protect the airway but have no role in sound production.

Fig. 21.13 ► **Cavity of the larynx**
Midsagittal section viewed from the left side.

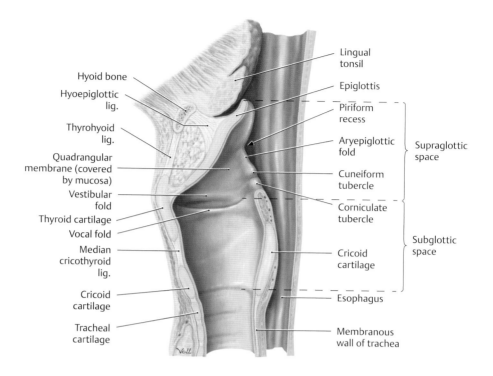

Hyoid bone

Hyoepiglottic lig.

Thyrohyoid lig.

Quadrangular membrane (covered by mucosa)

Vestibular fold

Thyroid cartilage

Vocal fold

Median cricothyroid lig.

Cricoid cartilage

Tracheal cartilage

Lingual tonsil

Epiglottis

Piriform recess

Aryepiglottic fold

Cuneiform tubercle

Corniculate tubercle

Cricoid cartilage

Esophagus

Membranous wall of trachea

Supraglottic space

Subglottic space

Fig. 21.14 ► **Vestibular and vocal folds**
Coronal section, superior view.

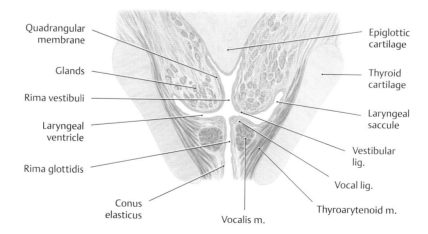

Quadrangular membrane

Glands

Rima vestibuli

Laryngeal ventricle

Rima glottidis

Conus elasticus

Vocalis m.

Epiglottic cartilage

Thyroid cartilage

Laryngeal saccule

Vestibular lig.

Vocal lig.

Thyroarytenoid m.

Fig. 21.15 ▶ **Laryngeal muscles**
The laryngeal muscles move the laryngeal cartilages relative to one another, affecting the tension and/or position of the vocal folds.

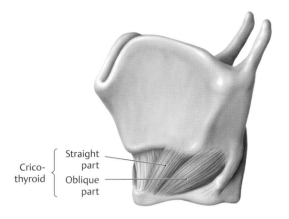

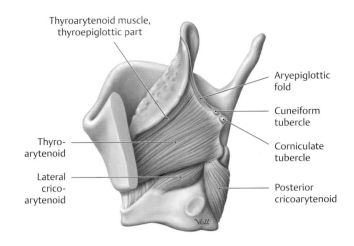

A Extrinsic laryngeal muscles, left lateral oblique view. *Removed*: Epiglottis.

B Intrinsic laryngeal muscles, left lateral view. *Removed:* Thyroid cartilage (left lamina). *Revealed:* Epiglottis and external thyroarytenoid muscle.

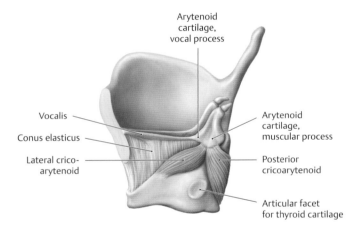

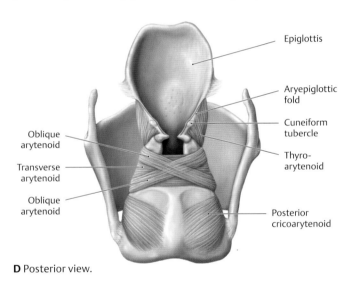

C Left lateral view. *Removed*: Thyroid cartilage (left lamina) and epiglottis.

D Posterior view.

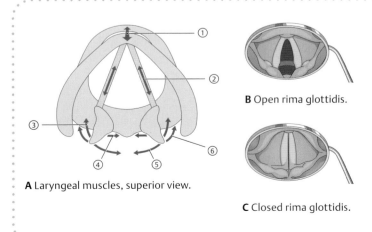

A Laryngeal muscles, superior view.

B Open rima glottidis.

C Closed rima glottidis.

Table 21.7 ▶ **Actions of the Laryngeal Muscles**		
Muscle	**Action**	**Effect on Rima Glottidis**
① Cricothyroid m.*	Tightens the vocal folds	None
② Vocalis m.		
③ Thyroarytenoid m.	Adducts the vocal folds	Closes
④ Transverse arytenoid m.		
⑤ Posterior cricoarytenoid m.	Abducts the vocal folds	Opens
⑥ Lateral cricoarytenoid m.	Adducts the vocal folds	Closes
* The cricothyroid m. is the only extrinsic laryngeal muscle.		

21.6d Muscles of the Larynx

The larynx has extrinsic and intrinsic muscle groups.

— Extrinsic muscles are attached to the hyoid bone and move the larynx and hyoid bone together. These include the suprahyoid muscles (see **Table 19.9**), which elevate the larynx, and the infrahyoid muscles (see **Table 21.3**), which depress the larynx.

— Intrinsic muscles move the laryngeal cartilages, which changes the length and tension of the vocal ligaments and size of the rima glottidis (**Table 21.7**; **Fig. 21.15A, B, C,** and **D**).

  • The **posterior cricoarytenoid muscle** is the only muscle that abducts the vocal folds and opens the rima glottidis.

  • The **cricothyroid muscle**, innervated by the external branch of the superior laryngeal nerve, is the only intrinsic muscle that is not innervated by the inferior laryngeal nerve (a continuation of the recurrent laryngeal nerve).

21.6e Neurovasculature of the Larynx (Figs. 21.16 and 21.17A and B)

— The superior and inferior laryngeal arteries are branches of the superior and inferior thyroid arteries, respectively. Veins of the larynx follow the laryngeal arteries and join the thyroid veins.

— The superior and inferior laryngeal branches of the vagus nerve (CN X) provide all of the motor and sensory innervation of the larynx.

  • The superior laryngeal nerve splits into an internal sensory branch, which supplies the mucosa of the vestibule and superior surface of the vocal folds, and an external motor branch, which innervates the cricothyroid muscle.

  • The **inferior laryngeal nerve**, a continuation of the recurrent laryngeal nerve, supplies the mucosa of the infraglottic larynx and innervates all intrinsic muscles of the larynx except the cricothyroid.

Recurrent laryngeal nerve paralysis with thyroidectomy

The recurrent laryngeal nerves in the neck are vulnerable to damage during thyroidectomy because they run immediately posterior to the thyroid gland. Unilateral damage results in hoarseness; bilateral damage causes respiratory distress and aphonia (inability to speak). Aspiration pneumonia may occur as a complication.

Fig. 21.16 ▶ **Arteries and nerves of the larynx, thyroid, and parathyroids** Anterior view.

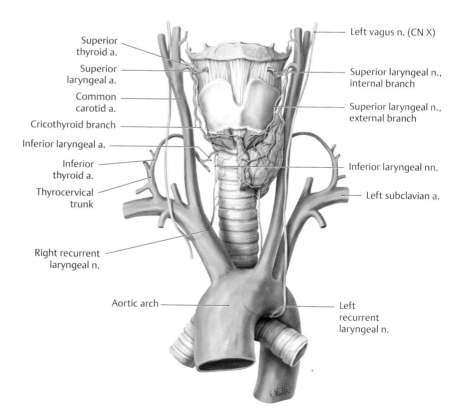

Fig. 21.17 ▶ **Neurovasculature of the larynx**
Left lateral view.

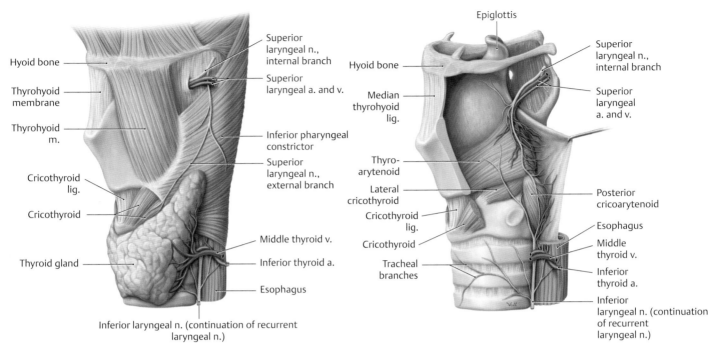

A Superficial layer.

B Deep layer. *Removed:* Cricothyroid muscle and left lamina of thyroid cartilage. *Retracted:* Pharyngeal mucosa.

21.6f The Trachea

The trachea, the extension of the airway inferior to the larynx, extends from the inferior border of the cricoid cartilage to the level of the T4–T5 intervertebral disks in the thorax, where it bifurcates into the two primary bronchi of the lungs (see Section 5.8).

21.7 Thyroid and Parathyroid Glands

The thyroid and parathyroid glands are endocrine glands that reside in the anterior cervical region.

21.7a The Thyroid Gland

The **thyroid gland**, the largest endocrine gland in the body, secretes **thyroid hormone**, which regulates the rate of metabolism, and **calcitonin**, which regulates the metabolism of calcium (**Fig. 21.18A**).

— The thyroid lies deep to the sternohyoid and sternothyroid muscles (infrahyoid muscles) and anterolateral to the larynx and trachea between C5 and T1 vertebral levels.
— The thyroid has right and left (lateral) lobes connected by a narrow **isthmus** anterior to the second and third tracheal rings.
— A **pyramidal lobe**, present in ~50% of the population, is a remnant of the embryonic thyroglossal duct that extends from the isthmus toward the hyoid bone.

— A fibrous capsule encloses the thyroid gland. The pretracheal fascia of the neck lies outside the thyroid capsule.

▮ Thyroglossal duct cyst

A thyroglossal duct cyst is a fluid-filled cavity in the midline of the neck, just inferior to the hyoid bone. It results from the proliferation of epithelium left behind from the thyroglossal duct during the descent of the thyroid gland from its embryonic origin on the tongue to its postnatal position in the neck. The cyst can enlarge and press on the trachea and esophagus, in which case it can be surgically removed.

21.7b The Parathyroid Glands

Parathyroid glands, small, ovoid endocrine glands that lie on the posterior surface of the thyroid gland, secrete **parathormone**, which regulates the metabolism of phosphorus and calcium (**Fig. 21.18B**).

— There are normally four glands, two superior and two inferior, although the number can range from two to six glands.
— The superior parathyroid glands are constant in position near the lower border of the cricoid cartilage. The position of the inferior parathyroid glands may vary, ranging from the lower pole of the thyroid gland to the superior mediastinum.

21.7c Neurovasculature of the Thyroid and Parathyroid Glands

- The superior thyroid artery, a branch of the external carotid artery, and the inferior thyroid artery from the thyrocervical trunk supply the thyroid gland (see **Fig. 21.16**). The inferior thyroid artery is usually the main supply to the parathyroid glands.
- **Superior** and **middle thyroid veins** drain into the internal jugular veins; **inferior thyroid veins** drain into the brachiocephalic veins in the mediastinum (**Fig. 21.19**). Venous drainage from the parathyroid glands joins the thyroid veins.

- Lymphatic vessels of the thyroid may drain directly into the superior and inferior deep cervical nodes or indirectly, passing first through prelaryngeal, pretracheal, and paratracheal nodes.
- The parathyroid glands drain with the thyroid into the inferior deep cervical and paratracheal lymph nodes.
- Cardiac and superior and inferior thyroid sympathetic plexuses arise from the superior, middle, and inferior cervical sympathetic ganglia to supply vasomotor innervation to the thyroid and parathyroid glands.
- The thyroid and parathyroid glands are under hormonal control and therefore lack secretomotor innervation.

Fig. 21.18 ▶ **Thyroid and parathyroid glands**

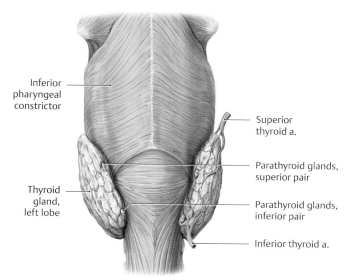

Cricothyroid lig.

Thyroid gland, right lobe

Thyroid gland, isthmus

Thyroid cartilage

Thyroid gland, pyramidal lobe

Cricothyroid

Thyroid gland, left lobe

Trachea

A Thyroid gland. Anterior view.

Inferior pharyngeal constrictor

Thyroid gland, left lobe

Superior thyroid a.

Parathyroid glands, superior pair

Parathyroid glands, inferior pair

Inferior thyroid a.

B Thyroid and parathyroid glands, posterior view.

Fig. 21.19 ▶ **Veins of the larynx, thyroid, and parathyroid glands**
Left lateral view. *Note:* The inferior thyroid vein generally drains into the left brachiocephalic vein.

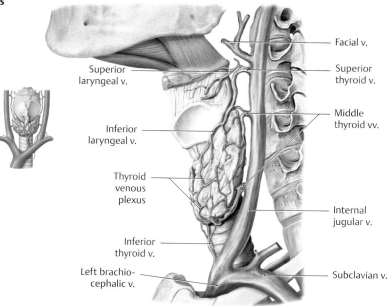

Superior laryngeal v.

Inferior laryngeal v.

Thyroid venous plexus

Inferior thyroid v.

Left brachio-cephalic v.

Facial v.

Superior thyroid v.

Middle thyroid vv.

Internal jugular v.

Subclavian v.

21.8 Topography of the Neck

The regions of the neck, defined by muscular and skeletal boundaries, are largely descriptive rather than functional, but they are useful for understanding the topographic relationships in the neck, which often play a significant role in medical practice (**Table 21.8**; **Figs. 21.20A** and **B** and **21.21A, B,** and **C**).

- The **anterior cervical region** (anterior triangle) extends from the midline of the neck to the anterior border of the sternocleidomastoid muscle.
  - The region is further divided into **submandibular, submental, muscular,** and **carotid triangles**.
  - The anterior region contains most of the cervical viscera, which includes the lower pharynx, esophagus, larynx, trachea, thyroid, and parathyroid glands.
- The **sternocleidomastoid region** is a narrow area defined by the anterior and posterior borders of the sternocleidomastoid muscle.
  - Inferiorly, the sternal and clavicular heads of the muscle define the small **lesser supraclavicular fossa**.
  - This region contains parts of the major vascular structures of the neck.
- The **lateral cervical region** (posterior triangle) extends from the posterior border of the sternocleidomastoid muscle to the anterior border of the trapezius muscle.
  - The posterior belly of the omohyoid muscle divides this region into **omoclavicular** and **occipital triangles**.
  - The scalene muscles, and cervical and brachial plexuses are located in this region.

- The **posterior cervical region** extends from the anterior border of the trapezius muscle to the posterior midline of the neck.
  - It contains the trapezius and suboccipital muscles, the vertebral artery, and posterior branches of the cervical plexus.
- The **root of neck**, a transition area for structures passing between the thorax and neck, is enclosed by the superior thoracic aperture, which is formed by the manubrium, the first ribs and their costal cartilages, and the first thoracic vertebra.
  - It contains the trachea, esophagus, common carotid and subclavian arteries, brachiocephalic veins, vagus and phrenic nerves, the sympathetic trunk, the thoracic duct, and the apex of each lung.

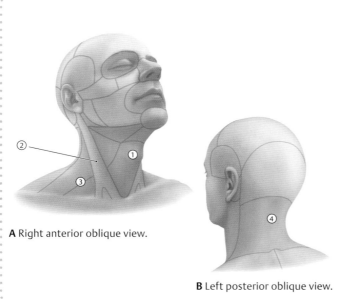

A Right anterior oblique view.

B Left posterior oblique view.

Table 21.8 ▸ Regions of the Neck

Region	Divisions	Contents
① Anterior cervical region (triangle)	Submandibular (digastric) triangle	Submandibular gland and lymph nodes, hypoglossal n. (CN XII), facial a. and v.
	Submental triangle	Submental lymph nodes
	Muscular triangle	Sternothyroid and sternohyoid muscles, thyroid and parathyroid glands
	Carotid triangle	Carotid bifurcation, carotid body, hypoglossal (CN XII) and vagus (CN X) nn.
② Sternocleidomastoid region *		Sternocleidomastoid, common carotid a., internal jugular v., vagus n. (CN X), jugular lymph nodes
③ Lateral cervical region (posterior triangle)	Omoclavicular (subclavian) triangle	Subclavian a., subscapular a., supraclavicular l.n.
	Occipital triangle	Accessory n. (CN XI), trunks of brachial plexus, transverse cervical a., cervical plexus (posterior branches)
④ Posterior cervical region		Nuchal muscles, vertebral a., cervical plexus

* The sternocleidomastoid region also contains the lesser supraclavicular fossa.

Fig. 21.20 ► **Cervical regions**

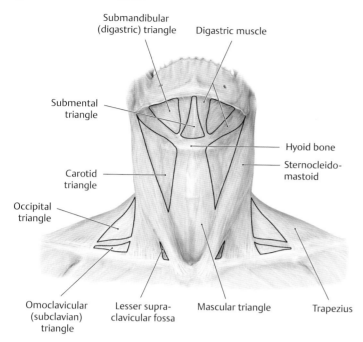

Submental triangle
Submandibular (digastric) triangle
Digastric muscle
Carotid triangle
Hyoid bone
Sternocleido-mastoid
Occipital triangle
Omoclavicular (subclavian) triangle
Lesser supra-clavicular fossa
Mascular triangle
Trapezius

A Anterior view.

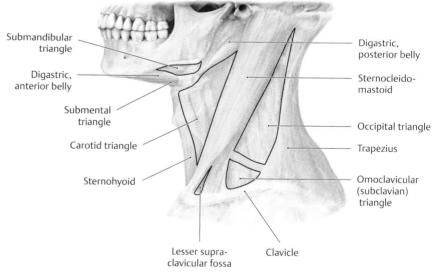

Submandibular triangle
Digastric, anterior belly
Submental triangle
Carotid triangle
Sternohyoid
Digastric, posterior belly
Sternocleido-mastoid
Occipital triangle
Trapezius
Omoclavicular (subclavian) triangle
Lesser supra-clavicular fossa
Clavicle

B Left lateral view.

Fig. 21.21 ► **Topography of the anterior cervical region**
Anterior view.

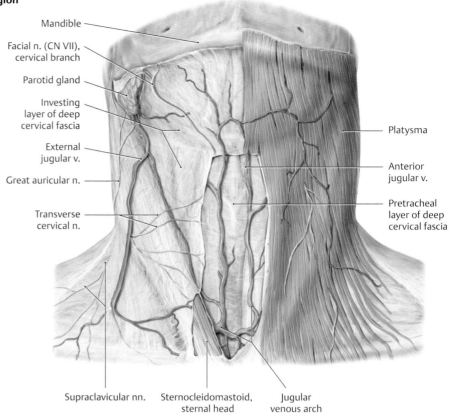

Mandible

Facial n. (CN VII), cervical branch

Parotid gland

Investing layer of deep cervical fascia

External jugular v.

Great auricular n.

Transverse cervical n.

Platysma

Anterior jugular v.

Pretracheal layer of deep cervical fascia

Supraclavicular nn.

Sternocleidomastoid, sternal head

Jugular venous arch

A Superficial dissection.

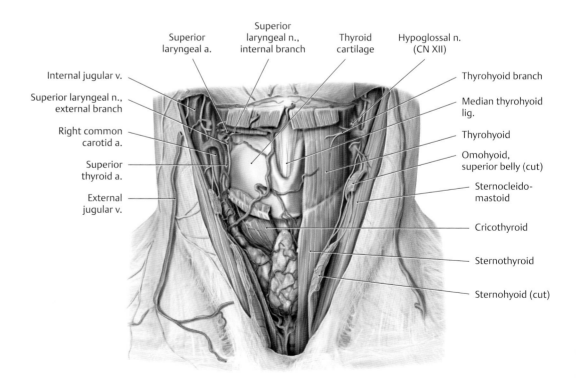

Superior laryngeal a.

Superior laryngeal n., internal branch

Thyroid cartilage

Hypoglossal n. (CN XII)

Internal jugular v.

Superior laryngeal n., external branch

Right common carotid a.

Superior thyroid a.

External jugular v.

Thyrohyoid branch

Median thyrohyoid lig.

Thyrohyoid

Omohyoid, superior belly (cut)

Sternocleido-mastoid

Cricothyroid

Sternothyroid

Sternohyoid (cut)

B Deep dissection.

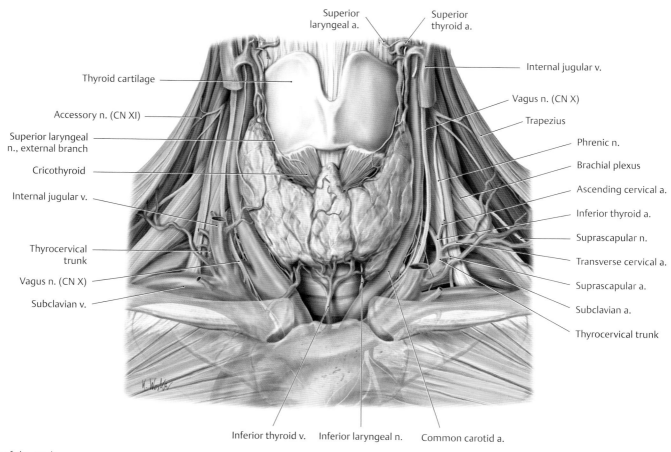

Superior laryngeal a.

Superior thyroid a.

Thyroid cartilage

Accessory n. (CN XI)

Superior laryngeal n., external branch

Cricothyroid

Internal jugular v.

Thyrocervical trunk

Vagus n. (CN X)

Subclavian v.

Internal jugular v.

Vagus n. (CN X)

Trapezius

Phrenic n.

Brachial plexus

Ascending cervical a.

Inferior thyroid a.

Suprascapular n.

Transverse cervical a.

Suprascapular a.

Subclavian a.

Thyrocervical trunk

Inferior thyroid v.   Inferior laryngeal n.   Common carotid a.

C Root of the neck.

Review Questions: Head and Neck

1. Which bone of the skull contains the optic foramen, foramen ovale, and foramen spinosum?
   A. Frontal
   B. Temporal
   C. Sphenoid
   D. Ethmoid
   E. Occipital

2. The internal jugular vein
   A. is located within the carotid sheath
   B. receives venous drainage from the brain
   C. is a tributary of the brachiocephalic vein
   D. receives blood from the facial vein
   E. All of the above

3. The following structure runs within the falx cerebri.
   A. Inferior sagittal sinus
   B. Transverse sinus
   C. Sigmoid sinus
   D. Cavernous sinus
   E. 3rd ventricle

4. The vertebral artery
   A. ascends through the transverse foramina of all seven cervical vertebra
   B. arises from the first part of the axillary artery
   C. terminates by joining with the posterior cerebellar artery
   D. supplies branches to the thyroid gland
   E. supplies the posterior cerebral circulation

5. A patient is taken to the emergency department after his wife noticed something wrong with the left side of his face during breakfast. He is found to have a problem with the nerve exiting the stylomastoid foramen, a disorder called Bell's palsy. Which of the following problems is this patient likely to have?
   A. He is unable to open his left eye.
   B. He is unable to raise his eyebrow on the left side.
   C. He is unable to protrude his tongue to the right.
   D. He is unable to chew.
   E. He is unable to feel pressure on his left cheek.

6. A patient came into the ER with a broken mandible resulting from an overswung bat. Which nerve is most likely affected by this injury?
   A. Lingual nerve
   B. Hypoglossal nerve
   C. Zygomatic branches of facial nerve
   D. Inferior alveolar nerve
   E. Chorda tympani nerve

7. The muscle of mastication that inserts into the condylar process of the mandible and its articular disk and the capsule of the temporomandibular joint (TMJ) is the
   A. medial pterygoid muscle
   B. lateral pterygoid muscle
   C. temporalis muscle
   D. masseter muscle
   E. buccinator muscle

8. A patient develops acromegaly secondary to a tumor in his pituitary gland secreting growth hormone. A transsphenoidal resection of the tumor is scheduled. During this process, part of the inferior and posterior nasal septum is removed. Which bone forms this part of the nasal septum?
   A. Vomer
   B. Ethmoid
   C. Palatine
   D. Temporal
   E. Sphenoid

9. The lacrimal gland is innervated by
   A. the facial nerve (VII)
   B. the postganglionic neurons with the cell bodies in the pterygopalatine ganglion
   C. the parasympathetic neurons
   D. the lacrimal nerve
   E. All of the above

10. A 2-year-old boy seen by his pediatrician was noticeably irritable and tugging at his ear. When his mother asked him in a normal tone to sit quietly, he covered his ears screaming in pain and asked her not to shout at him. On exam he was found to have a fever, and his tympanic membrane was red and bulging. He was diagnosed with otitis media and started on antibiotics. The child's extreme sensitivity to sound (hyperacusis) suggests that the infection affected the stapedius muscle. The nerve that innervates this muscle is a branch of what nerve?
    A. Maxillary division of trigeminal nerve
    B. Mandibular division of trigeminal nerve
    C. Facial nerve
    D. Glossopharyngeal nerve
    E. Vagus nerve

11. The innervation for the sternothyroid muscle is the
    A. ansa cervicalis
    B. facial nerve
    C. hypoglossal nerve
    D. accessory nerve
    E. recurrent laryngeal nerve

12. A patient was having an animated discussion with his friends when he started coughing after swallowing a piece of chicken. He soon became unable to speak or cough. Two paramedics who were taking a break at the same fast-food restaurant quickly came to his help, and one stood behind the man and performed forceful abdominal thrusts (Heimlich maneuver). After several attempts of not being successful at dislodging the aspirated food, the paramedics decide to perform an emergency airway. Where is the most superior site to perform this procedure so that the airway is secured below the vocal folds?
    A. Superior to the hyoid bone
    B. Between the hyoid bone and the thyroid cartilage
    C. Between the thyroid cartilage and the cricoid cartilage
    D. Between the thyroid cartilage and the arytenoid cartilage
    E. Superior to the manubrium in the jugular fossa

13. A patient is found to have a nodule in his neck. His calcitonin level is elevated, and a biopsy reveals medullary carcinoma of the thyroid. A thyroidectomy is performed. After surgery the patient's voice is found to be hoarse. What nerve was most likely injured during surgery?
    A. The glossopharyngeal
    B. The hypoglossal
    C. The ansa cervicalis
    D. The recurrent laryngeal
    E. The phrenic

14. A child who has been vomiting is diagnosed with an obstruction in his gastrointestinal tract. He becomes severely dehydrated, and a sunken anterior fontanelle is felt. What is the youngest age at which this sign no longer would appear in a dehydrated child?
    A. 1 month
    B. 3 months
    C. 6 months
    D. 12 months
    E. 24 months

15. The jugulodigastric lymph nodes that lie near the facial and internal jugular veins are also known as
    A. parotid nodes
    B. superior deep cervical nodes
    C. inferior deep cervical nodes
    D. retroauricular nodes
    E. lateral cervical nodes

16. A patient develops severely elevated intracranial pressure due to a brain tumor obstructing the flow of cerebral spinal fluid (CSF). A shunt is placed to relieve this pressure because the CSF is blocked from being returned to the venous system. Where would this resorption normally take place?
    A. At the choroid plexus
    B. At the interventricular foramen
    C. At the cerebral aqueduct
    D. At the lateral apertures
    E. At the arachnoid granulations

17. The vagus nerve (cranial nerve X)
    A. leaves the skull through the carotid foramen
    B. innervates the carotid sinus
    C. is transmitted through the superior orbital fissure
    D. innervates all of the muscles of the soft palate
    E. None of the above

18. A 40-year-old obese woman has frequent headaches. Upon eye exam, she is found to have papilledema (swelling of the optic disc). It is suspected that she has elevated intracranial pressure. CT scan is negative for any strokes or tumors. She is diagnosed with idiopathic intracranial hypertension (pseudotumor cerebri). One complication of this disorder is downward displacement of the brainstem, which leads to stretching of the abducent nerve. How would you diagnose if this complication occurred in this patient?
    A. She would be unable to move her eyes laterally.
    B. She would be unable to move her eyes medially.
    C. She would be unable to move her eyes superiorly.
    D. She would be unable to move her eyes inferiorly.
    E. She would be unable to rotate her eyes internally.

19. A 61-year-old firefighter was trapped for 12 hours in a collapsed building following an earthquake. Although he suffered a fractured tibia, the emergency room physician was also concerned about a deep scalp laceration that extended across the top of the patient's head. Infection from this laceration could spread
    A. to dural venous sinuses through emissary veins
    B. into the neck in the loose areolar tissue
    C. laterally beyond the zygomatic arches
    D. to the epidural space
    E. All of the above

20. A dentist who specializes in relief of facial pain is experimenting with a procedure to inject anesthetic into the pterygopalatine fossa through a lateral approach. The needle passes through the mandibular notch of the mandible, traverses the infratemporal fossa, and enters the pterygomaxillary fissure. Which of the following structures would be at risk during the procedure?
    A. Maxillary artery
    B. Mandibular division of the trigeminal nerve (CN III)
    C. Pterygoid venous plexus
    D. Otic ganglion
    E. All of the above

21. Which of the following drains into the inferior meatus of the nasal cavity?
    A. Nasolacrimal duct
    B. Frontal sinus
    C. Ethmoid sinus
    D. Sphenoid sinus
    E. Maxillary sinus

22. Which of the following vessels accompanies the optic nerve through the optic canal?
    A. Supratrochlear artery
    B. Supraorbital artery
    C. Ophthalmic artery
    D. Ophthalmic vein
    E. Ophthalmic nerve

23. The nerve that innervates the middle ear muscle that changes the shape of the tympanic membrane is the
    A. optic nerve
    B. oculomotor nerve
    C. trochlear nerve
    D. trigeminal nerve
    E. facial nerve

24. The branches of the cervical plexus
    A. originate from the anterior rami of C1 through C4
    B. innervate the sternocleidomastoid
    C. carry preganglionic fibers that synapse in parasympathetic ganglia of the head
    D. include only cutaneous nerves
    E. include the greater occipital nerve

25. Intubation is necessary during surgery because, due to muscle relaxants and other drugs administered during the procedure, patients are unable to fully relax the vocal folds. Paralysis of which muscle prevents the relaxation of the vocal folds?
    A. Thyroarytenoid muscles
    B. Posterior cricoarytenoid muscles
    C. Cricothyroid muscles
    D. Transverse arytenoid muscles
    E. Lateral arytenoids muscles

26. All of the innervation of the larynx, both sensory and motor, is supplied by
    A. the vagus nerve
    B. the glossopharyngeal nerve
    C. the recurrent laryngeal nerve
    D. the superior laryngeal nerve
    E. None of the above

27. Which is the only laryngeal cartilage to completely encircle the airway?
    A. Thyroid
    B. Cricoid
    C. Epiglottic
    D. Arytenoid
    E. Corniculate

28. A patient is in a knife fight and receives a stab wound between the sternocleidomastoid muscle and the superior belly of the omohyoid muscle. Profuse bleeding ensues due to penetration of the common carotid artery. Which structure within the same fascial sheath may also have been injured?
    A. External jugular vein
    B. Phrenic nerve
    C. Internal jugular vein
    D. Superior thyroid artery
    E. Sympathetic trunk

29. A diabetic patient complains a severe photophobia (sensitivity to bright lights) in her right eye. When light is directly shined in her right eye her pupil does not constrict. The physician decides that, given her diabetes, she has a third cranial nerve neuropathy that involves the periphery of this nerve. Which ganglion is most likely involved in her physical findings?
    A. Superior cervical
    B. Pterygopalatine
    C. Ciliary
    D. Otic
    E. Trigeminal

30. A patient with a long history of tobacco use goes to the dentist for a cleaning. The dentist notices a lesion on her patient's lateral part of the body of the tongue and refers him to an otolaryngologist (ENT). The ENT biopsies the lesion and determines that the patient has squamous cell carcinoma of the tongue. A CT of the patient's head and neck demonstrates metastasis to the patient's lymph nodes. The primary group of lymph nodes for the drainage of this patient's cancer is
    A. superior deep cervical
    B. inferior deep cervical
    C. anterior superficial cervical
    D. submandibular
    E. submental

31. All of the following bones form a part of the nasal walls or floor except
    A. Frontal
    B. Ethmoid
    C. Maxilla
    D. Vomer
    E. Palatine

32. The action of the medial pterygoid muscle is to
    A. elevate the mandible
    B. tense the soft palate
    C. elevate the soft palate
    D. elevate the hyoid bone
    E. retract the mandible

33. A 63-year-old patient complains of difficulty speaking, chewing, and swallowing. On physical exam, you see that the patient's tongue is atrophied, and when asked to stick out his tongue and say "ahh," the patient's tongue deviates to the left. Upon obtaining a medical history and physical exam, you find that the patient underwent recent surgery on his common carotid artery. Damage to which nerve has most likely caused the observed deficits?
    A. Right glossopharyngeal nerve
    B. Right hypoglossal nerve
    C. Left hypoglossal nerve
    D. Right lingual nerve
    E. Left lingual nerve

34. The mandibular division of the trigeminal nerve (V_3) passes through the foramen ovale into the
    A. infratemporal fossa
    B. pterygopalatine fossa
    C. orbit
    D. nasal cavity
    E. oral cavity

35. A patient with hypertension and a long history of smoking suffers a series of transient ischemic attacks (TIAs). Upon evaluation a carotid bruit is heard. Further testing reveals severe stenosis of his internal carotid artery due to atherosclerosis. The TIAs were due to embolism of the atherosclerotic plaque. Which of the following is the first branch of the internal carotid artery likely to be affected by an embolism?
    A. Superior thyroid
    B. Lingual
    C. Facial
    D. Maxillary
    E. Ophthalmic

36. A patient has thrombophlebitis of the right cavernous sinus due to a facial skin infection. The infection traveled via the angular vein to the superior ophthalmic vein and into the cavernous sinus. Which of the following is an additional symptom that this patient might exhibit?
    A. Jugular venous distension on the right
    B. Inability to smile
    C. Inability to chew on the right
    D. Loss of vision in the right eye
    E. Loss of sensation to the right cheek

37. Which of the following artery is a branch of the internal carotid artery?
    A. Posterior cerebral artery
    B. Occipital artery
    C. Labyrinthine artery
    D. Ophthalmic artery
    E. Middle meningeal artery

Answers and Explanations

1. **C** The sphenoid forms the posterior orbit and the floor of the middle cranial fossa between the frontal and temporal bones. Foramina of the sphenoid include the optic foramen, foramen ovale, foramen rotundum, foramen spinosum, and superior orbital fissure (Section 17.1a).
    A The frontal bone forms the forehead, the roof and superior rim of the orbit, and the floor of the anterior cranial fossa.
    B The temporal bone forms part of the middle and posterior cranial fossa. Its foramina include the internal and external acoustic meatuses, carotid canal, and stylomastoid foramen.
    D The ethmoid bone forms part of the anterior cranial fossa, medial walls of the orbit, and parts of the nasal septum and lateral nasal walls.
    E The occipital bone forms most of the posterior cranial fossa. Its foramina include the foramen magnum, condylar canals, and jugular foramina.

2. **E** The internal jugular vein is located within the carotid sheath (A), contains venous drainage from the brain (B), is a tributary of the brachiocephalic vein (C), and receives blood from the facial vein (D) (Section 17.4).
    A The internal jugular vein runs within the carotid sheath with the common carotid artery and vagus nerve. B, C, and D are also correct (E).
    B Cerebral venous drainage flow primarily to the internal jugular veins. A, C, and D are also correct (E).
    C The internal jugular veins join the subclavian veins to form the brachiocephalic veins. A, B, and D are also correct (E).
    D The facial vein is a tributary of the internal jugular vein. A through C are also correct (E).

3. **A** The inferior sagittal sinus runs in the inferior edge of the falx cerebri and ends as the straight sinus (Section 18.1c).
    B The transverse sinus runs along the posterolateral margins of the tentorium cerebelli.
    C The sigmoid sinuses run in grooves of the occipital and temporal bones.
    D The cavernous sinuses lie lateral to the sella turcica between the meningeal and periosteal dura.
    E The 3rd ventricle lies between the right and left thalami of the diencephalon.

4. **E** The right and left vertebral arteries join to form the basilar artery. Together these arteries supply the posterior circulation of the brain (Section 18.2c).
    A The vertebral artery ascends through the transverse foramina of C1–C6 vertebrae.
    B The vertebral artery is a branch of the subclavian artery.
    C The vertebral artery terminates by joining with the contralateral vertebral artery to form the basilar artery.
    D The vertebral artery has no branches in the neck.

5. **B** CN VII, the facial nerve, exits the stylomastoid foramen and is responsible for the muscles of facial expression, including the occipitofrontalis muscle, which elevates the eyebrows (Section 18.3).
    A The levator palpebrae superioris muscle elevates the eyelid and is innervated by CN III, the oculomotor nerve. In addition to the levator palpebrae superioris the occipitofrontalis muscle assists in raising the eyebrow, but because CN III is not affected the patient is able to open his eye. He is not, however, able to close his eye completely due to the paralysis of the orbicularis oculi muscle.
    C CN XII, the hypoglossal nerve, innervates most of the tongue musculature. A left-sided hypoglossal injury would lead to the inability to protrude his tongue to the right.
    D The muscles of mastication are innervated by the mandibular division of CN V, the trigeminal nerve. Although his ability to chew is unaffected, the patient does have some trouble eating because of paralysis to the buccinator muscle, which assists in positioning food in the oral cavity.
    E Sensation to the cheek is conveyed through the maxillary division of the trigeminal nerve.

6. **D** The inferior alveolar nerve courses within the mandibular canal of the mandible and would be injured in this patient (Section 18.3).
    A The lingual nerve courses through the infratemporal fossa and into the floor of the mouth.
    B The hypoglossal nerve courses anteriorly below the angle of the mandible before entering the mouth at the posterior border of the mylohyoid muscle.
    C Zygomatic branches of the facial nerve pass lateral to the masseter muscle as they cross the cheek.
    E The chorda tympani travels with the lingual nerve in the infratemporal fossa and floor of the mouth.

7. **B** The lateral pterygoid muscle inserts into the condylar process of the mandible and its articular disk and the capsule of the temporomandibular joint (TMJ) (Section 19.2).
A The medial pterygoid inserts into the pterygoid tuberosity on the medial surface of the angle of the mandible.
C The temporalis inserts into the apex and medial surface of the coronoid process of the mandible.
D The masseter inserts into the masseteric tuberosity at the angle of the mandible.
E The buccinator inserts into the angle of the mouth and obicularis oris.

8. **A** The vomer makes up the inferior and posterior parts of the nasal septum (Section 19.7a).
B The ethmoid bone, through its perpendicular plate, makes up the superior and posterior parts of the nasal septum.
C The palatine forms the posterior palate and does not contribute to the nasal septum.
D The temporal forms the base and lateral side of the skull and does not contribute to the nasal septum.
E Although some of the sphenoid bone will be removed as a part of the procedure, it does not contribute to the nasal septum.

9. **E** The lacrimal gland is innervated by visceral motor fibers (preganglionic parasympathetic [C]) of the greater petrosal branch of the facial nerve (A). The postganglionic neuron is the zygomatic branch of the maxillary nerve (V_2), which has its cell body in the pterygopalatine ganglion (B) and is then distributed to the lacrimal gland. The lacrimal nerve (D) provides sensory innervation to the lacrimal gland, conjunctiva, and upper eyelids (Section 18.3).
A The lacrimal gland is innervated by visceral motor fibers (preganglionic parasympathetic of the greater petrosal branch of the facial nerve). B through D are also correct (E).
B The zygomatic branch of the facial nerve carries postganglionic parasympathetic fibers from the pterygopalatine ganglion to the lacrimal gland. A, C, and D are also correct (E).
C Parasympathetic fibers of the zygomatic nerve innervate the lacrimal gland. A, B, and D are also correct (E).
D The lacrimal nerve provides sensory innervation to the lacrimal gland, conjunctiva, and upper eyelids. A through C are also correct (E).

10. **C** The stapedius nerve arises from the facial nerve in the facial canal to innervate the stapedius muscle, which dampens sound waves transmitted through the middle ear (Section 20.2b).
A The maxillary nerve is distributed to the orbit, nasal cavity, and oral cavity, but it has no branches in the middle ear.
B The mandibular nerve innervates the tensor tympani, which tenses the tympanic membrane.
D The glossopharyngeal nerve transmits sensation from the tympanic cavity and pharyngotympanic tube and joins with sympathetic fibers of the internal carotid plexus to form the tympanic plexus.
E The vagus nerve transmits sensation from the external surface of the tympanic membrane.

11. **A** The ansa cervicalis innervates all of the infrahyoid muscles except the thyrohyoid (Sections 21.2 and Table 21.3a).
B The cervical branch of the facial nerve innervates the platysma
C The hypoglossal nerve innervates all of the tongue muscles, including the genioglossus, hyoglossus, and intrinsic tongue muscles.
D The accessory nerve innervates the trapezius and the sternocleidomastoid muscles and contributes to the pharyngeal plexus that helps to control the pharyngeal muscles.
E The recurrent laryngeal nerve, a branch of the vagus nerve, innervates the intrinsic muscles of the larynx.

12. **C** An emergency tracheotomy (or cricothyrotomy) is performed to secure an airway in a patient with respiratory failure who does not have time to have a procedure performed in the operating room. The quickest access to secure an airway is by incising the cricothyroid membrane (Section 21.6b).
A Superior to the hyoid bone is superior to the vocal folds and is also a difficult access site given the presence of the mylohyoid muscles.
B The thyrohyoid membrane is between the hyoid bone and the thyroid cartilage and is superior to the vocal folds.
D Between the thyroid and arytenoid cartilages is too posterior to access the airway and is also at the level of the vocal folds.
E Superior to the manubrium in the jugular fossa is a potential site for an airway (tracheostomy) but is more inferior to the cricothyroid membrane. Also, incising the tracheal cartilage or trying to access the airway between the tracheal cartilages is too difficult without the benefit of being in the operating room. Another benefit of a cricothyrotomy versus a tracheostomy is that there are fewer structures at risk for injury such as blood vessels, the recurrent laryngeal nerve, the thyroid gland, and the esophagus.

13. **D** The recurrent laryngeal nerve is a branch of the vagus nerve, which travels in the tracheoesophageal groove, lateral and posterior to the thyroid gland. Injury to this nerve causes hoarseness, among other complications (Sections 21.6e and 18.3).
A, B, C, and E The glossopharyngeal nerve, hypoglossal nerve, nerves of the ansa cervicalis, and the phrenic nerve do not travel close enough to the thyroid gland to be at risk during careful thyroid surgery.

14. **E** The anterior fontanelle is the fibrous area at the junction of the frontal and parietal bones. It closes between 18 and 24 months of age (Section 17.1c).
A, B, C, D The anterior fontanelle remains open until 18 to 24 months.

15. **B** The superior deep cervical nodes lie between the jugular and facial veins and the anterior belly of the digastric (Section 17.5).
    A The parotid nodes are superficial nodes that overlie the parotid gland on the side of the face.
    C The inferior deep cervical nodes lie in the neck near the inferior part of the internal jugular vein.
    D The retroauricular nodes are superficial nodes that lie along the posterior margin of the auricle.
    E The lateral cervical nodes are superficial nodes that lie along the external jugular vein in the neck.

16. **E** The CSF is reabsorbed into the venous system by the arachnoid granulations, which protrude into the superior sagittal sinus (Section 18.2b).
    A The choroid plexus is the site of CSF production in each of the four ventricles (the two first and second [lateral], the third, and the fourth).
    B The interventricular foramen is the communication between the lateral ventricles.
    C The cerebral aqueduct is the communication between the third and fourth ventricles.
    D The lateral apertures are the communication between the fourth ventricle and the subarachnoid space.

17. **E** None of the answers above describes the vagus nerve correctly (Section 18.3).
    A The vagus nerve leaves the skull through the jugular foramen with the glossopharyngeal and spinal accessory nerves.
    B The carotid sinus is innervated by the glossopharyngeal nerve.
    C The oculomotor nerve (III), trochlear nerve (IV), abducent nerve (VI), ophthalmic nerve (V_1), and ophthalmic vein are transmitted through the superior orbital fissure.
    D The vagus nerve innervates all of the muscles of the soft palate except the tensor veli palatini, which is supplied by the mandibular division of the trigeminal nerve.

18. **A** The abducent nerves innervate the lateral rectus muscles, which move the eyes laterally (Section 18.3).
    B Medial movement of the eyes is controlled by the oculomotor nerves via the medial rectus muscles.
    C Superior movement of the eyes is controlled by the oculomotor and trochlear nerves via the superior rectus and inferior oblique muscles.
    D Inferior movement of the eyes is controlled by the oculomotor nerves via the inferior rectus and the superior oblique muscles.
    E Internal rotation of the eyes, also called intorsion or rotation along the long axis of the eye, is controlled by the trochlear nerves via the superior oblique muscles. This movement is normally prevented by the action of the inferior oblique muscles.

19. **A** Emissary veins communicate with veins of the scalp and can carry infections intracranially to the dural venous sinuses (Section 19.1).
    B The attachment of the occipitofrontalis muscle to the skull prevents infections of the scalp from spreading into the neck.
    C The attachment of the epicranial aponeurosis to the zygomatic arches prevents further lateral spread of infection.
    D Spread of infection intracranially occurs through the emissary veins, which communicate with the dural sinuses, not with the epidural space.
    E Not applicable.

20. **E** The infratemporal fossa contains the maxillary artery and many of its branches, the mandibular nerve, the pterygoid plexus, and the otic ganglion, as well as the medial and lateral pterygoid muscles (Section 19.5).
    A The infratemporal fossa contains the maxillary artery, but choices B, C, and D are also correct (E).
    B The infratemporal fossa contains the mandibular nerve, but choices A, C, and D are also correct (E).
    C The infratemporal fossa contains the pterygoid plexus, but choices A, B, and D are also correct (E).
    D The infratemporal fossa contains the otic ganglion, but choices A, B, and C are also correct (E).

21. **A** The nasolacrimal duct drains tears from the medial corner of each eye into the inferior meatus (Sections 19.7a and 20.1b).
    B The frontal sinus drains into the middle meatus through a frontonasal duct.
    C The ethmoid sinus drains into the superior and middle meatuses.
    D The sphenoid sinus drains into the sphenoethmoidal recess in the posterosuperior part of the nasal cavity.
    E The maxillary sinus drains into the middle meatus.

22. **C** Only the ophthalmic artery and optic nerve enter the orbit through the optic canal (Sections 17.1d and 20.1e).
    A The supratrochlear artery is a branch of the ophthalmic artery in the orbit that supplies the scalp.
    B The supraorbital artery is a branch of the ophthalmic artery in the orbit that supplies the scalp.
    D The ophthalmic vein enters the orbit through the superior orbital fissure.
    E The ophthalmic nerve (CN V_1) enters the orbit through the superior orbital fissure.

23. **D** The mandibular division of the trigeminal nerve innervates the tensor tympani muscle, which lessens damage from loud sounds by tensing the tympanic membrane (Section 20.2b).
A The optic nerve carries sensory innervation from the neural retina to the lateral geniculate nucleus.
B The oculomotor nerve innervates most of the extraocular muscles of the eye and the intrinsic muscles of the eye.
C The trochlear nerve innervates the superior oblique extraocular muscle of the eye.
E The facial nerve innervates the stapedius muscle, which dampens the vibrations of the stapes on the oval window.

24. **A** The cervical plexus originates from the anterior rami of C1–C4 (Section 21.3a).
B The accessory nerve (CN XI) innervates the sternocleidomastoid.
C Only the oculomotor, facial, and glossopharyngeal nerves carry preganglionic parasympathetic nerves that synapse in the head.
D The cervical plexus has both sensory and motor components. The sensory nerves of the plexus, the lesser occipital, great auricular, transverse cervical, and supraclavicular nerves innervate the skin of the anterior and lateral neck and lateral scalp. The ansa cervicalis, the motor part of the plexus, innervates most of the infrahyoid muscles.
E The greater occipital nerve is supplied by the posterior rami of spinal nerves C1–C3 and is therefore not a branch of the cervical plexus.

25. **B** The only muscles that relax the vocal folds are the posterior cricoarytenoid muscles. Note that there are other results of anesthesia that also necessitate intubation (Section 21.6d).
A The thyroarytenoid closes the vocal folds.
C The cricothyroid muscles do not have direct actions on the vocal folds.
D The transverse arytenoid muscles close the vocal folds.
E The lateral arytenoid muscles close the vocal folds.

26. **A** All of the innervation of the larynx, both sensory and motor, is supplied by the superior and inferior (recurrent) laryngeal branches of the vagus nerve (CNX) (Section 21.6e).
B The glossopharyngeal nerve (IX) innervates the tympanic cavity and pharyngotympanic (auditory) tube; the pharynx (sensory and motor), the tonsils, palate, posterior one third of the tongue (sensory and taste), and the stylopharyngeus muscle. It also innervates the carotid body and carotid sinus.
C The recurrent laryngeal nerve is a branch of the vagus nerve that innervates all of the muscles of the larynx except the cricothyroid and carries sensation from the lower half of the larynx (from the vocal cords downward).
D The superior laryngeal nerve innervates the cricothyroid muscle, which helps to tense the vocal folds and provides sensation to the upper half of the larynx (above the vocal cords).
E Not applicable.

27. **B** The only laryngeal cartilage to completely encircle the airway is the cricoid cartilage (Section 21.6a).
A The U-shaped thyroid cartilage has two laminae that join in the anterior midline to form a laryngeal prominence.
C The epiglottic cartilage, a single leaf-shaped cartilage, forms the anterior wall of the laryngeal inlet at the root of the tongue.
D Paired arytenoid cartilages articulate with the superior borders of the cricoid laminae. Their vocal processes attach to the thyroid cartilage through the vocal ligaments.
E Corniculate cartilages appear as small tubercles within the aryepiglottic fold.

28. **C** The common carotid artery, internal jugular vein, and vagus nerve are contained within the carotid sheath (Section 21.1).
A The external jugular vein is not within the carotid sheath.
B The phrenic nerve lies on the anterior scalene muscle behind the carotid sheath.
D The superior thyroid artery is a branch of the external carotid artery and does not travel in the carotid sheath.
E The sympathetic trunk lies behind the carotid sheath.

29. **C** Parasympathetic fibers of the oculomotor nerve (CN III) synapse in the ciliary ganglion and are responsible for pupil constriction (Section 20.1e).
A The superior cervical ganglia are sympathetic ganglia and not involved in the constriction of the pupils.
B The pterygopalatine ganglia are parasympathetic ganglia involved in lacrimation.
C The otic ganglia are parasympathetic ganglia involved in saliva production by the parotid glands.
E The trigeminal ganglia are sensory ganglia of the trigeminal nerve involved in sensation of the face and parts of the oral cavity.

30. **D** The submandibular lymph nodes are the primary nodes of the lateral part of the body of the tongue (Section 19.8c).
A The superior deep cervical nodes are the primary nodes of the root of the tongue.
B The inferior deep cervical are the primary nodes of the medial parts of the body of the tongue.
C The anterior superficial cervical nodes are the primary nodes of the skin anterior muscles of the neck and are not the primary lymph nodes of any part of the tongue.
E The submental nodes are the primary nodes of the apex and frenulum of the tongue.

31. **A** The ethmoid, maxilla, vomer, palatine, lacrimal, nasal, and inferior nasal concha form the bony skeleton of the nasal cavity (Section 19.7a).
B The ethmoid forms the cribriform plate at the roof of the nasal cavity, the superior and middle nasal concha of the lateral walls, and part of the nasal septum.
C The maxilla forms the anterior part of the palate on the floor of the nasal cavity.
D The vomer forms part of the nasal septum.
E The palatine bone forms the posterior part of the palate on the floor of the nasal cavity.

32. **A** The medial pterygoid muscle forms a sling with the masseter muscle to elevate the mandible (Section 19.2 and Table 19.3).
B The tensor veli palatini tenses the soft palate.
C The levator veli palatini elevates the soft palate.
D The suprahyoid muscles, including digastric, geniohyoid, stylohyoid, and mylohyoid, elevate the hyoid. The medial pterygoid can only elevate the hyoid secondarily by first elevating the mandible.
E The posterior part of the temporalis muscle retracts the mandible.

33. **C** The hypoglossal nerve (CN XII) innervates all muscles of the tongue except for the palatoglossus. When damaged, muscles on the affected side atrophy and fail to contribute to protrusion of the tongue. This causes the tongue to deviate to the side of the lesion (left side in this patient). The nerve is at risk during surgery on the common carotid artery because of its proximity to the carotid bifurcation (Section 18.3).
A The stylopharyngeus is the only muscle innervated by the glossopharyngeal nerve.
B Damage to the left hypoglossal nerve would cause atrophy of the left side of the tongue and deviation to the right side with protrusion.
D The lingual nerve, a branch of the mandibular division of the trigeminal nerve, transmits sensation from the anterior tongue. It also carries parasympathetic fibers via the chorda tympani to the submandibular and sublingual glands and taste from the anterior tongue.
E The lingual nerve, a branch of the mandibular division of the trigeminal nerve, transmits sensation from the anterior tongue. It also carries parasympathetic fibers via the chorda tympani to the submandibular and sublingual glands and taste from the anterior tongue.

34. **A** The mandibular division enters the infratemporal fossa where it sends motor branches to muscles of mastication and sensory branches to the tongue, mandibular teeth, oral cavity, and skin of the lower and lateral face (Section 18.3).
B The maxillary division of the trigeminal nerve passes through the foramen rotundum to the pterygopalatine fossa.
C The ophthalmic branch of the trigeminal nerve passes through the superior orbital fissure to the orbit.
D The maxillary branch of the trigeminal nerve innervates the nasal cavity.
E The lingual nerve passes from the infratemporal fossa into the oral cavity.

35. **E** The internal carotid arteries do not have branches in the neck. The ophthalmic arteries are the first major branches of the internal carotid arteries (Section 18.2c).
A The superior thyroid is a branch of the external carotid artery.
B The lingual artery is a branch of the external carotid artery.
C The facial artery is a branch of the external carotid artery.
D The maxillary artery is a branch of the external carotid artery.

36. **E** The cavernous sinus contains the oculomotor, trochlear, abducent, and ophthalmic and maxillary divisions of the trigeminal nerve. The maxillary division of the trigeminal nerve supplies sensation to the cheek (Section 18.1c).
A Jugular venous distension is caused by a decrease of venous return to the heart.
B The inability to smile is caused by a lesion to the facial nerve.
C The inability to chew is caused by a lesion to the mandibular division of the trigeminal nerve.
D Loss of vision is caused by a lesion to the optic nerve, which does not travel through the cavernous sinus. Note that there are additional causes of loss of vision, none of which are related to the cavernous sinus.

37. **D** The ophthalmic artery is the first major branch of the internal carotid artery in the anterior cranial fossa (Section 17.3b).
A The posterior cerebral is the terminal branch of the basilar artery.
B The occipital artery is a branch of the external carotid artery.
C The labyrinthine artery is a branch of the basilar artery.
E The middle meningeal artery is a branch of the maxillary artery, which is a branch of the external carotid artery.

Index

Note: Italicized page numbers represent clinical applications. Illustrative and tabular material is indicated by "f" and "t" respectively immediately following the page number.